YOUR FAMILY DOCTOR

Volume One: Reference Volume
Guide to Current Medical Practice

Your Family Doctor

Volume One: Reference Volume
Guide to Current Medical Practice

How your body works
Index of symptoms
Understanding medical terms
A–Z Medical Reference Guide

Volume Two: Practical Volume
Guide to First Aid, Safety, Care of the Sick, Pregnancy, Childbirth and Child Care, and Fitness

First Aid
Family safety
Care of the sick at home
Professional care for the sick
Pregnancy and childbirth
The healthy child
Age-by-age charts
Taking care of your own body
Physical fitness and exercises
Mental fitness

GUILD PUBLISHING

The Home Medical Encyclopaedia

YOUR FAMILY DOCTOR

DR JAMES BEVAN

With a Foreword by Lord Hunt of Fawley, Past President
The Royal College of General Practitioners

Volume One: Reference Volume
Guide to Current Medical Practice

The publishing staff of Mitchell Beazley and World Book-Childcraft International involved in the production of this book were:

Managing editors:	Michael Darton Dominic Miccolis (U.S.A.)
Editors:	Charles Boyle Loraine Fergusson Fern Fraser Cynthia Hole Margaret Kennedy Lloyd Lindo John Moore Martyn Page Hal Robinson
Assistant editors:	Ruth Binney Sarah Gratton Janet Proffitt
Editorial assistants:	Rosemary Bevan Sara Binney Amanda Marshall Valerie Nicholson Janet Peterson (U.S.A.) Kathy Phillips
Senior designers:	Peter Laws William Hammond (U.S.A.)
Assistant designers:	Jeremy Bratt Lisa Tai
Design associate:	Peter Wrigley
Picture researchers:	Brigitte Arora Sue Pinkus Paddy Poynder
Photographer:	John Watney
Production manager:	Graham Darlow
Production control:	John Hodgson Barbara Podczerwinski (U.S.A.)
Production assistant:	Moira Fox

Your Family Doctor

Filmset in Great Britain by Filmtype Services Ltd. Scarborough
ISBN 085533 295 6
(Library of Congress Catalog Number 79-56907)
Printed and bound in Spain
by TONSA, San Sebastian
Dep. Leg. S.S. 360-80

The general editor and publishers wish to acknowledge and thank the following consultants and contributors who helped in the production of this book:

Foreword:
Rt Hon. Lord Hunt of Fawley, C.B.E., D.M., F.R.C.P., F.R.C.S., F.R.C.G.P.

Emeritus editors:
Lt Gen. Sir James Baird, K.B.E., (late R.A.M.C.), M.D., F.R.C.P. (Lond.), F.R.C.P. (Edin.). Medical Adviser, Council of Postgraduate Medical Education; late Director General, Army Medical Services; Physician to British Army of the Rhine; Commandant, Royal Army Medical College

Dr Philip Evans, C.B.E., M.Sc., M.D., F.R.C.P. Late Physician-Paediatrician to H.M. the Queen; late Director, Paediatric Department Guy's Hospital and Physician, Hospital for Sick Children, Great Ormond St, London

Sir Francis Avery Jones, C.B.E., M.D., F.R.C.P. Consulting Physician, Central Middlesex Hospital, London; Hon. Consulting Physician, St Bartholomew's Hospital, London; Consulting Gastroenterologist, St Mark's Hospital, London, and to the Royal Navy

Sir Henry Osmond-Clarke, K.C.V.O., C.B.E., F.R.C.S. (Eng.), F.R.C.S.I. Late Orthopaedic Surgeon to H.M. the Queen; Consulting Orthopaedic Surgeon, the London Hospital and King Edward VII Hospital for Officers, London; Hon. Consultant in Orthopaedics to the Royal Air Force; past President, British Orthopaedic Association

Mr George Pinker, F.R.C.S. (Ed.), F.R.C.O.G. Obstetrician and Gynaecologist, St Mary's, Middlesex, and Samaritan Hospitals, Hospital for Women, Soho, and King Edward VII Hospital for Officers, London; Hon. Consultant, Royal Women's Hospital, Melbourne, Australia

Rt Hon. Lord Smith of Marlow, K.B.E., M.S., F.R.C.S. President, Royal Society of Medicine; past President, Royal College of Surgeons; late Surgeon, St George's Hospital, London; Hon. Surgeon to the Army and Prince Alfred Hospital, Sydney, Australia

Contributing Consultants:
Miss Christine Bruell, R.S.C.N.
Prof. Alain Enthoven (U.S.A.), M.A. (Stanford), B. Phil. (Oxon), Ph.D. (M.I.T.)
Mrs Dorothy Macdonald, M.C.S.P.
Dr Keith Manley (U.S.A.), M.D., M.R.C.P.
Mrs Betty Parsons
Lady Riches, S.R.N.
Mr Edward Sturges

Authenticating consultants:
Dr Ian Anderson, M.B., B.S.
Dr Art Boylston, M.D., M.R.C. Path.
Dr Alan Galbraith, M.B., B. Chir., D.C.H., D.R.C.O.G.
Dr Sally Newton, M.B., B.S.
Dr Jack Donald Singer, M.D.

Specialist consultants:
Dr J.H. Baron, D.M., F.R.C.P. Senior Lecturer and Consultant, Royal Postgraduate Medical School and Hammersmith Hospital, London

Dr Peter Beck, M.D., F.R.C.P. Physician, University Hospital of Wales

Dr Hamish Cameron, M.R.C.P., M.R.C. Psych., D.P.M. Consultant Child Psychiatrist, St George's Hospital, London

Mr Anthony Catterall, M.Chir., F.R.C.S. Orthopaedic Surgeon, Royal National Orthopaedic and Charing Cross Hospitals, London

Mr Alasdair Fraser, M.B., F.R.C.O.G. Obstetrician and Gynaecologist, St Mary's Hospital, London

Dr R.P. Goulden, M.B., Ch.B., D.Phys.Med. Chief Medical Adviser, N.E.M. Insurance Association Ltd.

Mr Eric Gustavson, M.B., F.R.C.S. Plastic Surgeon, University College Hospital and Hospital for Sick Children, London

Mr Michael Laurence, M.B., F.R.C.S. Orthopaedic Surgeon, Guy's Hospital, London

Mr Bruce Mathalone, M.B., B.Chir., F.R.C.S. (Eng.), F.R.C.S. (Ed.), D.O. Ophthalmic Surgeon, Westminster Group of Hospitals and Royal Eye Hospital, London

Dr Dowling Munro, M.D., F.R.C.P. Consultant Dermatologist, St Bartholomew's Hospital, London

Dr Graham Petrie, M.B., M.R.C.Psych., D.P.M., D.R.C.O.G. Psychiatrist, Cambridge Area Teaching Hospitals

Mr David A.S. Roberts, B.D.S. (Hons), L.D.S. R.C.S. Dental Surgeon

Mr John Stephen, M.A., Ch.M., F.R.C.S. (Ed.), F.R.C.S. (Eng.). Consulting Surgeon, St Mary's Hospital, London

Mr Gerald Walsh-Waring, M.B., B.S., F.R.C.S. ENT Surgeon, St Mary's Hospital, London

Preface
by James Bevan

This book is the outcome of the past twenty years of my professional life in general practice. It has developed out of my experience in dealing with my patients, their disorders and their needs. It contains the kind of advice that I find I am constantly asked for, explanations about diseases, and the treatments that I commonly recommend.

I wanted to go further than this. Many of my patients are afraid to remain at home during any lengthy illness or disability because they are unsure of being properly cared for by their family. Moreover their relations, also uncertain of what to do in the circumstances, generally come to me for advice. Often nursing at home needs simple skills that are easy to learn once they have been demonstrated. The later sections of this work are intended to teach these skills, through a combination of text and pictures.

Another frequent request is for an explanation of the more positive aspects of remaining healthy and keeping fit. In this way illness can often be prevented. This work contains sections on how to look after yourself and how to keep fit as well as listing the common disorders that affect each age group, together with the symptoms they cause and how to detect them.

I have not tried to tell you how to diagnose your own disorders. Diagnosis must at all times depend on the professional knowledge and experience of your own doctor. On the other hand this book will help you to decide when to consult the doctor and how to explain simply and clearly the symptoms of the disorder.

It will assist your doctor to know how you look after yourself and make it easier for the doctor to suggest any necessary changes in your way of life to help improve your health.

Although I have written a comprehensive alphabetical encyclopaedia section to the book, many of the names of the diseases and disorders may be strange to you. I have devised a means for you to find out about any of the disorders from which you might be suffering. Apart from the many cross-references throughout this section there is a revolutionary form of atlas-index, the Index of Symptoms, that will simplify your use of this book.

Your Family Doctor has been written to help you care for yourself and your family safely and comprehensively.

James Bevan

Foreword

by the Rt Hon. Lord Hunt of Fawley, CBE, DM, FRCP, FRCS, FRCGP

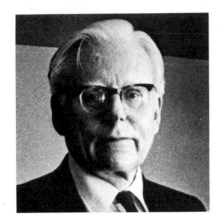

This large, accurate and comprehensive medical encyclopaedia, created here in Britain, deserves to be very successful. Around the world it will find many grateful readers, not least in developing countries where medical libraries are few or non-existent, where not many people can afford to buy medical books, and where even doctors and nurses may be scarce.

Where nursing and medical help is readily available, however, readers of these volumes must not feel that they can dispense with expert advice and care. That may be dangerous, leading to delay in obtaining proper treatment of a serious illness or accident. This work is not intended to be a "do-it-yourself" manual. It is to help readers to *understand* medical terms and disorders, so that they can describe accurately their symptoms to a doctor and better appreciate the doctor's explanation and treatment. The book should be read in a spirit of co-operation with all members of the nursing and medical professions and their ancillary services. The clear explanations and advice should help everyone to obtain rapid and accurate diagnosis and treatment for both trivial and serious conditions.

Your Family Doctor also answers a great number of questions which people are likely to ask about how they can keep themselves and their families healthy (mentally and physically), about first aid, nursing at home, and when patients should be admitted to hospital. The large number of illustrations are particularly valuable.

As in all encyclopaedias, the articles in the A–Z section of the book have to be in strict alphabetical order. This sometimes causes some unusual juxtapositions; one cannot help smiling to find "Black Death" next to "Black Eye"! However, the alphabetical section is quick and convenient to use.

Families will find these volumes a great support on many anxious occasions. Few parents could remember the wealth of detail they contain about children; the Age-by-age charts should be particularly useful. Older people, their relatives or companions, and their nurses should find this encyclopaedia equally helpful in a great many ways.

We must congratulate and thank the authors and publishers for appreciating the need for such a work, and for their diligence and enthusiasm in providing it.

Contents – Volume One

How your body works

Section contents

Introduction

This section is designed to tell a reader exactly how the body works, in words and pictures, with diagrams and captions. Every part of the body is examined and explained, either as part of one of the systems of the body or as a specific organ. The composition of each is clearly shown and the function described in detail.

The body is made up primarily of cells, of which there are many kinds. There are as many as 10 million million cells in the adult human body. The first pages of the section describe these "building blocks of life", and include information on structure and function, and on heredity, which is governed by the contents of most human cells.

The bones and joints make up the framework of the entire human body. There are about 206 bones in an adult, 22 of which alone form the skull. The joints are commonly thought only to exist to enable movement, but in fact many of them do not themselves move. The body has evolved clever systems of avoiding friction in those joints that do move.

Movement, digestion, respiration, blood circulation, and other internal systems, are all made possible by the muscles.

The heart is the body's engine, and pumps blood around the circulation system through the arteries. It is the blood that exchanges carbon dioxide for life-giving oxygen in the lungs, during the process of respiration. The movement of air in and out of the lungs helps in the production of speech, although speech also involves other organs in the throat and mouth.

The mouth is also the beginning of the digestive system, which consists of a tube about 33 feet long, all the way to the anus.

On the way, many processes, including those within the stomach, absorb and make use of substances in the food swallowed.

The brain interprets and remembers anything felt, smelled, heard, tasted, or seen, through the nervous system. The association centres and motor areas of the brain co-ordinate the movements and chemical reactions of the body, including the hormones secreted by the endocrine glands.

Finally, in this section the process of reproduction is fully explained.

A collection of cells

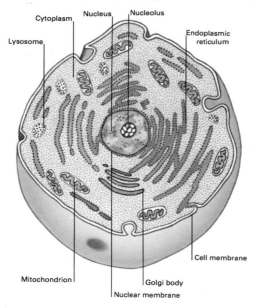

Cytoplasm • Nucleus • Nucleolus • Endoplasmic reticulum • Lysosome • Cell membrane • Mitochondrion • Golgi body • Nuclear membrane

All plants and animals are composed of microscopic "building blocks" called cells. Most cells measure only a few thousandths of a millimetre across. An adult human's body contains about 10 million million cells. Each human being starts life as a single cell, a fertilized egg, which divides during embryonic development. In the course of this reduplication, specialized cells do various jobs.

Cells group together to form tissues; tissues combine to compose body organs; and collections of organs make up the body systems. For example, the lining of the stomach is a tissue, and the stomach an organ that is part of the digestive system.

The cells in the body's tissues and organs vary greatly in size, shape, and appearance, but all cells are built to the same basic plan. Every cell has an outer membrane enclosing a jelly-like substance, the cytoplasm, in which substances are found that provide food, energy, building materials, and waste products for removal, plus many tiny bodies (organelles). The membrane is also involved in cell operations by assisting the minute-by-minute passage of selected materials in and out of the cell. The close positioning of membranes of adjacent cells helps to ensure communication of chemical information between cells.

Of all the bodies within the cytoplasm the most prominent is the nucleus, a spherical structure vital to life. The nucleus directs all the activities of the cell because it is the store of cell information. This information is stored in strands called chromosomes, within the nucleus. Nearly all human cells contain forty-six chromosomes arranged in twenty-three pairs. The chromosomes are "chains" of genes, units made of deoxyribonucleic acid (DNA), a remarkable substance that has the ability to duplicate itself. This duplication ensures human reproduction and cell replacement processes, which continue throughout life.

The DNA in the genes works by directing the production of proteins, molecules essential for cell survival. The manufacture of proteins is assisted by the nucleolus, a centre inside the nucleus, and by minute structures called ribosomes. The ribosomes lie outside the nucleus on the endoplasmic reticulum, a network of tubes running through the cytoplasm from the wall of the nucleus to the cell membrane. Both nucleolus and ribosomes contain a different nucleic acid, ribonucleic acid (RNA), which helps to control the build-up of raw materials into proteins. Once made, the proteins act as building materials, as chemical messengers (hormones), and as enzymes, the biological

All body cells have the same basic constituents. The cell is enclosed in a membrane and comprises the cytoplasm and nucleus. The cytoplasm contains organelles vital to cell activity, such as mitochondria, for energy production, and the endoplasmic reticulum, running from membrane to nucleus, that bears ribosomes essential to protein building. Instructions for protein manufacture are given by the DNA of the nucleus.

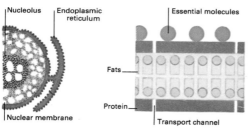

Nucleolus • Endoplasmic reticulum • Nuclear membrane • Essential molecules • Fats • Protein • Transport channel

In the nucleus, information is housed in the chromosomes. The nucleolus aids protein synthesis. Substances pass in and out of pores in the membrane.

The cell membrane consists of two layers of protein enclosing a layer of fats. Special areas in the membrane allow molecules to enter and leave the cell.

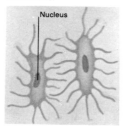

Nucleus

Cells called osteoblasts make the hard substances in bone. The minerals are moulded by the cells' long cytoplasm-filled arms.

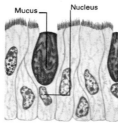

Mucus • Nucleus

Goblet cells form part of a mucous membrane. They secrete mucin, which combines with water to form slippery mucus.

catalysts that direct chemical reactions within all cells. Proteins arc "packaged" for removal from the cell in collections of minute tubes, the Golgi bodies.

Cells contain other vital organelles. The sausage-shaped mitochondria provide the cell with energy by breaking down substances passed to the cell in the blood. In round structures called lysosomes, large molecules are fragmented for use in the cell.

The variations between cells reflect the tasks of different cells. Some of the cells nearest to the "basic" design include the hexagonal liver cells, which perform many complex chemical reactions. Other simple cells are those that provide support and lining in many tissues. Often these column-shaped cells produce the sticky substance mucus and are edged with minute hair-like projections (cilia), which can waft substances along. The fat cells found beneath the skin and around many organs are simple cells whose cytoplasm is packed with globules of fat. The fat is used to provide insulation and energy. Red blood cells, which carry oxygen and carbon dioxide round the circulation, are unusual in having no nuclei in their mature form. In contrast, many of the white blood cells, part of the body's defence system against disease, have very large nuclei.

Three of the most specialized sorts of cells are muscle cells, nerve cells, and reproductive cells. Muscle cells are greatly elongated and have the power of contraction made possible by special proteins that can slide over one another. Because muscle contraction is energy-intensive, muscle cells have huge numbers of mitochondria.

Nerve cells are also elongated but have membranes specialized for transmitting the electrical impulses of nerve messages. Each nerve cell ends in a cell body bearing projections that lie close to similar projections on adjacent nerve cells. Messages "jump the gaps" with the aid of chemicals made in the nerve cells.

Reproductive cells, sperm from the male and eggs from the female, are unique in containing only half the usual number of chromosomes. This is necessary so that the number can be restored to forty-six when sperm and egg combine at fertilization.

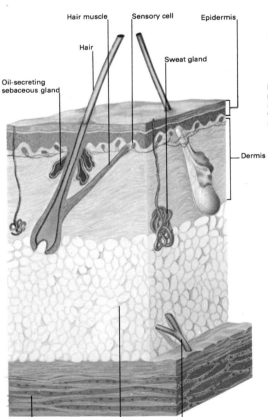

Hair muscle | Sensory cell | Epidermis
Hair
Oil-secreting sebaceous gland
Sweat gland
Dermis
Skeletal muscle | Fat cells | Blood vessel

The skin (left) contains cells with many different functions. The epidermis waterproofs; the dermis and muscle layers support. Hairs and sweat glands aid temperature control; fat cells insulate and store fuel; sensory cells detect touch, temperature, pressure, and pain.

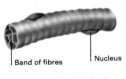

Band of fibres | Nucleus

Elongated cells of skeletal muscle look striped because they contain filaments that move to make the muscle contract.

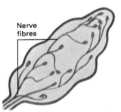

Nerve fibres

Cold is detected in the skin by end bulbs of Krause (above) made of nerve fibres enclosed within a thin covering membrane.

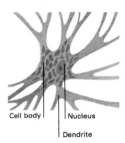

Cell body | Nucleus
Dendrite

The transmission of impulses between nerve cells is achieved with the help of outgrowths (dendrites) from each cell body.

Spherical fat cells can expand to accommodate large stores of energy-rich fats. They have small nuclei.

Mature red blood cells, flattened concave discs that have no nuclei, carry oxygen and carbon dioxide.

Bones and joints

The body's skeleton is its internal support system. Its bones also surround and protect vital organs and, together with the muscles, make movement possible. Some bones have the additional job of making blood cells.

Bone is a living tissue that is both rigid and resilient. Most bones are first formed as cartilage, a gristle-like elastic substance. The cartilage is then invaded by bone-building cells, which harden it by depositing calcium salts. Even when fully formed, many bones retain some cartilage at their ends to aid binding between bones or joint articulation.

In a mature bone the cells at the centre are arranged in a lattice to give lightness, whereas those toward the outside are densely packed for strength. The bone cells in the outer area are grouped in rod-shaped units, each penetrated by blood vessels that supply nutrients. Meshed between the rods are supple fibres that give bone its elasticity.

There is an average of 206 bones in the human skeleton, divided into two groups. The skull, spine, and rib-cage make up the axial skeleton. The limbs, shoulder (pectoral) girdle, and hip (pelvic) girdle compose the appendicular skeleton. The twenty-two skull bones form a protective vault for the brain and sockets for the eyes, ears, and organs of smell. The only skull bone that can move is the lower jaw. Teeth are embedded in this bone, and in the upper jaw.

Beneath the skull is a total of thirty-four vertebrae, which make up the spine (backbone) and encase the spinal cord. Toward the base of the spine, five vertebrae are fused together to form the sacrum, with the fused bones of the coccyx beneath them. The twenty-four curved rib bones are attached to the spine. At the front of the body the top ten rib pairs are attached to the breastbone (sternum). The rib-cage protects the heart, lungs, and large blood vessels; it can move in and out during breathing.

Lying over the upper part of the rib-cage at the back of the body are the shoulder blades (scapulae). The collarbones (clavicles) link the shoulder blades with the breastbone and give support to the shoulders. The upper arm bone (humerus) fits into a socket in the shoulder blade.

The bones of the arms and shoulder girdle are designed for dexterity. In contrast, those of the hip girdle and legs are constructed for

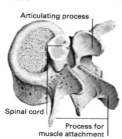

A lower back spine bone (above), turned side-on shows the processes designed for articulation and muscle attachment.

Articulating process

Spinal cord

Process for muscle attachment

Fused joint | Bone marrow

The flat bones of the skull (above) are connected by fused unmovable joints. Red blood cells are made in the marrow of skull bones, long bones, and vertebrae.

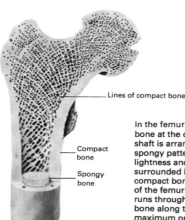

Lines of compact bone

Compact bone

Spongy bone

In the femur (left) the bone at the centre of the shaft is arranged in a spongy pattern for lightness and is surrounded by strong, compact bone. At the head of the femur compact bone runs through the spongy bone along the lines of maximum pressure and stress.

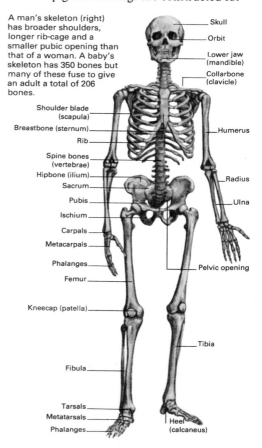

A man's skeleton (right) has broader shoulders, longer rib-cage and a smaller pubic opening than that of a woman. A baby's skeleton has 350 bones but many of these fuse to give an adult a total of 206 bones.

Skull

Orbit

Lower jaw (mandible)

Collarbone (clavicle)

Shoulder blade (scapula)

Breastbone (sternum)

Rib

Spine bones (vertebrae)

Hipbone (ilium)

Sacrum

Pubis

Ischium

Carpals

Metacarpals

Phalanges

Femur

Kneecap (patella)

Humerus

Radius

Ulna

Pelvic opening

Tibia

Fibula

Tarsals

Metatarsals

Phalanges

Heel (calcaneus)

weight-bearing and walking. The pelvic girdle also encloses and supports the organs of the lower abdomen. It is made up of three fused bones on each side of the body. Each hip-bone (ilium) is bound to the sacrum of the spine, and the two pubic bones are united at the front of the body. Each ischial bone of the girdle joins with the base of the hip-bone and the pubic bone. The upper leg bone (femur) forms a ball-and-socket joint at the junction of the three bones.

Joined to the strong upper bones of each limb are paired parallel bones – the radius and ulna in the forearm, the tibia and fibula in the lower leg. The wrist and the ankle are composed of a number of small bones. The framework of the hand is made up of meta-carpals; the foot is composed of metatarsals. The fingers and toes are constructed of bones called phalanges, those of the fingers being much longer than those of the toes.

Movements of the skeleton are made possible by the joints formed wherever two bones meet. The joints that allow most freedom of action are those at the shoulder and hip. Here a ball at the end of the limb bone fits into a socket on the girdle. At knee and elbow, hinge joints permit the limbs to bend in one direction only. The elbow also has a pivot joint enabling the arm to twist.

Other mobile joints include the ellipsoid joints between the hand's phalanges and metacarpals, which permit circular movement. The saddle joint of the thumb enables the thumb to touch each finger in turn.

Some joints are designed for only restricted motion or none at all. Discs of cartilage between the vertebrae permit only slight movement of the spine. The fused jigsaw-like joints between the skull bones eliminate all movement; their purpose is protection rather than mobility.

The detailed structure of each joint depends on the job it has to do. Wherever freedom of action is possible, the ends of each bone are capped with cartilage to cut down friction. A freely movable joint is lubricated with liquid produced by the capsule surrounding it. A large joint, such as the knee, also has a fluid-filled cavity (bursa) to the front that acts as a shock absorber. Joint strength is enhanced by ligaments and by tendons, which are extensions of the muscles whose action makes joints move.

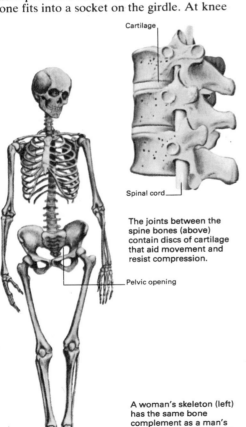

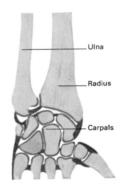

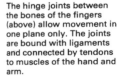

The joints between the spine bones (above) contain discs of cartilage that aid movement and resist compression.

At the gliding joints between the carpal bones of the wrist (above) the surfaces of the bones slide over one another.

The hinge joints between the bones of the fingers (above) allow movement in one plane only. The joints are bound with ligaments and connected by tendons to muscles of the hand and arm.

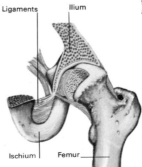

A woman's skeleton (left) has the same bone complement as a man's but its wider pubic opening assists childbirth.

The ligaments that bond the ball-and-socket joint of the hip (left) also carry nerves and blood vessels to the joint.

Muscles

Muscles are the motive force that makes possible the wide range of human movements. The activities of muscles are also essential for digestion, respiration, blood circulation, and other vital internal mechanisms. All muscles operate by shortening in length (contracting), and all muscle contraction is controlled by messages received from the nervous system.

There are three types of muscles: skeletal muscles, smooth muscles, and cardiac muscle. Skeletal muscles are those that allow body movement. They are also called voluntary muscles because their actions can be consciously controlled by the brain. Smooth muscles are found in the intestines, arteries, bladder, and other internal organs. Cardiac muscle, found only in the heart, is the driving force of the heartbeat. Both smooth and cardiac muscles act involuntarily, under the influence of the automatic (autonomic) section of the nervous system.

More than 600 skeletal muscles, arranged in layers, cover the bones. Many of these muscles are attached directly to bones by fibrous extensions known as tendons. Other skeletal muscles are linked to neighbouring

muscles or to the skin. At the joints between bones, skeletal muscles can produce bending, straightening, and turning movements; or they can move the limbs to and from the side of the body. In the face, skeletal muscles attached to the skin control facial expressions such as smiling and frowning.

Most skeletal muscles are positioned and operate in pairs. In the arm, for example, the biceps muscle at the front of the upper arm links the radius bone of the forearm with the bones of the shoulder and upper arm. The triceps muscle at the back of the upper arm links the ulna of the forearm with the shoulder and upper arm bones. When the forearm is raised, operating the elbow joint, the biceps contracts and the triceps relaxes. When the arm is straightened at the elbow, the biceps relaxes and the triceps contracts.

A skeletal muscle is made up of many bundles of long, straight fibres up to 30 cm (12 inches) long. Every fibre is composed of smaller units known as myofibrils. If viewed under a microscope, the fibres and myofibrils appear to have crosswise stripes. For this reason, skeletal muscle is often called striped or striated muscle. The stripes are created by

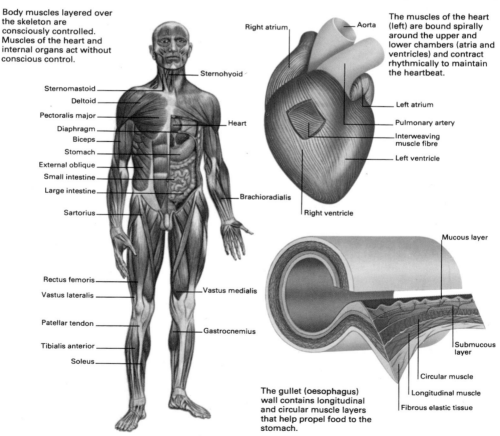

Body muscles layered over the skeleton are consciously controlled. Muscles of the heart and internal organs act without conscious control.

Sternomastoid
Deltoid
Pectoralis major
Diaphragm
Biceps
Stomach
External oblique
Small intestine
Large intestine
Sartorius

Sternohyoid
Heart

Brachioradialis

Rectus femoris
Vastus lateralis

Vastus medialis

Patellar tendon
Tibialis anterior
Soleus

Gastrocnemius

Right atrium
Aorta

The muscles of the heart (left) are bound spirally around the upper and lower chambers (atria and ventricles) and contract rhythmically to maintain the heartbeat.

Left atrium
Pulmonary artery
Interweaving muscle fibre
Left ventricle

Right ventricle

Mucous layer

Submucous layer

Circular muscle
Longitudinal muscle
Fibrous elastic tissue

The gullet (oesophagus) wall contains longitudinal and circular muscle layers that help propel food to the stomach.

overlapping strands of protein inside the myofibrils. To make a skeletal muscle contract, nerve messages are sent to the muscle fibres. When a message reaches a fibre a chemical is released that makes the protein strands in the myofibrils slide over each other, so reducing the fibre's length.

The cardiac muscle of the heart has cross-striations like those of skeletal muscle, but its fibres are branched and its actions cannot be voluntarily controlled. Cardiac muscle is exceptional because it has a built-in rhythm of contraction. In the body this rhythm is regulated by the autonomic nervous system to produce a regular, co-ordinated pumping action. During a heartbeat, the muscle relaxes as the heart fills with blood, then contracts to pump blood out of the heart.

The muscle of the internal organs is called smooth muscle because its unbranched fibres are not striped like those of voluntary and cardiac muscle. Smooth muscle is composed of fibres rarely more than 0.5mm (0.02 inches) long. These fibres are generally grouped in bundles or sheets. The body's largest concentration of smooth muscle is in the tube that forms the intestine. Here

smooth muscles are arranged and work in a paired way comparable to the action of skeletal muscles. Circular muscles lie around the intestinal tube, and longitudinal muscles run along its length. By alternate contraction and relaxation of the two sets of muscles, a wave-like motion called peristalsis is created that pushes food along the tube.

Elsewhere in the body, groups of smooth muscle fibres act without the need for pairing. In the skin, a bundle of smooth muscle fibres is attached to the tissues that surround the base of each hair. When the body is cold the fibres contract, making the hair stand up.

It is sometimes possible for the brain to override the instructions of the autonomic nervous system in the control of smooth muscle activity. The smooth muscle surrounding the exit to the bladder, for example, is normally kept contracted, closing the outlet. When the bladder is full, involuntary nerve messages instruct the muscle to relax so that urine can be passed. With training, nerve signals from the brain can cancel this command until urination is convenient.

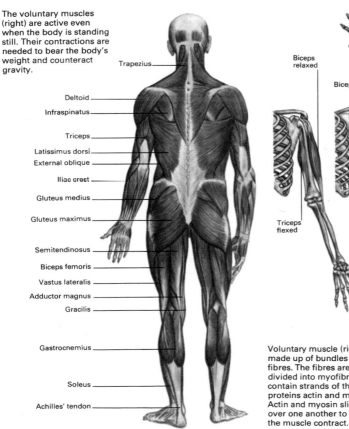

The voluntary muscles (right) are active even when the body is standing still. Their contractions are needed to bear the body's weight and counteract gravity.

Trapezius
Deltoid
Infraspinatus
Triceps
Latissimus dorsi
External oblique
Iliac crest
Gluteus medius
Gluteus maximus
Semitendinosus
Biceps femoris
Vastus lateralis
Adductor magnus
Gracilis
Gastrocnemius
Soleus
Achilles' tendon

Voluntary muscle (right) is made up of bundles of fibres. The fibres are divided into myofibrils that contain strands of the proteins actin and myosin. Actin and myosin slide over one another to make the muscle contract.

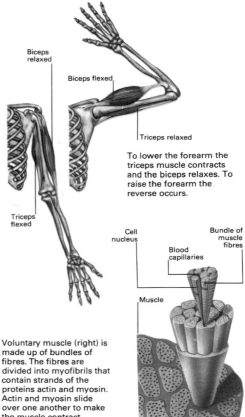

Biceps relaxed
Biceps flexed
Triceps relaxed

To lower the forearm the triceps muscle contracts and the biceps relaxes. To raise the forearm the reverse occurs.

Triceps flexed

Cell nucleus
Blood capillaries
Bundle of muscle fibres
Muscle

The heart

The blood circulation is the body system that carries essential supplies of food and fuel to every living cell and exchanges them for potentially harmful waste products. The adult circulation consists of thousands of miles of tubing containing about 4.7 litres (8.3 pints) of blood. The blood is kept flowing round the body by the pumping action of the heart.

Blood is made up of a pale yellow liquid (plasma) containing dissolved nutrients and wastes, plus blood cells, hormones, and other substances. Most numerous of these cells are the disc-shaped red blood cells (corpuscles). Their colour comes from the presence of the substance haemoglobin, which combines with oxygen. When red corpuscles filled with oxygen approach body cells, the oxygen is delivered in exchange for the waste product carbon dioxide. Other two-way transporting of materials takes place between the body cells and the plasma, and all unwanted substances are carried away in the blood for excretion by the kidneys, lungs, skin and liver. Plasma also contains white blood corpuscles, which help to fight infection, and platelets, which are involved in blood clotting.

In its passage through the body, blood is carried in tubes known as arteries and veins. Most arteries transport oxygen-rich (oxygenated) blood, whereas most veins transport carbon dioxide-rich (deoxygenated) blood. The largest artery is the aorta, which arises directly from the heart. The aorta and other large arteries have thick walls lined with muscle. Blood flow is assisted by the contraction of this muscle and the impetus given by the heartbeat. The "push" from the heart can be felt as the pulse where large arteries run near the body surface.

As they penetrate the tissues, arteries split into narrow branches called arterioles, which in turn divide into capillaries. It is across the very thin capillary walls that the blood gives

Aortic semilunar valve
Aorta
Superior vena cava
Pulmonary artery
Pulmonary semilunar valve
Right atrium
Left atrium

Blood flow in the heart is ordered by valves. The tricuspid valve controls flow from right atrium to right ventricle; the mitral valve flow from left atrium to left ventricle. Valves also guard the entrances to the aorta and pulmonary artery.

Right ventricle
Tricuspid valve
Left ventricle
Mitral valve

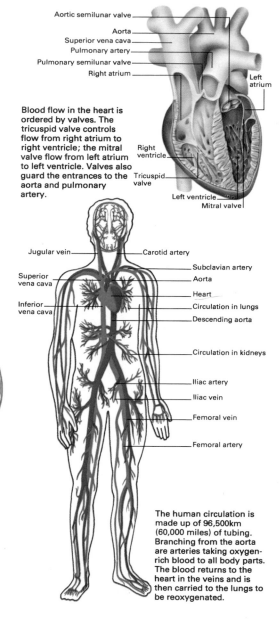

Fibrous covering
Smooth muscle
Connective tissue
Lining cells

Vein

Artery

Muscle
Valve

The walls of arteries and veins comprise the same four tissues, but arteries have more muscle to withstand more blood pressure. Blood flow in veins is aided by nearby muscles; valves prevent backflow.

Jugular vein
Carotid artery
Subclavian artery
Superior vena cava
Aorta
Heart
Inferior vena cava
Circulation in lungs
Descending aorta
Circulation in kidneys
Iliac artery
Iliac vein
Femoral vein
Femoral artery

The human circulation is made up of 96,500km (60,000 miles) of tubing. Branching from the aorta are arteries taking oxygen-rich blood to all body parts. The blood returns to the heart in the veins and is then carried to the lungs to be reoxygenated.

up its oxygen and nutrients and receives carbon dioxide and wastes. Deoxygenated blood in the capillaries flows into narrow veins (venules) and then into veins. The two largest veins, the venae cavae, return this blood to the heart. Veins have thin walls compared with those of arteries, and blood moves through the veins much more slowly. Blood flow in the veins is assisted by the action of muscles in surrounding tissues, and backflow is prevented by one-way valves.

The deoxygenated blood delivered to the heart along the veins is no use to body cells until it has been recharged with oxygen. To ensure reoxygenation, the circulation has a second "loop". In this part of the system, blood rich in carbon dioxide travels from the heart along the pulmonary artery to the lungs, where carbon dioxide is exchanged for oxygen breathed in. The pulmonary artery is the only artery to carry deoxygenated blood. The newly oxygenated blood is carried back to the heart along the pulmonary vein, the only vein to transport oxygenated blood.

The heart is a muscular organ about the size of a clenched fist. The structure and action of the heart are designed to serve the two loops of the circulation. Inside, the heart is divided vertically by a muscular wall. On each side of this wall is an upper chamber (atrium) and a thicker, lower chamber

(ventricle). Blood moves through each side of the heart systematically. Deoxygenated blood is delivered into the right atrium. It then enters the right ventricle, from where it is pumped out into the pulmonary artery and to the lungs. Oxygenated blood returning in the pulmonary veins flows into the left atrium. This blood enters the left ventricle and is then pumped into the aorta for circulation.

The flow of blood in each side of the heart is controlled by a series of valves. The pumping action of the heart is achieved by the contraction of the cardiac muscle of which the heart is largely composed. The rhythm of the heartbeat is regulated by bursts of electrical impulses sent out by a concentration of specialized heart tissue called the pacemaker.

Under the influence of the pacemaker, the heart of an adult at rest beats at a rate of 70 to 80 beats a minute. The pacemaker also helps to ensure the correct sequence of activities during each heartbeat; first the two atria contract, followed rapidly by the ventricles. The powerful contraction of the ventricles pushes blood into the aorta and pulmonary artery. This period of contraction (systole) is followed by a period of relaxation (diastole), during which the heart refills. The complete sequence is accompanied by electrical activity of the muscle, which can be monitored as an electrocardiogram (ECG).

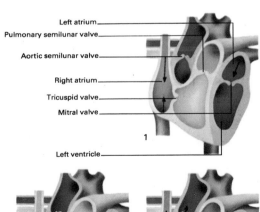

Left atrium
Pulmonary semilunar valve
Aortic semilunar valve
Right atrium
Tricuspid valve
Mitral valve
1
Left ventricle

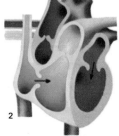
2

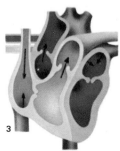
3

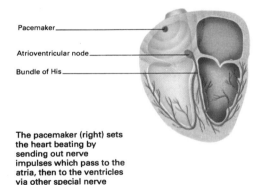

Pacemaker
Atrioventricular node
Bundle of His

The pacemaker (right) sets the heart beating by sending out nerve impulses which pass to the atria, then to the ventricles via other special nerve tissues.

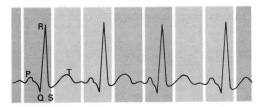

R
P T
Q S

As a heartbeat begins (1) right and left atria fill with blood. The atria contract (2) forcing blood into the right and left ventricles.

The ventricles then contract strongly (3) so that blood is pushed into the aorta and pulmonary artery.

An electrocardiogram (ECG) records the waves of nerve impulses of each heartbeat. The P wave starts just before the atria

contract, the QRS wave indicates the contraction of the ventricles, and the T wave the recovery period before the next contraction.

9

Respiration

Respiration is the process of breathing and the mechanism by which all cells in the body release energy from the materials they consume. The two sorts of respiration are closely linked. To produce energy, cells use oxygen and generate carbon dioxide and water. The movement of air in and out of the lungs makes oxygen available to the body and removes carbon dioxide and water.

Air enters the respiratory system through the mouth and nose, where it is warmed and moistened. Air breathed in through the nose is filtered by the coarse hairs that line the nostrils, which trap large dust particles. Smaller particles are trapped in a sticky fluid (mucus) produced by the cells lining the passage between nose and mouth. This mucus is continuously moved away by the beating of minute hair-like projections (cilia).

From the mouth, air travels through the throat (pharynx), voicebox (larynx), and windpipe (trachea). At the entry to the windpipe is a flap, the epiglottis, which closes to prevent choking when food is swallowed. At its base the windpipe divides into two tubes or bronchi, and one bronchus enters each lung. Both windpipe and bronchi are stiffened by rings of cartilage. As in the nose, the windpipe and bronchi produce dust-trapping mucus and have cilia to move this mucus up to the mouth.

Within each lung the bronchi split successively into smaller bronchi and then into many thousands of even narrower tubes called bronchioles. The bronchioles branch through the lungs and lead into millions of air sacs (alveoli) of the lung tissue. It is in the air sacs that gases are exchanged. Each air sac is surrounded by small blood vessels (capillaries) carrying blood from the heart containing carbon dioxide and water. Oxygen from the air breathed in passes into the blood and carbon dioxide and water vapour are

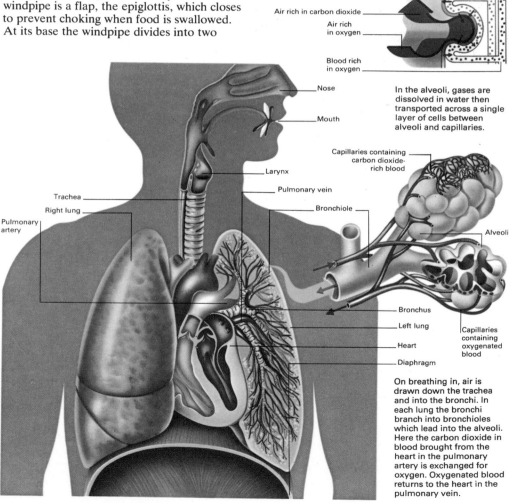

Blood rich in carbon dioxide
Layer of cells
Film of water
Air rich in carbon dioxide
Air rich in oxygen
Blood rich in oxygen

In the alveoli, gases are dissolved in water then transported across a single layer of cells between alveoli and capillaries.

Nose
Mouth
Larynx
Pulmonary vein
Trachea
Right lung
Pulmonary artery
Capillaries containing carbon dioxide-rich blood
Bronchiole
Alveoli
Bronchus
Left lung
Heart
Diaphragm
Capillaries containing oxygenated blood

On breathing in, air is drawn down the trachea and into the bronchi. In each lung the bronchi branch into bronchioles which lead into the alveoli. Here the carbon dioxide in blood brought from the heart in the pulmonary artery is exchanged for oxygen. Oxygenated blood returns to the heart in the pulmonary vein.

released into the air sacs of the lungs to be breathed out. The blood in the capillaries, now rich in oxygen, flows into the pulmonary vein and back to the heart for redistribution.

The lungs are enclosed in a bony cage made up of the ribs, breastbone, and backbone. The floor of the cage is formed by a sheet of muscle called the diaphragm. When a person breathes in, the muscles of the diaphragm contract, pulling the diaphragm downward. At the same time the rib-cage is pulled up and out, by the contraction of the muscles between the ribs, and air rushes in. When a person breathes out, the diaphragm and rib muscles relax and the chest subsides.

Respiration takes place ten to fifteen times a minute and is normally unconsciously controlled by a collection of cells in the brain called the respiratory centre. After air has been breathed out, carbon dioxide builds up again in the bloodstream. The cells in the respiratory centre are extremely sensitive to carbon dioxide concentrations. When the carbon dioxide in the blood reaches a certain level, messages are sent from the respiratory centre to the diaphragm and rib muscles stimulating them to contract. This once more initiates breathing in. As the lungs expand during inspiration, cells (stretch receptors) in the lung walls send signals back to the respiratory centre. The centre responds by instructing the muscles of ribs and diaphragm to relax so that breathing out takes place.

Respiration is not always a quiet process. The presence of many dust particles in the nose can trigger off sneezing. Irritants or too much mucus in the windpipe and bronchi cause coughing. Speech is also a special sort of "noisy" breathing. The sounds of speech are produced in the voicebox (larynx) and moulded into words in the mouth.

The larynx consists of a box of cartilage. Across the inside of the box are firm membranes, the vocal cords. The cords are made to move by the action of muscles attached to the cartilages of the larynx. During normal breathing, the vocal cords are held apart. For speech the cords are pulled together after a breath in, so that during breathing out the air is forced between the cords, making them vibrate. The tighter the cords are pulled together, the higher is the pitch of the sound produced. For loud sounds the air is forced through the cords faster than it is for soft sounds. The movements of the lips and of the tongue against the teeth and roof of the mouth achieve articulation. The resonance of spoken sounds and the characteristics of every individual voice are created by the cavities of the sinuses, nose, throat, and chest.

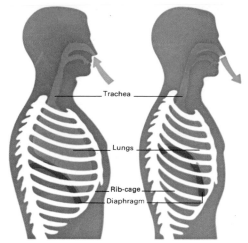

Trachea

Lungs

Rib-cage

Diaphragm

Breathing in is an active process. Air is drawn in as the rib-cage expands and the diaphragm contracts.

Breathing out is passive: the lungs recoil, the diaphragm relaxes, and the rib-cage subsides.

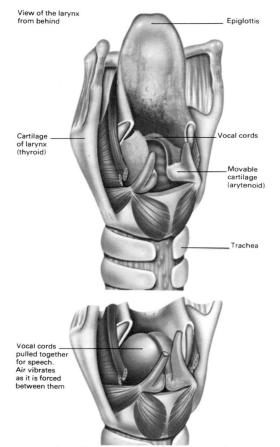

View of the larynx from behind

Epiglottis

Cartilage of larynx (thyroid)

Vocal cords

Movable cartilage (arytenoid)

Trachea

Vocal cords pulled together for speech. Air vibrates as it is forced between them

In normal breathing, the epiglottis is held upward and the vocal cords, joined to movable cartilages, are wide apart. In swallowing, the epiglottis is lowered. For speech the vocal cords are drawn close together.

11

The digestive system

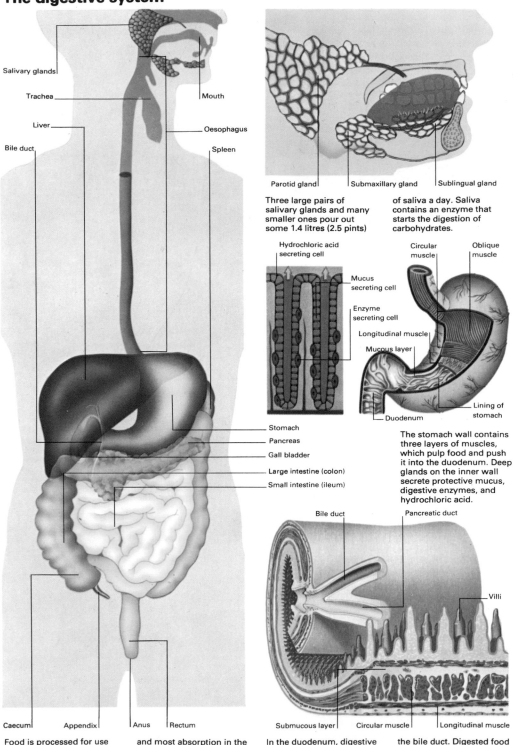

Salivary glands

Trachea

Liver

Bile duct

Mouth

Oesophagus

Spleen

Parotid gland | Submaxillary gland | Sublingual gland

Three large pairs of salivary glands and many smaller ones pour out some 1.4 litres (2.5 pints) of saliva a day. Saliva contains an enzyme that starts the digestion of carbohydrates.

Hydrochloric acid secreting cell

Mucus secreting cell

Enzyme secreting cell

Circular muscle

Oblique muscle

Longitudinal muscle

Mucous layer

Lining of stomach

Duodenum

Stomach

Pancreas

Gall bladder

Large intestine (colon)

Small intestine (ileum)

The stomach wall contains three layers of muscles, which pulp food and push it into the duodenum. Deep glands on the inner wall secrete protective mucus, digestive enzymes, and hydrochloric acid.

Bile duct

Pancreatic duct

Villi

Caecum | Appendix | Anus | Rectum

Submucous layer | Circular muscle | Longitudinal muscle

Food is processed for use as it passes along the digestive tract. Most food breakdown occurs in the stomach and duodenum, and most absorption in the jejunum and ileum. Water is absorbed in the caecum and colon, while wastes are passed at the anus.

In the duodenum, digestive juices are made by glands on the inner wall. More juices enter from the gall bladder and pancreas via the bile duct. Digested food is absorbed by the villi. Amino acids and sugars enter the blood, fats the lymph vessels.

Proteins, carbohydrates, fats, and liquids supply the body with energy and building materials. But these foods are of no use until they have been broken down into substances that can be absorbed into the blood circulation and transported via the liver to all body cells. This breakdown and absorption are the functions of the digestive system.

The digestive system consists of a tube about 10 metres (33 feet) in length that runs from the mouth to the anus. Within the tube many secretions are produced to aid the digestive process. These secretions include enzymes, which are biological catalysts that help to speed essential chemical reactions.

Food starts its journey through the digestive system in the mouth. There it is broken up by the teeth and moistened by secretions released from the salivary glands. Saliva also starts digestion, because it contains an enzyme that begins breaking down carbohydrates. The tongue and the teeth form each mouthful of food into a ball (bolus) and the tongue pushes it to the back of the mouth to be swallowed.

After leaving the mouth, food passes down the oesophagus (gullet) and into the stomach. Some food stays in the stomach for up to four hours. During this time it is churned and mixed with secretions produced by the cells of the stomach lining. These secretions include the enzyme pepsin, which begins breaking down proteins; hydrochloric acid, which sterilizes food and provides the right environment for stomach enzymes to work; and the sticky fluid (mucus) that protects the stomach cells from digesting themselves.

Digestion in the stomach converts food into a thick sludge called chyme. The chyme passes into the duodenum, the first part of the small intestine. The small intestine is a tube about 6.4 metres (21 feet) long, named for its width rather than its length. In passing down the small intestine – and the large intestine that follows it – food is moved along by peristalsis, rhythmic, wave-like contractions of the muscles in the intestine wall.

In the 25cm (10 inches) duodenum, many digestive juices are poured onto the chyme. The duodenum wall secretes alkaline juices that neutralize the acid from the stomach and contain enzymes and protective mucus. Further enzyme-containing juices enter the duodenum from the pancreas. The two sets of enzymes digest proteins, carbohydrates, and fats. Fat digestion is assisted by bile, which is made in the liver. Bile contains no enzymes but breaks fats into small globules that are easier for the enzymes to work on.

By the time it leaves the duodenum, most food has been broken down into absorbable fragments. Proteins have become amino acids; carbohydrates are now glucose; and other simple sugars and fats have been converted to glycerol and fatty acids. Some of these substances are absorbed in the duodenum, but most are taken up in the 2.5m (8 feet) jejunum and 3.6m (12 feet) ileum.

The inner wall of the small intestine is folded into millions of finger-like projections called villi, which provide a large surface area for absorption. Within each villus are small blood vessels (capillaries) and narrow branches of the lymphatic system. Amino acids and sugars are absorbed into the capillaries, while glycerol and fatty acids enter the lymphatic vessels, which drain into the bloodstream. Nutrients from digested food are then transported in the blood to the liver for storage until required by body cells.

Digestion in the small intestine takes four to five hours. The liquid remaining after absorption passes into the large intestine (colon), which includes the appendix, an organ with no apparent useful function. Movement of the remnants of digestion through the large intestine takes fifteen hours or more. In this time more than half the water contained is absorbed into the blood. The colon is also filled with bacteria. Some of these can break down the plant carbohydrate cellulose into usable sugars whereas others make vitamin B.

The faeces (stools), the final products of digestion, leave the large intestine via the anus. Water makes up 75 per cent of the stools. The remaining 25 per cent consists of worn-out digestive cells, dead bacteria, and undigested plant fibres. The urge to defecate occurs when the rectum fills with faeces.

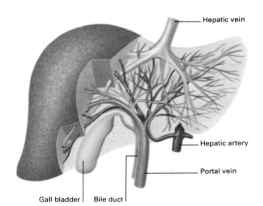

— Hepatic vein

— Hepatic artery

— Portal vein

Gall bladder | Bile duct |

Digested food reaches the liver in the portal vein and oxygen in the hepatic artery. Essential substances such as sugars, vitamins, and minerals are extracted for storage and spent blood leaves in the hepatic vein. Bile formed in the liver is stored in the gall bladder until needed for digestion.

The urinary system

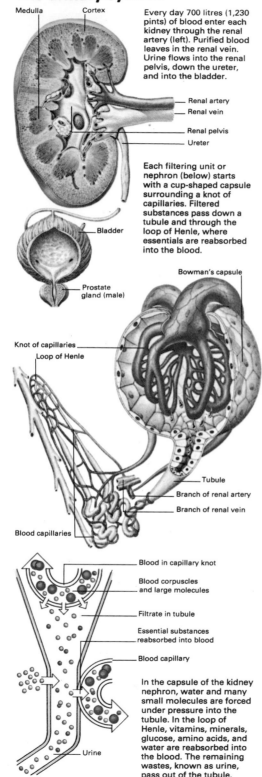

Medulla   Cortex

Every day 700 litres (1,230 pints) of blood enter each kidney through the renal artery (left). Purified blood leaves in the renal vein. Urine flows into the renal pelvis, down the ureter, and into the bladder.

— Renal artery
— Renal vein
— Renal pelvis
— Ureter

Each filtering unit or nephron (below) starts with a cup-shaped capsule surrounding a knot of capillaries. Filtered substances pass down a tubule and through the loop of Henle, where essentials are reabsorbed into the blood.

— Bladder

— Prostate gland (male)

Bowman's capsule

Knot of capillaries
Loop of Henle

— Tubule
— Branch of renal artery
— Branch of renal vein

Blood capillaries

Blood in capillary knot

Blood corpuscles and large molecules

Filtrate in tubule

Essential substances reabsorbed into blood

Blood capillary

In the capsule of the kidney nephron, water and many small molecules are forced under pressure into the tubule. In the loop of Henle, vitamins, minerals, glucose, amino acids, and water are reabsorbed into the blood. The remaining wastes, known as urine, pass out of the tubule.

— Urine

The urinary system filters soluble waste products from the blood. It consists of two kidneys, two ureters, the urinary bladder, and the urethra. The kidneys are about 11cm (4½ inches) long and about 6cm (2½ inches) wide. They lie in the upper part of the abdomen at the back. The ureters are tubes about 25cm (10 inches) long that drain urine from the centre of the kidneys, the renal pelvis, to the bladder. The bladder lies in the lower abdomen at the front of the body. The urethra is the tube through which urine is passed to the outside.

The renal pelvis is funnel-shaped; its widest part is in the centre of the kidney. As the renal pelvis narrows, it projects from the kidney and becomes the top of the ureter. The widest part of the renal pelvis is surrounded by the renal medulla, which is in turn surrounded by the renal cortex. The renal cortex is covered by tough fibrous tissue that forms the protective outer layer of each kidney.

Blood is brought to the kidneys by the renal arteries and, after filtration, is returned to the circulation through the renal veins. The blood vessels join the kidneys close to each renal pelvis.

The functional units of the kidney are microscopic filters. The renal cortex contains about one million of these filters. Each consists of a cup-shaped capsule (Bowman's capsule) that encloses a knot (glomerulus) of blood capillaries. Blood from the renal artery is pumped into the glomerulus by blood pressure. Water, sugar, salts, urea (a waste product of the breakdown of proteins), and other small molecules pass through the capillary walls into the Bowman's capsule. Blood cells and large molecules, such as whole proteins and fats, remain in the blood.

Filtered fluids pass from the Bowman's capsule into a coiled tube, the nephron, that leads through the renal medulla to the renal pelvis. Each nephron has a U-shaped loop, the loop of Henle, half-way along its length. The whole tube is closely surrounded by blood capillaries. As the filtered fluid passes through the tube, substances that the body needs, especially water, essential salts, and sugar, are reabsorbed from the fluid in the tube into the surrounding blood capillaries.

The concentrated fluid (urine) that results from the filtration and reabsorption processes collects in the renal pelvis before passing through the ureter to the bladder. A circular ring of muscle at the top of the urethra keeps urine in the bladder until voluntarily relaxed.

The nose, mouth, and throat

The nose has two primary functions: (1) to filter, warm, and humidify air before it reaches the lungs; and (2) to smell.

The internal surface of the nose is covered with tiny hairs (cilia) that are surrounded by sticky, fluid mucus. Both cilia and mucus remove dust particles and water droplets from the air that is breathed through the nostrils. At the top of the nasal cavity there are two areas of tissue in which the cells are sensitive to smell. When a substance is trapped in the mucus by the cilia, it causes a chemical change to affect the sensitive cells. The cells react by sending a nerve impulse to the brain that is interpreted there as a smell.

The mouth is the beginning of the digestive tract. The teeth, the tongue, and the salivary glands prepare food for digestion. The saliva contains enzymes that start the process of digestion. The organs of taste (taste buds) are located in tiny projections (papillae) on the surface of the tongue. Each taste bud consists of a cluster of receptor cells that react to a chemical change by sending a nerve impulse to the brain, where it is interpreted as a taste.

When food is swallowed, a flap of cartilage (the epiglottis) folds down to cover the opening to the trachea (windpipe). This action prevents food from going down into the lungs.

The vocal cords are located in the trachea, just below the epiglottis. Sound is produced when air from the lungs passes between vocal cords that have been voluntarily tensed. The sounds of the human voice are controlled by the movements of the vocal cords in combination with movements of the tongue and lips.

The back of the nose and mouth is lined with pads of spongy tissue made of lymphoid tissue. These pads include the adenoids in the nose, the tonsils at the back of the mouth, and a similar pad of lymphoid tissue on the back of the tongue. Invading bacteria are collected and destroyed by the cells (lymphocytes) that are concentrated in lymphoid tissue. A large number of lymph glands in the tissues at the top of the throat and below, in the neck, support this defence mechanism.

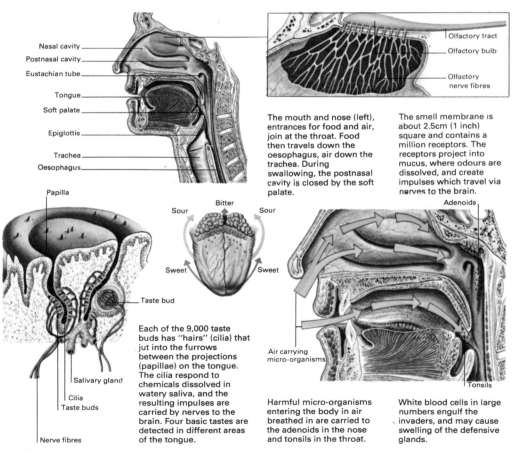

Nasal cavity
Postnasal cavity
Eustachian tube
Tongue
Soft palate
Epiglottis
Trachea
Oesophagus
Papilla

Olfactory tract
Olfactory bulb
Olfactory nerve fibres

The mouth and nose (left), entrances for food and air, join at the throat. Food then travels down the oesophagus, air down the trachea. During swallowing, the postnasal cavity is closed by the soft palate.

The smell membrane is about 2.5cm (1 inch) square and contains a million receptors. The receptors project into mucus, where odours are dissolved, and create impulses which travel via nerves to the brain.

Bitter
Sour
Sour
Sweet
Sweet
Adenoids

Taste bud
Salivary gland
Cilia
Taste buds
Nerve fibres

Air carrying micro-organisms
Tonsils

Each of the 9,000 taste buds has "hairs" (cilia) that jut into the furrows between the projections (papillae) on the tongue. The cilia respond to chemicals dissolved in watery saliva, and the resulting impulses are carried by nerves to the brain. Four basic tastes are detected in different areas of the tongue.

Harmful micro-organisms entering the body in air breathed in are carried to the adenoids in the nose and tonsils in the throat.

White blood cells in large numbers engulf the invaders, and may cause swelling of the defensive glands.

15

The eye and ear

The eyes and ears are organs vital to the body's interpretation of its environment. The eyes detect light rays; the ears pick up sound waves. The ears also contain the organs of balance.

Each eye is a spherical structure protected at its back and sides by the bones of the skull and at the front by two lashed eyelids. The outer covering of the eye, the sclera or "white", is both protective and structural. Light penetrates the sclera only at the front of the eye, where the outer surface bulges into the transparent cornea, a delicate structure covered with a thin defensive membrane, the conjunctiva. Under each upper eyelid is a tear-secreting lacrimal gland whose constant activity keeps the conjunctiva moist and free from infection.

Light entering the eye passes through the cornea and then through a watery fluid, the aqueous humour, in the front of the eye. Behind the fluid is the iris, a ring of muscle with a central hole, the pupil. The cornea focuses light rays so that they pass through the pupil. The iris determines how much light enters the eye. In dim light its muscles relax to let in more light; in bright light its muscles contract to reduce pupil size and restrict light entry.

The fine focusing of light is achieved by the lens, a soft, transparent structure lying behind the iris. The lens is held in place by ligaments attached to internal eye muscles. The actions of these muscles produce changes in the shape of the lens so that close and distant objects can be focused upon. For viewing near objects the muscles make the lens shorter and fatter; for viewing distant objects the lens becomes longer and thinner. This process is known as accommodation.

From the lens, light passes through the thick jelly (vitreous humour) that fills the centre of the eye. The light is projected onto the retina, a light-sensitive layer inside the sclera from which it is separated by the choroid, a dark layer of tissue rich in blood vessels. The retina contains two sorts of light-receptor cells: rods, which detect shades of black and white; and cones, which are sensitive to colour. In response to light, the rods and cones generate nerve impulses that pass along the optic nerve to the brain to be interpreted as vision. The concentration of cones is densest at a single spot called the

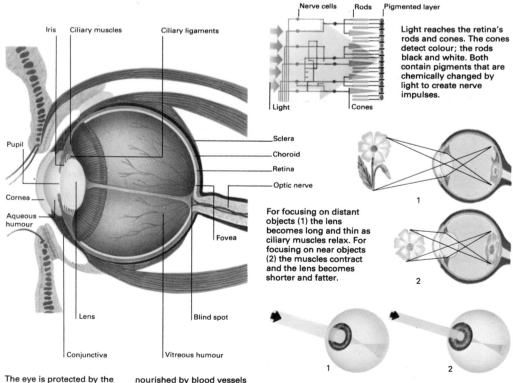

Nerve cells   Rods   Pigmented layer

Light   Cones

Light reaches the retina's rods and cones. The cones detect colour; the rods black and white. Both contain pigments that are chemically changed by light to create nerve impulses.

Iris   Ciliary muscles   Ciliary ligaments

Pupil

Cornea

Aqueous humour

Lens

Conjunctiva

Sclera
Choroid
Retina
Optic nerve

Fovea

Blind spot

Vitreous humour

For focusing on distant objects (1) the lens becomes long and thin as ciliary muscles relax. For focusing on near objects (2) the muscles contract and the lens becomes shorter and fatter.

1

2

1

2

The eye is protected by the covering conjunctiva and sclera. Light is focused by the cornea and lens onto the retina, which is nourished by blood vessels in the choroid. Impulses created on the retina leave the eye along the optic nerve.

The pupil, a hole in the centre of the iris, adjusts by reflex to control the amount of light entering the eye. The pupil becomes wider in dim light (1) and becomes smaller in bright (2).

fovea. Where the optic nerve leaves the back of the eye there are no rods or cones; this is called the blind spot.

The ears, like the eyes, are enclosed deep in the bone structure of the skull. Each ear is divided into outer, middle, and inner sections. The only visible part is the flap of cartilage (pinna) of the outer ear, which helps to collect sounds and concentrates them into a tube, the auditory canal. At the end of the canal is a thin membrane, the eardrum (tympanic membrane). When sounds reach the eardrum, they make it vibrate. These vibrations are transmitted and amplified through the middle ear by a chain of three small bones, the hammer (malleus), anvil (incus), and stirrup (stapes). The cavity of the middle ear, in which the bones are contained, is joined to the throat by the Eustachian tube. The tube ensures that the air pressure in the middle ear remains the same as that on the outer side of the eardrum. The middle ear also connects with the air cells in the mastoid bone behind the ear.

The stirrup, the last of the middle ear bones, rests against a membrane, the oval window, that leads to the cochlea, the part of the inner ear concerned with hearing. The cochlea is a spiral, fluid-filled tube divided internally along its length by a strip of tissue, the basilar membrane. The vibrations carried by the middle ear bones are transported in the fluid as pressure waves. These waves make special hair-bearing cells on the basilar membrane vibrate according to the loudness and pitch of sound. Their vibration sets up nerve impulses that are then carried to the brain along the auditory nerve, to be interpreted there as hearing. The hair-bearing cells and the membrane on which they are found are known as the organ of Corti.

The inner ear also contains the organs of balance which, like the cochlea, consist of fluid-filled chambers. Three of these, the semicircular canals, are set in planes at right angles to one another. At the ends of the chambers are collections of fine hairs. As the head moves, the fluid in each canal starts to move accordingly, and stimulates the hairs to generate nerve messages. Even when the head is still, body posture is detected by two further chambers, the utricle and saccule. Impulses from these chambers travel to the area of the brain responsible for balance.

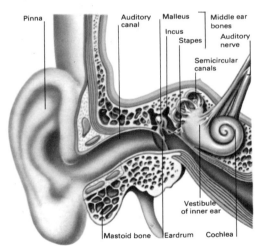

Sounds received by the ear's pinna pass along the auditory canal to the eardrum. Vibrations are carried by three bones to the cochlea, from which nerve impulses are sent to the brain.

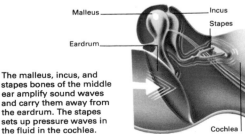

The malleus, incus, and stapes bones of the middle ear amplify sound waves and carry them away from the eardrum. The stapes sets up pressure waves in the fluid in the cochlea.

The spiral cochlea is divided internally into three compartments. Within the central one lies the organ of Corti. This has hairs that vibrate in response to sounds and create nerve impulses that travel via the auditory nerve to the brain for analysis.

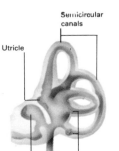

The semicircular canals detect body movement in three planes as the fluid they contain stimulates hair-like receptors. Utricle and saccule register the position of the head.

The brain

The brain is an organ constructed to receive, process, and store the information that floods into it from inside and outside the body, and to issue "instructions" for body action. It is the seat of human consciousness, intellect, memory, emotions, and personality. The brain is a delicate structure weighing about 1,380gm (3lb) in a man, and 1,250gm (2lb 12oz) in a woman; it is protected by covering membranes (meninges) and by the bones of the skull.

More than 30,000 million nerve cells (neurons) make up the brain. To accommodate these cells the surface of the brain is much folded. Most of the brain is symmetrically divided into right and left halves, linked by nerve tissue. Each half is made up of three main areas: the hind-, mid-, and forebrain. Different parts of each area have distinct functions that are carried out by the nerve cells that compose them. Lying deep within the brain are cavities (ventricles) filled with fluid.

The hindbrain, at the brain's base and joined to the spinal cord, is composed of two parts: the brainstem and the cerebellum. The brainstem controls essential life-supporting functions, such as respiration and heartbeat, and acts on the huge inflow of information it receives about the state of the body. Running through the brainstem is the reticular formation that helps to determine the whole level of brain activity and, for example,

whether a person is asleep or awake. The reticular formation also has an influence on the emotions. The cerebellum, just behind and above the brainstem, controls the co-ordination of body movements, posture, and balance, although it has no power to initiate movements.

Composing the midbrain are the hypothalamus, thalamus, pituitary gland, and limbic system. The hypothalamus is responsible for controlling the basic drives that ensure human survival: hunger, thirst, and sex. In addition, the hypothalamus helps to regulate body temperature and governs the activity of the pituitary gland, the gland that produces many hormones which control other glands in the endocrine system. Encircling the hypothlamus is the limbic system, which is involved in the expression of emotions such as anger and fear, in mood changes, and in the power of human memory. The limbic system also serves to integrate messages from the higher centres of the forebrain, while the thalamus acts as a relay station for information transfer between sense organs and the forebrain.

The forebrain or cerebrum, making up 70 per cent of the brain, is composed of two cerebral hemispheres linked by a bundle of nerve fibres, the corpus callosum. Each hemisphere is composed of an outer cortex (grey matter), containing millions of nerve cells, and an inner layer (white matter),

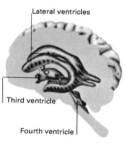

Four cavities (ventricles) in the brain contain a clear fluid that flows out of the fourth ventricle in the brainstem to lubricate the surfaces of brain and spinal cord. This cerebrospinal fluid is made by cells in the brain and acts to cushion the brain against injury.

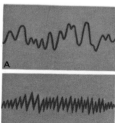

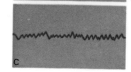

An electroencephalogram (EEG) is a trace of the electrical activity of the cells in the brain's cortex. The trace is obtained by placing electrodes on the scalp. In deep sleep (A), the waves are large and well spaced. When the body is awake but relaxed (B), the waves become sharper and more frequent; and are very fast and close together during physical exertion (C).

The brain's three main areas reflect its evolution. The hindbrain (brainstem and cerebellum) is less advanced than the midbrain (consisting of thalamus, hypothalamus, pituitary, and limbic system). Most advanced are the cerebral hemispheres of the forebrain.

consisting largely of nerve fibres that carry messages in and out of the cortex. The cortex is the brain's chief receiver, processor, and storer of information, and the main issuer of instructions for action.

The nerve fibres entering and leaving the cerebral hemispheres from all parts of the body cross over in the brainstem. This means that the left hemisphere serves the right side of the body, and the right hemisphere the body's left side. The two hemispheres are not, however, exactly the same. In most people the left hemisphere is the "logical" brain, the right hemisphere usually acts as the "artistic" brain, directing visio-spatial and musical skills.

Each cerebral hemisphere is divided into four lobes, which are known to perform specific tasks. Largest of these lobes are the frontal lobes at the front of the hemispheres. One area toward the back of each lobe (the

motor cortex) is responsible for directing voluntary movements. The rest of each frontal lobe is involved in personality development and the ability to form abstract concepts.

Behind the frontal lobes are the parietal lobes, which are primarily responsible for receiving sensations of touch and body position. The occipital lobes at the back of the hemispheres are the receivers and analysers of visual information. And the senses of hearing and smell are made possible by the temporal lobes that form the sides of each hemisphere.

To ensure that information reaching the four lobes of each hemisphere is properly integrated, the cerebral cortex contains groups of nerve cells which make up association areas. These areas allow the brain to create a total "picture" of the body's state and environment.

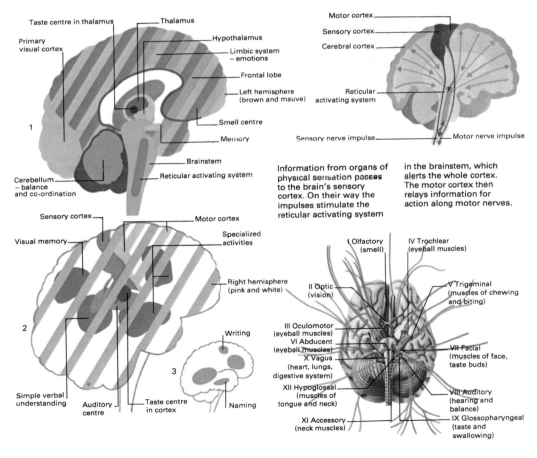

Information from organs of physical sensation passes to the brain's sensory cortex. On their way the impulses stimulate the reticular activating system in the brainstem, which alerts the whole cortex. The motor cortex then relays information for action along motor nerves.

Many of the brain's functions have been "mapped." Indicated here are the major activities governed by the left hemisphere, shown from inside (1) and outside (3), and of the right hemisphere (2) shown from the outer aspect.

Arising from the underside of the brain are 12 pairs of cranial nerves that receive and relay information to and from many organs.

Nerves carrying incoming messages are shown in green; those sending out instructions are shown in orange.

19

The nervous system

The function of the nervous system is to receive and respond to information from the body's environment. The system also co-ordinates and controls body activities. It is made up of millions of nerve cells, or neurons, each consisting of a cell body with an extension called an axon. In some cells, the axon may be lengthy. Nerve fibres are formed when the axons of many neurons group together.

The nervous system is in two parts. The central nervous system (CNS) comprises the brain and spinal cord. The peripheral nervous system spreads out from both brain and spinal cord, all over the body, carrying information to and from the central nervous system.

In the peripheral system, 31 pairs of spinal nerves branch from the spinal cord, and 12 pairs of cranial nerves arise from underneath the brain. There are also autonomic nerves, situated outside the spinal cord.

Most of the spinal and cranial nerves have sensory and motor components. Sensory nerves convey information from the sense organs to the central nervous system. They also monitor such internal conditions as muscle tension, and the oxygen content of the blood. Some of them, such as the optic and auditory nerves, are partly under conscious control. Motor nerves transmit instructions to the muscles, to carry out the movements desired, and are thus totally under conscious control.

The autonomic nerves work unconsciously to regulate such functions as heartbeat, respiration, and digestion. There are two kinds: sympathetic and parasympathetic. The sympathetic nerves prepare the body for immediate action; the parasympathetic nerves relax the body after exertion and keep the body functioning at a reduced level during sleep.

The messages that move along the nerves depend on electrically charged particles (ions) of sodium and potassium, which pass through the covering membrane and cause an electric charge to pass through the nerve fibre. The charge is then transmitted to the adjacent nerve cell body, and so on to its destination.

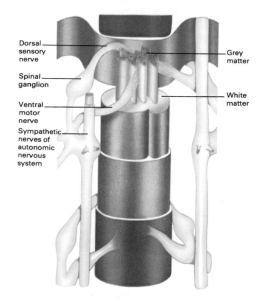

Dorsal sensory nerve
Spinal ganglion
Ventral motor nerve
Sympathetic nerves of autonomic nervous system
Grey matter
White matter

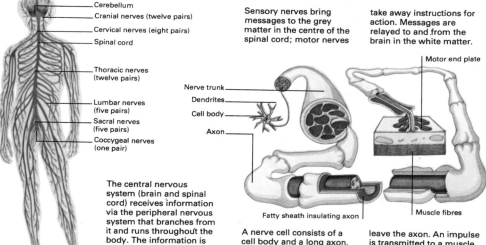

Cerebrum
Cerebellum
Cranial nerves (twelve pairs)
Cervical nerves (eight pairs)
Spinal cord
Thoracic nerves (twelve pairs)
Nerve trunk
Dendrites
Cell body
Lumbar nerves (five pairs)
Sacral nerves (five pairs)
Coccygeal nerves (one pair)
Axon
Motor end plate
Fatty sheath insulating axon
Muscle fibres

Sensory nerves bring messages to the grey matter in the centre of the spinal cord; motor nerves take away instructions for action. Messages are relayed to and from the brain in the white matter.

The central nervous system (brain and spinal cord) receives information via the peripheral nervous system that branches from it and runs throughout the body. The information is used for making conscious and unconscious decisions, resulting if necessary in orders for body actions.

A nerve cell consists of a cell body and a long axon. Impulses are transmitted as electrical charges created when sodium ions enter and potassium ions leave the axon. An impulse is transmitted to a muscle by a chemical transmitter substance that stimulates the muscle fibres to contract.

20

Endocrine glands

Endocrine glands are collections of tissue that control body functions by producing hormones. The endocrine glands release hormones directly into the blood.

The chief endocrine gland is the pituitary, situated beneath the brain, and divided into two lobes. The front (anterior) lobe produces a group of stimulating (tropic) hormones that are carried to other endocrine glands – the thyroid, adrenals, and sex glands – to trigger hormone production.

Other anterior pituitary hormones exert their influence directly. They include prolactin, which maintains milk production from the breasts, and growth hormone. The back (posterior) lobe of the pituitary produces two hormones: vasopressin (ADH), which is carried to the kidneys to help control body water content, and oxytocin, which assists the contraction of the womb during labour and encourages the flow of milk into the breasts after the birth of a baby.

Each of the adrenal glands, sited over the kidneys, is divided into an outer (cortex) and inner (medulla) region. The medulla makes the hormones adrenaline (epinephrine) and noradrenaline (norepinephrine), which help to prepare the body for "fight or flight" in response to threats. The hormones of the cortex include steroids involved in the body's metabolism of sugars and proteins, and in balancing body water content.

The thyroid gland lies below the voicebox or upper part of the windpipe. It secretes hormones that control the rate at which cells use nutrients. Attached to the back of the

thyroid are the four small parathyroid glands whose hormones regulate the amounts of calcium and phosphate in the blood, an activity vital to bone building.

The amount of glucose in the blood is governed by cells in the pancreas, situated beside the duodenum. The endocrine cells of the gland are clustered in small masses and make two hormones: glucagon, which raises blood glucose levels; and insulin, which decreases them. The sex glands – ovaries in a female and testes in a male – produce hormones that control the production of mature sex cells and help to determine a person's total sexual make-up.

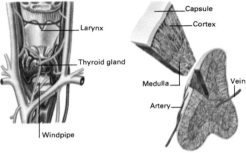

Hormones of the thyroid gland contain the mineral iodine. They help to control the rate at which the body burns and stores sugars.

The adrenal gland's cortex makes steroid hormones. The medulla's hormones prepare the body for "fight or flight".

Labels: Larynx, Thyroid gland, Windpipe; Capsule, Cortex, Medulla, Vein, Artery

The pituitary (right) is the most important endocrine gland. Hormones from the front (anterior) part of the gland control the activity of many other glands. The pituitary itself is governed by the hypothalamus of the brain.

Labels (body diagram): Brain, Pituitary gland, Thyroid gland, Parathyroid glands, Adrenal glands, Pancreas, Kidney, Ovaries in female, Testes in male

The endocrine glands produce hormones, chemical messengers that travel in the blood and influence a wide variety of body activities over long periods.

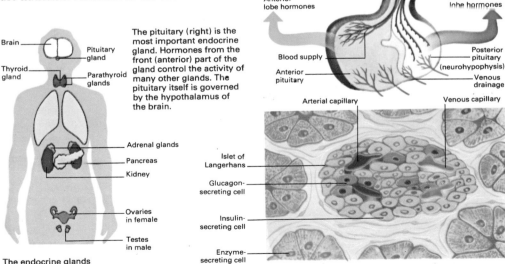

Labels: Anterior lobe hormones, Blood supply, Anterior pituitary, Arterial capillary; Posterior lobe hormones, Posterior pituitary (neurohypophysis), Venous drainage, Venous capillary; Islet of Langerhans, Glucagon-secreting cell, Insulin-secreting cell, Enzyme-secreting cell

Groups of cells in the Islets of Langerhans in the pancreas make two hormones that regulate body sugars. Insulin decreases the amount of sugar in the blood; glucagon increases it. The remainder of the gland secretes digestive enzymes.

Reproduction

The biological purpose of the sex organs is the reproduction of the human race. To make this possible, a male's reproductive system must be able to make sex cells (sperm) and place them inside the female. The female's system must be able to release mature female sex cells (eggs or ova). The sperm enter and fertilize the eggs, and the developing baby (foetus) is nurtured within the female until it is born.

In a mature man sperm are made in the two testes (testicles), organs filled with many coiled tubes. The testes are suspended in a sac, the scrotum, outside the body. The

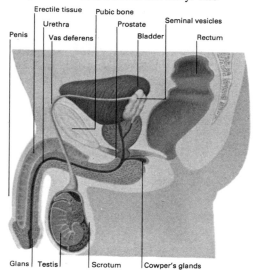

In the male, sperm are made in the testes. They pass along the vas deferens to be stored in the seminal vesicles. Prostrate, and Cowper's glands make fluids that compose semen.

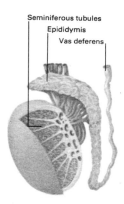 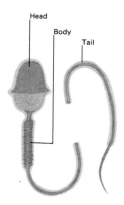

Sperm are made in the coiled seminiferous tubules of the testis, then matured in the adjoining epididymis.

The miscroscopic sperm has a head containing genetic material, a "body" that provides energy, and a whiplash tail for movement.

scrotum lies behind the penis, the organ sensitive to sexual arousal through which the sperm are transmitted to the female. Sperm are made continuously in the testes and stored in the seminal vesicles, two small structures next to the prostate gland. During sexual intercourse, some 250 million tadpole-like sperm are released (ejaculated) from the penis, together with secretions from several sex glands, including the prostate and the seminal vesicles. The mixture of sperm and fluids is known as semen.

All the reproductive organs of the female body are internal. Eggs are produced in a pair of organs, the ovaries. The ovaries are connected to the womb (uterus), the area of foetus development, by the fallopian tubes. The womb opens through a narrow orifice (the cervix), into the vagina, the cavity into which the penis is placed during intercourse. Surrounding the entrance to the vagina, on the outside of the body, are two pairs of skin folds. The larger pair (labia majora) lie outside the smaller (labia minora). Behind these folds is the clitoris, an organ of sexual arousal equivalent to the penis.

Puberty, the start of sexual development, begins in boys at the age of twelve or thirteen. The hypothalamus in the base of the brain stimulates the pituitary gland to secrete two hormones. These hormones act on the testes, to make them release male hormones (androgens), the most important of which is testosterone. This hormone brings about the enlargement of the sex organs, the start of sperm production, and the appearance of secondary sexual characteristics. Among these characteristics are the growth of hair on the body and face, the deepening of the voice, and increased development of bones and muscles. Maturation to manhood is not usually complete until about age twenty.

Girls start to mature sexually about two years earlier than boys. The pituitary, under the influence of the hypothalamus, secretes the identical hormones, which act on the ovaries and stimulate them to produce the two hormones oestrogen and progesterone. Oestrogen brings about enlargement of the sex organs, and controls the development of the female secondary sexual characteristics. These include the growth of the breasts, the widening of the hips, and the appearance of hair in the armpits and pubic region. The whole body grows rapidly and maturity is usually reached by the age of sixteen.

A girl experiences her first menstrual period before the time that ovulation begins. Menstruation, a bleeding from the womb, takes place about every 28 days and lasts for four or five days. It is closely controlled by hormones. In the ovary, each egg develops in a sac called a follicle. As the egg is prepared for release, the follicle produces the hormone oestrogen, which starts the build-up of the lining of the womb in preparation for receiving a fertilized egg. Once the egg has left the ovary the empty follicle secretes more oestrogen, plus a second hormone, progesterone. Together oestrogen and progesterone aid further thickening of the womb lining. If the egg is not fertilized, the follicle degenerates, hormone output ceases, and the womb lining is shed as the menstrual

period. If the egg is fertilized, it makes yet another hormone that keeps the womb lining developing to nurture the embryo.

In a man, the production of sex hormones and sperm continues from maturity for the rest of life, although there is a gradual decline from the 40s and 50s onward. In a woman, however, ovulation becomes less frequent as she becomes older, and the ovaries less responsive to the pituitary hormones. Eventually, the ovaries do not respond at all and menstruation ceases (the menopause). This commonly occurs during the mid-40s.

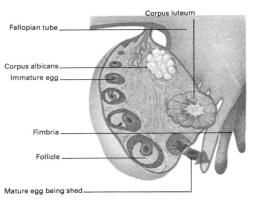

The ovaries of a baby girl contain thousands of immature eggs. After puberty, one egg ripens and is shed each month, leaving a corpus luteum, which makes hormones essential to the early stages of pregnancy. Fertilization usually occurs in the fimbria of the fallopian tubes.

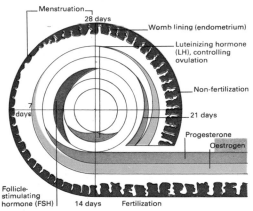

In the female, eggs are made in the ovaries and move through the fallopian tubes to the womb, where they will develop if fertilized. During intercourse the male penis is placed in the vagina.

Hormones regulate the menstrual cycle. The egg matures under FSH influence, oestrogen starts the build-up of the womb lining, and LH controls egg release. Progesterone completes the womb lining. If the egg is not fertilized, hormone production stops and menstruation occurs.

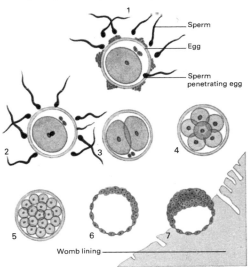

After fertilization (1), the egg divides (2-5) to form a ball of cells. A fluid-filled cavity then develops inside the structure (6), which enters the womb lining (7) a week after fertilization. When implanted in the womb lining, the structure develops into the embryo.

Index of Symptoms

Section contents

Introduction

The Index of Symptoms has been designed to be an easy-to-use reference guide to the A-Z section that follows it. Organization of this index enables a user quickly to relate a given set of symptoms to the various conditions and disorders described in the A-Z section.

The index is divided into two parts: the first part is pictorial, the second part is diagrammatic.

Each page of the pictorial part contains an illustration or illustrations of a portion of the human body. Placed around each illustration are lists of the titles of relevant articles in the A-Z section.

The first section on every page informs the user of the titles of general articles in the A-Z section that may give background information about the part of the body illustrated.

Each of the other lists on the page is headed by a specific symptom and informs the user of the title of every article related to that symptom in the A-Z section. The lists have been enclosed by boxes to enhance usefulness. Lines drawn from the boxes to specific sites on the illustration indicate where in or on the body each symptom may occur.

The diagrammatic part of the index, Charts of related symptoms, is designed to direct a user to appropriate articles in the A-Z section when two or more symptoms occur simultaneously. Information as to the best immediate course of action is included. This part of the index has its own introduction, explaining how, using these charts, the appropriate articles in the A-Z may be quickly identified.

The user should keep in mind throughout that the information contained in the Index of symptoms **is not intended to replace the knowledge or expertise of a trained doctor. It is not intended to be, and should under no circumstances be used as, a means of self-diagnosis.** This is no substitute for the background, training, and experience of a doctor.

However, an understanding of various disorders and their symptoms can help a patient to communicate more accurately with his or her doctor when a medical problem does arise. And this is the strength of the Index of Symptoms and the accompanying A-Z section.

The eye

General articles
Blindness
Eye
Eye disorders

Blurred vision
Alcoholism
Amblyopia
Astigmatism
Cataract
Conjunctivitis
Detached retina
Diabetes
Eclampsia
Glioma
Glaucoma
Iritis
Longsightedness
Melanoma
Migraine
Multiple sclerosis
Myopia
Retinitis
Retrobulbar
  neuritis
Tears

Double vision
Diplopia
Head injury
Multiple sclerosis
Strabismus

**Impaired colour
  perception**
Colour blindness

**Intolerance of
  light**
Conjunctivitis
Encephalitis
Hay fever
Iritis
Measles
Meningitis
Migraine

**Spots in front of
  eyes**
Detached retina
High blood
  pressure
Migraine
Retinitis

Squint
Strabismus

Blindness
Blindness
Cataract
Detached retina
Diabetes
Glaucoma
Migraine
Night blindness
Retrobulbar
  neuritis
Snow blindness
Stroke
Ulcer

Watering eyes
Allergy
Blepharitis
Common cold
Conjunctivitis
Dacryocystitis
Ectropion
Entropion
Hay fever
Stye
Tears

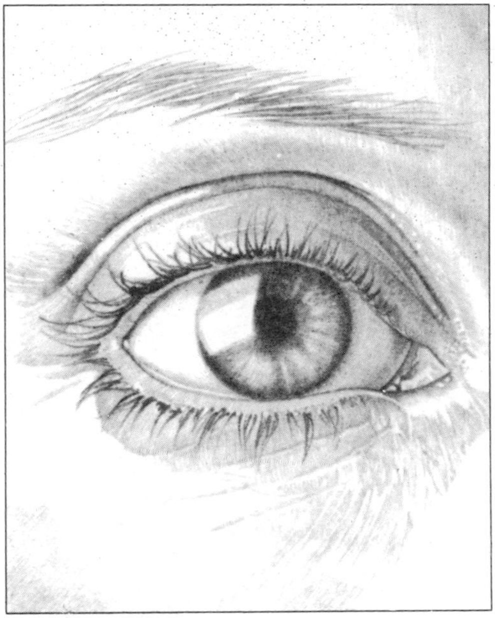

Red or pink eye
Allergy
Chemosis
Conjunctivitis
Glaucoma
Hay fever
Iritis
Marijuana
Measles
Red eye

Yellow eyes
Jaundice

Conjunctivitis
Allergy
Conjunctivitis
Hay fever
Measles
Smoking

Lump on lid
Chalazion
Melanoma
Mole
Papilloma
Rodent ulcer
Stye
Wart
Xanthelasma

Cysts on lid
Chalazion
Stye

Gritty feeling
Allergy
Blepharitis
Chalazion
Chemosis
Conjunctivitis
Hay fever
Iritis
Stye
Ulcer
Xerophthalmia

Protruding eyes
Iritis
Oedema
Proptosis
Thyrotoxicosis

Black eye
Bruise

Lids, drooping
Bell's palsy
Horner's
  syndrome
Myasthenia gravis
Ptosis
Stroke

Lids, sore
Allergy
Blepharitis
Chalazion
Ectropion
Entropion
Hay fever
Stye

Lids, swollen
Allergy
Angioneurotic
  oedema
Blepharitis
Ectropion
Entropion
Hay fever
Nephritis
Oedema
Stye

Lids, twitching
Anxiety

The neck and throat

General articles
Larynx
Lymph gland
Neck
Parathyroid gland
Pharynx
Swallowing
Throat
Thyroid gland
Tonsil

Adenoids
Adenoids
Adenoidectomy
Mucus
Snoring
Tonsil

Stiff neck
Stiff neck

Boils
Abscess
Boils

Lump on neck, stiff
Boils
Sebaceous cyst
Stiff neck
Whiplash injury

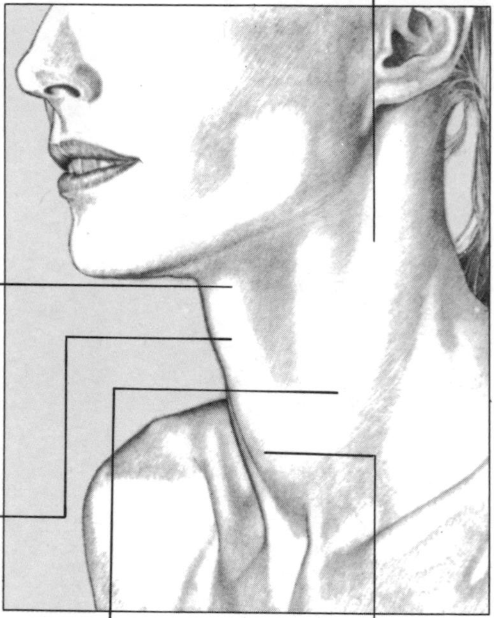

Swallowing, difficult
Achalasia
Bulbar paralysis
Dysphagia
Oesophagus

Swallowing, painful
Pharyngitis
Quinsy
Sore throat
Tonsillitis

Altered voice
Laryngitis
Larynx
Muscular disorders
Neurological disorders

Cough
Cough
Laryngitis
Mucus
Pharyngitis
Sinusitis

"Lump in throat"
Globus hystericus
Goitre
Laryngitis
Lymph gland
Pharyngitis

Hoarseness
Laryngitis
Pharyngitis
Smoking

Swollen glands
Glandular fever
Goitre
Hodgkin's disease
Leukaemia
Lymph gland
Lymphosarcoma
Tuberculosis

Goitre
Goitre
Myxoedema
Thyrotoxicosis

Loss of voice
Aphasia
Aphonia
Laryngitis
Larynx
Mute

Neck, swollen
Goitre
Lymph gland

Swollen and painful glands
Glandular fever
Lymph gland
Mumps
Tonsil

Sore throat
Glandular fever
Pharyngitis
Quinsy
Sore throat
Tonsillitis
Vincent's angina

See also
Head and face
Mouth

The mouth

General articles
Jaw
Salivary glands
Taste
Teeth

Bad breath
Abscess
Appendicitis
Bad breath
Gastritis
Gingivitis
Indigestion
Liver disorders
Pyorrhoea
Sinusitis
Smoking
Sore throat
Stomach disorders
Stomatitis
Tonsillitis
Tooth decay
Trench mouth
Vincent's angina
Uraemia

Cleft palate
Cleft palate

Dentures
Dentures

Teeth
Hutchinson's
  teeth
Teeth

Teeth, clenched
Abscess
Hysteria
Mumps
Tetanus
Tonsillitis

Teeth, discoloured
Tetracycline
Tooth decay

Teeth, painful
Abscess
Gingivitis
Impacted
Toothache
Tooth decay

Gums, pain in
Abscess, tooth
Cancer
Gingivitis
Leukaemia
Plaque
Pyorrhoea
Vincent's angina

**Gums, spongy and
  ulcerated**
Diabetes
Gingivitis
Leukaemia
Plaque
Scurvy
Stomatitis

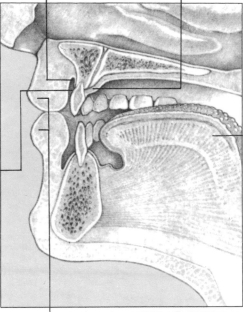

Lips
Chapping
Cold sore

Lips, blue
Cyanosis

**Lips, crack at
  corner of mouth**
Anaemia
Cheilosis
Deficiency
  diseases

Teeth, loose
Abscess
Gingivitis
Plaque
Scurvy
Teeth

Inner cheek
Cancer
Leukoplakia
Lichen planus
Measles
Moniliasis
Stomatitis
Syphilis
Ulcer

Ulcers
Aphthous ulcer
Cold sore
Herpes simplex
Moniliasis

Gums, bleeding
Deficiency
  diseases
Haemophilia
Leukaemia
Scurvy
Stomatitis
Trench mouth

Taste, bitter
Gastritis
Pyrosis
Stomatitis
Vomiting

Taste, loss of
Common cold
Head injury
Stomatitis

Tongue
Taste
Tongue

**Tongue,
  discoloured**
Furred tongue
Gastritis

Tongue, red
Addison's anaemia
Deficiency
  diseases
Glossitis
Scarlet fever

Tongue, sore
Glossitis
Moniliasis

Tongue, white
Furred tongue
Gastritis
Glossitis
Leukoplakia
Moniliasis

The head and face

General articles
Cranium
Headache
Salivary glands

Scalp, itching
Anxiety
Dandruff
Eczema
Nit
Ringworm
Seborrhoea

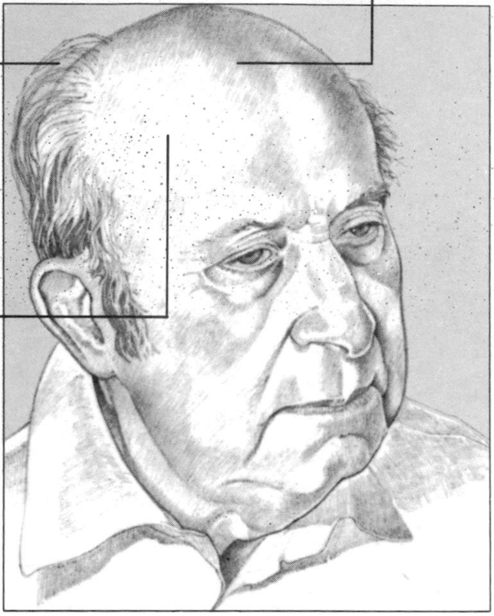

Scurf
Dandruff
Eczema
Psoriasis
Ringworm
Seborrhoea

Birthmarks
Birthmark
Haemangioma
Mole

Headache
Allergy
Altitude sickness
Anxiety
Diabetes
Eye disorders
Hangover
Headache
Migraine
Sinusitis

Hair, grey or white
Alopecia
Senility

Pain in forehead
Headache
Migraine
Neuralgia
Shingles
Sinusitis
Tension
Tumour

Baldness
Alopecia
Baldness
Eczema
Ringworm
Sebaceous cyst

Habit spasm
Anxiety
Spasm
Tic
Trigeminal
  neuralgia

Fainting
Adolescence
Arteriosclerosis
Diabetes
Epilepsy
Fainting
Menstruation
Pregnancy and
  childbirth

Hangover
Alcoholism
Hangover
Headache
Migraine

Concussion
Concussion
Headache
Head injury

**Paralysis or
  weakness**
Bell's palsy
Mastoid
Motor neuron
  disease
Muscular disorders
Myasthenia gravis
Poliomyelitis
Polyneuritis
Stroke

Dizziness
Arteriosclerosis
Concussion
Dizziness
Ear disorders
Epilepsy
Ménière's disease
Migraine
Vertigo

Head, lumps
Bruise
Dermoid cyst
Head injury
Hives
Osteoma
Paget's disease of
  bone
Rickets
Sebaceous cyst
Wart

See also
Neck and throat
Mouth
Ear; nose
Eye

Skin, pigment abnormalities
Freckles
Leprosy
Liver spot
Mole
Vitiligo

Skin, unusually brown
Addison's disease
Chloasma
Sunburn

Skin, unusually blue
Blue baby
Emphysema
Exposure
Heart disease

Skin, unusually pale
Anaemia
Bleeding
Fainting
Kidney disorders
Myxoedema
Pallor
Shock

Skin, unusually red
Acne
Birthmark
Boils
Bruise
Burn
Erysipelas
Fever
German measles
Hot flush
Lupus
  erythematosus
Measles
Menopause
Polycythaemia
Rosacea
Roseola
Seborrhoea

Face, rash
Allergy
Chickenpox
German measles
Measles
Roseola
Scarlet fever
Typhoid fever

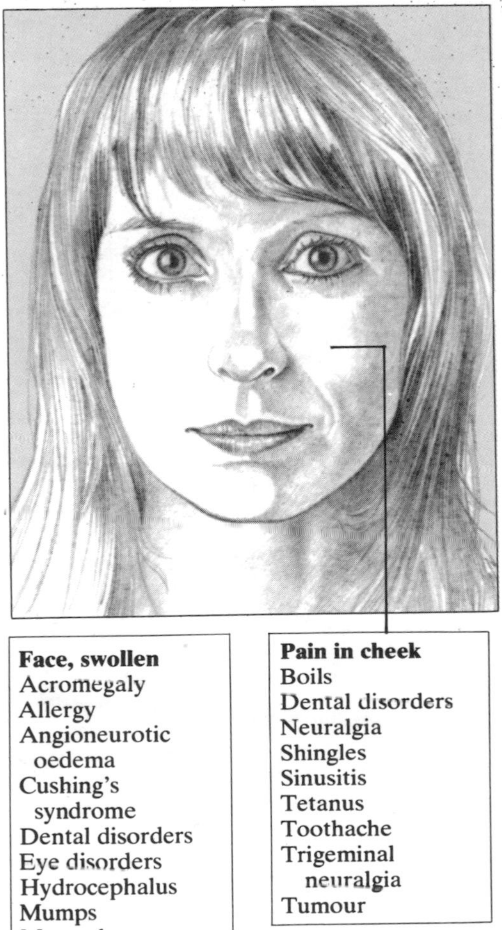

Face, greasy
Acne
Rosacea
Seborrhoea

Face, lumps
Abscess
Angioneurotic
  oedema
Boil
Bruise
Cyst, dermoid
Cyst, sebaceous
Dental disorders
Eye disorders
Hodgkin's disease
Insect bite
Lymph gland
Mumps
Osteitis
  deformans
Salivary glands
Sialolithiasis
Sinusitis
Tumour
Warts

Face, spots
Acne
Adolescence
Birthmark
Blackhead
Boils
Folliculitis
Impetigo
Insect bite
Papule
Pimple
Pustule
Rodent ulcer
Shingles
Wart

Face, swollen
Acromegaly
Allergy
Angioneurotic
  oedema
Cushing's
  syndrome
Dental disorders
Eye disorders
Hydrocephalus
Mumps
Myxoedema
Nephrotic
  syndrome
Paget's disease of
  bone
Sinusitis

Pain in cheek
Boils
Dental disorders
Neuralgia
Shingles
Sinusitis
Tetanus
Toothache
Trigeminal
  neuralgia
Tumour

Skin, unusually yellow
Jaundice
Pernicious anaemia

The ear

General articles
Deafness
Ear
Ear disorders
Mastoid

Buzzing and ringing
Labyrinthitis
Ménière's disease
Otitis
Otosclerosis
Tinnitus

Deafness
Common cold
Deafness
Influenza
Ménière's disease
Mumps
Mute
Occupational
  hazards
Otosclerosis
Otitis
Scarlet fever
Wax

Discharge
Boils
Mastoiditis
Otitis
Otorrhoea
Wax

Dizziness
Concussion
Dizziness
Ménière's disease
Vertigo

Earache
Boils
Common cold
Earache
Mastoiditis
Mumps
Occupational
  hazards
Otitis
Pharyngitis
Sinusitis
Tonsillitis

Itching
Chilblains
Dermatitis
Eczema
Otitis

Lumps on ear
Pimple
Rodent ulcer
Sebaceous cyst
Tumour

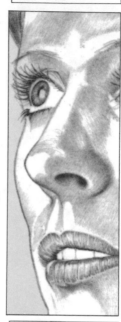

Blisters
Chilblains
Impetigo
Shingles

Boil
Boils
Carbuncle
Otitis

Mastoiditis
Mastoiditis

See also
Face

The nose

General articles
Nose
Smell, sense of

Red nose
Chapping
Common cold
Influenza
Rhinophyma

Blocked
Adenoids
Common cold
Polyp
Rhinitis

Catarrh
Adenoids
Allergy
Catarrh
Common cold
Influenza

Snoring
Adenoids
Catarrh
Deviated nasal
  septum
Polyp
Snoring

Bleeding
Blood disorders
High blood
  pressure
Nosebleed
Puberty

Running nose
Allergy
Catarrh
Common cold
Deviated nasal
  septum
Hay fever
Measles
Polyp
Sneezing
Vasomotor
  rhinitis

Sneezing
Allergy
Catarrh
Common cold
Influenza
Sneezing

Cold
Common cold
Measles

Loss of smell
Catarrh
Common cold
Head injury
Influenza
Smell, sense of
Stuffy nose

Swollen
Abscess
Boils
Cellulitis
Rhinophyma

See also
Head and face

The female breast

General articles
Breast
Breast disorders
Cancer
Nipple
Palpation

**Menstrual
changes**
Fibroadenosis
Mastitis
Menstrual
problems
Palpation
Pregnancy and
childbirth

Painful breast
Abscess
Breast disorders
Fibroadenosis
Lactation
Mastitis
Menstrual
problems
Pregnancy and
childbirth

Size changes
Cancer
Contraception
Fibroadenosis
Mammoplasty
Pregnancy and
childbirth

Tenderness
Abscess
Lactation
Menstrual
problems

Blushing, flushing
Flush
Hot flush
Menopause

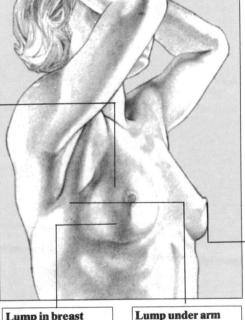

Lump in breast
Abscess
Cancer
Breast disorders
Cyst
Fibroadenosis
Lipoma
Palpation

**General
lumpiness**
Abscess
Cancer
Cyst
Lactation
Lipoma
Mastitis
Menstrual
problems

Lump under arm
Lymph gland

Nipple, bleeding
Breast disorders
Cancer
Nipple
Pregnancy and
childbirth

**Nipple,
discharging**
Breast disorders
Cancer
Colostrum
Eczema
Lactation
Paget's disease of
nipple
Witch's milk

Nipple, inverted
Cancer
Nipple

Nipple, sore
Eczema
Lactation
Pregnancy and
childbirth

Nipples, tingling
Lactation
Menstrual
problems

The chest

General articles
Arteriosclerosis
Heart disease
Lung disorders
Smoking
Sternum
Valvular disorders

Breathlessness
Anaemia
Anxiety
Asthma
Atelectasis
Breathlessness
Emphysema
Heart failure
High blood
  pressure
Lung disorders
Myocarditis
Obesity

**Irregular
  breathing**
Asthma
Cheyne-Stokes
  breathing

Pain on breathing
Bornholm disease
Embolism
Empyema
Pleurisy
Pneumonia
Tietze's syndrome
Tracheitis

Tightness in chest
Angina pectoris
Asthma
Breathlessness
Coronary heart
  disease
Emphysema
Heart failure

Heartburn
Hiatus hernia
Indigestion

Chest pain
Abscess
Angina pectoris
Cancer
Coronary heart
  disease
Hiatus hernia
Indigestion
Pericarditis
Pleurisy
Tietze's syndrome

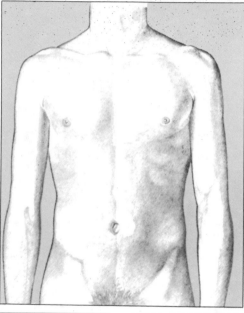

Cough
Bronchiectasis
Bronchitis
Bronchial
  pneumonia
Cough
Croup
Laryngitis
Pneumonia
Smoking
Tracheitis
Tuberculosis
Whooping cough

Wheezing
Asthma
Breathlessness
Heart failure

Lumps
Breast disorders
Lipoma
Tumour
von
  Recklinghausen's
  disease

Cyst
Lipoma
Sebaceous cyst

Heart attack
Coronary heart
  disease
Heart attack

**Irregular
  heartbeat**
Extrasystole
Palpitation
Stokes-Adams
  attack

Palpitations
Fibrillation
Indigestion
Palpitation
Tachycardia

Pain, ribs
Bornholm disease
Calculus
Gallstone

Pain, side
Pleurisy
Shingles

The abdomen

General articles
Abdominal pain
Colon
Gall bladder
Liver
Stomach
Stomach disorders

Liver
Cirrhosis
Hepatitis
Jaundice
Liver

Gall bladder
Biliary colic
Gall bladder
Gallstone

**Pain, top right
and middle**
Abdominal pain
Appendicitis
Cholecystitis
Duodenal ulcer
Gall bladder
Gallstone
Gastritis
Pancreatitis
Peptic ulcer

Pain, abdominal
Aneurysm
Colic
Colitis
Crohn's disease
Food poisoning
Gastroenteritis
Intestinal
  obstruction
Intussusception
Munchausen's
  syndrome
Pancreatitis
Peritonitis
Pleurisy
Stomach disorders
Volvulus
Vomiting

Gas
Belching
Flatus
Gall bladder
Gastritis
Hiatus hernia

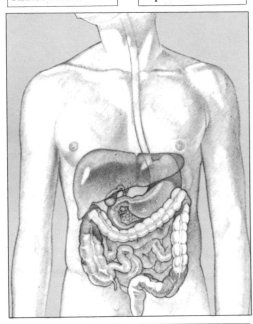

Pain, low
Appendicitis
Colitis
Diverticulitis
Diverticulosis
Dysmenorrhoea
Ectopic pregnancy
False labour pains
Pregnancy and
  childbirth
Salpingitis

Hiccup
Hiatus hernia
Hiccup
Uraemia

Indigestion
Cirrhosis
Dyspepsia
Gastritis
Heartburn
Hiatus hernia
Peptic ulcer

Colon
Coeliac disease
Colitis
Colon
Colostomy
Digestive system
Diverticulitis
Diverticulosis
Hernia

Internal parasites
Worms

Stomach
Cancer
Diet
Digestive system
Peptic ulcer
Stomach disorders

Vomiting
Acidosis
Anxiety
Appendicitis
Cancer
Cholecystitis
Diabetes
Food poisoning
Gall bladder
Gallstone
Gastroenteritis
Kidney disease
Ménière's disease
Meningitis
Migraine
Motion sickness
Peptic ulcer
Poisoning
Pregnancy and
  childbirth
Pyelonephritis
Vomiting
Whooping cough

Vomiting, black
Blood, vomiting of

Vomiting, blood
Blood, vomiting of
Gastritis
Nosebleed

**Vomiting, after
  food**
Anorexia nervosa
Peptic ulcer
Pyloric stenosis
Pylorospasm

Vomiting, at night
Hiatus hernia
Peptic ulcer

See also
Chest
Urinary system
Anus and rectum

33

The urinary system

General articles
Bladder
Bladder disorders
Cystitis
Kidney
Kidney disease
Urinary
  abnormalities
Urine

**Urine flow,
  dribble**
Bladder disorders
Incontinence
Prostate problems
Urinary
  abnormalities

**Urine flow,
  frequent**
Alcohol
Anxiety
Bladder disorders
Cystitis
Diabetes
Kidney disease
Nephritis
Nephrotic
  syndrome
Nocturia
Polyuria
Pregnancy and
  childbirth
Prostate problems
Pyelonephritis
Urinary
  abnormalities

**Urine flow,
  hesitant**
Anxiety
Bladder disorders
Prostate problems

**Urine flow,
  incontinent**
Enuresis
Epilepsy
Incontinence
Neurological
  disorders
Stress
  incontinence
Stroke

Stone
Calculus
Colic
Dysuria

Loin ache or pain
Abscess
Backache
Calculus
Kidney disease

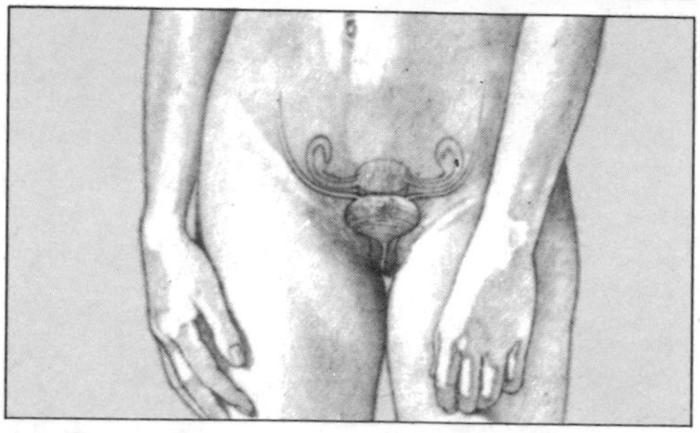

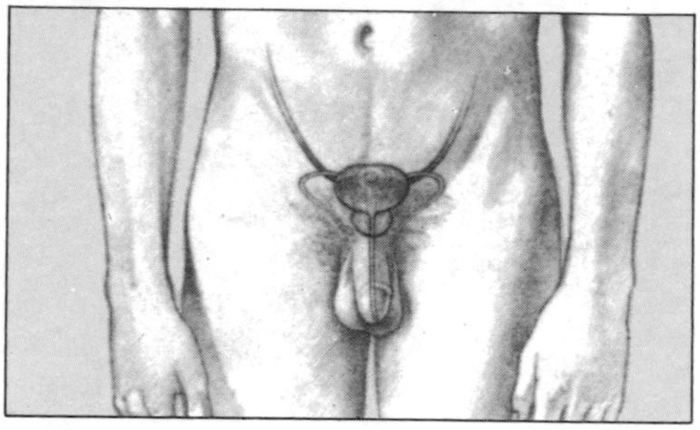

Urine, blood in
Bladder disorders
Calculus
Cystitis
Haematuria
Haemoglobinuria
Kidney disease
Nephritis
Prostate problems
Schistosomiasis
Urethritis
Urinary
  abnormalities

Urine, dark
Bladder disorders
Cystitis
Haemoglobinuria
Hepatitis
Jaundice
Melanuria
Oliguria
Porphyria
Urinary
  abnormalities

Urine, smoky
Calculus
Cystitis
Haematuria
Kidney disease
Pyelitis
Urinary
  abnormalities

**Urine flow,
  infrequent**
Dehydration
Fever
Kidney disease
Oliguria
Pre-eclampsia

**Urine flow, with
  pain**
Bladder disorders
Calculus
Cystitis
Dysuria
Prostate problems
Pyelonephritis
Tenesmus
Urinary
  abnormalities
Venereal diseases

**Inability to pass
  urine**
Anuria
Anxiety
Pregnancy and
  childbirth
Prolapse
Prostate problems
Retention
Strangury
Tenesmus

See also
Reproductive
  systems

The anus and the rectum

General articles
Anus
Constipation
Diarrhoea
Haemorrhoid
Rectum
Skin diseases

Faeces
Constipation
Diarrhoea
Faeces

Faeces, black
Cancer
Melaena
Peptic ulcer

Faeces, greasy
Coeliac disease
Crohn's disease
Gall bladder
Hepatitis
Sprue

Faeces, red
Cancer
Haemorrhoid
Diverticulitis
Diverticulosis
Dysentery
Intussusception

Faeces, white
Coeliac disease
Jaundice
Steatorrhoea

Pain at base of back
Abscess
Bedsore
Coccyx
Ischiorectal abscess
Pilonidal sinus
Pregnancy and childbirth

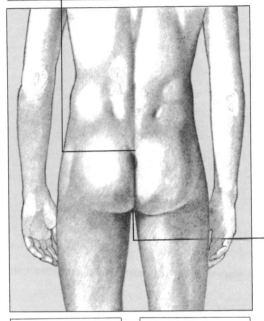

Diarrhoea
Coeliac disease
Cholera
Colitis
Cystic fibrosis
Diarrhoea
Diverticulitis
Diverticulosis
Dysentery
Food poisoning
Gastroenteritis
Hepatitis
Ileitis
Sprue
Steatorrhoea
Thyrotoxicosis
Typhoid fever

Constipation
Anxiety
Cancer
Constipation
Diverticulitis
Diverticulosis
Haemorrhoid
Hirschsprung's disease
Intestinal obstruction
Myxoedema
Pregnancy and childbirth

Bleeding
Colitis
Diverticulitis
Diverticulosis
Dysentery
Fissure
Haemorrhoid
Pilonidal sinus
Polyp
Schistosomiasis

Itching
Haemorrhoid
Moniliasis
Scabies
Worms

Pain in anus
Abscess
Cancer
Fissure
Fistula
Haemorrhoid
Proctalgia
Proctitis
Tenesmus

Piles
Cirrhosis
Constipation
Haemorrhoid
Pregnancy and childbirth

Protrusion from anus
Haemorrhoid
Intussusception
Polyp
Prolapse
Wart

Lump
Haemorrhoid
Intussusception
Pilonidal sinus
Polyp
Rectum

Worms
Worms

See also
Abdomen

The female reproductive system

General articles
Gynaecological
 disorders
Menopause
Menstrual
 problems
Pregnancy and
 childbirth
Premenstrual
 tension
Sexual problems
Vagina
Vulva
Womb

Cervix
Cervical cancer
Cervical erosion
Cervical smear
Cervicitis
Contraception
Pregnancy and
 childbirth

Fallopian tube
Ectopic pregnancy
Fallopian tube
Fertilization
Ovulation
Ovum
Salpingitis
Sterilization

**Bleeding after
 menopause**
Cervical cancer
Cervical erosion
Cervicitis
Menopause

Pain in midcycle
Menstrual
 problems
Ovulation

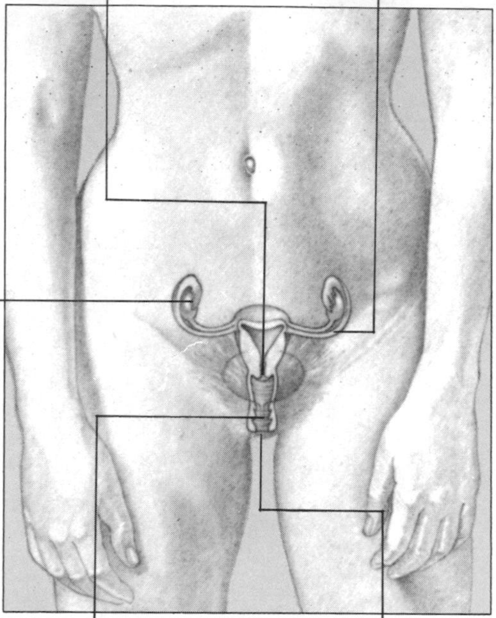

Fertility
Fertility
Infertility
Pregnancy and
 childbirth
Sterility

**Periods, flooding
 or heavy**
Adolescence
Abortion
Endometritis
Fibroid
Menorrhagia
Menstrual
 problems
Salpingitis

Ovary
Corpus luteum
Fertilization
Graafian follicle
Oophoritis
Ovulation
Ovum

Periods, irregular
Adolescence
Anxiety
Menopause
Menstrual
 problems

Venereal disease
Gonorrhoea
Syphilis
Urethritis
Venereal diseases

**Periods,
 nonexistent**
Haematocolpos
Infertility
Menarche

Vulva
Clitoris
Labium
Vulva

Intercourse, pain
Dyspareunia
Hymen
Sexual problems
Vaginismus

Vaginal discharge
Adolescence
Cervical cancer
Cervical erosion
Cervicitis
Endometritis
Gonorrhoea
Lochia
Ovulation
Salpingitis
Urethritis
Vaginitis
Venereal diseases

Periods, painful
Dysmenorrhoea
Endometriosis
IUD
Salpingitis

Vulva, sore
Dyspareunia
Vulvitis

Vagina
Contraception
Pregnancy and
 childbirth

Periods, stopped
Adolescence
Amenorrhoea
Anorexia nervosa
Contraception
False pregnancy
Menopause
Pregnancy and
 childbirth

Vulva, swollen
Bartholin's cyst
Menstruation
Prolapse

**Vaginal itching
 and irritation**
Gonorrhoea
Moniliasis
Trichomonas
Urethritis
Vaginitis
Venereal disease
Vulvitis

Ulcer
Chancre
Chancroid
Syphilis
Venereal diseases

Uterus
Contraception
Menstruation
Pregnancy and
 childbirth
Womb

See also
Abdomen
Urinary system

The male reproductive system

General articles
Epididymis
Penis
Prostate gland
Prostate problems
Scrotum
Sexual problems
Testis
Urinary
  abnormalities

Circumcision
Circumcision
Foreskin
Paraphimosis
Phimosis

Foreskin, tight
Paraphimosis
Phimosis

Testes, absent
Cryptorchidism
Testis

Testes, painful
Epididymitis
Hernia
Mumps
Orchitis
Testis
Venereal diseases

Scrotum, rash
Moniliasis
Ringworm

Scrotum, swollen
Cyst
Epididymitis
Hernia
Hydrocele
Mumps
Orchitis
Seminoma
Spermatocele
Tumour
Variocele

Sperm duct
Epididymis
Epididymitis

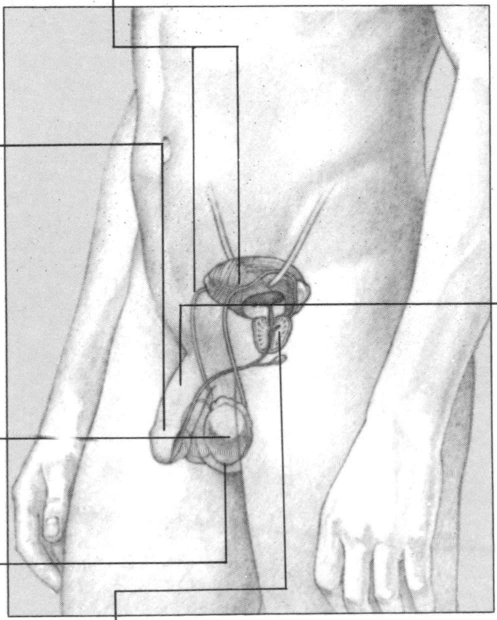

Prostate problems
Prostate problems

**Erection,
  problems with**
Alcohol
Anxiety
Depression
Diabetes
Drugs
Dyspareunia
Impotence
Priapism
Prostate problems
Sexual problems

Venereal disease
Gonorrhoea
Syphilis
Urethritis
Venereal diseases

Penis, ulcerated
Chancre
Chancroid
Cold sore
Syphilis
Ulcer
Venereal diseases

Penis, warts
Venereal diseases
Wart

Impotence
Anxiety
Depression
Impotence
Sexual problems

Infertility
Artificial
  insemination
Cryptorchidism
Fertility
Infertility
Impotence
Mumps
Prostate problems
Sterility

Penis
Erection
Foreskin
Urethra

Penis, blistered
Shingles

Penis, discharging
Balanitis
Gonorrhoea
Prostatitis
Urethritis
Venereal diseases

Penis, painful
Balanitis
Cystitis
Gonorrhoea
Priapism
Prostatitis
Ulcer
Urethritis
Venereal diseases

**Penis, shape
  abnormalities**
Congenital
  anomalies
Paraphimosis
Phimosis
Priapism

See also
Abdomen
Urinary system

The back, shoulder, arm, and hand

General articles
Armpit
Arthritis
Backache
Bone disorders
Elbow
Hand
Joint disorders
Muscular disorders
Nail
Neurological
  disorders
Pulled muscle
Rheumatic
  diseases
Scabies
Shoulder
Wrist

Shoulder
Arthritis
Dislocation
Frozen shoulder

Sacrum
Coccydynia
Myelocele
Pilonidal sinus
Sacrum
Spina bifida

Back pain
Ankylosing
  spondylitis
Backache
Depression
Dysmenorrhoea
Gall bladder
Osteoporosis
Peptic ulcer
Sciatica
Slipped disc
Spondylolisthesis

Stiffness
Ankylosing
  spondylitis
Arthritis
Rheumatic
  diseases
Stiffness

Elbow
Bursitis
Capsulitis
Elbow injuries
Humerus
Osteoarthritis
Rheumatic
  diseases
Rheumatic fever

Armpit, sweating
Bromhidrosis
Hyperhidrosis

Armpit, swollen
Boils
Carbuncle
Lymph gland

Wrist
Colles' fracture
Wrist drop

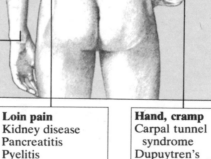

Arm, lumps
Bruise
Chondroma
Exostosis
Fibroma
Ganglion
Lipoma
Osteoma
von
  Recklinghausen's
  disease

Arm, painful
Causalgia
Cervical
  spondylosis
Fibrositis
Neuralgia
Osteomyelitis
Pulled muscle
Stiffness

Finger, blistered
Allergy
Blister
Hand-foot-and-
  mouth disease
Pompholyx

Finger, lumps
Heberden's nodes
Rheumatoid
  arthritis
Wart

Finger, painful
Arthritis
Chilblain
Polyneuritis
Raynaud's
  phenomenon
Rheumatoid
  arthritis
Whitlow

Loin pain
Kidney disease
Pancreatitis
Pyelitis
Shingles
Strain

Nails
Clubbing
Nail

Finger, stiff
Arthritis
Rheumatoid
  arthritis
Tenosynovitis

Hand, cramp
Carpal tunnel
  syndrome
Dupuytren's
  contracture
Scleroderma
Tetany

Hand, itching
Allergy
Dermatitis
Pompholyx
Scabies

Hand, shaking
Anxiety
Parkinson's
  disease
Thyrotoxicosis
Tremor

Paralysis of the arm
Hysteria
Motor neuron
  disease
Muscular disorders
Neurological
  disorders
Poliomyelitis
Stroke

Weakness
Cerebral palsy
Muscular disorders

The leg, hip, knee, and foot

General articles
Ankle
Arthritis
Foot
Hip
Joint disorders
Knee
Muscular
  disorders
Nail
Neurological
  disorders
Pulled muscle
Rheumatic
  diseases

Unsteadiness
Ataxia
Neurological
  disorders
Parkinson's
  disease

Limping
Claudication
Perthes' disease

Lumps
Bruise
Chondroma
Erythema
  nodosum
Exostosis
Fibroma
Osteoma
Varicose vein
von
  Recklinghausen's
  disease
Wart

**Pain in calf or
  thigh**
Buerger's disease
Causalgia
Claudication
Cramp
Osteomyelitis
Phlebitis
Sciatica
Tabes dorsalis
Tenosynovitis
Thrombophlebitis

Paralysis
Hysteria
Neurological
  disorders
Poliomyelitis
Stroke

Weakness
Cerebral palsy
Muscular disorders
Weakness

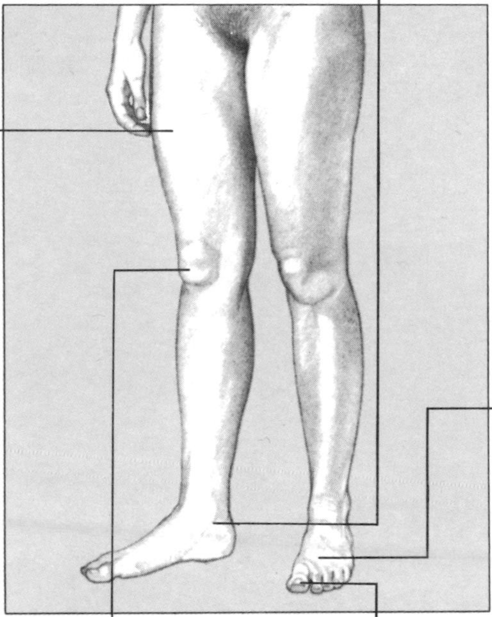

Knee, locked
Cartilage
Chondromalacia
Osteochondritis

Knee, painful
Arthritis
Chondromalacia
Rheumatic
  diseases
Sprain

Knee, swollen
Arthritis
Bursitis
Chondromalacia
Gout
Meniscus
Sprain

Achilles' tendon
Achilles' tendon
Tendinitis

Ankle, painful
Arthritis
Gout
Joint disorders
Pott's fracture
Rheumatic
  diseases
Sprain

Toes
Chilblains
Corn
Ingrowing nail
Pigeon toe
Ringworm

Foot, ulcerated
Diabetes
Gangrene

Foot, tingling
Chilblains
Polyneuritis
Tingling

Ankle, swollen
Ankles, swollen
Kidney disease
Oedema
Pre-eclampsia
Pregnancy and
  childbirth
Thrombophlebitis

Sciatica
Lumbago
Sciatica
Slipped disc

Hip, painful
Arthritis
Perthes' disease
Rheumatic
  diseases

Foot, blistered
Allergy
Blister
Chilblains
Hand-foot-and-
  mouth disease
Immersion foot
Pompholyx
Shingles

Foot, itching
Athlete's foot
Hyperhidrosis
Moniliasis
Pompholyx
Ringworm

Foot, lumps
Bunion
Corn
Hammer toe
Wart

Foot, painful
Arthritis
Buerger's disease
Callus
Chilblains
Foot disorders
Pregnancy and
  childbirth

Charts of related symptoms

Introduction
This section is most useful when two or more conditions occur at once. Beginning with a symptom that is most obvious and proceeding to less severe symptoms set out in parallel, a connection is established. When followed, this leads to brief advice on immediate action, on when to consult a doctor, and finally, the full list of relevant A–Z articles

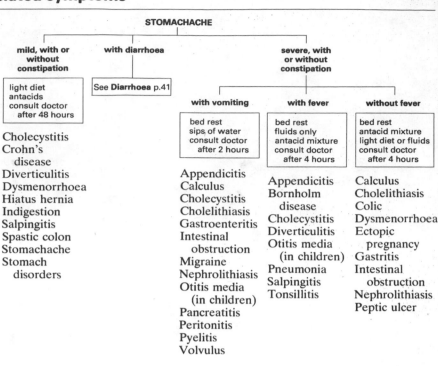

STOMACHACHE

mild, with or without constipation

light diet
antacids
consult doctor
after 48 hours

Cholecystitis
Crohn's
  disease
Diverticulitis
Dysmenorrhoea
Hiatus hernia
Indigestion
Salpingitis
Spastic colon
Stomachache
Stomach
  disorders

with diarrhoea

See **Diarrhoea** p.41

severe, with or without constipation

with vomiting

bed rest
sips of water
consult doctor
after 2 hours

Appendicitis
Calculus
Cholecystitis
Cholelithiasis
Gastroenteritis
Intestinal
  obstruction
Migraine
Nephrolithiasis
Otitis media
  (in children)
Pancreatitis
Peritonitis
Pyelitis
Volvulus

with fever

bed rest
fluids only
antacid mixture
consult doctor
after 4 hours

Appendicitis
Bornholm
  disease
Cholecystitis
Diverticulitis
Otitis media
  (in children)
Pneumonia
Salpingitis
Tonsillitis

without fever

bed rest
antacid mixture
light diet or fluids
consult doctor
after 4 hours

Calculus
Cholelithiasis
Colic
Dysmenorrhoea
Ectopic
  pregnancy
Gastritis
Intestinal
  obstruction
Nephrolithiasis
Peptic ulcer

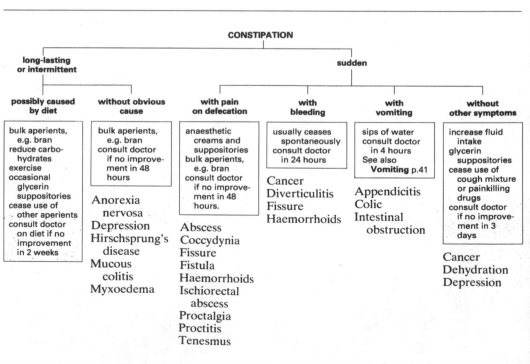

CONSTIPATION

long-lasting or intermittent

possibly caused by diet

bulk aperients,
  e.g. bran
reduce carbo-
  hydrates
exercise
occasional
  glycerin
  suppositories
cease use of
  other aperients
consult doctor
  on diet if no
  improvement
  in 2 weeks

without obvious cause

bulk aperients,
  e.g. bran
consult doctor
  if no improve-
  ment in 48
  hours

Anorexia
  nervosa
Depression
Hirschsprung's
  disease
Mucous
  colitis
Myxoedema

sudden

with pain on defecation

anaesthetic
  creams and
  suppositories
bulk aperients,
  e.g. bran
consult doctor
  if no improve-
  ment in 48
  hours.

Abscess
Coccydynia
Fissure
Fistula
Haemorrhoids
Ischiorectal
  abscess
Proctalgia
Proctitis
Tenesmus

with bleeding

usually ceases
  spontaneously
consult doctor
  in 24 hours

Cancer
Diverticulitis
Fissure
Haemorrhoids

with vomiting

sips of water
consult doctor
  in 4 hours
See also
  Vomiting p.41

Appendicitis
Colic
Intestinal
  obstruction

without other symptoms

increase fluid
  intake
glycerin
  suppositories
cease use of
  cough mixture
  or painkilling
  drugs
consult doctor
  if no improve-
  ment in 3
  days

Cancer
Dehydration
Depression

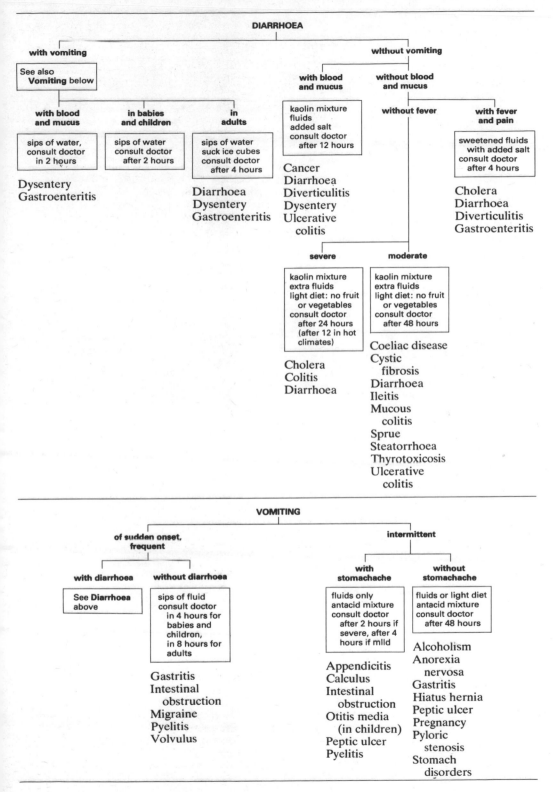

DIARRHOEA

with vomiting

See also
Vomiting below

with blood and mucus

sips of water,
consult doctor
in 2 hours

Dysentery
Gastroenteritis

in babies and children

sips of water
consult doctor
after 2 hours

in adults

sips of water
suck ice cubes
consult doctor
after 4 hours

Diarrhoea
Dysentery
Gastroenteritis

without vomiting

with blood and mucus

kaolin mixture
fluids
added salt
consult doctor
after 12 hours

Cancer
Diarrhoea
Diverticulitis
Dysentery
Ulcerative
    colitis

without blood and mucus

without fever

with fever and pain

sweetened fluids
with added salt
consult doctor
after 4 hours

Cholera
Diarrhoea
Diverticulitis
Gastroenteritis

severe

kaolin mixture
extra fluids
light diet: no fruit
    or vegetables
consult doctor
    after 24 hours
    (after 12 in hot
    climates)

Cholera
Colitis
Diarrhoea

moderate

kaolin mixture
extra fluids
light diet: no fruit
    or vegetables
consult doctor
    after 48 hours

Coeliac disease
Cystic
    fibrosis
Diarrhoea
Ileitis
Mucous
    colitis
Sprue
Steatorrhoea
Thyrotoxicosis
Ulcerative
    colitis

VOMITING

of sudden onset, frequent

with diarrhoea

See **Diarrhoea**
above

without diarrhoea

sips of fluid
consult doctor
    in 4 hours for
    babies and
    children,
    in 8 hours for
    adults

Gastritis
Intestinal
    obstruction
Migraine
Pyelitis
Volvulus

intermittent

with stomachache

fluids only
antacid mixture
consult doctor
    after 2 hours if
    severe, after 4
    hours if mild

Appendicitis
Calculus
Intestinal
    obstruction
Otitis media
    (in children)
Peptic ulcer
Pyelitis

without stomachache

fluids or light diet
antacid mixture
consult doctor
    after 48 hours

Alcoholism
Anorexia
    nervosa
Gastritis
Hiatus hernia
Peptic ulcer
Pregnancy
Pyloric
    stenosis
Stomach
    disorders

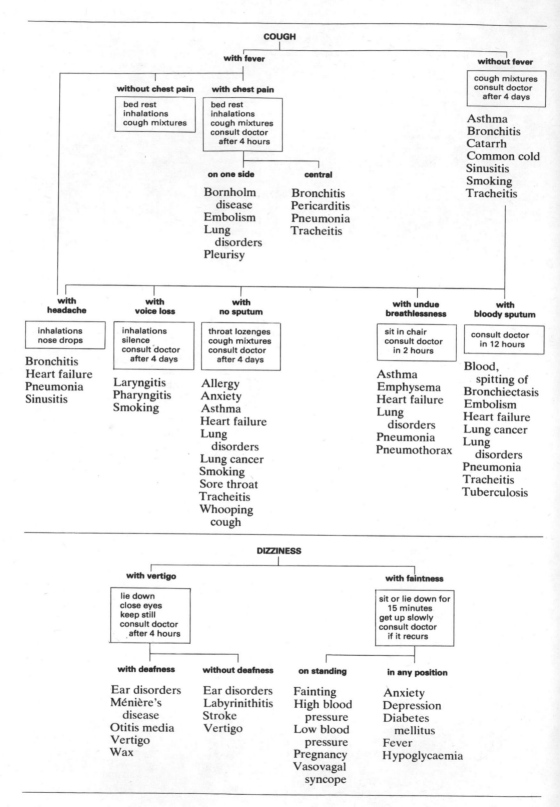

COUGH

with fever

without chest pain

bed rest
inhalations
cough mixtures

with chest pain

bed rest
inhalations
cough mixtures
consult doctor
after 4 hours

on one side

Bornholm
disease
Embolism
Lung
disorders
Pleurisy

central

Bronchitis
Pericarditis
Pneumonia
Tracheitis

without fever

cough mixtures
consult doctor
after 4 days

Asthma
Bronchitis
Catarrh
Common cold
Sinusitis
Smoking
Tracheitis

with headache

inhalations
nose drops

Bronchitis
Heart failure
Pneumonia
Sinusitis

with voice loss

inhalations
silence
consult doctor
after 4 days

Laryngitis
Pharyngitis
Smoking

with no sputum

throat lozenges
cough mixtures
consult doctor
after 4 days

Allergy
Anxiety
Asthma
Heart failure
Lung
disorders
Lung cancer
Smoking
Sore throat
Tracheitis
Whooping
cough

with undue breathlessness

sit in chair
consult doctor
in 2 hours

Asthma
Emphysema
Heart failure
Lung
disorders
Pneumonia
Pneumothorax

with bloody sputum

consult doctor
in 12 hours

Blood,
spitting of
Bronchiectasis
Embolism
Heart failure
Lung cancer
Lung
disorders
Pneumonia
Tracheitis
Tuberculosis

DIZZINESS

with vertigo

lie down
close eyes
keep still
consult doctor
after 4 hours

with faintness

sit or lie down for
15 minutes
get up slowly
consult doctor
if it recurs

with deafness

Ear disorders
Ménière's
disease
Otitis media
Vertigo
Wax

without deafness

Ear disorders
Labyrinithitis
Stroke
Vertigo

on standing

Fainting
High blood
pressure
Low blood
pressure
Pregnancy
Vasovagal
syncope

in any position

Anxiety
Depression
Diabetes
mellitus
Fever
Hypoglycaemia

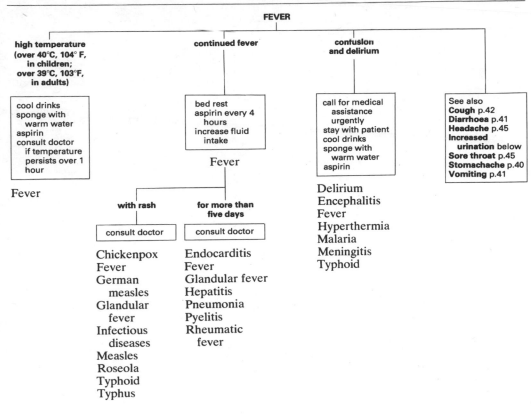

FEVER

high temperature (over 40°C, 104° F, in children; over 39°C, 103°F, in adults)

cool drinks
sponge with warm water
aspirin
consult doctor if temperature persists over 1 hour

Fever

continued fever

bed rest
aspirin every 4 hours
increase fluid intake

Fever

with rash

consult doctor

Chickenpox
Fever
German measles
Glandular fever
Infectious diseases
Measles
Roseola
Typhoid
Typhus

for more than five days

consult doctor

Endocarditis
Fever
Glandular fever
Hepatitis
Pneumonia
Pyelitis
Rheumatic fever

confusion and delirium

call for medical assistance urgently
stay with patient
cool drinks
sponge with warm water
aspirin

Delirium
Encephalitis
Fever
Hyperthermia
Malaria
Meningitis
Typhoid

See also
Cough p.42
Diarrhoea p.41
Headache p.45
Increased urination below
Sore throat p.45
Stomachache p.40
Vomiting p.41

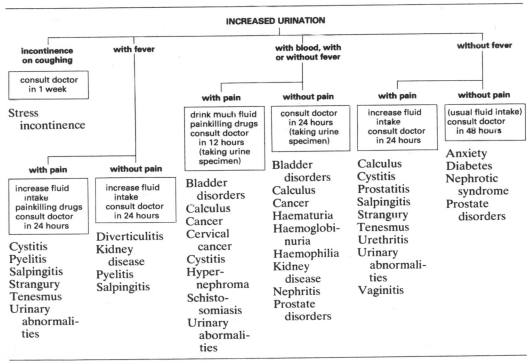

INCREASED URINATION

incontinence on coughing

consult doctor in 1 week

Stress incontinence

with pain

increase fluid intake
painkilling drugs
consult doctor in 24 hours

Cystitis
Pyelitis
Salpingitis
Strangury
Tenesmus
Urinary abnormalities

with fever

without pain

increase fluid intake
consult doctor in 24 hours

Diverticulitis
Kidney disease
Pyelitis
Salpingitis

with blood, with or without fever

with pain

drink much fluid
painkilling drugs
consult doctor in 12 hours
(taking urine specimen)

Bladder disorders
Calculus
Cancer
Cervical cancer
Cystitis
Hyper-nephroma
Schisto-somiasis
Urinary abormali-ties

without pain

consult doctor in 24 hours
(taking urine specimen)

Bladder disorders
Calculus
Cancer
Haematuria
Haemoglobi-nuria
Haemophilia
Kidney disease
Nephritis
Prostate disorders

without fever

with pain

increase fluid intake
consult doctor in 24 hours

Calculus
Cystitis
Prostatitis
Salpingitis
Strangury
Tenesmus
Urethritis
Urinary abnormali-ties
Vaginitis

without pain

(usual fluid intake)
consult doctor in 48 hours

Anxiety
Diabetes
Nephrotic syndrome
Prostate disorders

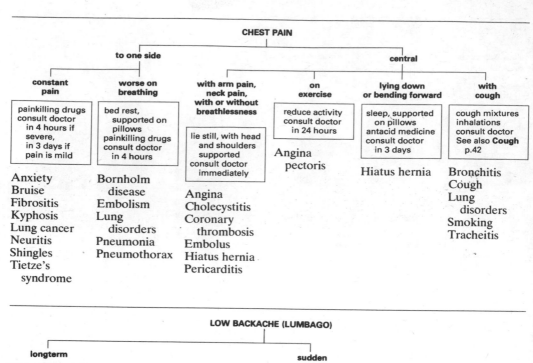

CHEST PAIN

to one side

constant pain

painkilling drugs
consult doctor
in 4 hours if
severe,
in 3 days if
pain is mild

Anxiety
Bruise
Fibrositis
Kyphosis
Lung cancer
Neuritis
Shingles
Tietze's
  syndrome

worse on breathing

bed rest,
supported on
pillows
painkilling drugs
consult doctor
in 4 hours

Bornholm
  disease
Embolism
Lung
  disorders
Pneumonia
Pneumothorax

central

with arm pain, neck pain, with or without breathlessness

lie still, with head
and shoulders
supported
consult doctor
immediately

Angina
Cholecystitis
Coronary
  thrombosis
Embolus
Hiatus hernia
Pericarditis

on exercise

reduce activity
consult doctor
in 24 hours

Angina
pectoris

lying down or bending forward

sleep, supported
on pillows
antacid medicine
consult doctor
in 3 days

Hiatus hernia

with cough

cough mixtures
inhalations
consult doctor
See also **Cough**
p.42

Bronchitis
Cough
Lung
  disorders
Smoking
Tracheitis

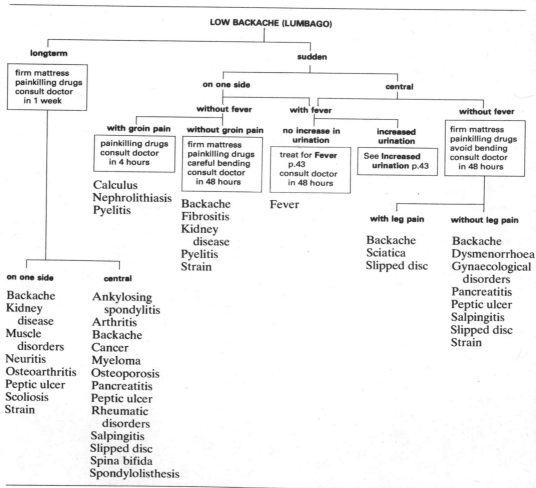

LOW BACKACHE (LUMBAGO)

longterm

firm mattress
painkilling drugs
consult doctor
in 1 week

on one side

Backache
Kidney
  disease
Muscle
  disorders
Neuritis
Osteoarthritis
Peptic ulcer
Scoliosis
Strain

central

Ankylosing
  spondylitis
Arthritis
Backache
Cancer
Myeloma
Osteoporosis
Pancreatitis
Peptic ulcer
Rheumatic
  disorders
Salpingitis
Slipped disc
Spina bifida
Spondylolisthesis

sudden

on one side

without fever

with groin pain

painkilling drugs
consult doctor
in 4 hours

Calculus
Nephrolithiasis
Pyelitis

without groin pain

firm mattress
painkilling drugs
careful bending
consult doctor
in 48 hours

Backache
Fibrositis
Kidney
  disease
Pyelitis
Strain

with fever

no increase in urination

treat for **Fever**
p.43
consult doctor
in 48 hours

Fever

increased urination

See **Increased
urination** p.43

with leg pain

Backache
Sciatica
Slipped disc

central

without fever

firm mattress
painkilling drugs
avoid bending
consult doctor
in 48 hours

without leg pain

Backache
Dysmenorrhoea
Gynaecological
  disorders
Pancreatitis
Peptic ulcer
Salpingitis
Slipped disc
Strain

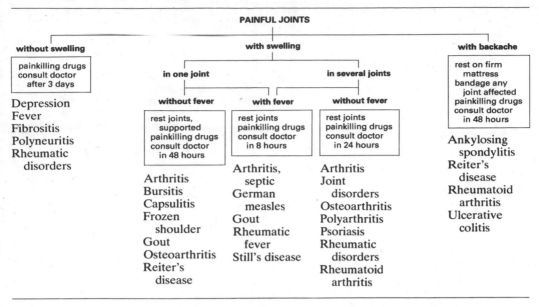

PAINFUL JOINTS

without swelling

painkilling drugs
consult doctor
after 3 days

Depression
Fever
Fibrositis
Polyneuritis
Rheumatic
disorders

with swelling

in one joint

without fever

rest joints,
supported
painkilling drugs
consult doctor
in 48 hours

Arthritis
Bursitis
Capsulitis
Frozen
shoulder
Gout
Osteoarthritis
Reiter's
disease

with fever

rest joints
painkilling drugs
consult doctor
in 8 hours

Arthritis,
septic
German
measles
Gout
Rheumatic
fever
Still's disease

in several joints

without fever

rest joints
painkilling drugs
consult doctor
in 24 hours

Arthritis
Joint
disorders
Osteoarthritis
Polyarthritis
Psoriasis
Rheumatic
disorders
Rheumatoid
arthritis

with backache

rest on firm
mattress
bandage any
joint affected
painkilling drugs
consult doctor
in 48 hours

Ankylosing
spondylitis
Reiter's
disease
Rheumatoid
arthritis
Ulcerative
colitis

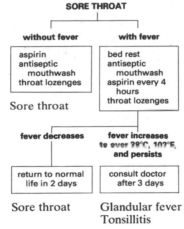

SORE THROAT

without fever

aspirin
antiseptic
mouthwash
throat lozenges

Sore throat

with fever

bed rest
antiseptic
mouthwash
aspirin every 4
hours
throat lozenges

fever decreases

return to normal
life in 2 days

Sore throat

**fever increases
to over 39°C, 102°F,
and persists**

consult doctor
after 3 days

Glandular fever
Tonsillitis

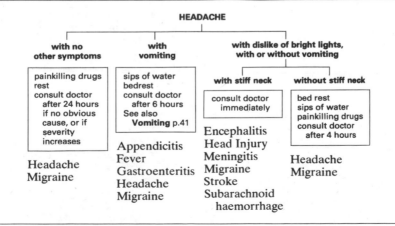

HEADACHE

**with no
other symptoms**

painkilling drugs
rest
consult doctor
after 24 hours
if no obvious
cause, or if
severity
increases

Headache
Migraine

**with
vomiting**

sips of water
bedrest
consult doctor
after 6 hours
See also
Vomiting p.41

Appendicitis
Fever
Gastroenteritis
Headache
Migraine

**with dislike of bright lights,
with or without vomiting**

with stiff neck

consult doctor
immediately

Encephalitis
Head Injury
Meningitis
Migraine
Stroke
Subarachnoid
haemorrhage

without stiff neck

bed rest
sips of water
painkilling drugs
consult doctor
after 4 hours

Headache
Migraine

45

Guide to current medical practice

Section contents

Introduction

This section comprises firstly a sort of glossary of word parts (linguistic elements) used in medical terms, and secondly a vast alphabetical compendium of information on all medical topics.

The glossary, entitled **Understanding medical terms**, begins on the next page and has a short introduction of its own. But it is essential to remember, in using the glossary, that it is not a dictionary of words but of word parts: very few of the elements cited and explained can actually stand on their own. With the word parts, however, a truly enormous number of combinations are possible. And the ordinary reader can then use the glossary to refer to the elements of any combination that he or she does not immediately understand.

The **A-Z of medicine and medical practice** is intended as a complete reference work in its own right. Under headings listed in alphabetical order, information is given on medical conditions; the systems, parts, and attributes of the body; and medical equipment, tests, substances, measurements, and studies.

The work has been thoroughly researched and checked by highly qualified experts in Great Britain and the United States, and care has been taken to provide up-to-date information.

The articles that are concerned with medical conditions generally contain the following information in this order. First, a definition describes the condition and outlines its degree of seriousness; a description of the symptoms then follows, with the causes of the condition. Treatment to remedy the situation is then discussed, and any precautions that could be taken to avoid the condition are given. Finally, further relevant information is given: whether or when to consult a doctor, the normal recovery time, and so on.

The articles that describe systems, parts and attributes (such as balance) of the body generally contain the following information in this order. The subject of the article is first located, and its function explained. A list of possible disorders follows, with treatments.

Other articles describe medical equipment, tests, and studies, or make up tables of useful statistical or reference information.

Cross-references to other relevant articles are included throughout.

Understanding medical terms

Few general dictionaries give complete coverage of medical terms. There are thousands of possible combinations of basic word parts (derived mostly from Greek or Latin) that a doctor can use to describe symptoms, disorders, and diseases. But any person who knows the meaning or meanings of the basic word parts can work out the meaning of even the most complicated medical term.

The following pages contain many such word parts, listed one by one in alphabetical order. The meaning of each word part as used in English is also given, and finally in each case there is an example of a medical term that contains the word part. By extension, recognizing and using the word parts, it is possible to "translate" other medical terms that contain them.

For instance: the medical term *cholecystitis* is made up of the parts *chole, cyst* and *itis.* These mean *gall, bladder,* and *inflammation.* So *cholecystitis* means *inflammation of the gall bladder.*

Element/derivation		Meaning	Example
(G = Greek; L = Latin)			
a, an	G	without; with no	amorphous: with no true form
ab	L	away from; off	abnormal: away (deviating) from the normal
ad	L	to; toward	adrenal: toward the kidney
aden, adeno	G	gland	adenitis: glandular inflammation
aemia *see* haem			
aesthe	G	feeling; sensitivity	anaesthesia: with no feeling
agogue, agogy	G	producing; promoting	galactagogue: causing the production of milk
alge, algia, algy	G	pain	analgesia: without pain
an *see* a			
andro	G	male; masculine	androgen: a male sex hormone
angi, angio	G	vessel (particularly blood vessel)	angiogram: X-ray record of a blood vessel
ante, ant	G	before; in front of	antecubital: in front of the cubitus (elbow)
anti, ant	G	against; countering	antipyretic: against a fever
apo	G	from; off; down	apoplexy: being struck down
arter, arteri, arterio	G	artery	arteriospasm: spasm of an artery
arthr, arthro	G	joint	arthritis: inflammation of a joint
asthenia, asthenic *see* a *and* sthenia			
ataxia, ataxy *see* a *and* taxia			
auto	G	self	autoplasty: grafting of tissue from another part of the same body
bi	L	two	bicuspid: (tooth) with two cusps
bili	L	bile	biliary: of bile
blast, blasto	G	the germ-plasm	blastogenic: originating in the germ-plasm
blephar, blepharo	G	eyelid	blepharitis: inflammation of the eyelid
bolus, bolism	G	lump	embolus: a lump inside (a vessel)
brachi, brachio	G	arm	brachial: of the arm
brachy	G	short	brachycephalic: short-headed
brady	G	slowness; slowing	bradycardia: slowing of the heart
bronch, bronchi, bronchio	G	bronchial tubes	bronchitis: inflammation of the bronchial tubes
capsul, capsulo	L	envelope of tissue	capsulitis: inflammation of a capsule (such as of the eye lens)
carcin, carcino	G	of cancer; cancerous	carcinogenic: causing cancer
cardi, cardio	G	heart	cardiomyopathy: sickness of the muscle of the heart
cata, cath	G	down	catalepsy: seizure in which the victim falls flat and remains rigid
cele, celo, cel	G	swelling; hernia	cystocele: swelling of the bladder
cephal, cephalo	G	head	acephalous: with no head

47

Element/derivation		Meaning	Example
cerebr, cerebro	G	brain	cerebrology: study of the brain
cervic, cervico	L	neck	cervicitis: inflammation of the neck of a structure (such as the womb)
chalasia	G	relaxing	achalasia: inability to relax the muscles
cheil, cheilo	G	lip	cheilitis: inflammation of the lips
cheir, cheiro, chiro	G	hand	cheirospasm: spasm of the hand muscles
chiro *see* cheir			
chol, chole, cholia, cholo	G	bile; gall	cholangitis: inflammation of the bile vessels
chondr, chondria, chondro	G	cartilage	chondroma: cartilage swelling
chord, chordo *see* cord			
cirrho	G	wasting	cirrhosis: wasting (of an organ)
coeli, coelio, coel	G	abdomen; cavity	coelioma: tumour of the abdomen
col, colo, colono	G	colon	colitis: inflammation of the colon
colp, colpo	G	vagina	colporrhaphy: stitching of the vagina
conidio, conio	G	dust	pneumoconiosis: respiratory disease caused by inhalation of dust
contra	L	against; countering	contraceptive: preventing conception
copr, copro	G	faeces; stools	coprolith: a solidified mass of faeces
cord, cordo	G/L	cord	cordectomy: removal of a vocal cord
cortico	L	of the cortex, the outer layer of an organ	corticotropin: causing growth of the cortex
cost, costo	L	rib	costal: of the ribs
cox, coxo	L	hip joint	coxalgia: pain in the hip joint
crani, cranio	G/L	skull	craniotomy: cutting the skull
cry, crymo, cryo	G	cold; freezing	cryosurgery: destruction of tissue by application of extreme cold
crypt, crypto	G	hidden	cryptogenic: of hidden origin
cubit, cubito	L	elbow	cubital: of the elbow
cuta, cuti, cuticul	L	skin	subcutaneous: under the skin
cyst, cysto	G	bladder	cystitis: inflammation of the bladder
cyt, cyte, cyto	G	cell	cytology: study of cells
dent, denti, dento	L	tooth	dentist
derm, dermato, dermis, dermo	G	skin	dermatitis: inflammation of the skin
dextr, dextro	L	right(-hand)	dextrocardia: having the heart on the right(-hand) side
di, dia	G	through	diathermy: heating through
di	G	two	dicephalous: having two heads
dipl, diplo	G	double	diplopia: double vision
dis	L	no longer in a state of	dislocation: no longer properly located
dorsa, dorsi, dorso	L	back	dorsalgia: pain in the back
duct	L	channel; tube	ovarian duct: tube from the ovary
duoden, duodeno	L	of the duodenum	duodenectomy: removal of the duodenum
dys	G	bad; abnormal; painful	dysentery: painful disorder of the intestines
ec, ecto, ectasia	G	out; outward; outer	ectopic pregnancy: a pregnancy in which the embryo grows outside the womb
ectomy (= ec + tomy)	G	cut out; removal	gastrectomy: removal of the stomach
em *see* en			
en, endo, em, ento	G	in; inside; within	endoscopy: looking inside
enter, entero	G	intestine	enteritis: inflammation of the intestine
ep, epi	G	upon; on the outside	epidermis: outermost layer of skin

Element/derivation		Meaning	Example
erythr, erythro	G	red	erythrocyte: red (blood) cell
esthe	G	feeling; sensitivity	anaesthesia: with no feeling
estro	G	stimulation; heat	oestrogen: a female sex hormone
ex	L	out; (to the) outside	exhale: breathe out
extra	L	beyond; extra	extrasensory: beyond the normal senses
fibr, fibro, fibros	L	fibre; fibrous tissue	fibrositis: inflammation of fibrous tissue
galact, galacto	G	milk	galactorrhoea: excessive milk production
gastr, gastro	G	stomach	gastritis: inflammation of the stomach
gen	G	originating; creating	cytogenic: forming a cell
gero, geronto, geria	G	old age	geriatric: pertaining to old age
gingiv, gingivo	L	gums	gingivitis: inflammation of the gums
gloss, glosso	G	tongue	glossitis: inflammation of the tongue
glyco	G	sugar	glycoprotein: a sugar and protein compound
gnosia, gnosis, gnostic	G	knowing; recognizing	prognosis: a forecast
gon, gono	G	seed; semen	gonorrhoea: a venereal disease
gonad, gonado	G	ovary or testis	gonadectomy: removal of ovary or testis
gram	G	record	cardiogram: record of the heart
graph	G	recorder	encephalograph: device for recording the electrical activity of the brain
gyn, gynae, gynaeco	G	female; feminine	gynaecomastia: having female breasts
haem, haema, haemat, haemato, (h)aemia, haemo	G	blood	haematuria: blood in the urine
hemi	G	half	hemiplegia: paralysis of one side of the body
hepat, hepato	G	liver	hepatitis: inflammation of the liver
heter, hetero	G	other; different	heteroplasty: grafting of tissue from another person
hidr	G	sweat	hyperhidrosis: excessive sweating
hist, histio, histo	G	tissue	histology: study of tissue
hom, homeo, homo	G	same; unchanging	homogeneous: of the same origin
hydr, hydro	G	water	hydrophobia: abnormal fear of water
hyper	G	over; excessive	hyperthyroidism: overactive thyroid gland
hypn, hypno	G	sleep	hypnosis: state of apparent sleep
hypo, hyp	G	under; too little	hypoglossal: under the tongue
hyster, hystero	G	womb	hysterectomy: removal of the womb
iatr, iatro, iatry	G	physician; treatment	iatrogenic: originating from the physician or from the treatment
ile, ileo	L	of the ileum (part of the small intestine)	ileocolitis: inflammation of the ileum and colon
ili, ilio	L	of the ilium (the hip bone)	iliac: of the ilium
infra	L	beneath	infracostal: beneath a rib or the ribs
inguin, inguino	L	groin	inguinal hernia: rupture in the groin
inter	L	between	intercostal: between the ribs
intra, intro	L	within; into	intravenous: into a vein
irid, irido, ir	G	of the iris	iridokeratitis: inflammation of the iris and the cornea
isch, ischo	G	suppression; retention	ischuria: retention of the urine
itis	G	inflammation	nephritis: inflammation of the kidney
kerat, kerato	G	the cornea; horn	keratosis: a horny growth; e.g. a wart
kin, kine, kino	G	movement	hyperkinetic: overactive in movement
koil, koilo	G	hollow; concave	koilonychia: a disease characterized by concave nails

Element/derivation		Meaning	Example
labi, labio, labr	L	lip	labial: of the lips
lact, lacti, lacto	L	milk	lactogenic: creating milk
laryng, larynge, laryngo	G	of the larynx	laryngitis: inflammation of the larynx
lepsy, lept	G	seizure; attack	narcolepsy: sudden onset of extreme drowsiness
leuc, leuk, leuko, leuco	G	white	leucocyte: white (blood) cell
lingu	L	tongue	lingual: of the tongue
lip, liparo, lipid, lipo, lipomata	G	fat; fatty	lipoma: fatty benign tumour
lith, lithia, litho	G	stone	lithotomy: cutting of a duct or organ to remove a stone
lob, lobo	G	lobe	lobotomy: incision into a lobe (of the brain)
lyo, lysis, lyso; lytic	G	dissolving; breaking down	haemolysis: breaking down of (red) blood cells
ma	G	swelling; tumour	carcinoma: cancerous tumour
macro	G	large	macrocyte: large cell
malacia, malaco	G	softness	osteomalacia: softening of the bones
mamm, mamma, mammo	G/L	breast	mammoplasty: plastic reconstruction of the breast
manu	L	hand	manual: using the hand
mast, masto	G	breast	mastectomy: removal of a breast
melan, melano	G	black	melanuria: dark pigment in the urine
meli, melit	G	sweetness	melituria: sugar in the urine
mening, meningo	G	the membranes round the spinal cord and the brain	meningitis: inflammation of the membranes around the brain
meno, mens, menstru	G/L	monthly	menopause: the end of menstruation
menstru see meno			
mes, meso	G	middle; medium	mesomorph: person of medium build
met, meta	G	with; alongside; just behind	metacarpals: bones of the hand, just behind the wrist (carpus)
metr, metria, metro	G	womb	metritis: inflammation of the womb
micro	G	small	microcephaly: small head
mon, mono	G	one; single	monocular: with one eye
morph	G	form; shape	endomorph: person of thin build
motor	L	causing movement	oculomotor nerve: the nerve that controls the eye muscles
muc, mucino, muco	L	of mucus	mucitis: inflammation of a mucous membrane
my, myo	G	muscle; muscular	myalgia: muscle pain
myco, myce, mycet, myceto	G	fungus	mycetoma: a fungal growth
myel, myelo	G	marrow; centre	myeloma: tumour of bone marrow cells
myo see my			
narco, narcotico	G	numbness	narcolepsy: sudden onset of extreme drowsiness
nas, naso	G	nose	nasopharynx: nose and pharynx (area)
necro	G	death; deadness	necrotic: concerned with death
neo	G	new	neoplasm: new growth of tissue
nephr, nephro	G	kidney	nephritis: inflammation of the kidney
neur, neuro	L	nerve	neurology: study of the nervous system
noct	L	night	noctambulism: sleep-walking
nyct, nycto	G	night	nycturia: urination at night
nymph, nympho	G	the labia minora or clitoris	nymphotomy: surgical cutting of the labia minora or the clitoris

Element/derivation		Meaning	Example
ocul, oculo	L	eye	oculist: eye specialist
odont, odonto	G	tooth	orthodontist: one who straightens teeth
odyn, odynia, odymo	G	pain	pleurodynia: pain in the chest wall
oedema	G	swelling	oedematogenic: causing oedema
oestro	G	stimulation; heat	oestrogen: a female sex hormone
olig, oligo	G	few; small; little	oligomenorrhoea: small menstrual flow
onco, oncus	G	swelling; bulge	oncology: study of tumours
onych, onychia, onycho	G	nail	onychopathy: nail disease
oo	G	egg; ovum	oogenesis: formation of the ovum
opathy see path			
ophthalm, ophthalmo	G	eye	ophthalmia: severe inflammation of the eye
opia, opic, opsis, opti, opto	L	eye	optic nerve: nerve from the eye to the brain
orchi, orchid, orchido, orchio, orcho	G	testis (testicle)	orchidectomy: removal of a testicle
orth, ortho	G	straight; correct; upright	orthoptics: straightening vision
oss, osseo, ossi, oste, osteo	G/L	bone	osteitis: inflammation of a bone
ostomy see stoma			
ot, oti, oto	L	ear	otorrhoea: discharge from the ear
ov, ovi, ovo	L	egg; ovum	oviduct: tube along which an ovum passes from the ovary
ovar, ovario	L	of the ovary	ovariectomy: removal of an ovary
pachy	G	thick	pachyderma: abnormal thickening of the skin
paed, paedia, paedo	G	child; boy	paediatrics: the treatment of children
palat, palato	L	of the palate	palatoplegia: paralysis of the palate
pan, pant, panto	G	whole; complete	pancarditis: inflammation of the entire heart
pancreat, pancreato,	G	of the pancreas; pancreatic duct	pancreatitis: inflammation of the pancreas
pant, panto see pan			
par, para	G	beside; beyond	paresthesia; beyond (normal) sensation
paresis, paretic	G	relaxation; weakness	myoparesis: weakness of a muscle
parous, parturi	L	bearing; giving birth	multiparous: having many children
path, pathe, patho, pathy	G	disease; ill condition	pathogen: disease-producer
pector, pectori	L	chest; breast	angina pectoris: pain in the chest
pelvi, pelvio	L	of the pelvis	pelvimetry: measurement of the pelvis
penia	G	lack; shortage	leucopenia: shortage of leucocytes (white blood cells) in the blood
pepsia; pepti	G	digestive juices	peptic ulcer: ulcer of the stomach
peri	G	round; around	pericardium: (sac) around the heart
periton, peritone, peritoneo	G	of the peritoneum (abdominal membrane)	peritonitis: inflammation of the peritoneum
pexia, pexis, pexy	G	fixing	orchiopexy: surgical fixing (by suture) of a testis
phaco, phako	G	lens; lens-shaped	phacometer: measure of focusing power
phage, phago, phagus, phagy	G	eating; consuming	phagocyte: cell that consumes other cells or micro-organisms
phako see phaco			
phall, phallo	G	penis	phallodynia: pain in the penis
pharyng, pharynge, pharyngo	G	of the pharynx (throat)	pharyngitis: inflammation of the throat

Element/derivation		Meaning	Example
phil, philia, philo	G	love	haemophilia: bleeding easily ("love of blood")
phleb, phlebo	G	vein	phlebitis: inflammation of a vein
phobe, phobia, phobic, phobo	G	abnormal fear; hatred	agoraphobia: fear of open spaces
phone, phonia, phonic, phono	G	sound	phonocardiograph: device to record the sound of the heart
phor, phore, phoresis, phoria	G	carry; conveying	oophoritis: inflammation of the ovary (egg-carrier)
phot, photo	G	light	photophobia: fear of light
phylac, phylactic, phylaxis	G	protection against infection	prophylaxis: preventive treatment
physo	G	air; gas	physometra: air or gas in the womb
plasm, plasmo, plasti, plasty, plasia	G	(basic) substance which can be added to or shaped	cytoplasm: basic contents of a cell
platy	G	broad	platyrrhine: broad-nosed
plegia, plegic, plexy	G	a stroke; paralysis	hemiplegia: paralysis of one side of the body
pleur, pleuro	G	membrane (pleura) around lungs in chest cavity	pleurisy: inflammation of the pleural membrane
pneuma, pneumato, pneumo, pneumon, pneumono	G	lung	pneumonectomy: removal of a lung
pod, podo	G	foot	podalgia: pain in the foot
polio	G	grey	polioencephalitis: inflammation of the grey substance of the brain
poly	G	many	polyarthritis: inflammation of many joints
post	L	after; behind	postnatal: after childbirth
pre	L	in front of; before	premolar: tooth in front of a molar
pro	G/L	before; forward	progeria: premature ageing
proct, procto	G	anus; rectum	proctitis: inflammation of the rectum
prostat, prostatico, prostato	G	of the prostate	prostatectomy: removal of part or all of the prostate
pseud, pseudo	G	false; imagined	pseudocyesis: false pregnancy
psych, psyche, psycho	G	mind	psychology: study of the mind
pulmo, pulmon, pulmono	G	lung	pulmonary: of the lungs
py, pyo	G	pus	pyogenic: forming pus
pyel, pyelo	G	kidney	pyelitis: inflammation of the kidney
pyresis, pyret, pyreto, pyrexia, pyro	G	fever; fire	pyretic: of fever
rachi, rachio	G	spine	rachiopathy: spinal disease
radi, radicul	L	root (of nerve or tooth)	radiculitis: inflammation of a nerve
ren, reno	L	of the kidney	suprarenal: above the kidney
retin, retino	L	of the retina	retinitis: inflammation of the retina
retro	L	backward; behind	retrobulbar: behind the eyeball
rhachi see rachi			
rhage see rrhage			
rhaphe see rrhaply			
rhin, rhino	G	nose	rhinitis: inflammation of the nose
rhoea see rrhoea			
rrhage, rrhagia, rrh	G	outflow	haemorrhage: outflow of blood
rrhaphy, rhaphe	G	suture; join	colporrhaphy: stitching of the vagina

Element/derivation		Meaning	Example
rrhine *see* rhin			
rrhoea	G	severe outflow; gush	diarrhoea: flow of faeces
sacr, sacro	L	of the sacrum	sacralgia: pain in the sacral region
salping	G	Eustachian or fallopian tube	salpingitis: inflammation of a fallopian tube
sapr, sapro	G	putrefaction	sapraemia: putrefactive bacteria in the blood
sarc, sarco	G	flesh	sarcoma: fleshy tumour
schisis, schisto, schiz, schizo	G	split; cleft; fissured	schizophrenia: "split mind"
scler, sclera, sclero	G	hardening	arteriosclerosis: hardening of the arteries
scope, scopic, scopy	G	view; look at	ophthalmoscope: instrument for looking at the eye
seba, sebi, sebo	L	fatty secretion of hair and skin	seborrhoea: excessive secretion of fatty substances from the skin
sect, section	L	cutting	Caesarian section
semeio	G	of symptoms	semeiotic: of symptoms
semi	L	half	semiconscious: half conscious
sepsis, septic	G	decay; putrefaction	septicaemia: pathogenic bacteria in the blood
sero	L	of serum (the liquid part of the blood)	serotherapy: treatment by injection of serum
sial, sialo	G	salivary gland	sialitis: inflammation of a salivary gland
sider, sidero	G	iron	sideropenia: iron deficiency
sinistr, sinistro	L	left(-hand)	sinistral: on the left
soma, somat, somato, somi, somia, some	G	body	psychosomatic: of both mind and body, or of one caused by the other
spasmo, spasti	G	of spasm	spasmogen: (substance) producing spasms
spermo, spermato, spermi, spermio, spermo	G	sperm; semen	spermatocele: swelling of a testicle
sphygm, sphygmo	G	pulse	sphygmomanometer: instrument for measuring the force of the pulse
spin, spina, spini, spino	L	spine	spinal: of the spine
splanchn, splanchno	G	visceral; intestinal	splanchnic: of the intestine
splen, spleno	G	spleen	splenomegaly: enlargement of the spleen
spondyl, spondylo	G	vertebra	spondyoarthritis: arthritis of the spine
state, stato, stasia, stasis	G/L	standing; still	venous statis: cessation of the blood flow through a vein
stear, stearo, steat, steato	G	fat	stcatoma: a fatty tumour
steat, steato *see* stear, stearo			
steno	G	contracted	stenosis: constriction (of a tube or vessel)
stern, sterno	G/L	of the sternum (breastbone)	manubrium sternum: the "handle" of the breastbone
steth, stetho	G	chest	stethoscope: device for listening to sounds in the chest
sthenia, sthenic	G	strength; ability	myasthenia: lack of strength in a muscle
stoma, stomat, stomato, stomy	G	mouth; opening	colostomy: making an opening in the body through which the contents of the colon may be emptied
strum, strumi	L	goitre; thyroid gland	strumitis: inflammation of the thyroid gland
sub	L	below; less than	sublingual: below the tongue
super, supra	L	above; more than	superovulation: producing more ova than usual
sy (syl, sym, syn)	G	with; together; the same	synergy: working together

Element/derivation		Meaning	Example
tacho, tacheo, tachy	G	speed; fast	tachycardia: fast heartbeat
tars, tarso	G/L	the margin of the eyelid; the instep of the foot	tarsomalacia: softening of the edge of an eyelid
taxia, taxy	G	co-ordination; voluntary movement	locomotor ataxia: disease in which co-ordination of the power to move is increasingly impaired
tel, tele, teleo	G	distance	telesthesia: sensation perceived as though from a distance
ten, teno	G	of a tendon	tenotomy: cutting of a tendon
thalam, thalamo	G	of the thalamus (part of the brain)	thalamectomy: surgical removal of part of the thalamus
thalass, thalasso	G	sea	thalassotherapy: treatment of disease by living near the sea, sea voyages, or sea bathing
therapist, therapeutic therapy	G	treatment for disease	hydrotherapy: treatment in (or with) water
therm, thermo	G	heat; warmth	thermalgia: sensation of burning pain
thoracic, thoraco	G	of the chest, thorax	thoracotomy: cutting into the chest
thrix see tricho			
thrombo, thrombus	G	blood-clotting	thrombus: a blood clot
thyro, thyroid	G	of the thyroid gland	thyroiditis: inflammation of the thyroid
tomy	G	cutting; separating	cystotomy: cutting into the bladder wall
tonia, tonic, toneum	G	stretched; strained	myotonic: being unable to relax a muscle
tonsill, tonsillo	G	of the tonsils	tonsillectomy
tox, toxic, toxico	G/L	poison	toxaemia: blood-poisoning
trache, trachea, tracheo	G	windpipe	tracheostomy: making an incision in the windpipe
trans	L	across; from one to another	transfusion: passing (blood) from one person to another
tricho, thrix	G	hair	trichoschisis: splitting of hairs
troph, tropho, trophy	G	nutrition; supply of material for growth	atrophy: lack of growth; wasting
tub, tubo	L	tube (usually uterine)	tubectomy: removal of the (uterine) tube
tympan, tympano	G	(ear)drum	tympanitis: inflammation of the middle ear
ultra	L	beyond	ultraviolet: electromagnetic radiation just beyond the visible spectrum
ur, ure, uret, uria, urico, urino, uro	G	urine	polyuria: frequent passing of urine
urethr, urethro	G	of the urethra	urethralgia: pain in the urethra
uter, utero	L	womb	uteritis: inflammation of the womb
uvul	G	uvula	uvulitis: inflammation of the uvula
vagin	L	vagina	vaginitis: inflammation of the vagina
vas, vasi, vaso	G	(blood-)vessel; sperm duct	vasectomy: removing part of the vas deferens (sperm duct)
vena, vene, veno	L	vein	venesection: cutting open a vein
vesic, vesica, vesico, vescula	G	bladder	retrovesicular: behind the bladder
vir, viro	L	virus	virology: study of viruses
xero, xer	G	dry	xerostomia: dryness of the mouth

Abdomen is the body cavity below the chest. It is bordered by the diaphragm above, the pelvis below, and the back muscles and spine behind. The abdomen contains various major organs, including the liver, spleen, pancreas, stomach, small and large intestines, kidneys, adrenal glands, and bladder. In a woman, the abdomen also encloses the reproductive organs; in a man, the abdomen contains the prostate gland.

All the abdominal organs are surrounded by a membrane called the peritoneum. The front and sides of the abdomen are covered by three layers of abdominal muscles. The abdominal aorta (a major artery that carries blood from the heart) and the major veins lie on the back wall of the abdomen.

See also ABDOMINAL PAIN.

A talk about Abdominal pain

Abdominal pain is any pain in the body cavity below the chest. The most common cause in both adults and children is INDIGESTION, as a result of eating too much or eating unsuitable food. Other causes range from the normal menstrual cramps experienced by many women to more serious ailments requiring prompt medical attention.

Q: *What are minor causes of abdominal pain?*

A: Indigestion is common and generally without serious consequence. It is often accompanied by HEARTBURN, belching, and a sensation of fullness or nausea. Sharp abdominal pain may also accompany diarrhoea or vomiting, but this usually settles within a few hours. In most cases, neither of these causes requires treatment by a doctor, except in an infant or anyone with a history of serious abdominal illness.

Q: *What are the more serious causes of abdominal pain?*

A: Sudden sharp pain that comes in waves (a condition known medically as COLIC) may be accompanied by vomiting, sweating, and the need to double up. Colic can be caused by several potentially serious disorders, such as intestinal obstruction; inflammation of the peritoneum

(PERITONITIS); or stones (*see* CALCULUS) in the gall bladder (biliary colic) or in the kidneys (renal colic). If such pain continues for more than one hour, a doctor must be consulted.

Continuous pain that comes on suddenly, together with slight fever, tenderness of the abdomen when touched, and sometimes vomiting and constipation, may be caused by inflammation of the appendix (appendicitis), gall bladder (acute cholecystitis), pancreas (pancreatitis), or in women a fallopian tube (salpingitis). In women, an ectopic pregnancy may also be a cause.

If any of the above symptoms continue for more than four hours, a doctor should be consulted.

Q: *What other disorders include abdominal pain as a symptom?*

A: Abdominal pain with backache and frequent, painful passing of urine suggests inflammation of the pelvis of the kidney (pyelitis), or of the bladder (cystitis). There may also be a fever. A doctor should be consulted within a day. Recurrent abdominal pain may be caused by a peptic ulcer, spastic colon, chronic cholecystitis, diverticulitis, or painful menstrual periods (dysmenorrhoea).

Q: *Are children especially subject to abdominal pain?*

A: No. The primary cause of stomachache in a child is muscle spasm. But a child with infection of the middle ear (otitis media) or inflammation of the tonsils (tonsillitis) may complain of a stomachache because

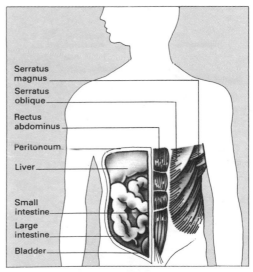

Serratus
magnus

Serratus
oblique

Rectus
abdominus

Peritonoum

Liver

Small
intestine

Large
intestine

Bladder

Abdomen has three layers of muscle outside the peritoneum and the internal organs.

Abortion

lymph glands near the intestine become tender and swollen. Pneumonia is also a disorder which may cause abdominal pain in children.

Q: *Can pain in the abdomen be a symptom of a disorder elsewhere in the body?*

A: Pain from a heart attack, pleurisy, or pneumonia can be experienced in the upper abdomen. But these disorders have other characteristic symptoms easily recognized by a doctor.

See also STOMACH DISORDERS.

Abortion is the termination of a pregnancy before the embryo or foetus can live independently of its mother. Popularly, the term abortion refers to the deliberate or induced termination of a pregnancy, whereas the spontaneous termination of a pregnancy is called a MISCARRIAGE.

Q: *Why might a doctor recommend a deliberate or induced abortion?*

A: A doctor might recommend an abortion if tests on the amniotic fluid show that there is a congenital abnormality, such as spina bifida or Down's syndrome (*see* GENETIC COUNSELLING). These tests involve inserting a needle into the uterus in the fourteenth week of pregnancy (amniocentesis) and removing some fluid. The doctor may also recommend an abortion if the mother's health, mental or physical, is seriously at risk if the pregnancy is allowed to continue.

Q: *How is a medically-induced abortion performed?*

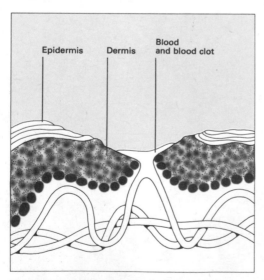

Epidermis   Dermis   Blood and blood clot

Abrasion is an injury to the surface layers of the skin exposing blood capillaries and nerves.

A: In early pregnancy, an abortion is generally performed using either minor surgery, such as D AND C (dilation and curettage), or a suction apparatus. When a pregnancy is several months old, a concentrated hormone and salt solution may be injected into the womb. This stimulates the womb to expel the foetus.

There are also various drugs, called abortifacients, that are sometimes used to induce abortion, but many of these contain the potentially dangerous drug ERGOT.

Rarely, a surgeon performs an operation to open the womb and remove the foetus.

Q: *Is an induced abortion dangerous to the woman?*

A: A medical abortion in early pregnancy, properly conducted, is a safe and minor operation. It can be performed in a clinic or with brief hospitalization.

An abortion performed by an unskilled person and without sterile conditions, exposes the patient to the risk of infection, haemorrhage, or even death.

The frequency of miscarriage is slightly increased in women who have had an abortion.

See also PREGNANCY AND CHILDBIRTH.

Abortion law in the United Kingdom allows a doctor to perform an abortion for any of four specific reasons only: (1) if the continuation of the pregnancy is likely to endanger the woman's life; (2) if pregnancy is more dangerous to her mental or physical health than a termination; (3) if there is a real likelihood that the baby will be congenitally deformed; or (4) if the continuation of the pregnancy may seriously affect the health of other children in the family, a social reason. The woman's own doctor and the operating surgeon have to sign a certificate, sent to the Department of Health and Social Security, stating for which reason the abortion is being done.

Abortus fever is another name for the infectious disease BRUCELLOSIS. It is also known as Rio Grande fever, undulant fever, Malta fever, or Mediterranean fever.

Abrasion is a minor injury in which the skin is scraped or grazed hard enough to make it bleed.

Treatment is to clean the wound immediately with cold water and to apply an antiseptic solution, if available. Apply a dry bandage. The dressing can be removed when a scab has formed, unless there is danger that clothing might rub against it.

See also First Aid, p.591.

56

Abscess is a localized collection of pus caused by bacterial infection. Bacteria that invade the body are attacked by white blood cells and reduced to pus, which is discharged through the skin. Pimples and boils are surface abscesses. An abscess commonly occurs under the skin and may be caused by an infection of any small gland in the skin (folliculitis), a minor abrasion, or a cut. Abscesses often occur in moist areas of the body, such as the groin or armpit, and are more frequent in persons with DIABETES.

Q: *What are some of the symptoms of an abscess?*

A: Pus forms and the surrounding tissues become red, swollen, and painful as the abscess stretches the area and tries to burst through the skin. Discomfort is relieved when the abscess bursts spontaneously or is lanced.

Q: *What is the treatment for an external type of abscess?*

A: The aim is to encourage the infection to reach the surface of the skin. The customary home treatment is a warm, moist compress. A medical objection to such treatment is that such a compress makes the surrounding tissue more prone to infection. Painkilling drugs, such as aspirin, may be used. The area may be rested, for example, by putting an arm in a sling when there is an abscess in the armpit. A dry dressing should be applied when an abscess comes to a head and discharges.

   The abscess may need to be lanced by a doctor if there is fever or pain, or if the surrounding skin becomes increasingly red and tender.

Q: *What other kinds of abscesses are there?*

A: There are internal abscesses, usually accompanied by fever, local pain, and a tired, rundown feeling. Such abscesses can occur around a tooth (gumboil), in the breast, in bone (in mastoiditis and osteomyelitis), in the liver (in amoebic dysentery), in the vagina (Bartholin's cyst), in the appendix (appendicitis), or in the anal area, between the rectum and the ischium (ischiorectal abscess). In all such cases, a doctor must be consulted.

   Another kind of abscess is the COLD ABSCESS, which may be caused by tuberculosis. A cold abscess is so called because it is slow-forming and without pain, redness, or heat.

   See also BOIL.

Accidental haemorrhage is a medical term for vaginal bleeding occurring after the 28th week of pregnancy. The blood comes from a normally positioned PLACENTA, the organ through which the embryo is nourished by the mother. When the placenta lies across the opening of the womb, obstructing normal delivery of the baby and causing bleeding before or during labour (placenta praevia), the bleeding is known as an inevitable haemorrhage. If this happens, a CAESAREAN SECTION is performed.

Accommodation is the adjustment made by the lens of the eye, by means of its muscles, in order to see clearly objects at various distances. The ability of the lens to focus in this way decreases with age, resulting in the condition called presbyopia. *See* EYE.

Acephalic describes a foetus without a head. Other parts of the body, such as the spine or feet, may also be malformed. A foetus that is born without a complete brain and spinal cord, and without the roof (vault) of the skull, is described as anencephalic. The baby may live for a very short time after birth. Approximately one anencephalic baby is born in every thousand births.

Acetabulum is the socket of the hip joint. It is a cup-shaped part of the pelvis into which the head of the thighbone fits. *See* p.4.

Acetaminophen is the U.S. name for PARACETAMOL.

Acetone is a chemical that is normally formed in the body only in very small amounts. Larger quantities are produced if there is a lack of insulin in the body. This may occur with diabetes, some severe illnesses, or starvation. The chemical can be detected in tests of the urine and blood, and there may be a characteristic odour of acetone (a fruity smell) on the breath.

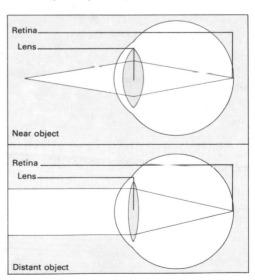

Retina
Lens

Near object

Retina
Lens

Distant object

Accommodation is adjustment of the lens in order to focus an image on to the retina.

Acetylcholine

Acetylcholine is a chemical that is produced in many nerve endings. It is essential for the transmission of nerve impulses. *See* p.20.

Acetylsalicylic acid is the chemical name for the painkilling drug aspirin. *See* ASPIRIN.

Achalasia is the failure to relax of an area of muscle in the digestive tract. It is caused by nerve damage and occurs most frequently in the oeosphagus (gullet). Difficulty in swallowing results; food may be held in the oeosphagus and cause it to expand. Vomiting then brings up the food. Pneumonia may follow if food spills into the lungs.

Q: How is achalasia treated?

A: Treatment is with drugs, stretching the muscle with an instrument, or by an operation.

Q: Where else can achalasia occur?

A: A similar condition occurs in the colon (large intestine) of infants. This is known as HIRSCHSPRUNG'S DISEASE, or megacolon.

Ache is any continuous pain that is not severe. Aches are usually caused by minor disorders, and can be treated with a mild painkiller.

Achilles' tendon is a thick band of connective tissue (tendon) that extends from the calf muscles to the heel bone (calcaneus). Contraction of the muscles attached to this tendon enables a person to stand on tiptoe. The tendon can be torn (ruptured), especially in middle-aged people, by sudden activity, often with little or no external sign of injury. The tear may have to be repaired by a simple surgical operation.

Achlorhydria is a condition in which there is an absence of free hydrochloric acid in the

gastric juice of the stomach. Hydrochloric acid kills bacteria and aids the absorption of iron and proteins. There are rarely any symptoms, and specific treatment for the disorder is not necessary. The condition is a result of chronic gastritis or pernicious anaemia. *See* PERNICIOUS ANAEMIA.

Achondroplasia is an abnormality in the growing areas of long bones such as the thighbone (femur) and upper armbone (humerus). It is caused by a defect in the process that converts cartilage into bone. The condition results in stunted growth, or dwarfism, and can normally be detected at birth. There is no treatment.

Q: Is achondroplasia hereditary?

A: Yes. It is inherited through a dominant gene or from a new gene change (mutation) in a parent.

Q: Are other physical or mental capacities affected?

A: No. Other systems are spared. Intelligence is usually normal.

Acidosis is a serious condition in which the body's acid-alkali balance is disturbed and the blood is more acid than normal. It results from a build-up of carbon dioxide in the blood, often associated with diabetes, kidney disorder, or starvation. It is treated by treating the underlying cause.

Q: Is acidosis associated with heartburn or indigestion?

A: No, not in the medical definition of the term. In popular usage, however, some people use acidosis to describe any minor stomach disorder, such as indigestion.

Acne is a skin disorder that usually affects the face. The neck, shoulders, and chest may also be affected. Acne is caused by oily secretions in the skin glands that clog the pores (tiny openings in the skin). In turn, pimples and blackheads form at the clogged pores. In its early stages, the condition is not associated with infection, but this may occur later, resulting in pustules. The role of infection in acne is not clear, but it makes scarring more likely to result. Acne occurs especially during adolescence.

Q: What causes acne in young people?

A: Acne in young people is simply a sign of the various hormonal changes that take place at puberty. One effect of these changes is an increase, and change, in the secretions from the glands. The occurrence of acne in teenagers is therefore the result of natural change. Time is needed for the body's adjustment, but measures may be taken to reduce the severity of the complaint.

Q: What precautions may minimize acne?

A: Some doctors advise against drinks

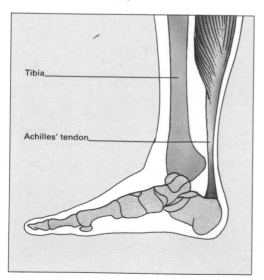

Tibia

Achilles' tendon

Achilles' tendon is the thick connective tissue that attaches the calf muscle to the heel bone.

that have a high sugar content, and such greasy foods as peanut butter, chocolate, and fried foods. Clean hair is also important, and the hair should be washed twice weekly or more. Spots should not be picked or squeezed, because this may lead to more severe inflammation. It is important to keep the face clean. Physical exercise is strongly recommended.

Q: *How effective against acne are unprescribed lotions and tablets?*

A: Most products sold as treatment for acne function reasonably well. Lotions, often containing sulphur, help to prevent greasy skin. Persons with severe acne should consult a doctor, who may prescribe special lotions or antibiotics. The antibiotics kill any infection present and have a beneficial, hormone-like effect on the skin.

Q: *Do weather conditions affect the severity of acne?*

A: Yes. The complaint tends to be aggravated by hot, humid conditions. Fresh air, sunshine, and plenty of exercise are all effective in combating acne.

Q: *Do people other than teenagers suffer from acne?*

A: Adults do not get acne as often as teenagers do. But the condition may affect many women before a menstrual period.

Acrocyanosis is a condition in which the fingers and toes turn blue. More common in women than in men, it is caused either by insufficient oxygen in the blood, or by low temperature. The result, in either case, is an extreme sensation of cold for the patient. The only treatment is to wear sufficient clothing to keep warm. Persons who suffer also from CHILBLAINS may be helped by drugs that dilate the blood vessels to improve circulation. Smoking may worsen the condition.

Acromegaly is a disorder in which the bones in the arms and legs get thicker and longer, as do those of the hands, feet, jaw, and skull. Facial features become coarser and the voice may become deeper. The disorder is caused by an excessive production of growth hormone by the pituitary gland, possibly because of a tumour.

In its early stages, acromegaly is almost undetectable. Advanced cases are accompanied by muscular weakness, impairment of vision, and reduced sexual desire.

Q: *Can any treatment halt the condition?*

A: Skilled medical and surgical care is necessary before too many of the changes become irreversible. X-ray therapy or surgery on the pituitary gland may be recommended.

See also GIGANTISM.

Acrophobia is an abnormal fear of heights. Occasionally it can be extremely severe and may be a symptom of depression.

ACTH (or corticotropin) is an abbreviation for adrenocorticotropic hormone. It is secreted by the pituitary gland at the base of the brain, and is responsible for the stimulation of the cortex (outer layer) of the ADRENAL GLANDS. It makes the adrenal cortex produce the hormones cortisol, corticosterone, and cortisone. Natural or synthetic preparations of ACTH have been used to treat various disorders, such as asthma, multiple sclerosis, and Bell's palsy. It is also used in a test of adrenal gland function.

Actinomycosis is a long-lasting disease caused by a fungus (*Actinomyces israelii*), which is normally present in the mouth and throat. Infection occurs most commonly in the jaw or neck, and sometimes in the lungs or intestine. Hard, slow-growing swellings form and eventually turn into abscesses. When the abscesses break down, pus is discharged through several openings in the skin. Doctors diagnose the condition by examining the pus under a microscope. Treatment with penicillin is usually effective if the drug is administered in large doses and over a long period of time. In some cases, however, the abscesses are removed by surgery.

Acupuncture is a method of pain relief and treatment in which the therapist inserts long needles in certain, precisely determined parts of the patient's body. Twirling the free ends of the needles (or sometimes passing a mild electric current through them) induces local anaesthesia, providing relief from pain. In

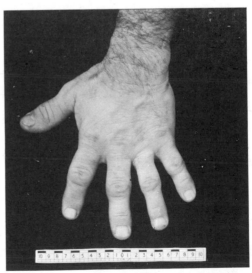

Acromegaly causes normal bone structures to become longer and thicker.

Acute yellow atrophy

China, surgery is performed using acupuncture as a local anaesthetic; the patient remains fully conscious during the operation. Its practitioners claim the anaesthetic is effective for complicated operations on the stomach, chest, neck, and head.

Q: *How does the therapist know where to insert the needles?*

A: The needles are located according to the symptoms, following the diagnosis of the practitioner. Many needle points have been charted on the body, and the insertion of needles in one place causes loss of sensation in another. The correct selection of points and the accurate insertion of the needles are essential to the effectiveness of the method.

Q: *Are there any advantages in using acupuncture for therapy?*

A: Until more medical evidence is available, the success of such treatment is impossible to judge. In any case, acupuncture is generally harmless with conditions such as hay fever, asthma, rheumatoid arthritis, and osteoarthritis.

However, the possible danger with serious, treatable disorders, such as early forms of cancer, is that any delay in seeking orthodox treatment may result in a worsening of the condition.

Q: *Is acupuncture generally available in the United Kingdom?*

A: No. Few doctors have been trained to use this technique; most practitioners are not medically qualified; many do not have any knowledge of orthodox medicine. So even apart from the general suspicion

with which acupuncture is regarded in Western countries, it is for these reasons that most doctors advise their patients not to seek help from an acupuncturist. Doctors are usually sympathetic, however, if their patient does try acupuncture when other forms of medical treatment seem to have failed.

Most reputable acupuncturists advise patients to discontinue treatment if there is little or no improvement after four or five sessions.

Q: *Why is acupuncture generally regarded with suspicion in Western countries?*

A: Because any scientific basis that it might have has not been demonstrated; neither is the principle fully understood.

Acute yellow atrophy is a very serious disorder that involves the death of large parts of the liver. Later, jaundice develops, with a high fever, confusion, vomiting, stomach pains, and bleeding through the skin. Acute yellow atrophy may be caused by severe viral infections (hepatitis) or by poisoning of the liver (as by swallowing chemicals such as carbon tetrachloride). Immediate hospitalization is necessary to provide intravenous therapy and high doses of corticosteroids. The death rate from this disorder is high.

Adam's apple is the cartilaginous structure in the front of the neck. It is part of the voice box (larynx), and is usually larger in men than in women. It grows larger in boys during puberty because of one of the effects of the male sex hormone TESTOSTERONE. As a result, vocal cords become longer, and the voice becomes deeper.

Addiction. See DRUG ADDICTION.

Addison's anaemia is another name for pernicious anaemia. See PERNICIOUS ANAEMIA.

Addison's disease is a rare condition that results from lack of production by the ADRENAL GLANDS of cortisol and aldosterone. It is caused by a disorder of the adrenal glands themselves or by the failure of the part of the pituitary gland that produces ACTH, the hormone that stimulates the adrenal glands, and is most common during middle age.

Q: *What are the symptoms of Addison's disease?*

A: Common symptoms may include weakness and dizziness caused by low blood pressure, vomiting, loss of weight, and a brownish colour of the skin and the membranes lining the mouth. It is difficult to diagnose the condition because it is slow to develop and there may be occasional, temporary improvements in the patient. Tests can reveal the low amount of adrenal hormones in the blood and a

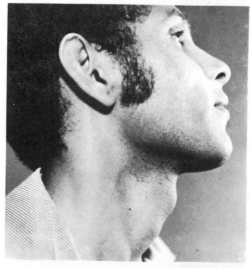

Adam's apple is a cartilaginous structure at the front of the throat.

disturbance in the balance of salts in the body fluids.

Q: *What is the usual treatment?*

A: Treatment following a correct, early diagnosis can be highly effective. The missing hormones are replaced and recovery is generally rapid.

Adenitis is inflammation of a gland or lymph node. Glandular fever is one example of adenitis.

Adenocarcinoma is a cancerous tumour that is situated in the tissue of a gland or duct.

Adenoidectomy is an operation for removal of the adenoids. *See* ADENOIDS.

Adenoids are the pad of tissue, resembling tonsil tissue, that forms a raised surface at the back of the nasal passage. It traps and destroys bacteria that enter the body through the nose, but is not essential for the body's defence against bacteria. It also helps the body to build up resistance (immunity) to future infections.

Q: *What can go wrong with the adenoids?*

A: In young children, between birth and the age of eight, the adenoids are proportionally larger than at any other age. This sometimes causes the nasal passage to become partly blocked, which may result in snoring, breathing through the mouth (because breathing through the nose is difficult), or the build-up of mucus (catarrh or post-nasal drip) in the nasal passage. The swelling or mucus may block the tubes that lead from the nasal passage to the middle ears (the Eustachian tubes), causing hearing difficulties. Ear infection (otitis media) may follow.

Q: *What treatment may be prescribed for such conditions?*

A: Antihistamine tablets and nasal drops can reduce congestion, but nasal drops should not be used for more than four days at a time. They may cause irritation and excessive dryness in the nose and make the condition worse. If deafness or infection in the middle ear persists, a doctor may recommend surgical removal of the adenoids (adenoidectomy). The operation is relatively simple and is often performed at the same time as the removal of the tonsils (TONSILLECTOMY). The adenoids grow again after removal, but seldom to the original size.

Adenoma is a usually non-cancerous (benign) tumour in glandular tissue. By itself, an adenoma causes no symptoms, although various disorders may result if the adenoma presses on a nearby part of the body.

Adenovirus is one of a group of viruses. Adenovirus infections are frequent and include common colds, conjunctivitis and various minor feverish respiratory illnesses.

Adhesion is a band that connects two sets of body tissues that are not normally connected. Adhesions form in some disorders, following injuries, or following surgery. The sticky healing fluid produced by the damaged internal tissue can solidify to form a band. This band then joins the injured tissue to any body structure or organ with which it comes in contact. Often this is a cavity wall, particularly in the abdomen. Usually this type of adhesion produces no problems. But if the structure so attached is normally free-moving, serious problems may result.

Adie's syndrome is a rare disorder that affects one or both pupils of the eyes. The disordered pupils adjust in size extremely slowly in response to changes of light and focusing. Tendon reflexes may be affected. The causes of the syndrome are not known; it occurs more often in women than in men.

A talk about Adolescence

Adolescence is the period of body growth and mental development between the onset of puberty and the attainment of physical and emotional adulthood. There is a general divergence between the timing of adolescence in young women compared with that in young men. Girls tend to reach puberty earlier and take less time from then on to reach adulthood, although their physical changes are greater. Adolescence in young women may be considered to last usually from about

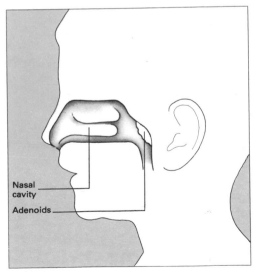

Nasal cavity

Adenoids

Adenoids at the back of the nose help trap and destroy bacteria, aiding resistance to infection.

Adrenal glands

age twelve to about age sixteen. In young men, the corresponding period is from about age thirteen to about age eighteen.

Q: *What physical changes take place during adolescence?*

A: In boys, the genitals increase in size; pubic hair then appears, then armpit hair and facial hair; the voice becomes deeper. In girls, the breasts develop; armpit and pubic hair appears; and menstruation begins.

Q: *What emotional and behavioural changes accompany these physical changes?*

A: Hormonal changes awaken sexual feelings, and most adolescents have some sexual encounters. Early experiences are likely to occur within a group of the adolescent's close friends.

Hormonal changes also account for the moodiness for which adolescents are well known. Inability or extreme reluctance to adjust to changes in outlook leads to depression and sometimes to a consequent apathy. Alternately, there are times when intense physical energy leads to unbounded enthusiasm for particular activities or causes, equally intensely felt.

There may also be a reaction against authority. In modern industrial societies, most adolescents are bound to their parents or guardians for material security. But the individual young person at this time experiences the desire to express his or her own personality, to form a definite character, and to feel as many new sensations as possible.

Some of the experimentation in various activities such as smoking and drinking alcohol that is common among many adolescents also represents a form of determined independence. But the desire for new experiences may, in some cases (as, for example, drug-taking), lead to addiction and eventual premature death.

Q: *How can parents prepare their child for adolescence?*

A: Children should be told frankly and sensibly about the coming changes in their body. Information about sex should be provided in a way that is easily understood and that leaves no questions unanswered. This information is best supplied by a parent, or someone with whom the child has an emotionally stable relationship. In many schools, children are taught about the dangers of casual sex, and of smoking, and alcohol and drug addiction.

Q: *How can parents help an adolescent child?*

A: Adolescents come under considerable pressure from the dictates of their own group which encourages them to conform. The bodily processes leading to physical maturity may also give rise to discomfort or embarrassment. One of the best ways that parents and other people can help is to provide understanding, sympathy, advice, and helpful discussion, on all the physiological and psychological problems that accompany this time.

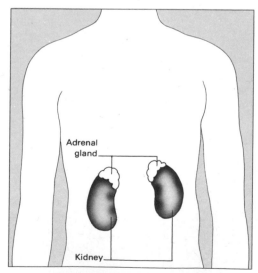

Adrenal glands produce many essential hormones including adrenaline.

Adrenal glands are two small glands that lie one above each kidney. They are also called suprarenal glands. Each is about 5cm (2 inches) in diameter. There are two main sections of the gland: the outer layer, known as the cortex, and the central part, or medulla. The gland acts as a hormone-producing centre. The medulla produces adrenaline and noradrenaline; the cortex, stimulated by another hormone (ACTH) from the pituitary gland, supplies the body with cortisol and aldosterone. For illnesses associated with disorders in the hormone production of the adrenal gland, *see* ADDISON'S DISEASE; CUSHING'S SYNDROME; PHAEOCHROMOCYTOMA.

See also p.21.

Adrenaline, or epinephrine, is a hormone secreted by the central part (medulla) of the ADRENAL GLANDS. It is the hormone that increases the heartbeat and blood pressure in response to stress or anxiety. The flow of blood to the muscles increases, the skin becomes paler, the pupils of the eyes dilate, and energy-producing glucose is released from the liver. These changes prepare the body for immediate action.

Q: Is adrenaline used as a drug?

A: Yes. Natural or chemically-produced adrenaline is injected to treat shock, acute allergy attacks, and asthma. It is also used to slow the absorption, and thus prolong the effect, of local anaesthetics.

Aerophagia is the nervous habit of swallowing excessive amounts of air. This may result in belching and swelling of the stomach. The habit is unconscious, and it must be made known to a person before the nervous tension causing it can be reduced.

Aetiology is the study of the causes or origins of disease. The aetiology of a disease includes not only its immediate cause, such as an infection, but also other contributing factors, such as family history and environment.

Afterbirth is the common name for the PLACENTA and associated membranes that are expelled from the womb, through the vagina, shortly after childbirth. Expulsion of the afterbirth, the third stage of labour, normally occurs within eight to ten minutes of the delivery of the baby. This is followed by a certain amount of bleeding from the womb.

See also PREGNANCY AND CHILDBIRTH.

Afterpains occur in childbirth once labour has ended. They are cramps in the womb as it contracts to return to its normal size. Pains are normally confined to the first forty-eight hours after childbirth, and often increase during breast-feeding. If the womb fails to contract and remains soft, prompt medical attention is needed.

See also PREGNANCY AND CHILDBIRTH.

Agammaglobulinaemia (also called hypogammaglobulinaemia) is a rare deficiency or virtual absence in the blood of the antibody proteins called GAMMA GLOBULINS. When the amount of these proteins is low, the body's natural ability to resist infection is weakened. Treatment is by injecting gamma globulin.

Agglutination is the clumping together of cells, bacteria, or particles within a fluid. Blood corpuscles clump together if they are mixed with other blood of an incompatible type. This example of agglutination is used in identifying blood groups.

Agnosia is a loss of the ability to interpret nerve messages from the senses. It accompanies some brain disorders, such as brain damage from a stroke or a tumour. The sensory organs themselves, such as those in the nose or ears, continue to function normally, but the brain cannot process the messages properly. In most instances only one of the senses is affected.

Agoraphobia is a fear of being in open spaces. It is the opposite of CLAUSTROPHOBIA (fear of closed spaces). Agoraphobia is sometimes strong and is usually uncontrollable.

It may be a symptom of depression or acute anxiety. The sufferer should consult a doctor because psychiatric help may be needed.

Agranulocytosis (or granulocytopenia) is an absence of, or deficiency in, white blood cells. It is a serious disorder because the body, lacking white blood cells, can no longer resist infection. The cause of agranulocytosis is not always known, but it most often follows the taking of certain drugs used to treat forms of cancer (such as leukaemia). The first signs of agranulocytosis may be infected ulcers on the mouth, throat, rectum, or vagina, accompanied by fever. The patient needs isolation in hospital and may require transfusions of white blood cells.

Air sickness. *See* MOTION SICKNESS.

Airway is a natural passage in the respiratory tract through which air passes in and out of the lungs during breathing. The principal airways are the windpipe (trachea) and the two bronchi. The term is also used for an artificial tube used to keep the natural breathing passage open, especially when anaesthetics are administered. Such a device is used during surgery on the windpipe (tracheotomy) to correct an obstruction to breathing.

Albino is a person whose body tissues lack the dark colouring matter (pigment) called melanin. Someone who has inherited this relatively rare condition (albinism) has white hair, milky-white skin, and pinkish irises. Albinism is usually caused by the absence of a specific enzyme resulting from a change in the genes; there is no treatment. Because of the absence of melanin, the skin and eyes of albinos are extra sensitive to the sun's rays,

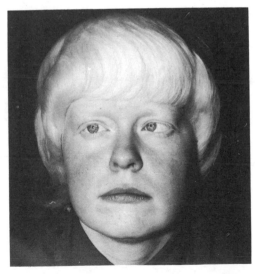

Albino persons lack the pigmentation needed to colour skin, hair, and sometimes eyes.

Albumin

and such individuals are advised to avoid direct sunlight and to wear dark glasses.

Albumin is a protein in blood plasma. It is essential for maintaining the correct balance of water in the body. During prolonged disease or when the body is suffering from starvation, the level of albumin decreases. Albumin in the urine (ALBUMINURIA) is usually a symptom of a disorder.

Albuminuria (proteinuria) is the abnormal excretion of the protein ALBUMIN in the urine. It can occur in kidney disease, in heart failure, and with a number of other disorders. Albuminuria should be investigated by a doctor; diagnosis is possible only by means of urine tests.

Q: Is albuminuria ever an urgent cause for treatment?

A: In pregnancy, albumin in the urine combined with high blood pressure (hypertension) and swelling, especially of the ankles, signals a serious malfunction.

See also ECLAMPSIA; PRE-ECLAMPSIA; PREGNANCY AND CHILDBIRTH.

Alcohol is one of a group of liquid organic chemicals of similar structure. Three alcohols only are of medical interest: ethyl alcohol (ethanol), the basic constituent of alcoholic drinks; methyl alcohol (methanol); and isopropyl alcohol (isopropanol). All alcohols are poisonous, but ethyl alcohol is less poisonous than the others.

Q: What are the medical uses of alcohol?

A: Ethyl alcohol hardens and cleans the skin, and is used for cooling the skin and as a rubdown to prevent bedsores.

Methyl alcohol is used as an antiseptic and as a cooling lotion to the skin. But it is extremely poisonous when drunk and can cause blindness, nerve inflammation (neuritis), and death.

Isopropyl alcohol is also used as a rubbing alcohol, but it has caused acute intoxication, convulsion, coma, and death in children after sponging for fever.

Q: Are alcoholic drinks dangerous?

A: Alcohol, taken in the form of alcoholic drinks, is the most commonly abused drug in the U.K. Alcohol is addictive, and its repeated use often results in the need to drink more and more to produce intoxication. Other symptoms of alcohol abuse are impaired co-ordination and, often, aggressive actions. Inflammation of the stomach lining (gastritis), vomiting, and "hangover" are almost inevitable. (*See* ALCOHOLISM.)

Contrary to popular opinion, alcohol acts as a depressant and reduces self-criticism and anxiety. The prolonged use of alcohol can cause damage to nerves (neuritis) and the liver (cirrhosis), produce mental deterioration (dementia), and increase a tendency toward inflammation of the pancreas (pancreatitis). Chronic gastritis may cause a loss of appetite (anorexia), leading to malnutrition. Alcoholic drinks are rich in calories, although they have little or no nutritive value. For this reason, heavy drinkers often have a weight problem.

Q: Is it safe to drink while taking medicines?

A: No. The effects of alcohol increase the power of drugs contained in, for example, some cough mixtures and sedative drugs such as sleeping pills, antihistamines, tranquillizers, and muscle relaxants. As a result, one drink may have the effect of several and can cause drowsiness and drunkenness. This is dangerous and can be fatal.

Q: When should alcohol be avoided?

A: Alcohol should not be taken by epileptics because it may bring on convulsions. It should be avoided by diabetics and by persons with gastritis and liver disease.

A talk about Alcoholism

Alcoholism is an addiction to ALCOHOL. Not everyone who drinks becomes an alcoholic, but there are familiar patterns of drinking that forecast an alcoholic future. Also, there is a greater incidence of alcoholism in certain occupations. Some families seem particularly susceptible to alcoholism, but this may be caused by an environment of heavy drinking.

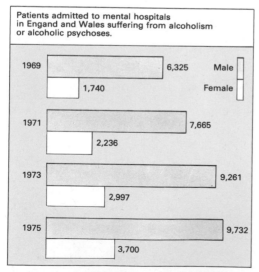

Patients admitted to mental hospitals in Engand and Wales suffering from alcoholism or alcoholic psychoses.

Year	Male	Female
1969	6,325	1,740
1971	7,665	2,236
1973	9,261	2,997
1975	9,732	3,700

Alcoholism may be associated with mental illness as well as with physical disorders.

Sometimes depression or other forms of mental illness may be the background for apparent alcoholism, but in individuals with such illnesses treatment of the depression may resolve the need to escape into excessive drinking.

Certain occupations are more disposed than others to heavy drinking, especially where social contact and stress are part of the job.

Q: *What are the danger signs that point to alcoholism?*

A: Some people reach for a bottle on waking and continue drinking throughout the day, either openly or secretly, by hiding bottles in unlikely but accessible places. A compulsive desire to drink before or during a stressful activity is also considered a danger sign. So is lying about the quantity consumed. Other people drink heavily for several days, to the exclusion of everything else, usually ending in hospital or a police cell.

Q: *What problems does alcoholism cause?*

A: Alcoholism is physically self-destructive, possibly giving rise to many other forms of illness: delirium tremens, convulsions, heart failure, muscle diseases (myopathy), cirrhosis, and neuritis. Alcoholics become inefficient at work and lose one job after another, often until they become unemployable. Marriages may not endure the strain, and children suffer emotionally and sometimes physically from dealing with a parent who is an alcoholic.

Q: *Is there satisfactory treatment for alcoholism?*

A: Doctors hold out hope for the person who really wants to stop drinking for his or her own self-esteem, if for no other reason. Alcoholics Anonymous (AA) and the National Council for Alcoholism are often able to give moral support. A person's local telephone directory or doctor's surgery will give information on how to contact AA. Hospitals can help with sedation during the initial "drying out" period, to prevent delirium tremens and to restore the patient's physical health. Some doctors believe that although an alcoholic can stop drinking, he or she cannot return to what may be called normal social drinking without the risk of becoming addicted once more; it is safer never to drink again.

Antabuse (disulfiram) is a drug that is sometimes given to encourage an aversion to alcohol. When taken in conjuction with alcohol, it causes acute vomiting, severe headache, and flushing. It is suc-cessful only if the patient takes it every day, and should be taken only under close medical supervision.

Aldosterone is a hormone released into the bloodstream by the ADRENAL GLANDS. It helps to control the balance of salts in the body. Excessive production causes high blood pressure (hypertension) due to retention of salt (Conn's syndrome).

See also ADDISON'S DISEASE.

Alimentary canal is the digestive tract, running from the mouth to the anus. It includes the mouth, pharynx (throat), oesophagus (gullet), stomach, small intestine, large intestine (colon), and rectum.

Alkali is a type of substance that neutralizes an acid. Most medicines used to relieve "acid stomach", heartburn, and indigestion contain varying amounts of alkalis.

Alkaloid is any one of a group of biologically active substances that contain nitrogen. Alkaloids are found in many plants, and are used to obtain such drugs as digitalis (from foxglove), atropine (from belladonna), and morphine (from the opium poppy). Most alkaloids have a bitter taste and may be highly poisonous if used incorrectly.

A talk about Allergy

Allergy is a condition in which the body reacts with unusual sensitivity to a certain substance or substances. These substances, which consist of proteins, are called antigens.

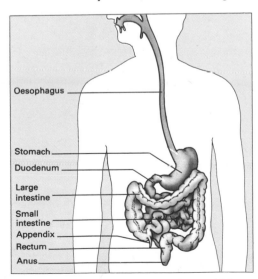

Alimentary canal is the passage down which food travels the entire length of the body.

Almoner

They stimulate the body to produce antibodies, which weaken or destroy the invading antigens. In some cases, when an antibody reacts with an antigen, the organic compound HISTAMINE is released from special body cells called mast cells. It is an excess of histamine that results in allergy symptoms.

Q: *What are the common allergy symptoms?*

A: A runny nose and watering or itching eyes are familiar to many persons who suffer each year from hay fever. In asthma, there is wheezing; with eczema and hives there is itching, redness, and lumps. Contact dermatitis, an inflammation of the skin, may occur possibly from wearing rubber gloves or touching a certain chemical, such as some kinds of soap. A reaction to antibiotics, particularly penicillin, may be in the form of a RASH.

Q: *Why are some people allergic to certain substances and others not?*

A: Partly this is due to hereditary factors; some families seem to be more liable to allergies than others, although particular allergies are not necessarily inherited. Sometimes emotional disturbances can have an aggravating effect on the underlying allergic condition, and can cause it to become worse in a way that is not fully understood.

Q: *How does a doctor determine the cause of an allergy?*

A: The doctor usually gets a detailed history from the patient to find the most likely source of the problem, and may then carry out a skin test. A weak solu-

tion of the substances that are suspected is injected into the skin. A red reaction indicates an allergy to that particular sub-stance. Sometimes a PATCH TEST is done for the same reason.

Q: *What treatment can be given for an allergy?*

A: When the cause of an allergy is known, the patient can undergo desensitization with injections of the allergen known to cause the symptoms. Beginning with a weak solution, the dose is gradually increased over a period of weeks until a strong solution is reached and the patient is immune to its effects.

   If the cause of the allergic reaction is not known, or if the reaction is already taking place, a doctor may prescribe ANTIHISTAMINE pills or corticosteroid nasal and lung sprays to control the symptoms.

Q: *Are there any dangerous allergic reactions?*

A: An allergic reaction to an insect sting or antibiotic drug, such as penicillin, is pot-entially dangerous and can even be fatal. A mild reaction usually causes a rash. But in a violent one, called ANAPHYLAXIS, the patient finds breathing increasingly difficult. This is an emergency condition and a doctor should be consulted urgently. Fortunately, the condition is not common.

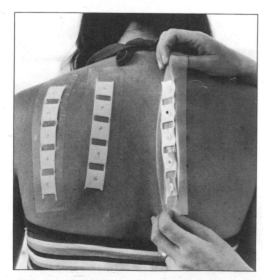

Allergy tests can be done by taping substances to the body and noting reactions.

Almoner. *See* MEDICAL SOCIAL WORKER.

Alopecia is the medical word for baldness. Total loss of hair (alopecia totalis) and patchy loss of hair (alopecia areata) may occur suddenly at any age. In some people, baldness is due to an abnormal reaction of the body to the hair substance itself. But in many other people the cause is not known. Common male baldness, or male pattern alopecia, results in full-scale loss of hair, usu-ally at the temples and the crown of the head; *see* BALDNESS.

Q: *What is the treatment for alopecia?*

A: In baldness associated with a sudden emotional shock or severe illness, the hair usually grows back. Sometimes cortisone creams and lotions are prescribed for alopecia areata only.

Altitude sickness, also known as mountain sickness, is a condition that some people experience after ascending rapidly to heights of more than about 2,500 metres (8,000ft). Others do not suffer until they reach an altitude of more than 4,000 metres (13,000ft). The condition occurs because the air at such altitudes contains less oxygen.

Q: What are the symptoms?

A: The symptoms include severe headache, shortness of breath, rapid heartbeat, weakness, and nausea with diarrhoea. Because not enough oxygen reaches the brain, the patient experiences mental confusion, and suffers from poor co-ordination and insomnia.

No one with heart or lung disease should consider journeys to high altitudes without first consulting a doctor.

Alveolus is a small, round body cavity. The term is usually used to describe the microscopic grapelike air cells of the lungs. The plural is alveoli. *See* p.10.

Alzheimer's disease is a form of presenile dementia, and is an abnormal degeneration of the brain that causes loss of memory, similar to that commonly associated with senility in the elderly. In many patients it is accompanied by hallucinations and by difficulty in remembering words (aphasia). It usually occurs in people between forty and sixty years old. The disease progresses slowly, but within a few years the patient becomes bedridden and helpless. The cause is not known, and so there is no treatment.

Amalgam is an alloy of mercury and one or more other metals. Dentists use an amalgam to fill a cavity in a tooth. *See* FILLING.

Amaurosis is the medical term for blindness in which the eye outwardly appears to be normal. It is usually caused by a disorder that affects the optic nerve, and may accompany the kidney disorder URAEMIA.

See also AMBLYOPIA; BLINDNESS.

Amblyopia is dimness of vision, although the eye outwardly appears to be normal. Causes vary; there may be poisoning due to nicotine, alcohol, or quinine, or there may be retention of poisonous waste products normally excreted by the kidneys (uraemia). The tendency for amblyopia to develop may be inherited. Treatment can be given once the cause is found. Tablets or injections of vitamin B complex are sometimes prescribed.

Amenorrhoea is the abnormal absence of menstrual periods in a woman. In the years during which a woman normally menstruates, pregnancy is the most common reason for periods to stop. But emotional stress in adolescents can cause amenorrhoea, as can depression or the semi-starvation of ANOREXIA NERVOSA. There are also physical causes, including endocrine disorders, heart disease, and diseases that affect the ovaries.

With any unexplained stoppage in the menstrual periods, a doctor should be consulted and the cause discovered before any treatment is given.

See also MENSTRUATION.

Amino acid is one of the basic nitrogen-containing substances that go into the making of proteins in living matter. There are more than 20 amino acids required for normal good health, but the human body is not able to make the eight essential ones. These are taken into the body in proteins from foods such as milk, meat, fish, eggs, and cheese.

See also PROTEIN.

Amnesia is the complete or partial loss of memory. General (complete) amnesia may be caused by an injury to the head. Or it can be caused by hysteria after something terrible has occurred and the patient cannot deal with the memory. If the cause is emotional, the forgotten memory can often be recalled when the patient is feeling secure, and especially when in the care of a psychiatrist who tries to bring the suppressed fears out into the open.

Q: What can cause partial amnesia?

A: Forgetting some things, such as names and places, and not others is commonly a sign of ageing, depression, or dementia. Certain disorders, such as alcoholism and thyroid deficiency (myxoedema), also can be a cause.

Amniocentesis is a method of extracting fluid from the bag of waters (amniotic sac) that surrounds a foetus during pregnancy. In early pregnancy the procedure is used to detect possible congenital abnormalities. The sac is punctured with a long needle (after the third month of pregnancy) after the woman has first been given a local anaesthetic. There is little danger to the foetus because the placenta is first located using ultrasound.

The fluid can be analysed for enzymes and

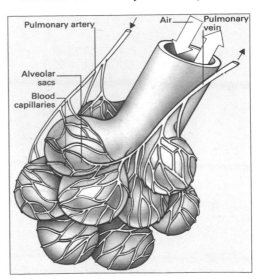

Alveoli in the lungs exchange the blood's carbon dioxide for oxygen from the air.

a culture can be made of the cells. If the foetus is found to have a severe disorder, the woman must decide whether to continue the pregnancy. Later in pregnancy the technique is used to test for anaemia due to Rhesus incompatibility (*see* BLOOD GROUPS), and also to test for lung maturity.

Amnion is the membrane lining the womb in which a foetus floats during pregnancy. It is made up of a tough layer of cells and, with the placenta, forms part of the afterbirth. *See* PREGNANCY AND CHILDBIRTH.

Amoebic dysentery is an intestinal disorder caused by the parasite *Entameba histolytica.* It is most common in the tropics and subtropics. *See* DYSENTERY.

Amphetamines are a group of drugs that stimulate the central nervous system. They cause a rise in blood pressure, a racing pulse, a feeling of excitement, sleeplessness, and loss of appetite. Amphetamines are used to treat chronic, recurrent drowsiness (narcolepsy) and excessive muscular and physical activity in children (hyperkinesis).

Q: Are amphetamines addictive?

A: Yes. The stimulative effects of amphetamines have led to abuse and addiction, particularly among adolescents. Doctors now prescribe amphetamines with greater caution and discretion, and supplies are also regulated by drug laws.
    See also DRUG ADDICTION.

Ampicillin is a broad-spectrum antibiotic drug which is used to treat infections of the respiratory tract, urinary tract, gastrointestinal tract, and ear, nose, and throat infections, enteric fevers, and gonorrhoea.

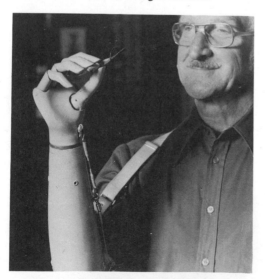

Amputation: the effects of losing a limb can now be minimized by the use of artificial limbs.

Q: What are the possible side effects of the use of ampicillin?

A: It may cause diarrhoea, nausea, and vomiting. Allergic reactions may also occur; a person allergic to penicillin will probably also be allergic to ampicillin. There is also a specific ampicillin allergy; if a skin rash develops, the patient should consult a doctor immediately. Also, because of the strong possibility of a rash, patients suffering from infectious mononucleosis (glandular fever) should not use ampicillin. There is a possibility that it may also reduce the effectiveness of oral contraceptives. Rarely, anaemia and liver disease may occur.

Ampule, or ampul, is a small, sealed, glass container for keeping a drug sterile.

Amputation is the surgical removal of a limb or other part of the body. The reasons for amputation are either damage or disease. When damage is so serious that repair or healing is impossible amputation may be a surgeon's only choice.

Q: What problems face a patient after the amputation of a limb?

A: Emotional stress is a serious problem after an amputation. Also, a patient may experience sensations as if the limb were still there. This can cause confusion and distress. A good rehabilitation programme therefore includes both physical and psychotherapeutic treatment.

Q: What about artificial limbs?

A: When performing an amputation, a surgeon normally tries to leave a stump of bone on to which an artificial limb can be attached.

Amyloidosis is a disorder marked by deposits of a waxy, clear substance (amyloid) in the tissues of the liver, spleen, kidneys, heart, or tongue. The deposits may be associated with chronic infections or inflammations, or some forms of cancer, but sometimes the cause is not known. Amyloid interferes with the normal functioning of the organ in which it is present. There is no known specific cure for the condition, which may progress and result in death. The only treatment is to deal with the cause, if known.

Amyotonia congenita is a group of congenital diseases characterized by muscular weakness.

A talk about Anaemia

Anaemia is any one of the disorders in which the blood has fewer than the normal number of RED BLOOD CELLS, or the red blood cells are deficient in HAEMOGLOBIN.

Q: What are the symptoms of anaemia?

A: Haemoglobin gives blood its red colour, and a person with anaemia may be noticeably pale, although various other disorders can also cause paleness. Other symptoms of anaemia include tiredness, headaches, dizziness, shortness of breath, and palpitations after only slight exertion.

Q: Is anaemia serious?

A: There are various types of anaemia. It may be only minor and give little cause for concern, or it may be a sign of a more serious condition. Therefore, a person should not ignore the symptoms, but should seek advice from a doctor.

Q: How is anaemia diagnosed?

A: Doctors diagnose anaemia by making a blood count. They take a small sample of blood from the patient and count the number of red blood cells in it. In a healthy person, each millilitre of blood contains between 5 million and 6 million red blood cells, which have a normal life of about three to four months and are replaced continually.

Q: What are the causes of anaemia?

A: Anaemia has three chief causes: (1) loss of blood through bleeding (haemorrhage); (2) failure of the body to make enough new red blood cells; or (3) haemolysis, the rapid destruction of the red blood cells in the blood.

O: What can prevent the body from making red cells?

A: Failure of red blood cell production can be caused by faulty diet. Lack of enough iron in the food a person eats leads to insufficient haemoglobin in the red blood cells. Lack of vitamin C (ascorbic acid) leads to the anaemia that accompanies scurvy. A deficiency of two essential B vitamins, folic acid and vitamin B_{12}, results in the production of fewer but larger than normal red blood cells (macrocytic anaemia). Small amounts of some elements in the diet to aid nutrition, such as copper and manganese, are needed for correct red blood cell formation. Lack of these elements may cause anaemia; treatment is to add the missing factor to the diet. In severe cases, a doctor may prescribe tablets or injections containing the missing factor.

Manufacture of red blood cells by the red bone marrow can also be slowed by the poisoning effect of an infection, by poisons such as lead, or by cancer. The anaemia is made worse if the cancer invades the bone marrow or begins there, as in LEUKAEMIA and MYELOMA. Treatment is to try to remove the cause, to prescribe a diet with additional vitamins, and to give blood transfusions if necessary.

Rapid destruction of red blood cells, called haemolytic anaemia, occurs in malaria and a few other diseases. It can also arise as a reaction to certain drugs, and in sickle cell anaemia, thalassaemia, and some other inherited disorders which result in abnormal red cells. Haemolytic anaemia can also arise from a blood transfusion with blood of the wrong type or incompatibility of RH FACTOR between a newborn child and its mother. Treatment is aimed at finding the cause, and blood transfusions may be given.

Complete failure to produce red blood cells, the disorder called aplastic anaemia, may occur suddenly for no apparent reason. Or it may be caused by sensitivity to a drug that results in destruction of bone marrow cells. Treatment is with corticosteroid drugs, blood transfusions, or, rarely, by bone marrow transplants.

Q: Should women routinely take iron tablets?

A: A well-balanced diet provides sufficient iron for a woman with normal menstrual periods. Such a woman needs about 60 mg of iron per month. If her periods are particularly heavy, or if she is pregnant, her iron intake may not keep pace with her loss and a doctor may prescribe additional iron.

A talk about Anaesthetics

Anaesthetics are drugs that cause a loss of

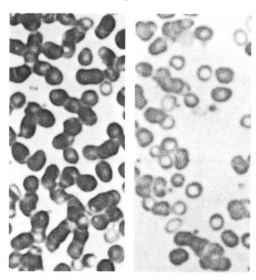

Anaemia is a condition in which blood that normally has many red cells (*left*) has few (*right*).

Anaesthetics

feeling. They are given before medical treatment that would otherwise cause pain. There are many anaesthetic drugs and they can be grouped according to the effect they are intended to have on the patient.

Q: What are the main types of anaesthetics?

A: A general anaesthetic, causing loss of consciousness as well as loss of feeling, is given in most surgical operations. Another group, called local anaesthetics, cause a loss of feeling only in the area to be treated. Dentists often use a local anaesthetic during the filling or extraction of a tooth. A third group are the surface anaesthetics, which remove feeling from a surface area such as an eye or the nose. They make possible medical examinations without pain to the patient.

Q: On what basis are different general anaesthetics given?

A: It is the task of an anaesthetist to decide which general anaesthetic is best for the patient. The anaesthetist reviews the patient's medical history and may order tests to help select the anaesthetic: the decision is made only after such preparation.

Q: Are the injections a patient receives when awake part of the anaesthetic?

A: To make the patient relaxed and drowsy, and to dry the mouth and lungs, a sedative injection is given one hour before the operation. Later, immediately before the general anaesthetic, an injection of a short period sleeping drug is given in a vein. This takes effect extremely quickly.

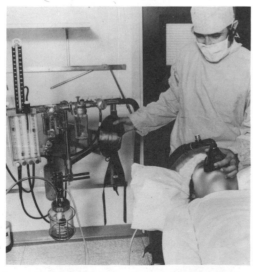

Anaesthetics: Boyle's machine is one of the most used and most essential tools in surgery.

Q: How is a general anaesthetic given?

A: When the patient is asleep after the intravenous injection, a small dose of a drug that relaxes the muscles is generally given. The drugs that continue the general anaesthetic are injected or given as gases either through a face mask or a tube inserted through the mouth or nose into the windpipe. The tube is attached to an anaesthetic machine, which ensures maximum control over the quantity and composition of anaesthetic and oxygen.

Q: What precautions are taken before the anaesthetic is administered, and after consciousness has been regained?

A: The patient is not allowed anything to eat or drink for at least four hours before the operation. This reduces the chances of vomiting and inhaling fluid into the lungs when the anaesthetic is being given.

After the operation, the anaesthetist remains with the patient until consciousness is regained.

Q: How do local anaesthetics differ from general anaesthetics?

A: A local anaesthetic is injected either into the tissues surrounding the area to be treated or next to the nerves serving the area. Adrenaline is sometimes added to the injection to increase the time for which the anaesthetic is effective.

Q: What are the various types of local anaesthetic?

A: There are four types of local anaesthetic. (1) The most common form of local anaesthetic is the type used for a dental injection, in which the loss of sensation affects only a limited area. (2) A local anaesthetic that affects a whole section of the body, such as an arm or a leg, produces what is called regional anaesthesia. The injection is given close to where the nerves leave the spinal cord. (3) When an injection is given around the spinal cord (epidural anaesthesia) or into the cerebrospinal fluid of the spinal cord (spinal anaesthesia), the body is anaesthetized below the site of injection. Epidural anaesthesia is often used during childbirth. (4) If sedative drugs are used with a local anaesthetic, the patient becomes peaceful and relaxed. This state, known as TWILIGHT SLEEP, is a condition favourable for performing examinations, such as that of the inner wall of the stomach (gastroscopy) using a fibrescope, which would otherwise need surgery.

Anaesthetic	Method	Comments
Barbiturates	Injection	Barbiturates produce rapid loss

Anaesthetic	Method	Comments
		of consciousness, and are effective for short periods. However, they do not cause a loss of pain. For this reason, a barbiturate is used only as a preliminary anaesthetic before a general anaesthetic is given.
Chloroform	Inhalation	Chloroform was once an extremely common anaesthetic, but it is rarely used in surgical procedures today. Chloroform may damage a patient's liver.
Cyclopropane	Inhalation	Cyclopropane is an effective anaesthetic, but it is not used as widely today as it once was because of its explosive properties. The recovery process from cyclopropane is speedy, but the patient may become considerably excited as he or she regains consciousness.
Ether	Inhalation	Ether was once widely used, but other drugs are considered safer.
Halothane (Fluothane)	Inhalation	Halothane is the most widely used anaesthetic today and is considered the most powerful. It is also safe for use in surgical procedures on persons suffering from asthma.
Nitrous oxide	Inhalation	A drawback of nitrous oxide is that it lacks strength, so large

Anaesthetic	Method	Comments
		amounts of the drug must be given to produce anaesthesia. It is sometimes known as laughing gas. Although the patient quickly becomes unconscious, anaesthesia may not be complete when it is used without oxygen. The patient may remain in an emotionally uninhibited state, which is often characterized by laughing or crying.

Local anaesthetics

Anaesthetic	Method	Comments
Procaine hydrochloride	Injection	This is the most widely used local anaesthetic. One disadvantage is that its effect wears off quickly. Adrenaline is sometimes mixed with the drug to make the effect last longer.
Lignocaine	Injection	These drugs are more poisonous to the body than

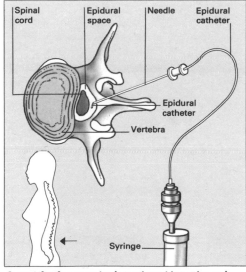

Anaesthetics may be introduced into the epidural space between spine and spinal cord.

Analeptics

Anaesthetic	Method	Comments
		procaine, and their use is regulated. One advantage over procaine is that the effect of these drugs lasts longer.
Cocaine Lignocaine	Direct application	Used for surface anaesthesia. A solution of the drug is applied directly to the area to be treated.

Analeptics are drugs that stimulate the central nervous system. They are used especially in the treatment of poisoning caused by a drug that has had a serious depressant effect on the nervous system. Analeptics such as caffeine and amphetamines help to restore a person to consciousness.

Analgesics are those drugs or medicines that relieve pain without loss of feeling or loss of consciousness. They work by altering the perception of pain by the pain receptors in the nerve endings of the affected area. The oldest of the common analgesic drugs is ASPIRIN. A more recent substitute for aspirin is PARACETAMOL, which is less irritating to the stomach.

Q: Are aspirin and paracetamol regarded as safe drugs?

A: The two drugs are medically safe enough to be readily available without prescription at a pharmacy. But doctors advise

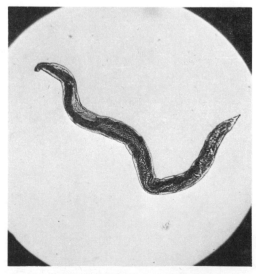

Ancylostomiasis is infestation of the small intestine with parasitic worms.

against excessive or prolonged use or large doses of these, or any other non-prescription analgesics, without discussion with your doctor.

Q: What types of pain need stronger analgesics?

A: With acute or persistent pain, a doctor's advice may well be essential. Doctors prescribe strong analgesics with caution, and dosages are carefully regulated because some analgesics can be addictive.

Anaphylaxis is a sudden, severe reaction. It is a reaction to the introduction into the body of any substance to which the body is hypersensitive. It may, for example, follow the injection of a drug, or an insect sting. The victim feels faint and becomes pale. The person may vomit and have no control over bowel movements. Wheezy breathing may occur; the patient may collapse into unconsciousness, which may be followed by death. These symptoms can occur in rapid succession.

Q: What is the treatment for anaphylaxis?

A: Emergency treatment is essential to save the patient's life. Skilled medical aid must be summoned immediately, and the patient hospitalized as soon as possible. The type of aerosol that asthmatics use may be helpful for assisting breathing until skilled help arrives.

Anasarca is the generalized swelling (oedema) of the body, especially in the legs and abdomen. It results from the accumulation of fluid in body tissues, often accompanying a kidney disorder. The condition was once known as dropsy.

Anastomosis is the connecting area between two tubes in the body. An artificial anastomosis may be created by surgery, for example, when the open ends of parts of the intestine are joined together after the removal of a diseased section between them.

Ancylostomiasis, also known as hookworm disease, is the infestation of the small intestine by small worms (*Ancylostoma duodenale* or *Necator americanus*). These worms, which grow up to 12mm (0.5 inches) long, enter through the skin, travel to the lungs and then to the intestine, and may leave an itching rash. Their eggs are excreted in the faeces, and end up living in soil as larvae until they can re-enter human skin.

Q: What are the symptoms of ancylostomiasis?

A: Symptoms of ancylostomiasis may be pain or diarrhoea, and a long infection can lead to anaemia with all the symptoms that accompany that disorder. If the disease is undiscovered in children, it may retard growth and mental development. Ancylostomiasis is diagnosed by examining the faeces for eggs, and is treated with drugs.

Q: In what parts of the world is ancylostomiasis most likely to occur?

A: It is more common where a hot climate and damp earth are favourable conditions for larvae to thrive, especially if there is poor sanitation as well. The worms usually enter the skin through bare feet that come into contact with larva-ridden soil.

Androgen is any of a group of substances that produce secondary sex characteristics in the male. TESTOSTERONE, the sex hormone produced by the testicles, is an androgen.

Aneurysm is a swelling of the wall of an artery, a vein, or the heart. Most aneurysms form as a result of the hardening of the arteries (arteriosclerosis). In the heart, an aneurysm may result from a heart attack (myocardial infarction). Accidents, such as a gunshot wound, or a weakness that has been present from birth may also cause aneurysms.

Q: Can an aneurysm be serious?

A: Yes. If an aneurysm bursts (ruptures), it is extremely dangerous. An aneurysm in the aorta, the major blood vessel leading from the heart, may partly rupture (dissecting aneurysm). It usually causes enough pain to act as a warning of impending complete rupture. If it ruptures in the brain, there is a stroke or brain haemorrhage (subarachnoid haemorrhage).

Q: Can a ruptured aneurysm be treated successfully?

A: If treatment can be given at once damage from the rupture may be controlled. A suspected rupture must be confirmed by an X-ray of the artery (arteriogram). Then a surgical operation is the only treatment.

Angiitis, or angitis, is inflammation of a blood vessel or lymph vessel. It may be caused either by infection (thrombophlebitis or lymphangitis) or by another type of disease, such as thromboangiitis obliterans or polyarteritis nodosa.

A talk about Angina pectoris

Angina pectoris was once the term for any pain in the chest, but it now refers to a specific condition that involves pain from the heart. The pain occurs because not enough oxygen reaches the heart muscle, especially during exercise. There is a tight feeling across the chest, which may later spread into the neck, jaw, shoulders, and to one or both arms as far as the hands. Occasionally, it may also spread to the upper abdomen. In most patients, however, pain is present only in some of these areas. Usually there is shortness of breath and a feeling of faintness.

Q: What disorders might be associated with angina pectoris?

A: Coronary heart disease (ARTERIOSCLEROSIS) is the cause of angina pectoris. The condition is not in itself a heart attack, but may be either a warning that one could occur, or the immediate result of one.

Q: How does a doctor distinguish between angina pectoris and other similar pain?

A: If angina pectoris is suspected, the doctor does a test called an ELECTRO-CARDIOGRAM (ECG), which may show abnormalities of the kind associated with the condition. This test provides the most reliable information if it is made during an exercise test.

Q: How is angina pectoris treated?

A: Overweight patients must lose excess fat, to reduce strain on the heart. Smoking must be discontinued, because nicotine contributes to hardening of the arteries. Regular exercise improves blood circulation to the heart. Before physical effort, drugs such as glyceryl trinitrate (nitroglycerine) help by causing the arteries to expand. Fast-acting capsules of amyl nitrate can be inhaled if pain occurs. Newer drugs called beta-blockers help to prevent pain by reducing the amount of oxygen that the heart muscle needs, and controlling the heart rate.

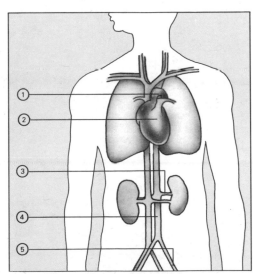

Aneurysms caused by a congenital weakness occur most commonly in these five sites.

Angiogram

Q: *Should a patient with angina pectoris become less active?*

A: No. The patient is usually encouraged to lead a normal life and gradually increase exercise. For personal safety, however, it is best to avoid periods of sudden great effort, heavy meals, and extreme variations of temperature.

Angiogram is a series of X-ray films of a blood vessel. A dye that X-rays or other radiation cannot penetrate is injected into a blood vessel, and X-ray pictures are then taken in rapid succession. The series of pictures show up the size and shape of veins or arteries in organs or tissue, and thereby reveal abnormalities such as arteriosclerosis.

Angioma is an abnormal growth of tissue formed by a group of small blood vessels. It may be present on the surface of the skin or internally, which may be flat, a port-wine stain, or raised. On the skin, an angioma is a soft, purplish mark, a strawberry naevus. If an angioma occurs in the brain, it can lead to serious conditions such as bleeding (sub-arachnoid haemorrhage) or a stroke. An angioma that bleeds in the intestine may cause black stools (melaena), the vomiting of blood (haematemesis), or anaemia.

Q: *What is the treatment for an angioma?*

A: Strawberry naevi usually disappear before puberty. If they do not, small ones can be cauterized and larger ones removed by plastic surgery. Port-wine naevi are more difficult to treat and often have to be hidden by cosmetics.

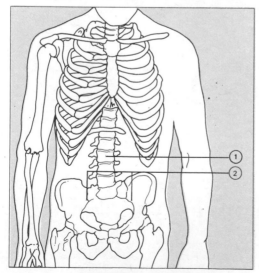

Ankylosing spondylitis usually begins in the lower spine (1) and sacroiliac joints (2).

Angioneurotic oedema (or angioedema) is a form of giant HIVES (urticaria) in which large, irritating swellings occur anywhere on or near the surface of the body. It is sometimes caused by an allergy to a specific food or to a drug. The condition is not usually considered to be serious unless it affects the mouth, throat, or larynx, where it may obstruct breathing. The usual treatment is immediate injection of adrenaline followed by antihistamines. In a more severe attack, a course of steroid drugs may be prescribed.

Ankle is the joint connecting the foot and the leg. The weight of the body is transmitted to the TALUS and the heel-bone (calcaneus) of the foot through the strong shin-bone (tibia). The outer side of the ankle is supported by the slender fibula bone. The ankle joint allows only up-and-down movements of the foot.

Q: *What can go wrong with the ankle?*

A: One of the commonest disorders is a sprained ankle, the tearing of the ligaments (bands of fibrous tissue) between the fibula and the side of the calcaneus bone. It is accompanied by pain, swelling, and tenderness. Treatment with painkilling drugs and bandaging, or strapping, for a few days helps it to heal.

A FRACTURE of the ankle may be a break of the fibula alone or of both the fibula and tibia. It is diagnosed by X-ray examination. Treatment consists in restoring the ends of the broken bones to their proper positions, which may require an operation, and then holding them there in a plaster-of-paris cast until they heal.

Ankles frequently swell because of excessive fluid in the tissues (oedema). Such swelling is common in hot weather, after a person has been standing for a long time, or during pregnancy. Resting with the feet raised generally reduces such swelling. Ankle sprains, varicose veins, obesity, and local infections may also cause ankle swelling.

Ankylosing spondylitis, also known as bamboo spine, is a condition in which the bones of the spine (vertebrae) fuse together. This causes stiffness and the spine can become bowed. Early symptoms are back-ache and stiffness in the morning. Ankylosing spondylitis occurs more often in men than in women and usually starts early in adult life. The symptoms gradually worsen but pain need not be continuous. The patient's eyes often become inflamed (iritis), and the joints can become swollen and tender (arthritis).

The cause of ankylosing spondylitis is not known.

Q: Can treatment arrest the progress of ankylosing spondylitis?

A: Yes, but only to the extent that a doctor can reduce the pain and stiffness associated with the disorder. Aspirin and some stronger antirheumatic drugs are prescribed for the pain or, if it is severe, radiotherapy may be used. It is important that the patient sleep on a firm mattress at night to prevent the spine stiffening in a bent position. Physiotherapy to keep the spine mobile and breathing exercises are essential aspects of the treatment.

Ankylosis is the stiffening of a joint or the fusing together of the bones that form it either through disease or by an operation. If it occurs naturally, the condition may be inherited or it may be discovered at birth. ANKYLOSING SPONDYLITIS is a disease in which the bones of the spine fuse together. Artificial ankylosis (ARTHRODESIS) is a way of stopping some painful joint conditions.

Anorectics are drugs that reduce the appetite. Most are AMPHETAMINES or related compounds that, because of their addictive properties, are now used only to treat extreme, life-endangering obesity. As a general rule, drugs should not be used to reduce weight.

See also WEIGHT PROBLEMS.

Anorexia nervosa is a severe loss of appetite, not due to any local disease. It is a form of mental illness, found most commonly in girls and women aged between twelve and twenty-one. It also occurs in older women and men.

The patient, if forced to eat, may vomit after the meal. Loss of appetite leads to loss of weight and, in women, menstrual periods may cease altogether (amenorrhoea). The weight loss may be accompanied by extreme wasting, and a growth of fine hairs on the skin. In men, the condition causes impotence.

Q: Can anorexia nervosa be detected in its early stages?

A: Early diagnosis is difficult. The patient, especially if an adolescent, commonly denies that anything is wrong, and continues to be cheerful and active. A young person may be deceptive about the quantity of food eaten, and may vomit in private after a meal. Patients tend to deny that they are wasting away and express a fear of being fat.

Q: How is anorexia nervosa treated?

A: Anorexia nervosa needs skilled psychiatric attention, which may begin with a term in hospital. It may be some years before normal health is regained.

Anosmia is the lack of a sense of smell. It occurs in the elderly, with nasal polyps and catarrh, and sometimes after a head injury. It may be accompanied by a loss of taste.

Anoxia is a lack of sufficient oxygen in the body.

Antacid is a substance that is used medically to neutralize the acid contents of the stomach. Most indigestion mixtures, powders, or pills contain antacids. The antacids may relieve pain, but some may have unpleasant side effects, such as diarrhoea or constipation. Prolonged use of antacids should be avoided, except under a doctor's advice.

See also ALKALI.

Antenatal, or prenatal, means before birth, and generally refers to the care given an expectant mother and her baby from the time the conception is confirmed until the beginning of labour. Such care is now considered almost as important as the delivery itself.

Anthelmintics are drugs that are used to treat disorders caused by infestations with worms.

Anthracosis is a form of PNEUMOCONIOSIS, a lung disorder once common among coal workers.

See also BLACK LUNG.

Anthrax is an infectious disease, now rare, that is transmitted to humans most commonly by farm animals. It can take the form of a characteristic boil on the skin or, if the germs are inhaled, it can cause pneumonia.

Q: What are the symptoms of anthrax?

A: Symptoms include a fever and the occurrence of a skin ulcer or boil. Anyone working with animals or animal products who develops an unusual boil should see a doctor at once. The boil, caused by *Bacillus anthracis*, is large with a black scab. It forms slowly on the skin and may spread to form more boils.

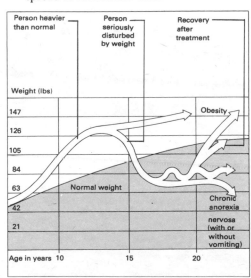

Anorexia nervosa is classically a hyperreaction to being overweight, and may be fatal.

Antibiotics

Q: *What is the treatment for anthrax?*

A: Immediate treatment with penicillin is usually effective. Unfortunately, anthrax bacilli form spores, a resistant form of the germ that is extremely difficult to destroy. Everything in contact with the patient must first be sterilized, and all contaminated animal products must be destroyed.

Antibiotics are drugs that are used to treat various types of bacterial infections. There are many types of antibiotics, and they work either by preventing the infection from growing, or by destroying it. Some antibiotics are produced by a mould or fungus; others are made synthetically.

Q: *What are the names of some of the antibiotics and what do they do?*

A: PENICILLIN, the first antibiotic (discovered by Sir Alexander Fleming in 1928), destroys multiplying bacteria by making their cell walls burst. There are also a number of newer forms of penicillin, such as ampicillin and amoxycillin

TETRACYCLINES, another important group, act by interfering with bacterial growth. They are broad-spectrum antibiotics, which means that they are active against many types of bacteria. Other antibiotics of this type include CHLORAMPHENICOL, used to treat typhoid fever, and streptomycin, used in the treatment of tuberculosis.

There are many other groups of antibiotics, each produced to combat specific diseases.

Q: *Are antibiotics safe?*

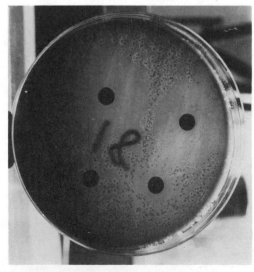

Antibiotics are shown here surrounded by clear areas of destroyed bacteria.

A: Antibiotics can save lives when prescribed with caution to treat bacterial infection. However, indiscriminate use of these drugs can have serious consequences, and cancel out their usefulness. In the years since 1941 (when antibiotics were first given to patients), a number of bacterial diseases have become resistant to the original antibiotics, but new ones are now available.

Some of the drugs, when taken over a long period, may produce unpleasant or damaging side effects. Certain antibiotics may become toxic when stale.

Sometimes, a patient has an allergic reaction to an antibiotic drug. This can be either the serious condition known medically as ANAPHYLAXIS, or a lesser condition that is still important to recognize. Patients who know they are allergic to an antibiotic drug should tell the doctor when being treated for any condition.

Antibody is a substance produced by the body in response to an infection. It combines with an antigen (the foreign substance that activated it) and puts it out of action. Antibodies are part of the development of natural IMMUNITY. They can be produced artificially by IMMUNIZATION.

See also ALLERGY.

Anticoagulants are drugs that interfere with the normal clotting ability of the blood. There are two main groups: direct-acting, such as HEPARIN, which is injected into a vein; and indirect-acting, such as coumarin, which is taken by mouth. Heparin acts quickly but the indirect-acting drugs take up to three days to work.

Q: *When are anticoagulants prescribed?*

A: They are given to prevent or help dissolve a blood clot, such as a blockage in the blood supply to the heart muscle (myocardial infarction) or in a leg vein (venous thrombosis). They may also be given before certain operations on the female reproductive system, to prevent the clotting in leg veins that tends to occur more frequently than in other operations.

Q: *Should a patient who uses anticoagulants observe special precautions?*

A: Patients taking anticoagulants require regular blood tests to ensure that the correct dosage is maintained. They should also carry a card naming the anticoagulant drug and stating the dosage, in case they are involved in an accident. Any other tablets or medicines should be avoided, until approved by a doctor or pharmacist, to ensure that they do not alter the anticoagulant effect.

Q: What are the signs of an overdose of anticoagulants?

A: Common indications are the appearance of unexpected bruising in various parts of the body, or bleeding in the urine.

Anticonvulsants are drugs used in the treatment of EPILEPSY to prevent the CONVULSIONS that accompany this disorder.

Antidepressants are drugs used in the treatment of mental DEPRESSION. There are two main categories: the monoamine-oxidase (MAO) inhibitor group and the tricyclic antidepressants. If the MAO INHIBITORS are prescribed, the patient is warned to avoid such foods as cheese, broad beans, alcohol, and some yeast extracts, whose chemical properties interact in a dangerous way with this group. The tricyclics are more frequently prescribed because they seem safer and often as effective as the MAO inhibitors, although they act more gradually. A third group, seldom used today, is AMPHETAMINES.

Antidepressants should be taken only under a doctor's supervision.

Antigen is a foreign substance in the body that stimulates the production of an ANTIBODY. Antigens may be bacteria, viruses, or any other physical agent, such as pollen.

See also ALLERGY; IMMUNIZATION.

Antihistamines are a group of drugs used to counteract histamine, the chemical in the body that is the main cause of allergic reactions. Antihistamines suppress the symptoms without treating the original cause.

Q: In what forms are antihistamines prescribed?

A: They can be obtained in many forms, such as tablets and capsules, injections, nose and eye preparations, and as cream for the skin.

Q: Do antihistamines have unpleasant or dangerous side effects?

A: Antihistamines are powerful drugs and should be used with care. Many of them cause drowsiness, and patients are warned to avoid taking them before driving a car. Others stimulate the brain, especially in children. Antihistamines often cause a dry mouth and, unless they are taken with food, they irritate the stomach.

See also ALLERGY.

Antinauseants are drugs used to prevent or relieve nausea. There are two main groups: (1) Anticholinergic drugs. These usually contain atropine, which acts on the nervous system to block secretions from the stomach and glands. They may produce blurred vision, a dry mouth, and a rapid heartbeat. Their use should not be prolonged, nor should they be given to patients with GLAUCOMA or to those

who may develop urine retention; (2) ANTI-HISTAMINES. These usually have a depressing effect on the brain, which produces drowsiness, but may occasionally cause stimulation in children, making them unable to sleep.

Both these types of drugs interfere with the ability to drive a car, and should not be taken with alcoholic drinks.

See also MOTION SICKNESS.

Antiperspirants are substances that reduce sweating. They are commonly used to avoid the bad odour associated with perspiration although, unlike deodorants in general, they actually prevent the formation of sweat.

Antipruritics are agents that prevent or relieve ITCHING (pruritus). There are many causes of itching, which should be diagnosed before treatment.

Antipyretics are agents (such as aspirin) that help to reduce a fever.

Antiseptic is a substance that prevents the growth of germs and infection. Carbolic acid (phenol) was the first antiseptic to be used, but this has given way to milder modern antiseptics such as cetrimide, alcohol, and iodine-containing compounds.

See also ASEPSIS.

Antiserum is a SERUM containing antibodies made from blood taken from a sensitized human being or animal. It can be injected to give temporary protection against a specific disease, for example, tetanus or diphtheria, in someone who has no immunity to the disease. The antiserum from animals, however, may itself cause an allergic reaction or even severe or fatal shock (anaphylaxis).

See also IMMUNIZATION.

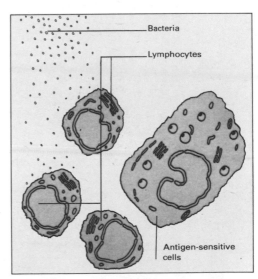

Bacteria

Lymphocytes

Antigen-sensitive cells

Antibodies are proteins produced by white cells in response to antigens such as bacteria.

Antispasmodics

Antispasmodics are drugs that prevent the contraction of smooth muscle. Antispasmodics are used to treat spastic colon, and bladder and gall bladder disorders.

Antitoxin is an ANTIBODY, formed in the body, that acts against a specific bacterial toxin (poison) by combining with it and neutralizing it.

See also IMMUNIZATION.

Antitussive is a drug used to stop coughing. There are two groups of such drugs, narcotic and non-narcotic. The narcotic drugs dull the nerves and relieve pain, but the patient may become dependent on them if they are used for a long period. CODEINE is the preparation most commonly used in prescription cough suppressants.

There are many non-narcotic cough suppressants available.

See also COUGH.

Antivenin is a SERUM used to treat poisoning by snake (or other animal) bite. It contains a high concentration of ANTIBODIES, and is injected around the area of the poisonous bite.

See also First Aid, p.514.

Antrum is a cavity within a bone. It is commonly used to describe the air spaces in the bones adjacent to the nose, the SINUSES.

Anuria is a serious disorder of the kidney in which no urine is produced. Without immediate treatment, anuria is fatal. The kidney failure can be caused by: (1) blockage by a stone (calculus) or tumour; (2) disease, such as acute nephritis; or (3) a drop in blood pressure during shock.

Hospitalization is urgent and requires skilled care. Fluids in the diet are restricted and given intravenously. Sometimes, an artificial kidney is used to allow the patient to get rid of the body's wastes and toxins.

See also DIALYSIS; KIDNEY DISEASE.

Anus is the opening at the lower end of the ALIMENTARY CANAL. It is kept closed by a ring of circular muscle called the sphincter. The anus is subject to three common disorders: (1) fissure, a small crack in the skin of the anus; (2) haemorrhoids (external piles), varicose veins outside the anus; (3) pruritus ani (itching), sometimes caused by a neurosis but often caused by a minor disorder of the anal skin (for example, as a result of worms).

The first two complaints may be treated by minor surgery and the last one by a suitable ointment prescribed by a doctor.

A talk about Anxiety

Anxiety is a feeling of fearful anticipation and worry, and is a response to possible danger. When fear is exaggerated or has no apparent cause, then, medically speaking, anxiety is an illness needing treatment.

Q: What are the symptoms of anxiety?

A: Anxiety is such a common problem that everyone has experienced it at some time and is familiar with the sweating, palpitations, trembling, nausea, and diarrhoea that may accompany the condition in various combinations. A medical check-up generally reassures the sufferer that there is not a more serious underlying cause.

Q: Can anxiety seriously affect a person?

A: Continued anxiety leads to fatigue and irritability. Sometimes there are sleepless nights (insomnia). Occasionally, anxiety shows itself in the form of a headache, a skin rash, an asthma attack, a peptic ulcer, or a spastic colon.

Children may regress to wetting the bed, or they may have bouts of vomiting, stomach pains, diarrhoea, and nightmares.

Q: Is there any way to get rid of these irrational feelings of fear?

A: Acute symptoms can be helped by TRANQUILLIZERS, but these do not cure the underlying condition and often give a false feeling of security. For some people, an honest discussion with a friend or a doctor may help immediately, but others may need psychiatric help for a longer period of time.

When the patient can be helped to cope with anxious feelings on a regular basis, a cure is in sight.

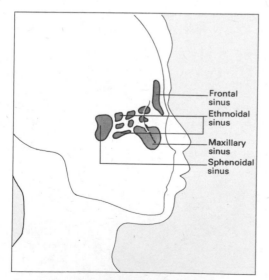

Frontal sinus

Ethmoidal sinus

Maxillary sinus

Sphenoidal sinus

Antrum is another name for the maxillary sinus, a bone cavity in the skull.

Aorta is the largest artery in the body, supplying blood to all the organs alongside its course. It starts at the left ventricle of the heart, then arches upwards and backwards, giving off branch arteries to the heart muscles, head, and arms. The aorta then runs down the back of the chest, in front of the spine and oesophagus (gullet), to reach the abdomen. There the aorta divides, just above the pelvis, into the common iliac arteries to the legs.

The most common disease that may affect the aorta is ARTERIOSCLEROSIS, which often also involves other arteries. An aortic ANEURYSM is usually fatal if it ruptures, but is is possible to replace the affected part with an artificial tube.

See also p.8.

Aortogram is an X-ray picture of the AORTA, taken after the injection of a special chemical into the blood vessels. It is a type of ARTERIOGRAM.

Aperient is an alternative word for a laxative, or a mild purgative. *See* LAXATIVES.

Apgar score is a rating system that assesses the vital functions in a baby during the first minute after birth. Five functions (heart rate, respiration, muscle tone, colour, and reflex response) are each assessed on a zero to two scale and totalled to a possible high of ten. Babies with a total score of eight to ten are given routine postnatal care. The lower the rating under seven, the more special is the attention needed to give the baby a normal start in life.

Aphakia is the condition of an eye in which the lens is absent. Aphakia may occur as a congenital abnormality, but it usually follows a CATARACT operation.

Aphasia is a condition in which an individual has lost the ability to speak and to understand speech. There is, commonly, also an inability to read and write. The complaint may be only temporary, following concussion, or permanent, after a stroke. Or it may occur briefly after a grand mal attack of epilepsy. Sometimes the condition is partial (dysphasia), and the person retains a usable capacity to write and understand writing.

Aphonia is loss of voice, and is usually a temporary condition. Speech remains possible, although it may be whispered instead of voiced. Aphonia may be the result of (1) inflammation of the larynx (laryngitis); (2) using the voice too much; or (3) radiotherapy for cancer of the vocal cord. Occasionally, hysteria may be the cause.

Aphrodisiac is a substance that increases sexual desire (libido). There are many substances that are said to have this property, but most of them are ineffectual, and their results often depend on how strongly the individual believes in them. Many so-called aphrodisiacs are harmless, but some may be poisonous, especially if taken in large amounts. Cantharides, a powder of the dried beetle Spanish fly, is highly dangerous when used as an aphrodisiac; consumption of cantharides can be fatal.

Alcohol, despite its initial effect of increasing self-confidence and releasing inhibitions, has an essentially depressant effect.

Patients suffering from impotence and other sexual problems should seek professional medical or psychiatric advice.

Aphthous ulcer is a small whitish sore, usually in the mouth, that is commonly called a mouth ulcer. *See* MOUTH ULCER.

Apicitis is an inflammation of the apex of a structure, and usually refers to a tooth.

Apoplexy (for EMERGENCY treatment, *see* First Aid, p.573) is a stoppage of the blood supply to the brain, and is more commonly known as a stroke. *See* STROKE.

Appendicectomy (or appendectomy) is the surgical removal of the APPENDIX, a structure without function attached to the first part of the large intestine. The operation is generally performed after diagnosis of APPENDICITIS, a painful inflammation of the appendix.

Q: How is the appendicectomy performed?

A: The appendix is removed under general anaesthesia, usually through a small diagonal cut in the lower right-hand side of the abdomen. Sometimes the surgeon makes a cut parallel to the middle line near the centre of the lower abdomen. With acute appendicitis the appendix may

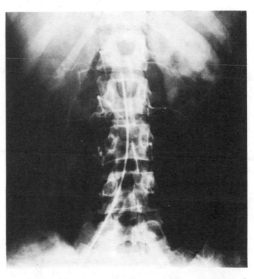

Aortogram: a catheter, shown above, is passed up the aorta and a chemical is injected.

Appendicitis

burst, and there is the slight risk that the operation itself may cause it to do so. If the appendix bursts and infection spreads to the lining of the abdomen (causing peritonitis), the surgeon leaves a tube in the wound to drain the infection to the surface; after about 48 hours the drain usually can be removed.

Q: *How long does recovery normally take after an appendicectomy?*

A: After the operation, recovery is usually rapid. The stitches are removed about five days later, and the patient is able to leave hospital within a week. Convalescence may take about a month or more while the various layers of tissue in the abdominal wall heal. In the past an appendicectomy was considered a risky operation, but today the success rate is nearly 100 per cent. About one person in ten has the operation.

Appendicitis is inflammation of the appendix, a structure attached to the first part of the large intestine. An early symptom is vague stomach pain around the navel, which becomes more severe and spreads within three or four hours to the lower right-hand part of the abdomen, sometimes with periods of griping pain (colic). A feeling of nausea is followed by vomiting, headache, and slight fever. The patient is usually constipated, although occasionally there may be diarrhoea. The stomach is tender, and touching it makes the pain worse.

Q: *If appendicitis is suspected, what should be done?*

A: Do not give the patient a laxative. If pain persists after a few hours, a doctor should be consulted. Failure to seek prompt medical attention may allow the appendix to burst, thus causing a serious infection of the abdominal lining (peritonitis). With acute appendicitis, the patient is admitted immediately to hospital for an APPENDICECTOMY, an operation to remove the appendix.

Q: *Does appendicitis affect certain age groups more than others?*

A: The complaint occurs rarely in children under the age of five, and rarely in adults after the age of fifty.

Appendix is any structure that is attached to a larger or more important part. The term usually refers to the vermiform appendix, which is a worm-shaped structure attached to the first part (caecum) of the large intestine, lying in the lower right side of the abdomen. It is, on average, about 8cm (3 inches) long although the size varies considerably. The appendix may also be in different positions; it can be tucked behind the caecum, or hang down into the pelvis. Inflammation of the appendix is called APPENDICITIS.

Appetite is a healthy and natural anticipation of food. It must not be confused with hunger, which is a stronger stimulus.

Many disorders result in or are accompanied by a loss of appetite. Anyone who undergoes a loss of both appetite and weight lasting for more than two weeks should consult a doctor. Some diseases, such as overactivity of the thyroid gland (thyrotoxicosis), increase the body's energy requirements and stimulate appetite.

Psychological conditions such as depression may cause either compulsive eating or loss of appetite. ANOREXIA NERVOSA, for example, occurring most often in adolescent girls, makes them unwilling to eat. A child's refusal to eat is commonly not a loss of appetite but a means of upsetting the parents.

It is possible to control appetite with the use of drugs, but this may be extremely dangerous and should be done only on a doctor's advice.

Aqueous humour is the watery fluid in the eye, in front of the lens. *See* HUMOUR.

Argyll-Robertson pupil is a disorder in which the process for focusing an eye works normally although the reflex response to light is absent. The pupil is commonly contracted and so may appear smaller than normal. The condition is generally a sign of one type of the venereal disease syphilis.

Armpit is the ordinary name for the axilla, the cavity below the shoulder joint. Strong muscles, attached to the chest and shoulder blade, form the front and back walls and help

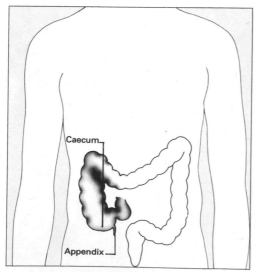

Caecum

Appendix

Appendix is a structure, about the size of a little finger, attached to the caecum.

to move the arm. The armpit contains sweat glands, lymph glands, and, in an adult, hairs.

Q: What can go wrong with the armpit?

A: Several common problems can arise there. Heavy perspiration (hyperhidrosis), occurring normally when a person is hot, active, and anxious, can be embarrassing to some people who suffer from the condition all the time. Treatment with a strong-acting deodorant and an antiperspirant preparation is often helpful. Newer treatments include operations to remove the areas of skin with excess sweat glands, or destroying them by freezing.

Other common disorders are abscesses. They may be a consequence of heavy sweating, or not washing the armpit, or too frequent shaving of the hair. They appear more often in persons with diabetes.

Some people have allergic reactions to deodorants, antiperspirants, and perfumes, each of which may produce an area of red, painful skin.

Pain in the armpit may be caused by boils, allergic skin problems, or swollen lymph glands. Swelling in the armpit may be caused by any condition causing enlargement of the lymph glands, such as local BCG innoculation or glandular fever.

Arrhythmia is an irregularity in the heartbeat and therefore the pulse rate. There are various causes for an irregular pulse. In sinus arrhythmia, a normal occurrence in young people at rest, the pulse rate increases or decreases with breathing. Breathing alters the amount of blood entering the heart and this changes the pulse rate.

See also FIBRILLATION; PAROXYSMAL TACHYCARDIA.

Arsenic is a metalloid chemical element. Its oxide, a greyish white powder, is extremely poisonous. Accumulation of arsenic in the body causes weakness, indigestion, diarrhoea, discoloration and peeling of the skin, mental disorders, and loss of sensation in the wrists and ankles. Acute arsenic poisoning causes death from vomiting and diarrhoea with acute abdominal pains.

Arteriogram is an X-ray picture of an artery. To take the picture, the radiologist first injects the artery with a substance that is opaque to radiation.

A talk about Arteriosclerosis

Arteriosclerosis is a disorder in which arteries become thick and hard and lose their supple,

elastic quality. This happens when fats are deposited in the vessel walls.

Q: What causes the deposits in the arteries?

A: The cause is not fully known, but it is believed to be part of the normal ageing process. Arteriosclerosis is more likely to occur or to be severe in any one of the following groups of people: the overweight; smokers; those with high blood pressure (hypertension); the inactive; those with diabetes; and those who have a family history of heart attacks that are connected with increased levels of LIPIDS and CHOLESTEROL in the blood.

Q: Is arteriosclerosis serious?

A: The exact degree of severity of the condition depends on which arteries are most involved. A narrowed artery to the heart muscle may cause ANGINA PECTORIS or a HEART ATTACK (myocardial infarction). If the arteries to the legs are involved, the patient feels pain in the calves when walking (intermittent claudication). Affected arteries to the brain may cause a succession of small strokes or a major one (*see* STROKE). Reduced flow of blood to certain areas of the brain may result in PARKINSON'S DISEASE.

Sometimes, when the artery is brittle, a piece of fatty substance (embolus) breaks away from the inside wall and enters the bloodstream. If the embolus is sufficiently large, it may block the bloodstream completely and cause a stroke. In one of the limbs, such an obstruction can be extremely serious and requires prompt

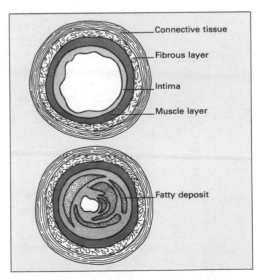

Arteriosclerosis, hardening of the arteries, develops when fat clings to the artery walls.

medical treatment before gangrene (tissue death) sets in below the blockage.

Q: Can a hardened artery be made to return to its normal size and suppleness?

A: No. If a limb artery has become blocked, after previous treatment has failed to improve circulation, the sclerotic (hardened) section has to be surgically replaced by a section of new artery, either natural or plastic (arterial graft).

Q: What is the treatment for arteriosclerosis?

A: Treatment of arteriosclerosis can only prevent the condition from becoming worse. Special drugs such as clofibrate tend to reduce cholesterol in the blood, and others reduce blood pressure. The patient must lose weight, stop smoking, take regular exercise, reduce the amount of cholesterol-containing foods in the diet, and keep diabetes under control. The same regimen should be followed to help to prevent arteriosclerosis.

Artery is one of the tube-shaped blood vessels that carry oxygenated blood from the heart to the body tissues. Arteries are thick-walled, flexible, and muscular.

See also p.8.

A talk about Arthritis

Arthritis is a general term for any condition in which joints become inflamed, usually accompanied by pain, swelling, and limited movement. Arthritis has many different

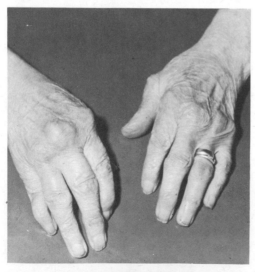

Arthritis is inflammation of the joints that produces the characteristic swelling.

forms, but the three most common forms are osteoarthritis, rheumatoid arthritis, and gout. Doctors are not always able to determine the cause of a specific arthritic complaint. In general, arthritis may be caused by infection in a joint, by degeneration of a joint as a person becomes older, or by a disorder of which arthritis is a symptom. The cause of the arthritis determines which course the affliction takes.

Q: What is osteoarthritis?

A: Osteoarthritis is the form of arthritis most common in elderly people. Time takes its toll of joints, which suffer from general wear and tear. The connecting surfaces of the joints become rougher as the cartilage lining the bone deteriorates. Osteoarthritis most commonly affects those joints that support weight, such as the knees, hips, and spine. For this reason, the condition can be worse in people who are overweight. The effects of the ageing process can be hastened if joints have been damaged earlier in life by an accident or injury.

Q: What measures can be taken by the osteoarthritis patient to relieve discomfort?

A: Aspirin is effective for reducing pain, but a doctor sometimes prescribes stronger drugs depending on the severity of the condition. A heating pad, or shortwave diathermy, often gives short-term relief. If the pain is in a weight-bearing joint (knee or hip), the use of a walker or a stick may help. Care should be taken when moving. The patient should lose weight, if necessary, and wear soft, rubber-heeled shoes. A living area can be modified to assist an arthritic person: handles near showers, baths, toilets, and beds are all useful aids. A straight-backed chair is easiest to use.

Q: Can a person become crippled with osteoarthritis?

A: Patients with osteoarthritis rarely become bedridden or crippled. The bulbous knobs that may develop on the fingers or toes can be painful and stiff, but serious crippling does not result. Pain flares up with sudden activity after rest, and a bad attack may last for several days. Osteoarthritis of a hip or a knee may prevent a patient from walking normally. If the joints in both legs are affected, the patient may become chairbound.

Q: What is rheumatoid arthritis?

A: Rheumatoid arthritis is painful swelling, usually of the smaller joints, together with the destruction of tissue around them. It most often begins in early adult life, and although an attack may subside, it usually flares up again later. The cause of this affliction remains unknown. There is a risk with rheumatoid arthritis of crippling or other physical deformity. In children, the condition is known as STILL'S DISEASE.

Q: *What is the treatment for rheumatoid arthritis?*

A: Treatment is aimed at providing relief from the symptoms. But the damage to the joints that accompanies the disorder cannot be repaired. Heat, in the form of shortwave diathermy and wax baths, can give short-term relief, and physiotherapy may ease the pain and keep the joints mobile. Salicylate drugs (a category that includes aspirin) and stronger antirheumatic drugs may be prescribed. Some deformities resulting from the disease can be remedied by surgery.

Q: *What is gout?*

A: Gout is a congenital disorder in which the body cannot rid itself of all the uric acid it produces. Excessive quantities of uric acid build up in the bones and joints, as well as in various tissues and cartilage, and this can cause extremely painful attacks of arthritis. A blood test reveals a high concentration of uric acid in the bloodstream. If diagnosis is made early, future attacks may be prevented by the regular use of drugs, such as allopurinol.

Q: *What other disorders cause arthritic symptoms?*

A: Joints may become infected as part of a generalized disease, often accompanied by a fever and a feeling of general illness. Bacterial arthritis is the invasion of joint areas by bacteria, causing swelling and inflammation. It occurs with tuberculosis and gonorrhoea. In children, rheumatic fever causes painful joints that become better, then worse over a period of weeks. This is an allergic reaction to streptococcus bacteria. Virus infections, such as rubella (German measles), mumps, and hepatitis, may sometimes produce inflamed joints. Arthritis may also be associated with the spinal disorder ankylosing spondylitis, with ulcers in the colon (colitis), or with inflammation of the urethra (Reiter's disease).

Q: *How effective are hydrocortisone injections for treating osteoarthritis?*

A: Hydrocortisone cannot cure osteoarthritis. It reduces the inflammation in a joint, and thereby relieves the pain. Treatment is highly effective for as long as the drug is present, but when the effect wears off, the pain may return. Too many injections are dangerous, because they damage the joint in some instances.

Q: *How can surgery help patients with osteo- and rheumatoid arthritis?*

A: A method of stopping pain in a stiff joint (such as the ankle) is by fusing its bones together in an operation (arthrodesis, or artificial ankylosis). Another possible operation is the replacement of the arthritic joint by an artificial one made of steel or plastic. This proves highly effective for an arthritic hip, knee, or fingers, but is still experimental for the elbow and ankle.

Arthrodesis is the deliberate fusing together of the bones of a joint by an operation (artificial ANKYLOSIS). It is used to relieve a painful condition, such as severe osteoarthritis or a joint damaged in an accident.

Artificial heart is a machine used during cardiac surgery to perform the functions of the real heart while the operation takes place. Investigations have been made into the possibility of using an artificial heart to rest a diseased one before a transplant takes place.

See also HEART-LUNG MACHINE; REPLACEMENT SURGERY.

Artificial insemination is a technique in which sperm is introduced into the neck of the womb (cervix) for the purpose of fertilizing an egg (ovum) by means other than sexual intercourse. This is normally done with a syringe. Artificial insemination is used in some cases of infertility.

Q: *How important is the timing of the insemination?*

A: The timing of the introduction of the

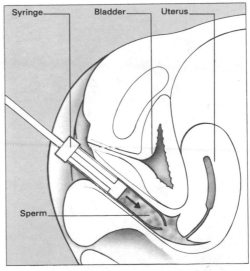

Syringe — Bladder — Uterus — Sperm

Artificial insemination is the introduction of healthy sperms into the vagina using a syringe.

Artificial kidney

sperm is critical; it should take place during ovulation (when an ovary releases an egg). The timing is estimated by following the woman's morning temperature charts, which show a sudden, slight increase in temperature on the day of ovulation.

Q: Who supplies the sperm for the insemination?

A: It is most common for the woman's husband to supply the sperm. This is known as AIH (artificial insemination by husband). The husband, although fertile, may not be able to have sexual intercourse. Or the quantity of sperm produced may be so small that the chances of conception are slight. In this case, sperm is collected and deep frozen until there is a sufficient amount.

Artificial insemination by donor (AID) is the provision of sperm by an unknown male. This is used when the husband is infertile but both partners want a baby of their own. The doctor chooses a man with qualities that are compatible with those of the future parents in vital respects, such as race and physical characteristics, absence of congenital abnormalities, and the correct blood group. The practice of artificial insemination is controversial in many countries on legal, religious, and moral grounds.

Artificial kidney is a machine that takes over the function of the natural kidneys when they are damaged by disease and cannot clean the blood of toxic substances. The poisonous substances produce URAEMIA, a serious condi-

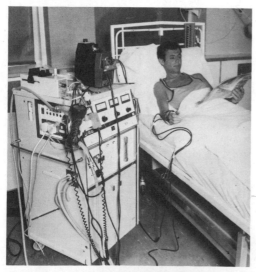

Artificial kidney filters out waste substances in the blood, just like a natural kidney.

tion that, if left untreated, leads to death.
See also KIDNEY DIALYSIS.

Artificial limb. *See* PROSTHESIS.

Artificial respiration (for EMERGENCY treatment, *see* First Aid, pp.518–523) is any means of inducing breathing in a person whose breathing has stopped. As a part of first aid, it is often the primary treatment. Techniques that are commonly used in artificial respiration include mouth-to-mouth resuscitation, the Holger Nielsen method, and the Silvester method, all of which are fully illustrated in the First Aid section of these books. An extreme emergency may require a TRACHEOSTOMY, an operation performed by a professional medical person in which a hole is made in the front of the neck into the windpipe (trachea).

Asbestosis is a form of the lung disease pneumoconiosis caused by inhaling asbestos fibres. *See* PNEUMOCONIOSIS.

Ascariasis is an infection of the bowels by roundworms (*Ascaris lumbricoides*). *See* WORMS.

Ascites is an accumulation of fluid in the abdominal cavity. *See* OEDEMA.

Ascorbic acid is the chemical name for vitamin C. *See* VITAMINS.

Asepsis is the condition of an environment that is free from infecting organisms. In operating theatres, for example, it is essential that there be no airborne infection. To achieve asepsis, the air is filtered and kept at a higher pressure than normal air pressure outside, so that the aseptic air cannot be contaminated by unfiltered air. Operating instruments, surgical clothes, and gloves are all sterilized beforehand, and surgeons scrub their hands and forearms before dressing. Complete asepsis is not possible in a situation where humans are present. In the pharmaceutical industry many drugs are prepared and packaged in closed chambers.

Aspergillosis is infection by any member of the genus of fungi called *Aspergillus*.

Asphyxia (for EMERGENCY treatment, *see* First Aid, pp.518–523) is a condition in which an interference with the breathing process has seriously affected or even stopped the action of the heart and lungs. It is most often caused by SUFFOCATION (choking or obstruction of the air passages). Asphyxia requires urgent treatment because brain damage begins about five minutes after the cessation of the oxygen supply to the brain.

Q: What are other causes of asphyxia?

A: Asphyxia can also result from a reduction of the oxygen content in the air, chest injury, paralysis of the lungs, bleeding into the lungs, narcotic drugs, deep anaesthesia, or electric shock.

Aspirin is the most widely used painkilling drug (analgesic). It is also used to reduce fever (as an antipyretic) and is beneficial in the treatment of diseases of the joints, such as rheumatoid arthritis, osteoarthritis, and rheumatic fever.

The usual dose of aspirin is effective for about six hours, after which time it is broken down by the liver or excreted in the urine. If there is no improvement in a condition within this time, it is of no use to continue treatment. If symptoms persist, a doctor should be consulted.

Q: *Is aspirin a harmless drug?*

A: When taken according to specified dosages, aspirin is an extremely safe drug. The availability of aspirin without prescription can, however, result in aspirin poisoning if the drug is swallowed by children, for whom it may be fatal; adults may also be poisoned by aspirin. Continued use of the drug can cause stomach ulceration and bleeding, which may result in anaemia. Also, people suffering from certain disorders should not take aspirin.

Q: *Which disorders indicate caution with aspirin?*

A: People who have peptic ulcers should not use aspirin without medical advice: internal bleeding often occurs and blood is vomited (haematemesis). People who suffer from persistent indigestion and patients taking anticoagulant drugs are also advised against taking aspirin. Mild sensitivity to aspirin may cause an itchy skin irritation (urticaria) or allergic asthma. In such cases, a doctor may recommend PARACETAMOL as a safe alternative painkiller.

Asthenia is a general condition of weakness, usually arising from muscular or psychological disorders.

A talk about Asthma

Asthma is a disorder in which the patient experiences difficulty in breathing, accompanied by a slight wheezing and a "tight" chest. Additional symptoms can be a dry cough and vomiting (usually in children). An asthma attack may start suddenly, and the fear and worry that this causes can prolong the attack.

Q: *What causes asthma?*

A: Asthma most often occurs as an ALLERGY. Many pollens, moulds, dusts (especially dust containing the house mite), and animal hair and dander can all cause asthma attacks. Asthmatic symptoms are sometimes associated with HAY FEVER. Infection in the respiratory system is another cause of asthma.

Exposure to cold, exercise, fatigue, irritating fumes, and certain emotional and psychological states can all trigger an asthma attack. Or these conditions may serve as secondary factors that increase the severity or frequency of attacks. Asthma from these causes may occur in people who have no history of allergic reactions, as well as in those who do.

Q: *How does asthma interfere with breathing?*

A: Air passes through the lungs via tubes (called bronchi) and smaller vessels (bronchioles). With asthma, the smaller bronchi and bronchioles become swollen and clogged with mucus, and the muscles surrounding the bronchioles contract so that the air that should pass through is unable to do so. The body reacts to the lack of oxygen, and the patient forces more and more air into the lungs. But, because of the blockages, there is difficulty in exhaling it. The wheezing noise is caused by air being forcibly exhaled through the narrowed bronchi.

Q: *How long does an asthma attack last?*

A: An attack of asthma may last for a few minutes, but most go on for several hours. A severe, prolonged attack (a form of asthma known as status asthmaticus) may last for a number of hours or even days. A person with status asthmaticus requires hospitalization.

Q: *What immediate help can be given to a person suffering from asthma?*

Age of child	Advised baby aspirin dose. Consult a doctor before giving a third dose.	Frequency
6 months		every 3 to 4 hours
1 year		every 3 to 4 hours
2 years		every 3 to 4 hours
3 years		every 3 to 4 hours
4 years		every 4 hours
5 years		every 4 hours

Aspirin dosage must be carefully controlled for children: 4 baby aspirins=1 adult aspirin.

Astigmatism

A: With more severe attacks, it is important that the patient sits upright, either in a chair or in bed and propped up by pillows. A table in front of the patient is useful, because this can be grasped and the arm muscles used to assist breathing. A patient is rarely hungry, but should be encouraged to drink large amounts of liquids. Antispasmodic inhalants from aerosol cans may be helpful in relaxing the muscles of the bronchioles.

Q: How does a doctor treat asthma between attacks?

A: When the cause is an allergy, ANTI-HISTAMINES are often prescribed. Other drugs that may be given are salbutamol and terbutaline. These can be taken in tablet form, or in an aerosol spray if an attack seems imminent. Aerosols are generally successful in treating asthma, but the consequences of overuse have proved fatal because aerosols contain the drug isoprenaline, which has a stimulant effect on the heart.

Two new inhalant drugs, disodium cromoglycate (Intal) and corticosteroid inhalant have also achieved some success in preventing asthmatic attacks.

Q: What is the treatment for severe asthma (status asthmaticus)?

A: An attack of status asthmaticus requires urgent hospital treatment. A slow injection of adrenaline may stop the attack quicker than any other treatment.

Patients can be taught how to administer the injection themselves so that time need not be wasted waiting for a doctor to administer the dose.

Q: Apart from taking the appropriate drugs, what other precautions can be taken to prevent an asthma attack?

A: Several simple measures can reduce the risk of attack. Most attacks occur at night, and so anxiety arising from the possibility can be lessened by taking a mild sedative at bedtime. A person with allergic asthma should sleep in a room without carpets or rugs. Blankets and pillows of synthetic fibre reduce the risk of house dust and mites. In dry climates, a humidifier can be used to increase the moisture content of the air in the room.

For patients in whom asthma is caused by respiratory infection, breathing exercises may be of value. A physiotherapist can teach the patient the most appropriate ones. These exercises are not only a psychological help in preventing an attack, but when minor respiratory infection does occur, the lungs should function more efficiently.

Q: Can asthma have any complications?

A: Because so much air is held in the lungs during an asthma attack, the air cells (alveoli) can become so stretched that the cell walls may tear. This damage causes a gradual loss of elasticity in the lungs and can lead to the condition known as EM-PHYSEMA. If the patient coughs too much, the surface of a lung may burst, causing the air to escape into the cavity that encloses the lung (pleural cavity). This condition is known as a pneumothorax.

Other complications can arise from the mucus secretions that do not drain properly during an asthma attack. This can lead to bronchitis and sometimes bronchial pneumonia. Frequent attacks may result in chronic bronchitis.

Q: What other disorders might be confused with asthma?

A: A disorder mistakenly known as cardiac asthma has symptoms similar to asthma (gasping for breath, a "tight" chest), but is actually a type of heart disease. Immediate medical attention is required.

Q: Can asthma be cured completely?

A: Asthma cannot be cured. The possibility of future attacks can be minimized by drugs and other preventives, but if a person is disposed to asthma, there is always a chance that an attack will occur.

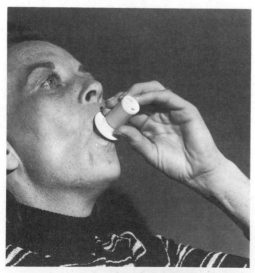

Asthma causes severe breathing difficulties: these may be relieved by means of an inhaler.

Astigmatism is a distortion in vision caused by an irregularity in the curvature of either the outer layer (cornea) of the eye, or the lens. Light rays passing through are not accurately focused on the retina at the back of the eye; the result is a blurring of vision. Astigmatism is found to a small degree in almost everyone. More serious cases can be compensated for by the use of spectacles.

Astringent is a substance that helps to stop the outflow of internal body fluids, especially of blood or mucus. Astringents may work in a number of ways: (1) by making the blood vessels smaller; (2) by helping the blood to coagulate; or (3) by removing the water that is essential to the formation of mucus. They are important in treating bleeding from the nose and throat, bleeding from surface wounds, and surface ulcers. The most common astringents are metallic astringents (for example, copper sulphate, silver nitrate, or calcium carbonate); adrenaline, natural and synthetic; vegetable astringents (such as witch hazel); and substances containing alcohol (for example, cologne or after-shave lotion).

Ataxia is an unsteadiness of movement when muscles fail to work together properly. Ataxia is the result of damage in the brain, especially in the cerebellum, the part of the brain that helps to control balance.

Atelectasis is either complete or partial collapse of a lung. The term refers to two distinct conditions. The first is the failure of the lungs to expand at birth, and the second is the collapsed (airless) condition of a segment of a lung. This collapse is generally caused by an obstruction in the tube (bronchus) leading to the lung, or by excessive secretion of mucus in the lung wall. Such a condition can occur in several respiratory disorders, particularly in pneumonia but also in bronchitis. Pressure from outside the lungs from a tumour or expanded blood vessel (aneurysm), for example, can also press on part of a lung and cause a collapse.

Q: What is the treatment for atelectasis?

A: If the cause of the collapse is a blocked bronchus, such an obstruction may be removed by using a special instrument called a bronchoscope. Atelectasis from other causes can often be corrected by vigorous exercises prescribed for the patient by a physiotherapist.

Q: Are there any possible complications of atelectasis?

A: If excessive amounts of mucus are the cause of the collapse, the mucus build-up can become infected.

Atheroma is a condition of the larger arteries in which areas of the arterial walls degenerate into fatty tissue. The condition is part of the blood-vessel disease ARTERIOSCLEROSIS.

Athlete's foot, or tinea (tinea pedis), is a surface infection of the foot caused by any of a number of fungi. It takes the form of small blisters between the toes. Pain and irritation accompany the infection and, if the surface of the skin breaks, bacterial infections may develop. The fungus grows on moist skin and is usually transmitted in places where many people walk barefoot, such as communal showers and swimming pools.

Q: How is athlete's foot treated?

A: Treatments are available from chemists without prescription in the form of lotions, ointments, and powders. Finding the most suitable treatment is largely a matter of trial and error. It is important that the infected area be kept dry. Care should be taken to wipe off all moisture after bathing or swimming. If home treatment fails a doctor should be consulted.

Q: Can similar infection occur elsewhere on the body?

A: Yes. Similar infection can appear between the legs (tinea cruris), on the face, under the arms, in the scalp, and especially in the beard area (tinea barbae).

Atopic describes a tendency to acquire allergies. Only the tendency is acquired, not any specific disorder. Hay fever, asthma, and eczema may be atopic allergies.

See also ALLERGY.

Atrium is the medical term for a cavity. It is used most often to describe each of the two blood-collecting chambers in the HEART.

Atrophy is the wasting away of tissue, of an organ, or of the entire body.

Atropine is an alkaloid drug that is extracted from several plants, including belladonna

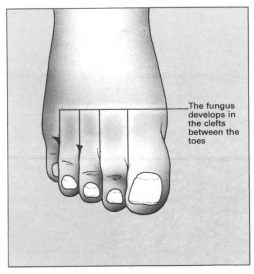

The fungus develops in the clefts between the toes

Athlete's foot is a fungal infection that can cause blisters to form between the toes.

Audiogram

(deadly nightshade). It has several applications. It is used as a stimulant for the respiratory and circulatory systems. Its effect of stopping the flow of secretions in the mouth makes it valuable as a pre-anaesthetic drug when the anaesthetic is to be inhaled. A weak solution of atropine is often applied to the eye to make the pupil dilate. This makes various eye examinations easier for the doctor. Atropine is also used to decrease involuntary muscle spasms in the intestine and bladder as part of the treatment for certain intestinal disorders.

Audiogram is a chart showing the results of a hearing ability test, recorded by a delicate instrument called an audiometer. The test is based on sounds of different frequencies and loudness.

See also DEAFNESS.

Aura is an awareness of an approaching attack of a disorder such as EPILEPSY or MIGRAINE. This awareness may be accompanied by unusual sensations of sight, smell, hearing, or taste.

Auricle is a term that is used to mean two separate and small parts of the body. It can be either (1) the external projecting part of the ear (also called the pinna); or (2) one of the ear-shaped appendages projecting from each ATRIUM of the heart. The terms auricle and atrium are often mistakenly used interchangeably.

Autism is a severe psychological condition in which experience centres entirely on the self and the person displays an apparent disregard of reality. It appears most often in childhood, usually before the age of three.

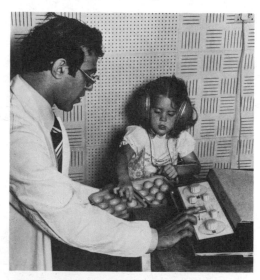

Audiogram: the doctor directs a controlled tone through the girl's headphones.

Early indications of autism include a vacant stare, a lack of response to affectionate gestures and an apparent insensitivity to pain, perhaps accompanied by acts of self-mutilation. Autistic children may respond with tantrums to changes in their physical surroundings, such as a rearrangement of furniture or toys. Many autistic children are mute, and in others the development of speech is severely restricted, perhaps to a meaningless repetition of a few words.

Q: Can autism be successfully treated?

A: The underlying reason for autism is not fully known, and so treatment is concentrated on the symptoms. In all cases, treatment is long and complex.

Q: Is an autistic person mentally retarded?

A: No. Mental functions are rarely impaired by autism.

Autoimmune disease is a disorder in which the body treats its own tissues as if they were infections and produces antibodies to destroy them.

Automatism is a state in which a person acts as if automatically, without conscious knowledge (or later memory) of what is happening. Although the person appears normal and functions normally, he or she does not manifest personality, and behaviour may be abnormal. The condition commonly represents a hysterical trance or may follow an attack of epilepsy. Sleepwalking is also an example of automatism.

Patients in this condition are not responsible for their actions, so it is most important that they are never left alone.

Autonomic nervous system is the part of the nervous system that controls involuntary functions in the body. These functions include gland activity; contraction of involuntary (smooth) muscles; and the action of the heart. Within the autonomic nervous system, there are two divisions: the sympathetic system and the parasympathetic system.

Q: What functions does the sympathetic system control?

A: The sympathetic system controls those activities that prepare the body for sudden activity. These include increasing the blood pressure and heart rate (sending blood to the muscles), increasing glucose production by the liver, reducing the secretion of saliva, causing the hairs on the skin to stand up, and dilation of the pupils of the eyes.

Q: What functions does the parasympathetic system control?

A: The parasympathetic system produces effects opposite to those of the sympathetic system. It is responsible for a reduction in blood pressure and the slowing of the heart rate, contraction of the pupils of the eyes, copious secretion of saliva, and increased activity in the stomach and intestines. Thus, after the sympathetic system speeds up the body's responses, the parasympathetic system is the means by which the body returns to its normal calm.

Axilla is the armpit. *See* ARMPIT.

B

Babinski's reflex, or sign, is the turning upward of the big toe and the spreading out of the other toes when the sole of the foot is stroked on the outer edge. Babinski's reflex in an adult indicates damage to the nervous system, such as occurs in a stroke. But it is a perfectly normal reaction in babies under the age of one year.

A talk about Baby care

Baby care. Much of baby care is routine and is best approached in an organized way. The key to this organization is to correctly equip and arrange well the baby's room. Bathing, changing, and feeding a baby should also follow a fixed routine wherever possible. More important than routine are love and affection. Common-sense is also essential, especially concerning safety for the child. Pets should be kept out of the baby's room, as should any member of the family with an infection.

Parents should remember that general advice of the type contained in this article often refers to the average baby. No individual baby is "average" in every respect. Slight variations from the average can be discussed with a doctor.

Q: *How should a baby's room be organized?*
A: The baby's room should be light, warm (21–24°C; 70–75°F), well aired, and close to the parent's bedroom. The cot must be stable so that it cannot easily be knocked over.

A clean sheet should cover a waterproof mattress. Light blankets should be available, but a pillow must never be used because it may smother a young baby.

A table provides an excellent surface for changing and dressing, and for the baby's bath. A nearby shelf should be cleared for nappies, plastic pants, baby powder, soap, towels, cotton wool balls or swabs, baby oil, cream or ointment for nappy rash, spare sheets, and clean clothing. A bucket is needed for dirty nappies, and an upright chair with supporting back is needed for feeding.

Q: *What routine should be followed when changing and bathing a baby?*
A: Clothes and nappies should be changed on a firm, flat surface for safety reasons. A newborn baby's neck muscles are too weak to support the head, which must be held while handling the baby. After removing a nappy, gently clean the area with water, soap and water, or baby oil, and rub in some cream to prevent soreness.

Before bathing the baby, test the water (with the elbow) to ensure a comfortable temperature. Always support the baby's head, while he or she enjoys the freedom of kicking in the water. Next take the baby out of the water, soap all over the body, particularly in the armpits and groin, and rinse thoroughly. Dry gently in a soft towel and powder the skin, particularly in the creases. The eyes, nose, and ears can be cleaned with cotton wool. Any flaking skin on the scalp can be rubbed with oil.

Q: *Do the baby's hair, nails, and mouth need any special care?*
A: The hair should be brushed twice daily with a soft brush; the nails are soft and can be pared back carefully using small scissors. The mouth should be cleaned with a piece of moist tissue paper.

Q: *What should a baby be fed?*
A: A baby needs food and water. Milk pro-

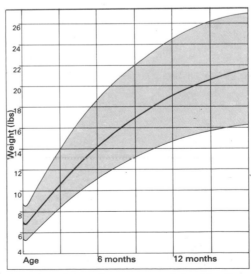

This chart shows the average weight gain of a baby, and normal maximum and minimum.

Bacillus

vides both, and mother's milk supplies, in addition, antibodies that help to protect against disease in the first few weeks of life. Also, mother's milk does not produce the intolerance or allergy that a few babies have to cow's milk.

If the mother is not breast-feeding, she feeds the baby on the bottle, as the doctor directs.

Solid foods need not be started until the baby weighs at least 10 pounds (4½ kilos) or is 2 to 4 months old. The first solids may be strained meat, creamed rice, banana fruit, vegetables, or cereal, which can be given for one meal a day. At first, portions should be small; too much may produce diarrhoea.

Q: *How much and how often should a baby be fed?*

A: Each day, a young baby requires 2½–3 ounces (70–85 grams) of milk for each pound (half-kilo) of body weight. In hot weather or during illness, there is a greater need for water (not food), and so extra water or juice should be given.

The baby should be fed every four hours for the first two weeks of life, but a rigid schedule need not be followed because the baby's hunger may vary.

Q: *How should a baby be fed?*

A: Feeding should take place in a comfortable chair. The temperature of a bottle-feed should be tested by sprinkling a little on the back of the hand or wrist. Bottle-fed babies must have the teat removed from the mouth from time to time to allow air to enter the bottle. Too small a hole in a teat causes excessive swallowing of air, and a hole that is too large feeds too quickly and may produce choking.

Half-way through and after each feed, the baby should be rested against the parent's shoulder, who should rub the child's back to produce burps, which are the sign of air escaping from the stomach.

Q: *What is the normal weight change in a baby?*

A: It is usual for a baby to lose a few ounces in the first week of life. Then an average gain of 5–7 ounces (150–200 grams) a week can be expected for the first three months, followed by a more gradual weight gain.

Q: *How much sleep does a baby need?*

A: A newborn baby requires 20–22 hours of sleep a day. The baby should be placed in the cot face down with the head turned to one side. Soft toys must not be left near the face.

Bacillus is a general term for any rod-shaped bacterium of class Schizomycetes, and for bacteria of the genus *Bacillus*. Most bacilli are harmless and found everywhere. Others cause disease, such as *Bacillus anthracis* (*see* ANTHRAX).

See also BACTERIA.

A talk about Backache

Backache is an extremely common complaint characterized by local or generalized pain anywhere in the spinal region from the neck to the buttocks. It may be caused by various disorders, but the most common are those associated with muscles, ligaments, bones, or nerves.

Q: *How does muscular strain cause backache?*

A: Any sudden strain on the back can cause small tears in the muscles. These tears are felt as local pain. The area is tender when touched and movement may be painful for several days while the tears heal.

Q: *Can pain all over the back be due to a muscular cause?*

A: Yes. Pain from generalized muscle ache (myalgia) can sometimes be caused by infection, which triggers off wide areas of muscle spasm. Generalized muscle disorders, particularly in elderly people, often start as backache between the shoulder blades. This may be a symptom of the old-age disorder polymyalgia rheumatica. *See* FIBROSITIS.

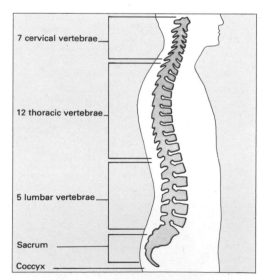

7 cervical vertebrae

12 thoracic vertebrae

5 lumbar vertebrae

Sacrum

Coccyx

Backache can be caused by disorders in any of the divisions of the spine or allied muscles.

Q: *How can backache be caused by ligament problems?*

A: Ligaments are just as susceptible to small tears as are muscles. The tears are again usually caused by unexpected strain, but the pain is more localized than muscular pain and tends to be present continuously. Slight movements can aggravate the tears and make the pain worse.

Q: *Can anything other than sudden strain cause pain in the ligaments?*

A: Yes. Prolonged strain is sometimes put on ligaments from a deformity or weakness that remains from an old fracture. A short leg or muscle weakness may also cause recurrent pain in the ligaments.

Q: *What bone disorders can cause backache?*

A: Several diseases of the vertebrae, including a SLIPPED DISC, cause backache. Old age can cause the bones to become brittle (osteoporosis). When this happens the vertebrae collapse slightly, causing compression of the nerves and strain in the ligaments. Both result in backache, and the condition gradually becomes worse. The vertebrae may also collapse, with identical effects, if cancer spreads to the bones.

In osteoarthritis (*see* ARTHRITIS), a roughening of the bone edges causes nerve irritation and backache. In young to middle-aged people, a disorder that causes vertebrae to fuse together (ANKYLOSING SPONDYLITIS) produces pain and a gradual stiffening of the back.

Q: *What nerve disorders can cause backache?*

A: A dull deep backache may begin several days before the onset of shingles. A tumour on the spinal cord sometimes causes backache. But the most common form of backache of this type is associated with the inflammation of a nerve (neuritis).

Q: *Apart from causes directly associated with the spine, what other disorders can result in backache?*

A: A low ache in the back often occurs in women before the onset of menstruation, or as part of a painful menstrual period (dysmenorrhoea). Other gynaecological disorders may also cause backache.

Pain from a kidney infection (such as pyelonephritis) often occurs in the loin. A dull ache high in the back may be a symptom of a chest disorder.

Q: *What is the treatment for backache?*

A: Painkilling drugs, such as aspirin or paracetamol, may be taken to relieve the pain due to a minor strain of a muscle or ligament. For more severe backache, a doctor may prescribe an antirheumatic drug such as phenylbutazone or indomethacin.

Treatment by physiotherapy may include exercises, massage, or local heat. Bone manipulation, sometimes carried out by an osteopath after X-ray examination, may help backache resulting from slipped disc or ligament problems. The spine may be carefully stretched using traction, but hospital treatment is not usually necessary.

Q: *What everyday precautions can relieve back problems?*

A: Correct posture, a firm mattress, and strengthening of the muscles by means of careful exercise can all help to relieve some types of backache. Maintaining correct body weight (by dieting if necessary) also helps to prevent backache, because being overweight puts extra strain on the spine. (*See* DIET.)

Bacteraemia (or bacteriaemia) is a medical name for a type of blood poisoning. *See* BLOOD POISONING.

Bacteria are a large group of microscopic, single-celled organisms, some of which can cause diseases in humans. There are three different types of bacteria: cocci (*see* COCCUS), which are spherical; spirochetes, which are rigid, flexible, or curved coils (*see* SPIROCHETE); and bacilli (*see* BACILLUS), which are rod-shaped.

Bacterial endocarditis is inflammation of the lining of the heart valves and the heart chambers. It is caused by a bacterial infection and

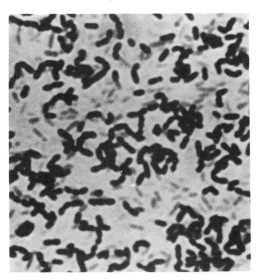

Bacteria can be identified through a microscope after they have multiplied.

91

Bad breath

is particularly likely to occur in persons who have some sort of heart valve deformity, either from birth (congenital deformity) or from damage caused by rheumatic fever. *See* ENDOCARDITIS.

Bad breath is known medically as halitosis. There are many causes but smoking and poor oral hygiene are probably the most common. Adequate dental care and cleaning the teeth after meals should correct most cases of bad breath. If bad breath continues even after such care, a doctor should be consulted.

Bagassosis is an asthma-like attack caused by inhaling the spores of a fungus that infects sugar cane. The attack comes several hours after contact, in a person who has worked with the cane for some months. Repeated attacks lead to fine scarring of the lungs and to the development of PNEUMOCONIOSIS. Apart from a change of job or environment there is no treatment.

Bag of waters is a common name for the protective fluid-filled sac that surrounds a foetus in the womb and breaks at the onset of labour. Its medical name is amniotic sac (*see* AMNION).

Balance. Body equilibrium or balance is controlled by the part of the brain called the cerebellum. Changes in body position are detected by the three semicircular canals of the inner ear; by the eyes; and by sensors in the body that send messages to the brain.

Q: What can go wrong with the sense of balance?

A: Various disorders can affect balance. Some are minor or only temporary. For example, some persons travelling by

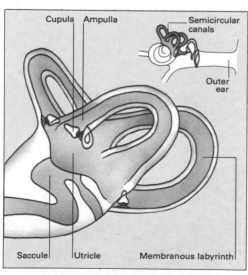

Balance is monitored by fluid within the ears' semicircular canals.

Cupula Ampulla

Semicircular canals

Outer ear

Saccule Utricle Membranous labyrinth

car, ship, or aeroplane experience MOTION SICKNESS. Middle ear infection, known medically as OTITIS MEDIA, can also upset the sense of balance by affecting the inner ear. Dizziness or giddiness, caused by an inadequate supply of blood and thus of oxygen to the brain, is the . sensation that precedes fainting. It may be due to emotional stress, or it may be a symptom of anaemia, heart disease, or a circulatory disorder. Vertigo, in which balance is so severely affected that the room seems to be spinning round, may be a symptom of MÉNIÈRE'S DISEASE or some other ear disorder.

Balanitis is inflammation of the end of the penis (the glans penis), accompanied by itching and a slight discharge. It is caused by a failure to keep the glans clean. For this reason, balanitis is more common in men and boys who have not had a circumcision, particularly if they suffer from PHIMOSIS (the inability to pull back the foreskin). Prevention and treatment depend on keeping the area washed and clean.

Baldness is the loss of hair that occurs naturally in many men as they grow older. Baldness usually begins at the temples or the crown of the head. A tendency to go bald is inherited and the age at which it begins, and the pattern it takes, are often similar in successive generations.

Q: Do women go bald?

A: All women experience partial hair loss as they grow older, but complete baldness in women is extremely rare.

Q: Is there any way of preventing baldness?

A: No. There is no way of preventing the onset of natural baldness. Wigs or hair transplants can disguise the condition.
    See also ALOPECIA.

Ballistocardiogram is a record of the movements of the body caused by the heartbeat. It is made by an instrument called a ballistocardiograph.

Bamboo spine is a common name for the condition known medically as ANKYLOSING SPONDYLITIS.

Banti's syndrome is a syndrome whose main signs are enlargement of the spleen and anaemia, usually caused by hepatic cirrhosis.

Barber's itch is a form of folliculitis that affects a man's face. *See* FOLLICULITIS.

Barbiturates are a group of sedative drugs derived from barbituric acid. Doctors use short-acting barbiturates, injected into a vein, as anaesthetics. Longer-acting barbiturates are occasionally prescribed as sleeping pills or used to reduce anxiety or to treat epilepsy.

Q: Can a person become addicted to barbiturates?

A: Barbiturates are mildly addictive, and they alter the normal pattern of sleep. Because of the dangers of DRUG ADDICTION and overdosage, doctors prefer to prescribe other kinds of sleep-inducing drugs.

Barbiturates should never be taken in combination with alcohol, because of the danger of possibly fatal consequences.

Barium is a metallic chemical element. The metal and its salts, particularly barium sulphate, show up clearly on X-ray photographs. A patient undergoing certain types of X-ray examinations may be asked to swallow a mixture of barium sulphate and water, called a barium meal, which is fairly tasteless unless artificially flavoured. A doctor can watch by X-rays the progress of the barium during and after it is swallowed, as it enters and leaves the stomach, and then as it moves through the small intestine to reach the colon (large intestine). A barium enema, a barium sulphate mixture passed into the rectum and colon, shows the outline of the colon.

Q: Why might a doctor ask for a barium test?

A: Barium investigations are used to help diagnose various conditions affecting the digestive tract.

Barotrauma is damage to a part of the body caused by high or low air pressure. It is particularly common in the middle ear when mucus blocks the Eustachian tube (the tube connecting the middle ear to the back of the throat), and after flying. The barotrauma causes pain in the ear and, in severe cases, may rupture the eardrum. A similar condition may occur in the nasal sinuses.

Bartholin's cyst is caused by a blockage of the duct of BARTHOLIN'S GLAND in the vagina. Its symptoms are a feeling of stretching and sometimes discomfort, particularly during intercourse (the condition called dyspareunia).

The usual treatment is surgical removal of the cyst in order to prevent repeated infections (Bartholin's abscesses).

Q: How soon after the operation can a woman resume intercourse?

A: A woman should not have intercourse for at least three weeks, and it may be a little painful for a further two months.

Bartholin's gland is one of a pair of lubricating glands at the entrance to the vagina. *See also* BARTHOLIN'S CYST.

Basal metabolic rate (BMR). The metabolic rate is a measure of the speed at which a person "burns" energy while at rest.

Measurement of BMR is seldom used now except in medical research.

Battered baby syndrome, also called child abuse or non-accidental injury, is a social problem that involves the physical ill treatment of children by their parents or guardians. It is usually discovered when a doctor examines a baby or child and finds evidence of repeated injuries for which the parents make apparently reasonable excuses.

All cases of child abuse should be reported to the appropriate authorities.

Q: Why do some parents abuse their children?

A: The causes of the problem are not always known. Most child abusers were themselves abused when they were children. The parents cannot cope emotionally with a crying, demanding child, and sometimes assault the child in an outburst of rage.

Q: What is the solution to the problem?

A: Family counselling by social workers and other experts can often reduce or eliminate the problem. They co-operate with various social and legal agencies to help the parents, who may also benefit from psychiatric therapy. In some cases, the child may have to be removed from the home, although generally this is only a temporary measure.

BCG vaccine (bacillus Calmette-Guérin) is a preparation of harmless TUBERCULOSIS vaccine which is used to give protection against the harmful, natural form of the disease. It was first used by Léon Calmette and Camille Guérin in Paris (1906). In countries where tuberculosis is still common, BCG is given in infancy. A skin test, the MANTOUX TEST, is carried out first to show whether natural immunity has already been acquired, and is repeated to ensure that it has worked.

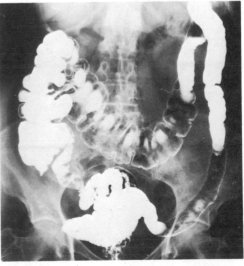

Barium is a radiopaque element the salts of which show up on X-ray photographs.

Bedbug

Bedbug (*Cimex lectularius*) is a small blood-sucking insect that can infest bedding. The insect is red-brown, oval, flat, and wingless. Its bite is painful and causes swelling, itching, and sometimes infection. It may transmit RELAPSING FEVER. A doctor can prescribe a cream containing a mild antiseptic such as cetrimide for treating bites. Also, the bedroom furniture should be disinfested.

Bedsore (known medically as decubitus ulcer) occurs in bedridden patients, the elderly or chronically ill, who are unable to move themselves and who have to lie in the same position for long periods of time.

Q: Where do bedsores form and what do they look like?

A: The parts of the body most likely to be affected are the pressure areas: the bone at the lower end of the spine (the sacrum), the buttocks, and the heels. The shoulder blades and elbows may also develop these sores. The area first becomes slightly red with cracked skin, which turns dark blue before ulcerating as dead tissues disintegrate.

Q: Can bedsores be prevented?

A: Yes. Patients who cannot move themselves must be moved every few hours so that the pressure areas are changed.

   Bedclothes must be kept clean, dry, and free from creases. Additional protection can be given to the pressure areas by using rubber rings, foam pads or, even better, real or artificial sheepskin.

Q: What is the treatment if an ulcer has formed?

A: The patient must not lie on the ulcer, and

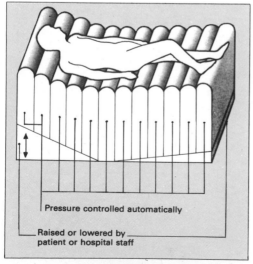

Bedsore problems in an incapacitated patient can be eliminated with a variable-pressure air bed.

this can be awkward. The ulcer should be cleansed with an antiseptic, such as hydrogen peroxide or cetrimide. There is some evidence that zinc salt tablets, in addition to vitamins, may aid recovery. The sores will heal, over a period of time, if they are carefully tended.

A talk about Bed-wetting

Bed-wetting (known medically as nocturnal enuresis) is a common problem of childhood, sometimes causing needless distress to parents and children. A calm, reassuring approach on the part of parents is the key factor in dealing with bed-wetting. Eventually, almost all children become dry.

Q: At what age does a child usually stop wetting the bed?

A: As the nervous system matures, the reflexes that control the bladder come under the voluntary control of the brain even while the child is asleep. This occurs at different ages in different children, but by the age of three or four most children are dry.

Q: What causes bed-wetting in an older child?

A: Usually the cause of such bed-wetting is emotional. In such a situation, it is wise to consult a doctor because the cause needs investigation. Some authorities state that the method by which a child is taught TOILET TRAINING is an important factor in bladder control at night.

   In some cases there is a physical cause. There may be a urinary infection, or there may be a structural defect in the urinary tract, present from birth. Rarely, there may be a disorder of the nerves that serve the urinary system.

Q: What should be done about bed-wetting?

A: The child should never be scolded or punished. The parents should be calm, rational, and understanding in dealing with the problem.

   The child should be given nothing to drink for about an hour or so before bedtime, and should empty the bladder just before going to bed. A doctor may be able to help by suggesting methods that other parents have found successful.

Bee sting (for EMERGENCY treatment, *see* First Aid, p.514) can have serious consequences in people who have an allergy to the bee's venom. Desensitizing injections may increase the time between a sting and the development of an allergic reaction, thus allowing more time for treatment. However, most people are not seriously allergic to bee venom and experience no serious complications from occasional bee stings.

The usual treatment is swabbing with an alkaline solution, such as sodium bicarbonate or dilute ammonia. Antihistamine drugs may be prescribed for severe cases. The sting may be removed with a pair of tweezers.

Behaviour therapy is a form of psychiatric treatment in which a patient's behaviour is modified by a system of rewards and punishments. This is usually used for individuals whose behaviour is socially unacceptable.

Belching, sometimes called burping, is the noisy emission of wind from the stomach via the oesophagus. It is common for babies to belch after a feeding, but adults also belch, especially if they have eaten too rapidly or taken carbonated drinks. Air swallowing (AEROPHAGIA) is a nervous habit that often results in belching.

Belladonna is an extract of the deadly nightshade plant. It contains ATROPINE, an alkaloid drug used in various forms to treat intestinal disorders and Parkinson's disease. It is also used in eye examinations to dilate the pupils. Large doses cause a dry mouth; an overdose may cause an excited, confused mental state and may have fatal consequences.

Bell's palsy is paralysis of the muscles of the face, caused by acute inflammation of, or damage to, the nerve that supplies them.

Paralysis usually occurs without apparent cause, although it may be associated with SHINGLES.

Q: *What are the symptoms of Bell's palsy?*

A: Facial features lose their symmetrical appearance, and the mouth droops at one corner. Paralysis of the muscles results in loss of control over saliva or tears, so that the patient may dribble or appear to cry.

Q: *What is the treatment for Bell's palsy?*

A: It is important that a doctor is consulted within 24 hours because immediate treatment with corticosteroid drugs may help. Many patients recover spontaneously; about 70 per cent recover completely within four to six weeks, and about 20 per cent make a partial recovery.

Bends, or caisson disease, is a disorder caused by the formation of nitrogen bubbles in the blood after a person changes too quickly from an environment of high atmospheric pressure to one at normal pressure. Symptoms of the bends include painful joints, tightness in the chest, vomiting, giddiness, abdominal pain, and visual disturbances. Sometimes the victim suffers from convulsions and paralysis may follow. In severe cases, the condition can be fatal.

Q: *How are the bends treated?*

A: The victim must be returned immediately to a high-pressure atmosphere, either at the original work site or in a recompression chamber. The patient is then brought back very slowly to normal atmospheric pressure. This allows enough time for the dissolved nitrogen to be safely reconverted to its normal gaseous form and breathed out via the lungs.

Q: *Can the bends cause permanent damage?*

A: Damage to the joints may leave permanent arthritis. The nervous system may also be damaged, causing paralysis or signs of a stroke.

Benign describes a condition that is usually nonrecurrent and seldom causes severe problems. It is the opposite of MALIGNANT.

See also TUMOUR.

Beriberi is a disease caused by a deficiency of vitamin B_1 in the diet. The disorder produces nerve degeneration (peripheral neuritis) and muscle disease (myopathy), particularly affecting heart muscle. Beriberi is commonly associated with alcoholism, because many alcoholics fail to eat a properly balanced diet.

Q: *What are the symptoms of beriberi?*

A: There are two kinds of beriberi, called dry and wet. Dry beriberi results in the loss of strength and of some feeling in the limbs due to nerve degeneration (neuritis). Wet beriberi is caused by accumulated fluid in the limbs (oedema) and in the abdomen (ascites) because of heart malfunction; neuritis is commonly present as well.

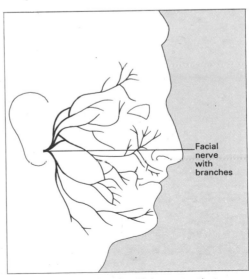

Bell's palsy, is a disorder of the nerve that controls the muscles of the face.

Beta-blockers

Q: *How is beriberi treated?*

A: Treatment with vitamin B$_1$ leads to rapid improvement of heart function, and reduction of the neuritis. Care should be taken to provide the patient with a more balanced diet.

Beta-blockers, or beta-adrenergic blocking agents, are drugs that act upon the sympathetic nervous system and reduce the stimuli that, under normal conditions, would cause an increase in both blood pressure and pulse rate. They are used in the treatment of high blood pressure and angina pectoris.

Biceps is a muscle with two heads. The biceps muscle of the upper arm (biceps brachii) is Y-shaped, the single muscle branching into two strands higher up. This muscle bends the arm at the elbow. The biceps muscle of the thigh (biceps femoris) flexes the knee.

Bile, or gall, is an alkaline liquid produced by the liver. The liquid is a dark yellow-green colour, and it contains CHOLESTEROL, bile salts, a dark orange pigment called bilirubin, some proteins, and urea. It passes down the common bile duct to enter the duodenum (the first part of the intestine). A branch joins the bile duct to the GALL BLADDER, in which bile can be stored until it is needed.

Q: *Why is bile needed?*

A: Bile helps to break down fats in food so that they can be absorbed, and it helps to neutralize the acidity of the stomach contents when they reach the duodenum. The presence of fats in the duodenum causes the release of a hormone that stimulates the contraction of the gall bladder and the production of bile.

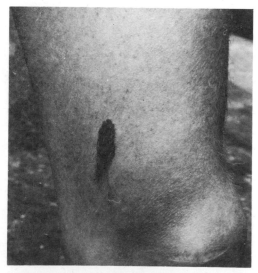

Birthmark of the common, small type needs no treatment unless it causes embarrassment.

Q: *Are there any bile disorders?*

A: The most familiar is obstructive JAUNDICE, in which a blockage of the bile ducts causes bilirubin to circulate in the blood, giving the skin a characteristic yellow colour.

  See also BILIARY COLIC; CHOLECYSTITIS; GALLSTONE.

Bilharzia is another name for the parasitic disease schistosomiasis. *See* SCHISTOSOMIASIS.

Biliary colic is an extremely severe pain in the upper right-hand part of the abdomen. The pain, which comes and goes, is often accompanied by sweating and vomiting. It is the result of a spasm of the gall bladder or of obstruction of the bile ducts, either of which is caused by one or more gallstones.

Q: *What is the treatment for biliary colic?*

A: Injections of antispasmodic drugs reduce the pain, which usually ceases altogether when the gallstone passes into the duodenum or lodges at the side of the bile duct. An X-ray of the biliary system is taken and the gallstone (and bladder if it is diseased) are removed by an operation.

Biopsy is the removal of a small piece of tissue for the purpose of examining it under a microscope to see whether disease is present.

  There are several ways in which a biopsy can be performed: (1) through a small cut in the skin; (2) by a tube passed through the mouth into the intestine to remove a small piece of intestinal lining; (3) through an instrument such as a sigmoidoscope or cystoscope; or (4) with a special needle to reach the liver or kidney.

Biotin, also known as vitamin H, is one of the VITAMINS of the vitamin B complex. It is found in many foods, but particularly rich sources are liver, kidney, milk, egg yolks, and yeast. Biotin deficiency occurs only in association with deficiency of others of the vitamin B group.

Birth control. *See* CONTRACEPTION.

Birth defects. *See* CONGENITAL ANOMALIES.

Birthmark, or naevus, is a blemish on the skin that is present at birth. Birthmarks do not usually cause problems, although there are some abnormal marks that may be a major cosmetic problem.

Q: *What are the main types of birthmarks?*

A: The most common birthmark is a simple skin discoloration (naevus pigmentosus), which may be any colour from light yellow to black. A mole is typical of this type of birthmark. It does not need treatment, unless it is irritated by clothing or is disfiguring.

  Rarer types of birthmarks are generally the result of having a cluster of blood vessels just below the surface of the skin.

Typical of this type is the strawberry naevus. It is a slightly raised reddish or purplish mark that appears most often on the face, head, neck, or arms. It grows rapidly for the first year after birth and then decreases in size. In most children it disappears by the age of five.

A port-wine stain is a complex, flat birthmark. It does not disappear but grows in proportion with the rest of the body. Like a strawberry naevus, it is caused by expanded blood vessels below the surface of the skin.

Q: Why should some birthmarks be removed?

A: If birthmarks of the port-wine stain type are large enough or serious enough to cause danger in case of injury, they may be removed by plastic surgery. In many cases, removal of a birthmark is not medically advised, but cosmetics can be used to reduce any embarrassment that the blemish might cause.

Bites (for EMERGENCY treatment, *see* First Aid, p.544), are punctures or other wounds on the skin caused by animals. The most common bites are those of dogs, snakes, spiders, and various insects. Most bites require only thorough cleansing with an antiseptic and dressing with a small bandage, if necessary. But some bites are serious (such as the bite of the black widow spider) and require specialized medical treatment.

See also RABIES; STING.

Black death is an old name for BUBONIC PLAGUE.

Black eye is a swollen bruise of the eyelids and eye socket. It is usually caused by direct injury, or it may be the result of a fractured skull. The dark colour of the skin results from the escape of blood into the eye socket and the thin tissue surrounding it. The blood tends to drain into the upper eyelid, which may bc difficult to open. It may also spread down the cheek. Cold packs applied with pressure as soon as possible after the injury cause the damaged blood vessels to contract, and reduce the swelling.

Blackhead, or comedo, is a plug of hardened secretion in the duct of an oil gland in the skin.

Black lung is the common name for the lung disorder anthracosis. The normal pink colour of the lungs is turned black by coal dust or smoke that is inhaled. Once a common disorder only among coal miners, anthracosis is now also found in city dwellers.

Q: What are the symptoms of anthracosis?

A: In the early stages the symptoms resemble those of bronchitis, with coughing and shortness of breath. If the cause is not removed, over a period of years the symptoms gradually get worse. Diagnosis is confirmed by an X-ray examination.

Q: What is the treatment for anthracosis?

A: The lung damage caused by the inhaled dust cannot be repaired, nor can it be treated directly. Breathing clean air halts the progress of the disease and may help to reduce the severity of the symptoms.

Blackout (for EMERGENCY treatment *see* First Aid, p.544) is a temporary loss of consciousness. It is most commonly a condition of FAINTING but may also occur during an epileptic seizure, during a mild stroke, or following heavy drinking.

Bladder is a hollow body structure that collects and stores urine. It is a strong, muscular organ that receives urine from the kidneys, and releases it to be passed out of the body through a tube called the urethra.

Q: How much liquid does the bladder hold?

A: In most adults, the bladder holds a little more than 475ml (one pint) of urine. This quantity may be much greater as a result of certain BLADDER DISORDERS. Between 1.2 and 1.4 litres (2½ and 3 pints) of urine are usually excreted each day.

Q: Is the bladder in a child weaker than in an adult?

A: No, but a child's bladder is smaller, and he or she often feels nervous when the bladder is full.

Bladder disorders. The following table lists some common disorders that affect the bladder, grouped according to their chief symptoms. The symptoms may also indicate other clinical disorders; this is not a complete list. A good medical history and physical

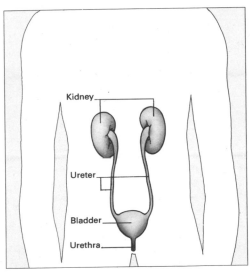

Bladder collects urine from the kidneys, before passing it out through the urethra.

Bland diet

examination by a doctor are essential for adequate diagnosis. Each disorder has a separate article in the A-Z section of this book.

Symptom	Disorder
Blood in the urine	CALCULUS (a stone in the kidney, ureter, or bladder)
	CYSTITIS (bladder inflammation)
	TUBERCULOSIS
	TUMOUR
Difficult urination	PROSTATE PROBLEMS
	STROKE (nerve damage affecting bladder control)
Frequent urination	CYSTITIS (bladder inflammation)
	DIABETES (glucose in urine; thirst)
	FIBROIDS (benign tumours in the womb)
	PROSTATE PROBLEMS
	STRESS INCONTINENCE
	STROKE (nerve damage affecting bladder control)
Painful urination	CALCULUS (a stone in the bladder)
	CYSTITIS (bladder inflammation)
	PROSTATE PROBLEMS
	URETHRITIS (inflammation of urinary tube)

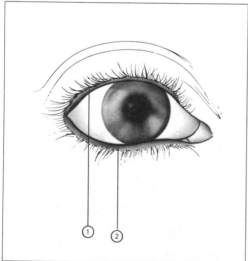

Blepharitis is inflammation of the eyelash follicles on both rims (1, 2) of the eyelid.

Bland diet is a non-irritating diet of foods such as milk, eggs, chicken, and fish, with little or no salt or spices and minimal roughage. A doctor may recommend a bland diet for a patient who is suffering or recovering from a gastrointestinal disorder.

Blastomycosis is a rare infection caused by a fungus. The infection occurs in the lungs causing a slow form of PNEUMONIA with pleurisy.

Bleeding (for EMERGENCY treatment, see First Aid, p.516) occurs from a broken blood vessel as in a cut or other wound, or from internal haemorrhaging (*see* HAEMORRHAGE). Blood in mucus that is coughed up, in vomit, or in the stools could be a symptom of an internal disorder, and should be reported to a doctor. *See* BLOOD, SPITTING OF; BLOOD, VOMITING OF; HAEMORRHOID.

Blepharitis is a disorder affecting the eyelids. Redness and inflammation of the eyelids, soreness, and stickiness are all symptoms. If the lids are infected, a STYE (an infected swelling of a hair follicle) may appear. The cause of blepharitis is often unknown, although it is sometimes the result of an allergy to dust, smoke, irritating chemicals, or even a particular cosmetic.

Q: *What is the treatment for blepharitis?*
A: The eyelids should be cleansed regularly with a warm solution of salt water. A mild antiseptic may be applied to the rims. A doctor may prescribe antibiotic or corticosteroid drugs, but continued treatment with these may cause a skin allergy.

Blindness is the loss of vision in one or both eyes. It may be present at birth, or it may occur suddenly in one or both eyes at a later stage in life. Commonly blindness involves a gradual deterioration of vision until the stage when no sight remains. It may be caused by various disorders affecting the eye itself, or may result from a disorder of the visual centre of the brain. The medical term for blindness in which the eye appears to be normal is amaurosis. Temporary blindness, commonly called a blackout, can occur with some minor disorders, such as fainting.

Q: *Why are some babies born blind?*
A: Congenital blindness is sometimes caused by infection of the mother by German measles (rubella) at some time during the first three months of pregnancy. The disease causes the lenses in the baby's eyes to be opaque. Other causes of congenital blindness are defects in the formation of the eye and various metabolic disorders.

Q: *What are the causes of gradual blindness?*
A: Any of the following disorders may cause

gradual blindness: pressure within the eyeball (GLAUCOMA); the formation of opaque patches in the eye lens (CATARACT); a retina damaged as a result of high blood pressure (hypertension), diabetes, or degenerative disease of the retina; pressure on the optic nerve from a tumour (for example, pituitary gland ADENOMA); or recurrent ulcers on the cornea, which may be caused by a form of conjunctivitis (TRACHOMA) common in the tropics. Treatment of the cause usually arrests the condition and, in some cases, may restore sight.

Q: *What causes sudden blindness?*

A: The retina, the part of the eye on to which light rays are focused, may become detached from the layer enclosing it (the choroid), and blindness can result. This retinal detachment may be caused by an accidental blow to the eye, or it may occur spontaneously in people with the vision defect myopia. Bleeding behind the retina or inflammation of the optic nerve (RETROBULBAR NEURITIS) may cause blindness in one eye. A blocked vein or artery supplying the eye can also result in sudden blindness.

   Sudden blindness in one eye occurs much more frequently than sudden blindness in both. Blindness occurring suddenly in both eyes is usually caused by a stroke that affects the visual centre of the brain.

Q: *What causes temporary blindness?*

A: Temporary blindness may be caused by a spasm of the arteries during a bad migraine headache, by high blood pressure (hypertension), by low blood pressure that precedes fainting, or by a small blood clot (embolus) which is passing through an artery that serves the eye.

Q: *How can a blind person lead a normal life?*

A: Family and friends should encourage the blind patient to make use of all available resources in making the adjustment to being blind. The patient can learn braille, and discussions with those who are already blind can help the patient to cope with fears and worry. For cases of total blindness, aids such as a white cane, guide dogs, talking books and other electronic machines can help to reassure a person that independence can be maintained. For those who are born blind, special schools are available for education and training.

   See also AMAUROSIS; COLOUR BLINDNESS; NIGHT BLINDNESS.

Blister is a raised area on the skin that contains fluid derived from blood serum. It generally forms as a result of skin irritation, from rubbing, or from pinching. Excessive heat also causes blistering. A blood blister is a purplish area beneath the skin caused by the bursting of blood vessels.

Q: *What is the best treatment for blisters?*

A: Normal blisters are most effectively treated by applying a mild antiseptic cream and by covering them with a clean, dry pad to prevent further rubbing. If a blister bursts, it should be kept as clean as possible with an antiseptic solution. A blood blister is best wrapped in a firm dressing with a little pressure, to prevent further bursting of blood vessels.

Blood is the body's "transportation system", the medium that carries oxygen and essential nutrients to all parts of the body. It also carries waste products, such as carbon dioxide, to the organs that eliminate them from the body.

Q: *What else does blood do?*

A: Heat from inner parts of the body is carried in the blood to the skin to keep the temperature of the body stable. The blood also carries defences against infection (antibodies) to all body tissues, and transports vital chemicals and hormones that are used in the control of body functions. (*See* ANTIBODY.)

Q: *How much blood does the body contain?*

A: In an adult of average size there is a little less than 4.7 litres (10 pints). The heart pumps about 4.2 litres (9 pints) a minute when the body is at rest.

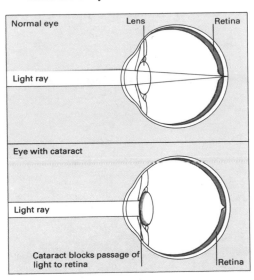

Normal eye — Lens — Retina — Light ray

Eye with cataract — Light ray — Cataract blocks passage of light to retina — Retina

Blindness may be caused by a cataract or by disorder of the retina.

Blood, spitting of

Q: *What is the composition of blood?*

A: A straw-coloured fluid called PLASMA makes up more than half the volume of the blood. Plasma carries red blood cells, white blood cells, blood platelets (essential for clotting), and fat globules. Various chemicals, hormones, proteins, and some gases are also present and are carried either in suspension or dissolved in the fluid. Normal blood is about 78 per cent water and 22 per cent solids.

See also BLOOD DISORDERS; BLOOD GROUPS; BLOOD PRESSURE; p.8.

Blood, spitting of (known medically as haemoptysis), is a symptom of bleeding somewhere in the respiratory tract. Blood may come from the nose, mouth, or throat (upper respiratory passages), the lower respiratory passages, or the lungs. The seriousness of the disorder depends on the cause.

Q: *What can cause the spitting of blood from the upper respiratory passages?*

A: The most common and least serious reason for blood in the sputum (the substance spat out) is that coughing has ruptured a small blood vessel in the mouth or throat. Any infection or damage in the mouth, throat, or back of the nose may also cause bleeding.

Q: *What causes the spitting of blood from the lower respiratory passages?*

A: Bleeding from this region is caused by damage or infection in the trachea (windpipe) or the bronchi (tubes to the lungs). If a bronchus has been subjected to repeated infection, scarring causes deformity that prevents mucous secretions from draining properly, causing bleeding. Damage to a bronchus from breathing in a foreign body, such as a peanut or piece of bread, also causes spitting of blood.

Q: *What causes bleeding from the lungs?*

A: Spitting of blood derived from the lungs may be the first symptom of lung cancer. An inefficiently functioning heart may cause congestion of blood in the lungs, resulting in a bright pink froth at the mouth. Certain other disorders, for example, PNEUMOCONIOSIS, result in a fine, general scarring of the lungs and also cause the spitting of blood.

Q: *When is medical treatment necessary?*

A: A small amount of blood in the saliva should not be cause for alarm. In most cases of haemoptysis, the cause is either obvious or can be easily explained. The unexpected coughing up of blood can be serious, and if the reason is not already known, a doctor should be consulted.

Blood, vomiting of (known medically as haematemesis), is a condition that can be serious. Acid in the stomach makes the colour of the blood dark, often black. For this reason vomited blood is sometimes described as "coffee grounds".

Q: *What causes vomiting of blood?*

A: The most frequent, and least serious, cause is blood that has been swallowed during a nosebleed. Another common cause of vomiting blood is acute gastritis that occurs after excessive alcohol intake or following a virus infection.

Vomiting blood is more serious if it involves bleeding from a PEPTIC ULCER in the stomach or duodenum, or cancer of the stomach. The vomiting of blood is only rarely associated with haemophilia, leukaemia, or other BLOOD DISORDERS.

Q: *What treatment can be given to someone who repeatedly vomits blood?*

A: The person should lie down. Cover him or her with a blanket or coat to treat for shock. Call a doctor or take the patient to hospital immediately.

Blood blister. *See* BLISTER.

Blood clot is a jelly-like mass of congealed blood. Clotting is the normal way the body stops bleeding and begins healing following injury. It involves complex chemical reactions between many substances that are present in the blood plasma. Absence of one of these substances results in the disorder HAEMOPHILIA. A clot in a blood vessel is called a thrombus.

Q: *When might a blood clot be harmful?*

A: A blood clot can block an artery or vein and stop the flow of blood (THROMBOSIS). Cerebral thrombosis is a blood clot in an

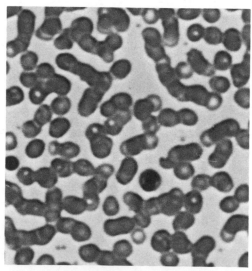

Blood contains microscopic cells of many varieties, as shown by this photomicrograph.

artery to the brain, which can cause a stroke. Thrombosis can occur in a leg or pelvic vein (deep vein thrombosis). If this clot dislodges and enters the bloodstream, it may block an artery in the lungs (pulmonary embolus).

Q: *Are some people more susceptible to blood clots than others?*

A: Patients with ARTERIOSCLEROSIS are more likely to get blood clots because the inner walls of the blood vessels are irregular. Blood clotting also occurs more easily if the circulation is slow, a condition in those with varicose veins. Other factors which increase the likelihood of blood clots are major injury to the body, the prolonged use of certain drugs such as birth control pills (*see* CONTRACEPTION), smoking, and prolonged bed rest.

Blood disorders. Disorders of the blood are generally categorized by doctors according to the nature of the complaint. There are (1) disorders of blood production; (2) disorders within the blood cells; (3) infections in the blood; and (4) disorders of the blood clotting mechanism.

The following table lists the most common disorders that are caused by blood disease or malfunction. The basic characteristic cited is not intended to denote symptoms, however, but to inform the reader who has heard the name of one of these disorders as to exactly what that condition means with respect to one of the above categories.

(Hodgkin's disease and lymphosarcoma are often considered to be blood disorders but are in fact more accurately regarded as disorders of the lymphatic system.)

Of the conditions listed below, most are serious and require immediate medical treatment. However, many characteristics cited here may also be indicative of some other clinical disorder. A good medical history and physical examination by a doctor are essential for adequate diagnosis of a problem. Each disorder listed here has a separate article in the A-Z section of this book.

Disorder	Basic characteristic
AGRANULOCYTOSIS	Reduced production of white blood cells
ANAEMIA	Reduced production or loss of red blood cells
BLOOD POISONING	Infection of blood stream by bacteria
CHRISTMAS DISEASE	Defective blood clotting
GLANDULAR FEVER (Mononucleosis)	Excess of large white blood cells
HAEMOPHILIA	Defective blood clotting
LEUKAEMIA	Uncontrolled and disorderly increase of white blood cells

Disorder	Basic characteristic
MALARIA	Parasitic infestation of red blood cells
MYELOMA	Cancer of the bone marrow
POLYCYTHAEMIA	Excessive production of red blood cells
PURPURA	Bleeding under the skin
SICKLE CELL ANAEMIA	Deformity of red blood cells in which the cells take on a sickle shape
THALASSAEMIA	Deformity of red blood cells
THROMBOCYTOPAENIA	Decreased production of blood platelets

Blood groups, or blood types, are classified according to the presence in the blood of particular antigens or proteins. A knowledge of a person's blood group is important when a blood transfusion is necessary, and in preventing problems with newborn children. There are various systems of blood grouping; the two most important are the ABO system and the Rhesus (Rh) system.

Q: *What is the ABO system?*

A: The ABO system distinguishes four blood groups: A, B, AB, and O. All blood can be classified in one of these groups. Group A blood contains proteins that react against the proteins of the red blood cells from group B or group AB. If a patient of group A is given a transfusion of group B or group AB blood, a serious reaction occurs. The situation is identical for group B blood with respect to A or AB transfusions.

Q: *What is the Rh factor?*

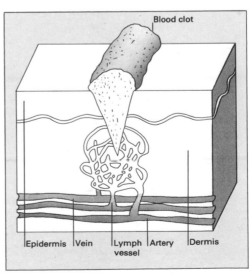

Blood clots form when blood contacts air or fluid from injured tissue.

Blood poisoning

A: The Rhesus system defines two blood types: blood in which the Rh factor is present (Rhesus positive, or Rh+), and that in which it is not (Rhesus negative, or Rh−). In Western countries, about 85 per cent of people are Rh+. See HAEMOLYTIC DISEASE OF THE NEWBORN; RH FACTOR.

The Rhesus system and the ABO bear no correlation whatsoever with each other, but for the sake of clarity the ABO and Rhesus classifications are generally combined when stating a blood group (for example, A+, O−, etc.).

Q: *Is one blood group more common than the others?*

A: Yes. Recent statistics show the following world incidence of blood groups: group O, 46%; A, 42%; B, 8%; AB 4%.

Blood poisoning (also called septicaemia or bacteraemia) is the presence of bacterial infection in the bloodstream. Once infection has arisen in the blood, it may increase locally or be carried with the blood to other parts of the body (*see also* TOXAEMIA). Frequent, intermittent high fever, shivering attacks, and occasionally red streaks leading from a wound and a rash are all symptoms. In extreme cases, abscesses may appear throughout the body, both on the skin and in internal organs such as the liver or brain (*see* PYAEMIA). Severe blood poisoning may be fatal if hospital treatment is delayed.

Blood pressure is a measure of the pressure exerted on the wall of any blood vessel, although it is generally recorded for an artery. Two measurements are taken, the highest and lowest values for pressure, which correspond to the two main stages in the pumping action of the heart.

Q: *How is blood pressure measured?*

A: Blood pressure is usually measured by an instrument called a sphygmomanometer. To measure the pressure, an inflatable cuff is placed around the patient's upper arm and a stethoscope is applied to the artery just below the cuff. By listening for changes in the sound of the pulse, a doctor knows how much to inflate the cuff to stop blood flowing in the arteries in the arm. Air is slowly let out of the cuff until the blood just starts flowing again. At this stage, the sphygmomanometer records what is called the systolic blood pressure. Further air is let out of the cuff until the sounds become muffled. The instrument then indicates the diastolic pressure. The higher, systolic pressure corresponds to the contraction of the heart muscle, and the diastolic pressure corresponds to relaxation of the heart. The two pressures are expressed in the following way: 120/80.

Q: *What is considered a normal blood pressure reading?*

A: A healthy (normal) blood pressure reading varies with age, activity, and altitude, and from person to person. Bearing in mind these qualifications, values between 100/60 and 145/90 are generally considered normal.

Q: *Are there any disorders that cause blood pressure to rise?*

A: HIGH BLOOD PRESSURE, also called hypertension, is itself a major disorder that requires treatment.

There are several other serious disorders that cause blood pressure to rise well above the normal level.

Q: *What causes low blood pressure?*

A: LOW BLOOD PRESSURE (hypotension) can result from shock and some diseases. It can cause FAINTING.

Blood transfusion is the transference of blood from one person to another. A patient is usually given a transfusion using blood supplied by a blood bank, where the blood has been stored under refrigeration after collection from the donor. Usually in a transfusion, the blood is allowed to flow slowly by gravity into a vein in the patient's arm.

Q: *When is a transfusion necessary?*

A: A transfusion may be carried out because a patient is extremely anaemic, either as a result of disease or from a loss of blood through bleeding. A transfusion may also be considered necessary in the treatment of acute shock.

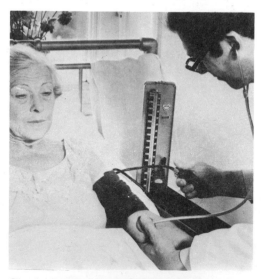

Blood pressure is measured by a piece of apparatus called a sphygmomanometer.

Q: Can a person's blood be completely replaced by a transfusion?

A: Yes. This type of transfusion (exchange transfusion) is sometimes necessary in newborn babies. *See* HAEMOLYTIC DISEASE OF THE NEWBORN.

Q: What precautions are taken before transfusing blood?

A: The blood of the donor must be tested to ensure that it is not anaemic, nor infected with hepatitis, malaria, or syphilis. A sample of the donor's blood is mixed (crossmatched) with a sample of the recipient's blood beforehand to make sure that the BLOOD GROUPS are compatible.

Blue baby is a baby born with a congenital heart defect that causes a bluish tinge to the skin. Because of the heart defect, some blood bypasses the lungs and thus misses the normal oxygenation process. Any complication in breathing makes the bluish tinge darker. In many cases, blue babies can be treated by surgery.

See also CONGENITAL HEART DISEASE.

Blurred vision is a common eye disorder. Frequently it is caused by longsightedness, shortsightedness, or astigmatism, all of which can be corrected by eyeglasses or contact lenses. In the elderly, the gradual onset of blurred vision can be caused by a cloudiness in the eye lens (cataract) or degeneration of the retina at the back of the eye.

Q: What can cause sudden blurred vision?

A: There are several possibilities, all of which should be considered by an eye specialist. Conjunctivitis is one of the most common. There are other more serious possible causes, including iritis or glaucoma, in which there is abnormally high fluid pressure inside the eyeball. Some drugs, including alcohol, also cause blurred vision.

Any case of persistent blurred vision should be discussed with a doctor.

Body odour. *See* BROMHIDROSIS.

Body temperature, even in a healthy person, varies slightly during the course of the day. It is lowest early in the morning and highest later in the afternoon. The highest "normal" temperature, taken using a thermometer placed in the mouth, is generally accepted as being 37°C (98.6°F). The temperature taken in the rectum is more accurate, but tends to be about 0.5°C (1°F) higher than the mouth temperature. The least accurate temperatures are those taken in the armpit or groin.

Q: What can cause variations in normal body temperature?

A: An unexpected variation in body temperature may be a sign of illness (*see* FEVER; HYPOTHERMIA), or may merely reflect normal changes taking place in the body. Children have a wider range, so a physically active day may raise their temperatures a degree or so above normal without any sign of illness.

Between puberty and the menopause, women experience a rise in body temperature midway through the menstrual cycle when ovulation takes place. This higher temperature continues as the basic normal one until menstruation. Such temperature measurement can be used to time the occurrence of ovulation and improve the chances of conception in a woman who wants to have a baby.

Boils, also called furuncles, are infections of the hair roots or sweat glands caused by the STAPHYLOCOCCUS bacteria. They commonly occur in the armpit, on the back of the neck, in the groin, or on the buttocks, but can appear elsewhere. A red, painful lump forms that gradually grows bigger and then breaks down to form pus in the centre. The pus normally discharges spontaneously. Sometimes a series of boils may appear.

See also ABSCESS.

Bone is the hard, rigid tissue that forms the body's skeleton. It supports the body and surrounds and protects its internal structures. Bone is made of tough fibres embedded with calcium-containing salts, which make up 95 per cent of its substance. Usually hollow, bone acts as a storage place for calcium and the soft, blood-forming tissue called marrow.

See also BONE DISORDERS.

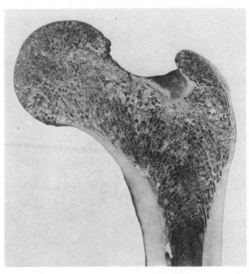

Bone is honeycombed in specific directions for maximum strength, as in the femur.

Bone disorders

Bone disorders. The following table lists disorders that affect bones, grouped according to cause. Each has a separate article in the A-Z section of this book.

Cause	Possible disorder
Congenital (present at birth)	OSTEOGENESIS IMPERFECTA (abnormally fragile bones)
Hormone imbalance	ACHONDROPLASIA (dwarfism caused by lack of growth hormone)
	OSTEOPOROSIS (softening of bone commonly following the menopause)
Infection	OSTEOMYELITIS (infection of bone)
Physical damage	FRACTURE (broken bone)
	PAGET'S DISEASE OF BONE (bone deformity of unknown cause)
Tumour	OSTEOMA (non-malignant tumour of bone)
	OSTEOSARCOMA (malignant tumour)
Vitamin deficiency	OSTEOMALACIA (bone softening in adults due to lack of calcium caused by vitamin D deficiency)
	RICKETS (bone softening in children due to lack of calcium caused by vitamin D deficiency)

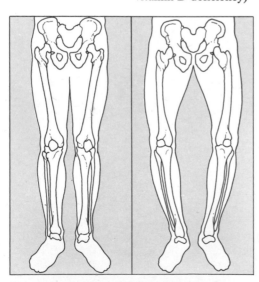

Bow-legs (right), a natural or bone condition, contrasted with normal legs (left).

Booster shot is an additional injection given some time after an initial injection to maintain a person's immunity to a disease. *See* IMMUNIZATION.

Bornholm disease is a name for epidemic pleurodynia. *See* PLEURODYNIA, EPIDEMIC.

Botulism is a rare, severe form of food poisoning. It occurs when food that contains a toxin produced by the organism *Clostridium botulinum* is eaten. Disturbances in vision and general weakness are the most common initial symptoms. Nausea, abdominal pain and diarrhoea also occur. The toxin attacks the central nervous system.

Prompt medical treatment is essential, because the disease develops rapidly and has a high mortality rate.

See also FOOD POISONING.

Bougie is a slender cylindrical instrument used for dilating body passages or canals such as the urethra.

Bowels is the popular name for the intestines. *See* INTESTINE.

Bow-legs (or genu varum) are legs that curve outward, so that when the feet are together there is a gap between the knees. Babies often have bow-legs when they begin to walk. The curvature corrects itself gradually, although sometimes over-compensation in the young child produces knock-knees (genu valgum), the inward curving of the legs at the knees.

By the age of 4 to 5 years, a child's legs normally become straight.

Q: Can older people develop bow-legs?

A: Yes. Legs that become bowed later in life may be caused by softening of the bones (OSTEOMALACIA or, in children, RICKETS) or, in elderly people, by PAGET'S DISEASE OF BONE and OSTEOARTHRITIS.

Brace is a support, made of metal and other materials, that is used in treating certain growth disorders. Children's teeth are commonly fitted with braces during the growing stage of the jaw to correct any developing irregularities.

Bradycardia is a slow pulse rate. As a medical disorder, bradycardia frequently follows virus illness such as influenza or infectious hepatitis. Bradycardia also occurs with the underactive thyroid disorder myxoedema, and with heartblock.

Braille is a system of writing or printing for the blind that uses tangible raised dots.

Brain is the large soft mass of nervous tissue enclosed by the skull that regulates and coordinates body activities. It is the primary part of the complicated and refined central nervous system, that controls all the actions of the body, voluntary, involuntary, and reflex. The central nervous system also includes the spinal cord. The largest part of the brain, the CEREBRUM, is the centre for voluntary muscular activity, for sensation, and for the highest mental functions as well as for innate instincts. The CEREBELLUM, at the back of the brain, is the centre that co-ordinates movements. Vital functions such as breathing, blood pressure, and hunger are controlled by the HYPOTHALAMUS.

See also p.18.

Brain disorders. The following table lists some disorders that affect the brain, along with basic characteristics of each condition. Each has a separate entry in the A-Z section of this book.

Disorder	Basic characteristic
ABSCESS	Collection of pus in brain tissue
ALZHEIMER'S DISEASE	Premature aging of brain cells, occurring in the middle aged
ANOXIA	Oxygen starvation to the brain during childbirth
BLOOD CLOT	Subdural haematoma pressing on brain
CEREBRAL HAEMORRHAGE	Rupture of blood vessel in brain
COMA	Prolonged unconsciousness
CONCUSSION	Temporary confusion following a blow to the head
DOWN'S SYNDROME (Mongolism)	Mental retardation that also produces Mongoloid features
ENCEPHALITIS	Inflammation of the brain by viral infection
EPILEPSY	Convulsions with or without loss of consciousness
GERMAN MEASLES (in pregnancy)	Possible mental retardation of the newborn
GLIOMA	Malignant tumour of the brain
HYDROCEPHALUS	Abnormal accumulation of cerebrospinal fluid within the skull, causing possible retardation
MENINGIOMA	Non-malignant tumour of the brain
MENINGITIS	Inflammation of the membranes that surround the brain
MULTIPLE SCLEROSIS	Destruction of material coating the nerves; poor muscle movement and co-ordination

Disorder	Basic characteristic
SPINA BIFIDA	Incomplete development of the vertebrae
STROKE	Rupture of blood vessel in brain or blockage of blood vessel to brain
SYPHILIS (final stage of infection)	Paralysis, loss of sense of position and balance
VITAMIN B DEFICIENCY	Temporary degeneration

Breakbone fever. *See* DENGUE.

Breast is the front of the chest. The same term is used, in the plural, to describe the mammary glands in women. Breast development is one of the secondary sexual characteristics that distinguish women from men. The function of breasts is to produce milk after childbirth to feed the baby. Each breast in an adult female contains 15 to 20 milk glands or lobes (surrounded by fatty tissue), each of which contains a duct (lactiferous sinus) that leads to the nipple. Breasts develop in girls at the onset of puberty in response to hormones produced by the ovaries and the pituitary gland. *See* ADOLESCENCE.

Q: Is it normal for one breast to be slightly larger than the other?

A: Yes. The difference is partly caused by a variation in the size of the underlying muscles that supply the shoulder. The muscles tend to be larger on the dominant side (for example, the right side of a right-handed person).

Q: When do the breasts produce milk?

A: Milk production is a response to special

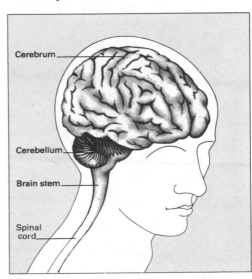

Brain is the controlling area for the entire nervous system.

105

hormones that are produced at the end of pregnancy. The start of milk production in the breasts coincides with the birth of the baby. Early milk is a thin white fluid (colostrum) that differs in composition from normal breast milk that is secreted later. *See* PREGNANCY AND CHILDBIRTH.

Q: *Do males ever grow female-type breasts?*

A: Such a condition (GYNAECOMASTIA) may occur in adolescent boys. A boy should be reassured that the condition will last only for three or four months. In an adult male, hormone imbalance or disease may cause female characteristics.

Q: *Is it natural for the breasts at times to feel different and change in size?*

A: Such changes accompany different stages of the menstrual cycle. Before menstruation, the breasts may feel "tight" and congested; some pain may be experienced, often accompanied by a tingling sensation in the nipples. These changes settle down as soon as the menstrual period begins.

Q: *Why do some women have bigger breasts than others?*

A: Differences in breast size and shape are largely due to inherited factors. Being overweight increases the size of the breasts with extra fatty tissue.

Breastbone, or sternum, is the central, vertical bone down the centre of the chest, to which most of the ribs are attached.

Breast disorders. The following table lists some disorders that can affect the female breast, and the basic characteristic of each condition. It should be noted that most lumps in the breast are benign (noncancerous) and respond rapidly to treatment. But if a woman does develop such a lump, she should consult a doctor as soon as possible. (*See also* PALPATION.) Hormonal changes caused by the menstrual cycle or taking birth control pills may cause breast pain or tenderness. (*See* CONTRACEPTION.) Each disorder listed here has a separate article in the A-Z section.

Disorder	Basic characteristic
ABSCESS of breast	Inflammation or rash
ADENOMA	Nonmalignant fibrous growth
CANCER of breast	Malignant tumour
CYST	Nonmalignant growth of tissue
MASTITIS	Inflammation
PAGET'S DISEASE OF THE NIPPLE	Inflammation of areola and nipple

Breast examination. *See* PALPATION.

Breast pump is a small suction device that helps to draw milk from a mother's breast if her baby cannot suckle efficiently. It may be made of plastic or glass and may be operated by hand or by electricity. A mother may need to use a breast pump if a distended breast causes pain, or if a baby has a cleft palate or is premature and therefore unable to suck efficiently.

Breath, bad. *See* BAD BREATH

Breathalyzer is an apparatus that is used to analyze exhaled air. The best known breathalyzer is the one used by civil authorities to ascertain whether or not the alcohol content of a motorist's blood is within the legal maximum. One simple type of breathalyzer is a tube containing bichromate crystals that change colour when alcohol-rich air is blown through them. A more complicated type used to measure basal metabolic rate analyzes exhaled air electronically.

Breath-holding attack occurs when a child stops breathing during a period of severe crying or in anger (*see* TEMPER TANTRUM). Such attacks occur most commonly in children between the ages of one and four years. An attack is preceded by a cry or wail, after which the breath may be held for as long as 20 to 30 seconds. The child may turn blue in the face and fall to the ground as if unconscious, making occasional convulsive movements. After recovery, the child may be confused for a further 10 to 15 seconds.

Q: *Is a breath-holding attack serious?*

A: Although these attacks are frightening to witness, they are not serious.

Breathing. *See* RESPIRATION.

Breathing disorders. *See* LUNG DISORDERS.

Breathlessness, known medically as dyspnoea, is a normal reaction to greater than usual exertion.

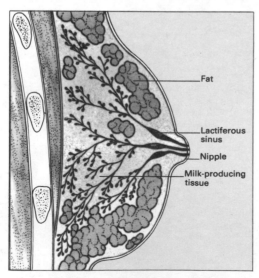

Breast disorders can affect any part of the milk-producing tissue and related breast structures.

Fat

Lactiferous sinus

Nipple

Milk-producing tissue

The normal result of physical exercise is an increase in the amount of carbon dioxide in the blood. Breathing rate automatically increases to get rid of the carbon dioxide through the lungs.

A wide range of lung disorders can be responsible for breathlessness, such as asthma, or pneumonia.

People with heart disorders often have difficulty with breathing. A moderate degree of anaemia also causes shortness of breath after exercise.

Breech birth is the delivery of a baby buttocks or feet first, rather than head first. *See* PREGNANCY AND CHILDBIRTH.

Brodie's abscess is an area of bone infection filled with pus, usually found in one of the long bones of the arm or the leg. *See* OSTEOMYELITIS.

Bromhidrosis is the medical name for body odour. An offensive smell is caused by the breaking down of stale sweat by bacteria on the skin. Sweat, especially in the armpits and groins, mixes with dead skin cells and decomposes. The odour produced varies from one person to another and depends also on the diet. Treatment is a daily bath or shower and a change of underwear, plus the use of an ANTIPERSPIRANT or DEODORANT.

Bronchial dilators are drugs that widen the airways to the lungs. They enlarge the bronchi and so improve the breathing of patients with bronchial asthma and other chronic chest disorders such as emphysema and bronchitis. Depending on the specific preparation, bronchial dilators may also increase the blood pressure, and the heart rate, and stimulate the respiratory centre in the brain.

Bronchial pneumonia, also called bronchopneumonia, is an infection of the lungs. This type of PNEUMONIA is localized mainly in the smaller branches of the bronchial tubes, called the bronchioles.

Bronchial pneumonia can be caused by the pneumoccocus or certain other bacteria or by viruses. The bronchioles become inflamed as they clog with pus and mucus, resulting in one or more of the following symptoms: coughing, chest pain, fever, blood-streaked sputum, chills, and difficulty in breathing.

Treatment is with antibiotic drugs and bed rest. Hospitalization is recommended for many patients, because special tests are necessary for complete diagnosis.

Bronchiectasis is a chronic disorder of the bronchi and bronchioles, the tubes that carry air in and out of the lungs. The tubes become weakened and stretched, and do not allow normal drainage of fluid secretions from the lungs. This inelasticity of the bronchi may result from an infection, following collapse of the lung (atelectasis), or be an abnormality present at birth.

Q: What are the symptoms of bronchiectasis?

A: Bronchiectasis may produce few symptoms. Sometimes the patient has a cough with thick phlegm, which occasionally contains blood. There may be a slight fever.

Q: How is bronchiectasis treated?

A: A doctor may prescribe antibiotic drugs at the beginning of any respiratory infection for a patient with a history of bronchiectasis. It is important to drain the secretions from the lung, and for this reason the patient is taught correct breathing and how to use POSTURAL DRAINAGE. If repeated infections still occur, the doctor may recommend a LOBECTOMY, an operation to remove the diseased area.

Bronchiole is any of the many narrow branches of the bronchi, the tubes that carry air to and from the lungs. *See* p.10.

A talk about Bronchitis

Bronchitis is inflammation of the bronchi, the air passages to the lungs. It may be either acute or chronic. Bronchitis often follows a common cold or any infection of the nose and throat.

Q: What are the symptoms of acute bronchitis?

A: There is a slight fever, 37.8 to 38.9°C (100 to 102°F) with a painful, dry,

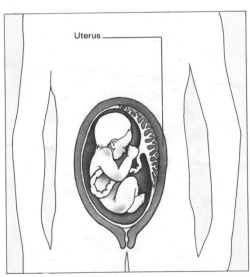

Uterus

Breech birth occurs when the baby's buttocks are born before the head.

cough that starts to produce thick, yellow sputum after two or three days. At this stage the fever often reduces and the pain from coughing diminishes. Even after the condition improves, a slight cough usually remains for another week or two.

Q: *What is the treatment for acute bronchitis?*

A: The patient needs bed rest in a warm, humid room with frequent steam inhalations from a vaporizer to soften the infected mucus in the bronchi. Hot drinks should be given; they help the patient cough up and spit out phlegm, and prevent dehydration. A sedative cough medicine may be taken at night to help the patient sleep. A cough syrup without a sedative may help during the day.

If the condition becomes worse and the fever increases, a doctor should be consulted. An antibiotic may be needed for the infection.

Q: *How soon after an attack of acute bronchitis may a person return to work?*

A: All crowded places should be avoided for at least ten days to allow the mucosal lining of the bronchi to heal before taking the risk of encountering new infection.

Q: *What causes chronic bronchitis?*

A: Chronic bronchitis is caused by repeated attacks of acute bronchitis. It is aggravated by smoking and by harmful environmental conditions, such as air polluted by chemicals, smoke, and dust.

Q: *What are the symptoms of chronic bronchitis?*

A: The main symptom is a cough which is

usually worse in the mornings, as the bronchi have not drained overnight. The patient produces clear, mucous sputum. The sputum becomes thicker and yellow if any infection occurs.

The constant, vigorous coughing may break the fine tissues of the lungs and produce a condition called EMPHYSEMA. A patient with emphysema tires quickly and becomes breathless after exercise. HEART FAILURE may occur.

Asthma, obesity, and smoking all complicate and aggravate chronic bronchitis. When these conditions are treated as well, the bronchitis usually also improves.

Q: *Can chronic bronchitis be treated?*

A: A close watch is kept for any colds or respiratory infections. The doctor usually prescribes antibiotics at the first sign of acute bronchitis to prevent the possibility of secondary bacterial infection and further damage to the bronchi and lungs. Breathing exercises, and sometimes POSTURAL DRAINAGE, can help to keep the bronchi clear. The doctor will also recommend stopping smoking and, if necessary, a change of working conditions.

Bronchogram is an X-ray picture that shows the structure of the lungs. It is taken after a dye (which is opaque to X-rays) has been introduced onto the lining of the windpipe (trachea), from where it spreads downward to the lungs.

Bronchopneumonia, is also called bronchial pneumonia. *See* BRONCHIAL PNEUMONIA.

Bronchoscope is a long thin tube, containing a light, used for examining the windpipe (trachea) and main breathing tubes (bronchi). It can also be used for removing objects that have been accidentally inhaled (such as peanuts) or for clearing mucus from the bronchi in a collapsed lung.

See also ATELACTASIS; FIBRESCOPE.

Bronchus is either of the two tubes that carry air in and out of the lungs. The bronchi branch from the lower end of the windpipe (trachea), one going to each lung. They are kept permanently open by rings of cartilage, and are lined with special hair-like cells that sweep dust and mucus upward toward the throat. The bronchi themselves divide further into narrower branches and finally into the extremely narrow bronchioles.

Brucellosis is an infectious disease, principally of cattle, goats, and pigs, but also occasionally of humans. It is caused by bacteria of the genus *Brucella,* which are found in the milk of infected animals. Human

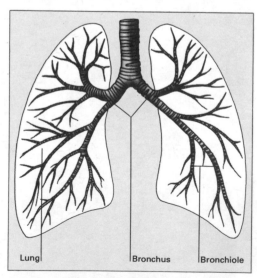

Lung | Bronchus | Bronchiole

Bronchus is one of the two main branches leading from the trachea to the lung.

beings contract the disease by consuming infected milk or meat, usually from cattle, or by handling diseased animals. In humans, brucellosis is more commonly known as undulant fever or Malta fever.

Recovery generally takes a long time; the patient continues to feel weak and unwell during this period.

Bruise is a visible, purplish mark beneath the surface of the skin, caused by the escape of blood from small blood vessels. Most bruises result from a blow or pressure, but sometimes a bruise occurs spontaneously in elderly people. The colour of the bruise fades away gradually, becoming purplish blue, brownish, and then yellow, before disappearing.

Bruises may be slightly painful, but they are not usually serious. But a bruise that appears with no apparent cause may be a sign of a disorder such as HAEMOPHILIA.

See also First Aid, p.578.

Bubo is a painful, swollen lymph node (a junction of the vessels of the lymphatic system), often containing pus. Buboes most commonly occur in the groin and armpit. They can accompany infectious diseases (for example, bubonic plague), and often develop in conjunction with VENEREAL DISEASES.

Bubonic plague is a form of PLAGUE in which the lymph nodes become painful, tender, and swollen, forming buboes. Early symptoms are a high fever, restlessness, and mental confusion, which lead to coma and death unless promptly treated. *See* BUBO.

Budd-Chiari syndrome is a blockage in the veins that carry blood from the liver, caused by clotting (thrombosis) or the presence of cancer cells. The condition greatly enlarges the liver, which becomes tender, and causes a build-up of fluid in the abdominal cavity (ascites).

Buerger's disease (known medically as thromboangiitis obliterans) is a rare condition of inflammation of the arteries and veins of the arms and legs. It is commoner in men, especially those who smoke. The symptoms vary in intensity. Commonly the disease produces tender, swollen areas over the inflamed veins and then coldness of the feet and hands. Pain occurs in the calves on walking (intermittent CLAUDICATION), due to arterial blockage. The poor circulation may result in GANGRENE.

Q: What is the treatment for Buerger's disease?

A: The patient, if a smoker, stops smoking; this often produces an immediate improvement. A doctor may prescribe drugs that dilate the blood vessels.

Bulbar paralysis is paralysis of the muscles of the tongue, lips, palate, and throat. The cause is either an infection or stroke interfering with the co-ordinating centres in the brain. The patient has difficulty in swallowing and speaking, and may inhale saliva and food.

Bulla is a medical term that may describe one of three things: (1) a large fluid-filled VESICLE; (2) a blister; or (3) a space within an organ, such as a lung.

Bunion is the swollen, inflamed condition of the saclike structure (BURSA) adjacent to the joint of the big toe. It causes a thickening of the toe and usually turns it in toward the other toes of the foot (hallux valgus). Loose shoes should be worn and special pads used to protect the bunion from irritation. Bunions may be removed surgically.

See also First Aid, p.579.

Burn (for EMERGENCY treatment *see* First Aid, p.524) is an area of tissue damage caused by heat (including friction and electricity) or cold, by a caustic chemical, or by radiation. Burns are classified according to the depth of the tissue damage.

First-degree burns produce a redness of the skin, and they heal without scarring.

Second-degree burns cause the destruction of deeper structures within the skin, resulting in blistering.

Third-degree burns destroy the full thickness of the skin, leaving an open area; sometimes the deeper tissues (fat or muscle) are also destroyed.

First- and second-degree burns tend to be more painful than third-degree burns, because the nerve endings are damaged but not completely destroyed. Extensive third-degree burns are a life-threatening emer-

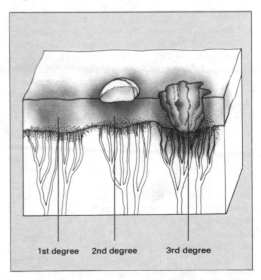

| 1st degree | 2nd degree | 3rd degree |

Burn can be classified as one that reddens skin (left), blisters skin (centre), or destroys it.

gency. Large areas of burnt skin cause the loss of body fluid into the surrounding tissues, which can lead to dehydration and the rapid onset of shock, particularly in children. For this reason, intravenous transfusions may be necessary as well as local treatment and painkilling drugs. Second- and third-degree burns often require a skin graft.

Bursa is a small sac-like structure, found mainly in joints, that protects bones and the tissues of muscles and organs where friction may occur (for example, in the elbows and knees). Bursae are filled with a thick compressible fluid.

Bursitis is inflammation of a BURSA. It is caused by excessive use, and is a painful condition, best treated by rest, use of a heating pad or hot water bottle, anti-inflammatory drugs, and sometimes an injection of a corticosteroid drug.

Byssinosis, also called Cotton workers' disease, or Monday fever, is an allergic reaction to cotton dust. The symptoms are coughing, breathlessness, and constriction in the chest. Symptoms initially occur only on the first working day of each week (hence "Monday fever"). Later, symptoms occur throughout the week, and eventually there is lung scarring, EMPHYSEMA, and PNEUMOCONIOSIS.

C

Cadmium is a metallic element. Both the metal and its compounds are poisonous. They are widely used in industry, for example, in batteries, electroplating, welding, and also ceramics. If cadmium salts are swallowed, violent diarrhoea and vomiting result. More serious poisoning results from prolonged breathing of cadmium oxide fumes. This may cause a cough, pains in the chest, and general weakness. Emphysema may result, causing further difficulty in breathing; it may be fatal if not treated swiftly.

Caecostomy is an artificial opening made by joining the first part of the large intestine (caecum) to the wall of the abdomen. It may be a permanent or temporary measure to treat a blockage of the colon if it is damaged by such conditions as ulcers (ulcerative colitis) or cancer, or after surgery.

Caecum is the sac-like first section of the large intestine, just beyond the point at which the lower part of the small intestine (ileum) joins the large intestine. Attached to the caecum is the vermiform APPENDIX.

See also p.12.

Caesarean section is the delivery of a baby through a surgical opening in the abdominal and uterine walls into the womb (uterus). This method may be preferable to natural birth through the vagina for various reasons: (1) if the mother's birth canal is too narrow for normal childbirth; (2) if a misplaced placenta blocks the exit from the womb (placenta praevia); (3) when the foetus is in an unusual position (for example, head up, feet down); (4) when signs of foetal distress or potential illness occur; or (5) when the mother is ill.

Q: *Can a woman who has had a Caesarean section have a normal delivery for her next baby?*

A: Yes, unless the reason for surgical delivery was a narrow birth canal or some permanent illness in the mother.

See also PREGNANCY AND CHILDBIRTH.

Caffeine is a stimulant alkaloid drug, present in coffee, tea, and some carbonated drinks. Caffeine increases the pulse rate and stimulates the production of urine from the kidneys. Excessive intake of coffee, and therefore of caffeine, may lead to insomnia, a rapid or variable pulse rate, and a feeling of anxiety and apprehension. A sharp reduction in caffeine intake may on the other hand produce acute withdrawal symptoms, such as headache, sweating, tremor, and an inability to concentrate.

Caisson disease. See BENDS.

Calamine lotion is a liquid preparation containing zinc oxide. It has a soothing effect when applied to inflamed or irritated skin.

Calcaneus. See HEEL.

Calciferol is vitamin D prepared chemically from ergosterol, a substance found in plants and animal tissues. It is used for treating disorders associated with low calcium levels in the body, such as RICKETS.

Calcification is the depositing of calcium salts in body tissues. It occurs normally in bone, especially after a fracture. The temporary build-up of calcium-containing tissue at the site of a bone fracture is called a CALLUS. Calcium compounds may also be deposited in other tissues after injury or infection, causing complications. Torn ligaments surrounding the hips and shoulders are areas most likely to be affected.

Calcium is a metallic element whose compounds occur in the body and are essential for good health. Ninety-nine per cent of body calcium is in the form of calcium phosphate, the chief mineral component of bones and teeth. Calcium is also present in the blood and is needed for the correct functioning of muscles and nerves. Lack of sufficient calcium in the body can lead to bone disorders such as RICKETS.

Children need between 0.3 and 0.5 grams of calcium daily; adults need 0.8 to 1.2 grams. Pregnant women and mothers who are breast-feeding should increase their calcium intake by about half as much again.

The absorption of calcium is controlled by vitamin D. Foods rich in calcium include bread and milk, and other dairy products.

Calculus is a stonelike mass that may form in ducts or hollow organs of the body, especially the gall bladder, kidneys, and ureters.

Calculi are composed mainly of crystalline substances: certain salts, cholesterol, and some protein. Because of their hardness, calculi can obstruct a duct or an organ, resulting in inflammation through infection.

Q: Why do calculi form?

A: Calculi formation may be due to a combination of factors, rather than to any one factor. Among such factors are local infection, high levels of calcium or other salts in the blood, and some conditions that cause a reduction in the flow of bodily fluids.

Q: What symptoms might indicate that calculi have formed?

A: Symptoms depend upon the part of the body involved. For example, calculi in the gall bladder (*see* GALLSTONES) may cause no symptoms, or may cause vomiting, jaundice, and severe pain (*see* COLIC) if they lodge in and obstruct the bile duct. The only way to determine if calculi have formed is to conduct tests, including X-rays, on parts of the body suspected to be involved (*see* CYSTOSCOPY).

Q: How are calculi treated?

A: Treatment depends upon the site of the calculi and on the severity of the symptoms. For most cases, however, surgical removal of calculi is necessary (*see* LITHOTOMY).

Caldwell-Luc operation is an operation to relieve chronic SINUSITIS by improving the drainage of the maxillary sinus. An opening is made through the upper jaw above one of the second molar teeth, and a second from the sinus to the nasal floor. This allows drainage of fluid from the sinus into the nose. Once the sinus has drained, the opening into the mouth is allowed to heal.

Callus is an area of skin that has become thickened and coarsened as a result of constant rubbing or pressure. The term callus also describes the temporary bone-like tissue that forms between the broken ends of a bone fracture as a normal part of the healing process (*see* CALCIFICATION).

Calorie is a unit of heat energy. In dietetics and medicine, calories are a measure of the energy content of foods. Some foods yield more calories than others when eaten and digested. Individual calorie requirements depend on a person's age, sex, build, and occupation. If a person takes in more calories than he or she needs, a weight gain results.

A talk about Cancer

Cancer is a condition in which certain body cells multiply without any apparent control and destroy healthy tissue and organs.

There are about 100 different types of cancer that affect human beings. The most common forms are breast cancer, skin cancer, lung cancer, and cancer of such digestive organs as the stomach and colon. But cancer can attack virtually any part of the body, including the organs that form blood.

Cancers are grouped into two main scientific classifications: carcinoma, or cancer of the epithelial tissue that forms skin and the linings of internal organs, and sarcoma, or cancer of connective tissue, such as cartilage and bone. Cancer of bone marrow and other blood-forming organs results in the production of cancerous white blood cells, the condition called leukaemia. Cancer of lymph glands and other lymphoid tissue is called malignant lymphoma. Both leukaemia and lymphoma are often classed as sarcomas, because blood and lymph are forms of connective tissue.

Q: How does cancer develop?

A: In a healthy human, new body cells are produced to enable growth and to replace cells that die through wear and tear. The

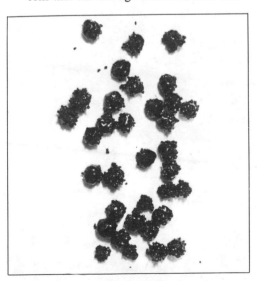

Calculus is a "stone" that forms in hollow organs: these are gallstones.

Cancer

new cells are formed when existing cells divide. Normally, the body cells divide at a controlled rate, producing just enough new cells to replace those that die. But cancer cells divide at an uncontrolled rate, forming a cluster of cells called a tumour. Benign tumours do not spread to other parts of the body; malignant (cancerous) ones do.

The spread of cancer (metastasis) occurs when some cancer cells break away from the tumour and travel through the lymphatic system or the bloodstream. These cancer cells may then lodge in other organs or tissues and cause new tumours to form. Once cancer has spread, it is very difficult to treat.

Cancer can also spread by invading tissues that surround the tumour. Once formed, cancerous tumours continue to grow.

Q: *What are the symptoms of cancer?*

A: Cancer has no symptoms in its early stages. But symptoms may appear before the cancer begins to spread. The sooner cancer is detected, the better is the chance of successful treatment.

There are seven possible warning signals that may indicate that the disease is developing:

(1) Any changes in bowel or bladder habits. These might indicate cancer of the colon, bladder, or prostate.

(2) A sore that does not heal. This could be a warning that mouth or skin cancer is developing.

(3) Unusual bleeding or discharge. Blood in the urine may be a symptom of bladder or kidney cancer; blood or mucus in the stools may indicate bowel cancer. Any unusual vaginal discharge or bleeding might be a sign of cancer of the reproductive organs.

(4) Thickening or lump in the breast or elsewhere in the body.

(5) Persistent indigestion or difficulty in swallowing. These may warn of stomach cancer or cancer of the oesophagus or throat.

(6) Obvious change in a wart or mole. Any sudden change in its size, shape, or colour could signal skin cancer.

(7) Nagging cough or chronic hoarseness. A persistent cough, especially if there is spitting of blood and a loss of weight, may be a sign of lung cancer.

Anyone developing any of these symptoms should consult a doctor at once. They do not necessarily indicate cancer, they are warnings of a possible danger. Only a doctor can diagnose cancer.

Q: *How is cancer treated?*

A: Surgery, radiation (radiotherapy), and drugs (chemotherapy) are the most common methods used to treat cancer. But treatment varies, depending on the kind of cancer. Surgery is used to remove most tumours, and usually the surrounding tissue, particularly for cancers of the breast, colon, lung, stomach, and womb. Some brain tumours can also be removed surgically. In addition, the patient may receive radiotherapy or chemotherapy before and after the operation.

Some forms of cancer, such as those involving the bladder, cervix, skin, and areas of the head and neck, can be treated with radiotherapy alone. The diseased area is exposed to radiation from X-rays or radioactive substances, such as cobalt 60. Radiation kills normal cells as well as cancerous ones, so care must be taken to administer radiation doses that do not endanger life.

Powerful anticancer drugs are particularly effective against leukaemia and lymphoma, but chemotherapy is also used against a variety of cancers. Like radiation, the drugs also kill normal cells and have side effects ranging from nausea to high blood pressure.

Researchers are looking for drugs that will be less harmful to healthy cells, as well as combinations of several anticancer drugs that selectively kill cancer cells.

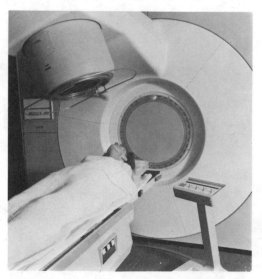

Cancer can be treated with a linear accelerator that disrupts a tumour without damaging skin.

Q: *What is a cancer patient's chance of survival?*

A: The sooner cancer is diagnosed and treated, the better are the chances of survival. Except for malignant pigment-cell tumours (melanomas), skin cancer is the easiest to treat, because it grows slowly and does not spread quickly to other parts of the body; 95 per cent of the patients recover. Lung cancer, because it is difficult to detect before it begins to spread, has a high death rate; only 10 per cent of the patients recover.

   If a patient remains free of cancer for five years after the end of treatment, it is likely that he or she is permanently cured. The five-year survival rate of breast or cervical cancer patients is 60%; of uterine cancer, 75%; of colon and rectum cancers, 45%; of prostate cancer, about 50%. There are several forms of leukaemia and lymphoma, and survival rates vary. But chances of surviving leukaemia have increased greatly since the 1960s. Patients with Hodgkin's disease, the most common form of lymphoma, have a survival rate of between 70 and 90 per cent.

Q: *Are there any known causes of cancer?*

A: Scientists have not found one single cause of cancer in humans, but they know that certain cancer-causing agents (carcinogens) increase the probability of cancer. Carcinogens damage body cells and can eventually cause at least one cell to become cancerous.

   Industrial chemicals, such as arsenic, asbestos, and some products of coal and oil, can create hazards for workers. Chemical carcinogens polluting air or drinking water can increase cancer risks for entire communities. Carcinogens have also been found in drugs and food supplies. They include chemicals used in food processing or agriculture. Some natural substances, such as moulds that grow on corn and peanut crops, are also suspected carcinogens. Diets that are high in fats may play a role in colon cancer. But the most common chemical carcinogen is the tar found in tobacco smoke. Cancer of the lungs, tongue, larynx and oesophagus are all more common in smokers of tobacco, including pipe smokers and cigar smokers.

   Overexposure to the ultraviolet rays in sunlight can cause skin cancer, particularly in people with fair, sensitive skin. Large doses of X-rays are also a cancer hazard, as are radioactive substances.

Q: *Can cancer be inherited?*

A: There is an inherited tendency for a few cancers, such as a rare eye cancer that occurs in children under three years of age. Also, cancer of the breast and colon occurs among members of the same family at a higher than average rate.

Q: *Does the body have any natural defences against cancer?*

A: Yes. The immune system that protects against invading bacteria and viruses also fights against cancer cells. This is probably why most people never develop the disease. On the other hand, some people may have a weak immune response to cancer cells, and therefore the disease is more likely to develop.

Q: *Can cancer be prevented?*

A: Avoiding known cancer-causing agents, such as tobacco smoke, can certainly reduce the risk. But should cancer develop, early detection and treatment is essential. Therefore, regular medical check-ups and alertness to the seven warning signs are the best defence against cancer.

   See also CERVICAL SMEAR; LEUKAEMIA; ONCOLOGY; PALPATION; RODENT ULCER.

Candida is a genus of yeast-like fungi. The species *Candida albicans* is the main infective agent in MONILIASIS (thrush).

Canine describes the four pointed teeth, of which the upper two are known also as the eyeteeth. *See* TEETH.

Canker sore is an alternative name for APHTHOUS ULCER. *See* MOUTH ULCER.

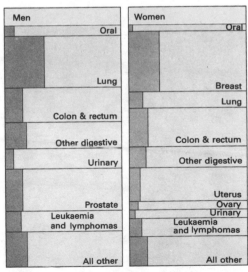

Types of cancer: coloured bands show frequency (height) and death rates (width).

Cannabis

Cannabis is another name for marijuana. *See* MARIJUANA.

Cantharides, also known as Spanish fly, is a poisonous substance made from the dried bodies of the beetle *Cantharis vesicatoria*. It has been thought by some to act as an APHRODISIAC, but it is more likely to cause diarrhoea and kidney damage. It is fatally poisonous if taken in large doses.

Capillary is the smallest type of blood vessel in the vascular system. Capillaries connect the smallest arteries with the smallest veins, and are so narrow that only one blood cell can pass along them at a time. The function of capillaries is to carry oxygen-containing blood to the tissues, to pass food substances to tissue cells, and to carry away waste products such as carbon dioxide. *See* p.8.

Capsulitis is inflammation of any membrane that encloses an organ. There are various forms of the disorder, but the most common affects the membranes of large joints, especially the hip and shoulder. The inflammation causes stiffness and pain when the joint is moved.

An affected joint should be rested, and a doctor may recommend painkilling drugs (analgesics) and antirheumatic drugs for the first few days. If capsulitis takes a long time to improve, the doctor may prescribe corticosteroid drugs, physiotherapy, or shortwave diathermy.

Carbohydrate is an organic substance that is an energy-producing constituent of many foods. Carbohydrates are rich in calories. The principal carbohydrates are sugars and starch. Common foods containing them include potatoes, cereals and cereal products (such as bread), and cane or beet sugar. During the digestion of such foods, the carbohydrates are broken down into the energy-producing sugar glucose (with water and carbon dioxide as waste products).

See also pp.12–13.

Carbolic acid, also known as phenol, is one of the oldest antiseptics. It was responsible for an important advance in sterile techniques in medicine during the nineteenth century.

Carbon dioxide is a gas that occurs in the atmosphere (0.035 per cent by volume) and is produced in body tissues as a waste product of energy-generating processes. Dissolved in the blood, carbon dioxide is carried to the lungs, and from there is breathed out as a gas. Some carbon dioxide also leaves the body in urine and in perspiration. If the level of carbon dioxide in the blood rises above normal, the brain automatically stimulates the lungs into working faster. The increase in breathing rate is necessary to rid the body of the extra carbon dioxide but it may be harmful in other ways (*see* ACIDOSIS). Solid carbon dioxide (dry ice) is used medically (CRYOSURGERY) to destroy warts.

Carbon monoxide is a poisonous, inflammable gas that is colourless and, when pure, odourless. It is present in the exhaust fumes from all internal combustion engines, in the gas produced from burning coke, and in sewers. Carbon monoxide is dangerous if inhaled because it is easily absorbed by haemoglobin in the blood, in preference to oxygen, preventing the blood from carrying oxygen. This results in ASPHYXIATION, which can cause death or, if the victim recovers, brain damage.

Q: What are the symptoms of carbon monoxide poisoning?

A: Symptoms vary greatly, but the victim normally has a pink or blotchy face and chest, and complains of dizziness, nausea, faintness, ringing in the ears, and throbbing temples. The pupils of the eyes become dilated, and the victim may lose consciousness.

Q: What action should be taken for carbon monoxide poisoning?

A: Remove the victim as quickly as possible from the source of the fumes. Fresh air and artificial respiration aid the recovery of the victim, but an oxygen mask is the best treatment. For EMERGENCY treatment, *see* First Aid, p.562.

Carbon tetrachloride is a clear, colourless liquid with anaesthetic and sleep-inducing (narcotic) properties. In these respects it resembles chloroform, but it is too poisonous to be used as an anaesthetic. The most com-

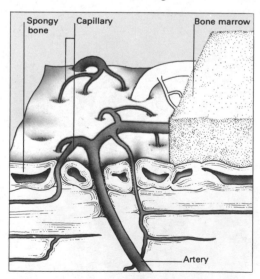

Capillary absorbs blood that is formed in the bone marrow and conveys it to the arteries.

mon uses of carbon tetrachloride today are in the chemical industry.

Q: What are the poisonous effects of carbon tetrachloride?

A: Small doses taken orally may cause giddiness, headache, and vomiting, and symptoms of severe kidney and liver damage may occur within weeks. The toxic effects are made worse if carbon tetrachloride is inhaled. Immediate treatment is to move the patient to fresh air and, if necessary, to give artificial respiration and call an ambulance (*see* First Aid, p.518).

Carbuncle is an inflamed bacterial infection of the skin. It is similar to a BOIL, except that a carbuncle tends to spread locally, sometimes forming clusters with several openings that discharge pus. Carbuncles occur most commonly on the back of the neck, buttocks, and thighs. The infection is usually treated with antibiotics, taken under medical supervision, but sometimes a doctor has to make an incision to drain a carbuncle.

Carcinogen is any substance that can cause cancer, for example, tobacco tar or asbestos. *See* CANCER.

Carcinoma is a type of cancer that forms in the epithelial tissue, which covers the inside and outside of various organs, most commonly on the skin and the intestine. *See* CANCER.

Cardiac describes anything pertaining to the HEART.

Cardiac arrest is the sudden stoppage of the heart. *See* HEART STOPPAGE.

Cardiac massage is the manipulation of the heart to restore and maintain the heartbeat. *See* First Aid, p.554; HEART STOPPAGE.

Cardiac murmur is a blowing or rasping noise that can be heard, using a stethoscope, as blood passes through the heart. This is a common condition that may or may not be a symptom of a disorder. *See* HEART MURMUR.

Cardiac pacemaker is a group of cells in the right ATRIUM of the heart that naturally generates and regulates the impulses that make the heart beat. The term also describes an artificial pacemaker that is used in the treatment of some heart conditions.

Cardiogram is a graph that records the electrical activity of the heart muscle. *See* ELECTROCARDIOGRAM.

Cardiology is the specialty of the study of the heart, its functions, and its disorders.

See also HEART; HEART DISEASE.

Cardiomyopathy is a general term for disorders of the heart muscle that commonly cause palpitations and an irregular pulse. There are various possible causes: (1) genetic factors, (2) infection caused by rheumatic fever or

viruses, (3) beriberi and other vitamin B deficiency disorders, and (4) excessive alcohol intake. Usually, however, the cause is unknown.

Cardioversion is the restoration of normal rhythm to a disordered heart by means of carefully controlled electric shocks. It may be done when the rhythms normally controlled by the CARDIAC PACEMAKER have been replaced by irregular rhythm, such as atrial FIBRILLATION.

Caries. *See* TOOTH DECAY.

Carotene is a yellow pigment present in many foods (for example, carrots, corn, and eggs). When such a food is digested, the carotene is stored in the liver until it is converted there into vitamin A.

See also VITAMINS.

Carotid artery is either of the two arteries that lead off the main artery from the heart (aorta) and supply blood to the neck, head, and brain. Each carotid artery divides into an internal and an external artery.

See also p.8.

Carpal tunnel syndrome is a tingling feeling in the fingers (except the little finger), which may also be weak. The sensation is particularly noticeable at night, and it may be strong enough to wake up a person.

Q: What causes carpal tunnel syndrome?

A: A ligament across the front of the wrist becomes swollen and compresses the nerve that supplies the fingers. The condition becomes worse with excessive use of the wrist, before the menstrual period (when fluid normally builds up in ligaments), and with mild arthritis. In

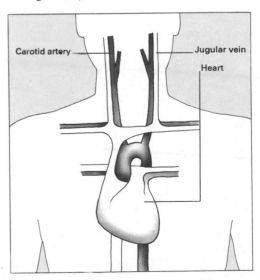

Carotid artery situated on each side of the neck is the main route for blood to the brain.

rare cases, it may result from hormone disorders and rheumatoid arthritis.

Q: *How is carpal tunnel syndrome treated?*

A: Resting the wrist and taking water-removing drugs (diuretics) should improve the condition. If these fail, a doctor may inject a corticosteroid drug into the ligament. Sometimes a minor operation is needed to divide the ligament and free the nerve.

Carpus is the medical name for the wrist. A carpal bone is any of the eight small bones in the wrist. *See* WRIST.

Carrier is an apparently healthy person who carries or passes on a disorder without developing its symptoms. This may occur with such diseases as typhoid, diphtheria, and streptococcal infections. A healthy person may also carry a GENE for a disorder, such as haemophilia, which can be passed on to some of the children. A disease-carrying organism, such as a mosquito, is also sometimes known as a carrier.

Car sickness. *See* MOTION SICKNESS.

Cartilage is dense, specialized, semi-transparent connective tissue that is capable of withstanding great pressure and tension. Cartilage forms part of the structure of the skeleton in some ribs and between vertebrae of the spine. It is also present in the nose, in the external ear (auricle), and as the gristle covering on joints that makes them move easily. In a developing foetus, cartilage is the major component of the skeleton, and bones are formed later when the cartilage becomes impregnated with deposits of calcium salts.

Q: *What is a torn cartilage?*

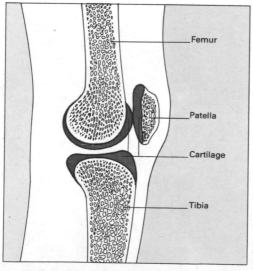

Cartilage in the knee allows the bones to move smoothly against each other.

Femur

Patella

Cartilage

Tibia

A: A torn cartilage commonly refers to a disorder of the knee. The cartilage tears away from the ligament that holds it in position, and a piece of cartilage may become free to move around in the knee joint. This can cause pain, swelling, and sometimes "locking" of the knee, in which it gets stuck in one position. Weight cannot be placed on the leg.

Q: *How is a torn cartilage treated?*

A: A minor tear can be treated effectively with a firm bandage around the knee and by taking as much rest as possible. More serious tears require the removal of the cartilage by an operation (meniscectomy). Osteoarthritis may affect the knee joint later in the patient's life.

Caruncle is a small fleshy lump. A caruncle sometimes appears at the outer opening of the urethra in women. A urethral caruncle may cause bleeding and pain on urination, and may be extremely sensitive to irritation. It is not serious in itself, and can be removed by a minor operation if it causes discomfort.

Castration is the surgical removal of the genital organs. The term is commonly taken to mean the removal of the testicles (ORCHIDECTOMY), although medically it also applies to the removal of the ovaries (OOPHORECTOMY). Castration may be necessary if the growth of a cancerous tumour is stimulated by sex hormones, as happens, for example, with cancer of the prostate or cancer of the breast. The removal of one, or both, testicles or ovaries is sometimes necessary if they have been seriously damaged by infection. In women, the ovaries may be removed at the same time as the womb (HYSTERECTOMY).

Q: *Does castration affect sexual desire and fulfillment?*

A: The operation in men reduces the sexual drive (libido). Intercourse is still technically possible but unlikely, and the semen does not contain sperm. Growth of body hair is reduced, but the depth of the voice remains unchanged. If a boy is castrated before puberty, secondary sexual characteristics (such as hair growth and deepening of the voice) do not develop.

Castration in women does not reduce a woman's ability to have sexual intercourse or her enjoyment of it, but the possibility of conception is permanently removed.

See also STERILIZATION.

Catalepsy, also called anochlesia, is a prolonged state of immobility in which the patient seems to be in a trance. It is normally associated with psychotic disorders such as SCHIZOPHRENIA, and sometimes accompanies HYSTERIA.

Cataract is an opacity in the lens of the eye. Cataracts cause a gradual, painless deterioration of sight, beginning with an inability to see detail clearly, and distortion of sight in the presence of bright lights.

Q: What causes cataracts?

A: Cataracts often develop in elderly persons as a result of degeneration of the tissue of the lens. Cataracts may be present at birth (congenital), and the most common reason for this is thought to be German measles (rubella infection) in the mother during early pregnancy. Injury to the eye later in life may also cause cataracts, or they may accompany a disease, particularly diabetes.

Q: How are cataracts treated?

A: If vision is seriously impaired, the lens is removed in an operation. After an initial period of adjustment, clear vision is usually restored with the assistance of strong spectacles or contact lenses.

Catarrh is an inflammation of the mucous membranes of the nose or throat that results in the discharge of excessive mucus.

Smoking and alcohol worsen the condition, as do many nasal sprays and drops. The condition can be improved by good hygiene and plenty of exercise.

Catatonia is a disorder in which a person appears to be in a stupor, and is usually rigid physically, being unable to move. It is usually considered to be a form of SCHIZOPHRENIA.

Catgut is a sterile strand of sheep's intestine used as a surgical LIGATURE.

Cathartic, or purgative, is a laxative that induces one or several watery bowel movements. Castor oil is an example.

See also LAXATIVES.

Catheter is a tube inserted into a body cavity to extract or inject fluids. It is usually made of flexible plastic or rubber.

CAT scanner is an abbreviation of computerized axial tomography scanner, a machine that passes X-rays through a patient's body from various angles. This technique enables a computer to build up a cross-sectional X-ray picture. The computer analysis itself needs expert interpretation.

Cat-scratch fever is a disorder thought to be caused by a virus transmitted by a scratch or bite of a cat. It develops seven to fourteen days after the scratch or bite. Inflammation of the affected area heals in a few days, but lymph glands in the area remain slightly swollen and tender. A mild fever and general feeling of being unwell may persist from two weeks to a month. There is no specific treatment for cat-scratch fever, which eventually cures itself, but a doctor may prescribe painkilling and antifever drugs.

Cauliflower ear is a misshapen ear often suffered by professional boxers as a result of repeated blows that cause bleeding into the tight membrane surrounding the cartilage of the ear. Its appearance resembles the shape of a cauliflower. Treatment is by plastic surgery.

Causalgia is severe burning pain in an area where nerves have been injured, particularly the palm of the hand or the sole of the foot. The surface skin often becomes thinner and reddish, and slight changes such as a cool breeze may aggravate the burning sensation. The patient may become emotionally disturbed. Causalgia is difficult to treat. If pain-killing drugs are not effective, a doctor may try local anaesthetic injections. In some cases, a surgeon may perform an operation to cut the damaged nerves.

Cautery is an artificial way of destroying tissue for medical reasons. It is done using heat, corrosive chemicals, electricity, or (the most recent method) a beam of laser light. Tissue may be cauterized to treat wounds that are likely to become infected or to destroy a lumpy scar, which may result from excessive reaction of tissue in a wound during healing. In surgery, an electric cauterizing needle is often used to stop bleeding from small blood vessels. Other examples of cautery are the use of silver nitrate to stop recurrent nosebleeds, and laser beams as the cauterizing agents in eye surgery. Cautery may be used to rid a patient of warts.

Cellulitis is a spreading of infection in the tissue under the skin, commonly associated with a small cut, abrasion, or boil. It occurs if

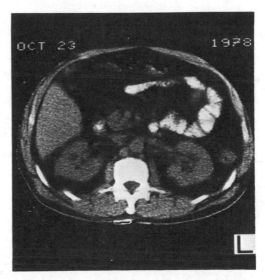

CAT scanner: cross-sectional X-ray, above, shows vertebra (white) and various organs.

117

Cellulose

the body's defence mechanisms fail to localize the infection. The tissue surrounding the infection becomes red, swollen, and tender, and this area tends to enlarge rapidly. Red lines spreading from the infection toward a local lymph gland are a sign that the lymph vessels have also become infected (lymphangitis). To treat cellulitis, a doctor usually prescribes a course of an appropriate antibiotic drug.

Cellulose is a carbohydrate that does not change chemically during the human digestive process. It is present in fibre-containing foods such as green vegetables and whole grain wheat bread. Cellulose aids the elimination of waste products from the intestine. For this reason, it is sometimes used in the treatment of constipation.

Celsius. *See* CENTIGRADE.

Centigrade, or Celsius, is a scale of temperature measurement in which 0° centigrade (written 0°C) is the freezing point of water at sea level, and 100°C is the boiling point of water at sea level. The other common system of temperature measurement is the FAHRENHEIT scale. The normal average human body temperature is 37°C (equal to 98.6°F).

Cerebellum is the part of the brain that lies behind and below the cerebral hemispheres of the brain. It is responsible for the co-ordination of voluntary movements throughout the body, and it is the centre that controls balance.

See also p.18.

Cerebral cortex is the ridged "grey matter" of the brain that forms the outer layer of each hemisphere of the CEREBRUM. The cerebral cortex receives and interprets nerve impulses from the sense organs. It is also concerned with higher mental functions, such as intelligence, memory, and perception.

See also p.18.

Cerebral haemorrhage is a form of apoplexy caused by the bursting of a blood vessel within the brain. This causes bleeding into the brain matter and damage to the surrounding tissue. For symptoms and treatment of a cerebral haemorrhage, *see* STROKE.

Cerebral palsy is a general term for various disorders resulting from damage to the brain. The damage to the brain may occur before, during, or shortly after birth.

However, whatever the origin of this brain damage, all conditions that may be categorized under the term cerebral palsy have several factors in common. There is always some loss of muscle control. Spasticity and/or paralysis may also result from the brain damage.

See also SPASTIC.

Q: What causes cerebral palsy?

A: There are several possible causes of cerebral palsy. Some of these causes are injury, improper development of the brain, and certain diseases. Furthermore, each of these causes may occur before birth, during the birth process, or shortly after birth. For example, before birth, brain damage to the unborn may result from a disease contracted by the mother during pregnancy, such as German measles. Improper development of the unborn's brain may result if the mother's diet during pregnancy is deficient in certain essential nutrients.

During the birth process, brain damage may result if the baby's head is too large to pass safely through the pelvis of the mother. Sometimes the birth process takes so long that the infant's brain cells are deprived of an adequate supply of oxygen. Without that supply, many of the infant's brain cells will die, resulting in permanent loss of function of the parts of the body controlled by those cells.

After birth, an infant can develop cerebral palsy as the result of brain damage caused by a blow to the head. An infant can also develop cerebral palsy as the result of certain diseases that damage his or her brain cells.

Q: What are some symptoms of cerebral palsy?

A: Some of the more common symptoms of cerebral palsy are lack of balance, clumsy walk, unclear speech, shaking, jerking movements, and convulsions. In some people with cerebral palsy, there is also

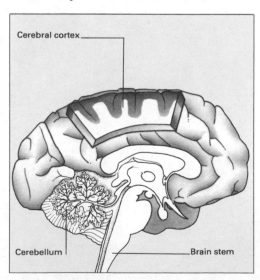

Cerebral cortex and cerebellum co-ordinate the body and control higher mental functions.

mental retardation, crippling, and/or severe hearing and sight problems. Symptoms of cerebral palsy are sometimes apparent at birth. However, in most cases, the symptoms of cerebral palsy are not evident until the child is more than six months old.

Q: *How is cerebral palsy treated?*

A: There is no known cure for cerebral palsy. Therefore, treatment for the condition is aimed at helping the patient make best use of his or her physical and mental abilities. Yet the degree of success of treatment of cerebral palsy is largely dependent upon the extent of brain damage involved.

In general, treatment for cerebral palsy usually includes physiotherapy, speech therapy, and/or drug therapy, and special education.

For many people with cerebral palsy, a doctor may prescribe braces and other devices that provide support and can also aid walking.

Cerebrospinal fever is an infection of the MENINGES, caused by the meningococcus.

Cerebrospinal fluid is a clear, watery fluid that surrounds the brain and spinal cord and helps to protect them from external shock. The fluid, under pressure, assists the supply of nutrients to the brain and the disposal of waste substances.

See also p.18.

Cerebrum is the largest part of the brain, situated beneath the roof of the skull. It consists of two hemispheres that are separated lengthwise by a furrowed division. The outer layer of each hemisphere is the CEREBRAL CORTEX, the section of the brain popularly known as "grey matter".

Within the cerebral hemispheres is white matter consisting of three kinds of fibres that connect the hemispheres, convey impulses to and from the cortex and the spinal cord, and connect different areas of the cortex with each other.

See also p.18.

Cerumen. *See* WAX.

Cervical refers to any cervix, or neck-like structure, for example, the upper seven bones of the spinal column (cervical vertebrae) or the neck of the womb (cervix uteri).

A talk about Cervical cancer

Cervical cancer is cancer in the neck of the womb (cervix). There are no symptoms in the early stages of the disease, but blood-stained discharge may occur later either between menstrual periods or after sexual intercourse.

Local pain may develop and there may be some difficulty in urinating. Sometimes, blood in the urine is a late symptom.

Q: *Can cervical cancer be detected early?*

A: If a regular CERVICAL SMEAR (Pap test) is done, as gynaecologists advise, cervical cancer can be detected at an early stage, although there are no external early symptoms. Diagnosis must be confirmed by further tests, such as biopsy. Immediate treatment following early detection is successful.

If cervical cancer remains undetected until it is in an advanced stage, then radiotherapy may be used alone or following removal of the womb (hysterectomy). Untreated, cervical cancer is fatal.

Q: *Are some women more likely than others to get cervical cancer?*

A: Yes. Research has shown that cervical cancer is most common in women who have had sexual intercourse from an early age, with several partners, and whose standards of hygiene have been generally low.

It is also more likely to occur in women who have had children. Cervical cancer is rare in women who have not had sexual intercourse.

See also CANCER.

Cervical erosion is the destruction by bacteria of an area of the surface wall of the neck of the womb (cervix). Natural healing of the disorder involves the downward growth of tissue cells from the endocervical canal. But it is not uncommon for healing to be incomplete and for the area to become ulcerated. This may cause an abnormal discharge from the vagina, and occasional bleeding, particularly after sexual intercourse.

Q: *What causes cervical erosion?*

A: Infection in the vagina, the stimulus to hormone production resulting from pregnancy, or the use of birth control pills may cause cervical erosion.

Q: *How is cervical erosion treated?*

A: Cervical erosion does not usually require treatment unless it causes a troublesome discharge, when antiseptic or antibiotic pessaries or creams may be used to kill the infection. If this fails, cautery of the damaged area is the usual treatment.

Q: *How soon after cautery can a women resume sexual intercourse?*

A: A women should not have sexual intercourse until a further physical examination confirms that the area has healed properly.

Cervical rib

Cervical rib is a small extra rib found in some persons. It is an appendage to the seventh cervical vertebra in the neck. The extra rib need not cause problems. But if it puts pressure on the adjacent nerves and blood vessels, there is pain in the arm and hand, and possibly symptoms similar to RAYNAUD'S PHENOMENON. If a cervical rib causes such symptoms, treatment is to remove it.

Cervical smear (Papanicolaou's test, or Pap test) is a test for the early detection of cancer cells on the neck of the womb (cervix). The test is painless and harmless, and entails the rubbing of a specially shaped piece of wood or plastic across the cervix. This removes some cells, which are examined using a microscope. The test is normally done during a routine gynaecological examination. If it reveals abnormal cells, CERVICAL CANCER may be present in an early stage.

Q: How are the results of the test diagnosed?

A: Cells taken in the test are studied (cervical cytology) and then classified into one of four groups: (1) class I cells are normal in structure; (2) class II cells are slightly abnormal, and the possibility of vaginal infection may be investigated; (3) class III cells are definitely abnormal but they are not cancerous; (4) class IV and V cells are cancerous, and the appropriate action should be taken immediately.

Q: How often should a cervical smear be done?

A: Regular gynaecological check-ups with smear tests are advised for all women over the age of about twenty and for younger women who are sexually active. A smear that is normal should be repeated in about a year. After a class II result, a repeat test is advised within three to six months. It is likely that a doctor will decide to repeat a class III smear result either at once or within a few weeks. Class II or class III results should not cause alarm, because the cell structures often return to normal. It takes several years for cervical cancer to develop from a class II result.

Cervical spondylosis is an arthritic condition of the upper spine and neck, or a traumatic condition associated with a prolapsed disc. It tends to become worse with time. A stiff neck may be the only symptom, although pressure on nearby nerves may cause pain and weakness in the arm and hand. Cervical spondylosis is most commonly part of the normal ageing process. It can begin earlier in life as the result of neck injuries.

Q: How is cervical spondylosis treated?

A: Heat applied locally to the area, massage, physiotherapy, and antirheumatic drugs all may be of assistance in treating the condition. If these are not successful, it may be necessary to immobilize the neck in a surgical collar. This must be worn at night and often during the day, especially if the patient is travelling in a car.

Cervicitis is the inflammation of the neck of the womb (cervix). The symptoms may be a thick discharge from the vagina, pain during sexual intercourse, bleeding after sexual intercourse, and backache. The cause of cervicitis often remains unknown, but it may be caused by cervical erosion, or by vaginal infections. The condition may also be a complication of childbirth if the cervix is torn.

Q: What is the treatment for cervicitis?

A: A doctor may prescribe antibiotic drugs and recommend abstinence from sexual intercourse and alcoholic drinks. A persistent case of cervicitis may be treated by destroying the infected area using CAUTERY or CRYOSURGERY. This causes a scab to form in place of the infected tissue. The scab falls off in about ten days, and is either dissolved or discharged through the vagina, perhaps with a little bleeding. Sexual intercourse must not take place for two weeks, or until a medical examination has been done to ensure that the cervix has healed properly.

Cervix is the neck or any part of an organ that resembles a neck. The cervix of the womb (uterus) is the narrow opening at the base of the womb that protrudes slightly into the vagina.

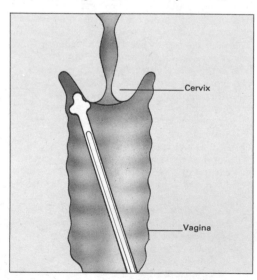

Cervical smear: cells taken from the cervix can reveal the presence of cancer.

Cestodiasis is the infestation of the intestine by WORMS of the subclass Cestoda (phylum Platyhelminthes). The most common parasitic worms in this group are tapeworms.

Cetrimide is an antiseptic substance that is used as a cream, solution, or ointment in the treatment of wounds or skin infections. It is also an ingredient of some shampoos and skin cleansers, although cetrimide is poisonous if swallowed.

Chafing is soreness caused by rubbing the skin, usually in fatty areas, on another skin surface, or on wet clothing. The most common areas of chafing are the groin, anal region, neck, wrists, and between the fingers and toes. If the chafed area is kept clean and dry, the irritation heals itself.

Chagas' disease is a disorder transmitted by the bloodsucking bite of a bug that carries the causative agent, *Trypanosoma cruzi*. It is one form of trypanosomiasis, a disorder that occurs also as SLEEPING SICKNESS. There is a red swelling around the site of the bite which, if on an eyelid, may cause the eye to close. The infection enters through the conjunctiva of the eye, the mucous membranes of the mouth or nose, or a skin abrasion. Symptoms of Chagas' disease are fever, general enlargement of the lymph glands, and a rapid heartbeat. A form of brain inflammation (encephalitis) may develop, with insomnia and irritability.

Q: What is the treatment for Chagas' disease?

A: There is no effective form of treatment, and the disorder has a high death rate, particularly among children.

Q: Is there a higher incidence of Chagas' disease in some countries?

A: Yes. Chagas' disease is most common in Central and South America, and it occasionally occurs also in the southwest United States.

Chalazion (meibomian or tarsal cyst) is a small hard growth on the eyelid similar to a sebaceous CYST. It forms when an oil-producing gland (a tarsal gland) becomes blocked with secretion. A chalazion is not painful, but if treatment is advised, an ophthalmic surgeon can remove it by cutting it away from the inner side of the eyelid.

See also STYE.

Chancre is a painless ulcer that is an early sign of the venereal disease SYPHILIS. It usually appears on the genitals, but may occur elsewhere depending on the site of the infection, for example, the lips or skin. A chancre appears about three weeks after infection and becomes an ulcerous sore that heals slowly during the next month. It may leave a small scar. It is important to consult a doctor about a possible chancre, to receive early treatment of the underlying disease.

Chancroid, also called soft chancre or soft sore, is a highly infectious venereal condition, which may accompany syphilis. It is caused by bacteria (*Haemophilus ducreyi*) and is most common in the tropics. About three or four days after contact with the infection, the patient develops a small red ulcerating sore on the genitals. This becomes painful and the local lymph glands swell and may discharge. Other symptoms may be a slight fever and a general feeling of being unwell.

Q: How is a chancroid diagnosed?

A: A venereologist examines the discharge from the ulcer or gland, and may do a special skin test. Additional tests may be done to ensure that other venereal diseases are not present.

Q: How is a chancroid treated?

A: A course of an appropriate antibiotic drug heals the chancroid effectively. The patient's sexual contacts should be examined for presence of the infection.

See also VENEREAL DISEASES.

Change of life is the time in a woman's life at which menstruation ceases permanently. *See* MENOPAUSE.

Chapping is a sore, inflamed condition of the skin caused by excessive exposure to cold or wet. Chapped skin should be protected by warm, dry clothing. Preventive measures include the use of water-repellent cream for outdoor activities, and nourishing hand and face creams.

Charleyhorse is a popular term for persistent pain and stiffness in a muscle, usually in the leg. *See* CRAMP.

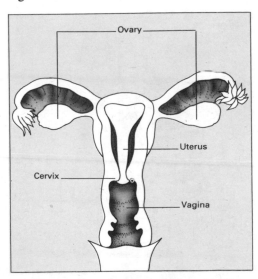

Cervix is the narrow entrance from the vagina leading to the uterus and the fallopian tubes.

Cheilosis

Cheilosis is a reddened condition of the lips, with scaling and cracks at the corners of the mouth, which may become infected. Cheilosis is often caused by poorly fitting dentures in the elderly, or, rarely, by a deficiency of the vitamin B complex.

Vitamin B tablets and antibiotic skin creams improve the condition.

Chelating agents are substances that combine chemically with heavy metals, such as lead and mercury. They are used, for example, to combat poisoning by such metals. There are various chelating agents, such as penicillamine and EDTA (ethylenediaminetetra-aceticacid).

Cheloid. *See* KELOID.

Chemosis is excessive swelling of the mucous membranes that line the eyelids (conjunctiva). It is most commonly caused by CONJUNCTIVITIS, or by contact with an irritating substance, for example, chlorine. It may be a temporary reaction, but if the condition does not improve within a few hours, a doctor should be consulted.

Chemotherapy is the treatment of disease by chemical agents that have a destructive (toxic) effect on the specific infecting organism, but are not harmful to the patient. The most common types of chemical-containing agents are: antibiotics (for example, penicillin and tetracyclines); antimalarials (for example, quinine); antifungals (for example, nystatin); antivirals (for example, idoxuridine); antiseptics (for example, chlorhexidine and hexachlorophene); and anticancer (cytotoxic) drugs (for example, methotrexate and cyclophosphamide).

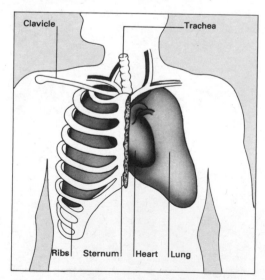

Chest, protected by the ribs, contains most of the respiratory organs, and the heart.

Chest (or thorax) is the upper part of the trunk of the body. It extends from the base of the neck to the diaphragm, which separates the chest from the abdomen. The framework of the chest consists of twelve pairs of ribs, which are connected to the spine at the back, and the intercostal muscles in between them. The upper seven pairs of ribs are connected at the front to the breastbone (sternum). The lower five pairs do not connect directly to the sternum; three pairs are connected indirectly by cartilage, and the other two pairs to the spine only. The intercostal muscles allow the lungs to expand during breathing.

The thoracic cavity enclosed by this frame contains the heart; the respiratory apparatus, including the two lungs in their surrounding membrane (pleura), the lower part of the trachea, and the bronchi; various glands; the oesophagus (gullet); the two vagus nerves and two phrenic nerves; and the major blood vessels. Movement of the diaphragm and intercostal muscles changes the volume of the thoracic cavity during breathing.

Cheyne-Stokes breathing is a breathing pattern which is first shallow and infrequent and then increases gradually in depth and speed before fading away again. Before the next cycle begins, breathing may stop for five to fifty seconds. Cheyne-Stokes breathing is often accompanied by alterations in the levels of consciousness, and it most commonly occurs in seriously ill patients with brain or heart disorders.

The condition is named after the Scottish and Irish physicians John Cheyne (1777–1836) and William Stokes (1804–78).

Q: Is Cheyne-Stokes breathing invariably associated with serious disorders?

A: No. This breathing pattern can occur in elderly people, especially when they have taken sleeping tablets, and the control of normal respiration is reduced.

Q: Is there any treatment for Cheyne-Stokes breathing?

A: If the breathing abnormality is associated with a heart or brain disorder, it improves when the cause is treated. Sometimes, a doctor prescribes the drug aminophylline.

A talk about Chickenpox

Chickenpox (or varicella) is a virus infection characterized by a rash of small red spots that first appear on the back and chest, and spread to cover the rest of the body. The rash is usually preceded for a few days by a slight fever, sore throat, and discharge of mucus from the nose. The spots develop quickly into clear, oval blisters of various sizes. These become milky in colour and within three or four days shrivel up as scabs, which may take another week to fall off. One or two more waves of rashes may occur in the next two to three days. During the acute stage of the disorder, which lasts for three or four days, the patient's temperature may rise as high as 39–40°C (102–104°F), and a doctor should be consulted. There is no vaccine against chickenpox.

Q: *Is chickenpox contagious?*

A: Yes. The first symptoms appear two to three weeks after contact with the disease. The contagious stage extends from about five days before the outbreak of the rash until six days after the first crop of blisters has appeared. It is advisable to isolate the patient once the spots appear.

Q: *How long is chickenpox likely to last?*

A: The acute illness lasts for between three and four days, but it is usually another seven to ten days before the spots have disappeared.

Q: *Are some people more likely than others to get chickenpox?*

A: Yes: children. Adults are less likely to catch chickenpox because, by the age of fifteen, about seventy-five per cent of children have had chickenpox, and it is unusual to get the disease a second time. People in poor health and the elderly should avoid contact with a child with chickenpox, because the infection may cause the related disorder SHINGLES (herpes zoster), which is more common in adults.

Q: *How is chickenpox treated?*

A: Calamine lotion has a soothing effect on the irritating spots, and a doctor may prescribe an antihistamine drug (also useful for its sedative effect) to reduce the irritation. It is most important to keep the patient from scratching the spots, because further infection can easily result if the skin is broken. For this reason, babies and small children may sometimes have to wear gloves. A doctor may prescribe aspirin, taken every four hours, to reduce the fever and headache. A child must be encouraged to drink plenty of liquids. Nightwear and bedclothes should be light and preferably made of cotton, because wool and synthetic fabrics are likely to be irritating to the skin.

Q: *Where else do spots occur apart from the back and chest?*

A: Spots may spread to the rest of the trunk and face, as well as to the limbs. Spots may also appear in the mucous membranes, such as those of the mouth and vagina, or in the ears.

Q: *Can complications result from chickenpox?*

A: Complications are rare, but chest infections such as bronchitis and pneumonia, sinusitis, and middle ear infection (otitis media) may occur. A more serious possible complication is encephalitis. These can all be treated effectively with prescribed antibiotics.

Q: *How long is it before a child is back to normal after chickenpox?*

A: A child may be irritable and unusually tired for about a week after the symptoms of chickenpox have disappeared, so it is important that he or she does not return to school too soon after the illness.

Chilblain, known medically as pernio, is a swollen, painful, reddened area occurring on the feet, toes, or fingers, and occasionally on the ears. The complaint occurs in cold, damp weather conditions. The cold damages small blood vessels and nerves in the skin. Some persons are more susceptible than others to such damage, and the condition is more common in women and children. A chilblain may cause aching, burning, and itching, especially when the body becomes warmer. Some chilblains form ulcers that may leave scars after healing.

Q: *How is a chilblain treated?*

A: Thick, woollen clothing should be worn in cold weather, with adequate covering of the head, legs, and arms, as well as the

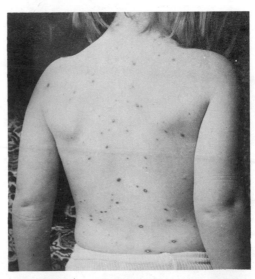

Chickenpox is a highly contagious viral disease that produces a characteristic itchy rash.

Childbirth

rest of the body. Drugs that cause an expansion in the blood vessels are sometimes prescribed. Corticosteroid creams are soothing for itching skin.

Childbirth is the process of having a baby. *See* PREGNANCY AND CHILDBIRTH. For EMERGENCY, *see* First Aid pp.540–543.

Childhood disorders. The following table lists some common illnesses and conditions pertaining specifically to children, or occurring more often in children than in adults, grouped according to symptom. The symptoms may also indicate other clinical disorders; this is not a complete list. A good medical history and physical examination by a doctor are essential for adequate diagnosis of a problem. Each disorder has a separate article in the A–Z section of this book.

Symptom	Disorder
Aching joints	EXHAUSTION
	INFLUENZA
	POLIOMYELITIS
	RHEUMATIC FEVER
Breathing difficulty	ASTHMA
	BRONCHITIS
	CROUP
	DIPHTHERIA
	ENLARGED ADENOIDS
	ENLARGED TONSILS
	WHOOPING COUGH (pertussis)
Convulsions	EPILEPSY
	FEVER (at the onset of illness)
	MENINGITIS
Cough	ASTHMA
	BRONCHITIS
	COMMON COLD
	CROUP
	CYSTIC FIBROSIS
	DIPHTHERIA
	INFLUENZA
	MEASLES
	PNEUMONIA
	TUBERCULOSIS
	WHOOPING COUGH (pertussis)
Diarrhoea	CYSTIC FIBROSIS
	FOOD POISONING
	GASTROENTERITIS
	INDIGESTION
	INFLUENZA
	MOTION SICKNESS
Painful ears	EARACHE
	TEETHING
	WAX (in ears)
Rash on the skin	ALLERGY, plant
	CHICKENPOX
	ECZEMA
	GERMAN MEASLES
	HEAD LICE

Symptom	Disorder
Rash on the skin (continued)	HIVES
	IMPETIGO
	INSECT BITES
	MEASLES
	NAPPY RASH
	PRICKLY HEAT
	RINGWORM
	SCABIES
	SCARLET FEVER
Reading difficulty	DYSLEXIA
	LEARNING DISABILITIES
	LONGSIGHTEDNESS (hyperopia)
	SHORTSIGHTEDNESS (myopia)
Red, inflamed eyes	ALLERGY
	CONJUNCTIVITIS
	MEASLES
	STYE
	TIREDNESS
	WEEPING
Runny nose	ALLERGY
	COMMON COLD
	INFLUENZA
	MEASLES
	WHOOPING COUGH (pertussis)
Sore throat	BRONCHITIS
	COMMON COLD
	DIPHTHERIA
	ENLARGED TONSILS
	GERMAN MEASLES (rubella)
	INFLUENZA
	MUMPS
	SCARLET FEVER
Stomachache	APPENDICITIS
	COLIC
	COMMON COLD
	CONSTIPATION
	FOOD POISONING
	INDIGESTION
	INTESTINAL OBSTRUCTION
	INTUSSUSCEPTION
	WORMS
Swollen glands	EARACHE
	GERMAN MEASLES (rubella)
	GLANDULAR FEVER
	MUMPS
Vomiting	GASTROENTERITIS
	INDIGESTION
	INFLUENZA
	MIGRAINE
	MOTION SICKNESS
	PNEUMONIA
	POLIOMYELITIS
	SCARLET FEVER
	WHOOPING COUGH (pertussis)

Chill is a shivering attack and the accompanying sensation of coldness. It is due to an irregular impulse to the part of the brain that regulates body temperature, and is a normal reaction to cold. A mild fever sometimes follows a chill, which may be the first indication of an impending infectious illness.

Chiropractic is an alternative, non-orthodox system of medicine in which diseases are thought to be caused by the improper functioning of the nervous system. A major aspect of treatment is spinal manipulation.

Chloasma is a patchy yellowish-brown discoloration of the skin of the face caused by a concentration of the pigment melanin. It often occurs in pregnancy, sometimes in women who take birth control pills, and in ADDISON'S DISEASE.

See also MELASMA.

Chloramphenicol is an antibiotic drug. It is used in the treatment of typhoid fever, some forms of meningitis, and as drops or ointments for skin, eye, or ear infections. It has wide applications but it is used only with extreme caution because it may cause serious and even fatal damage to the blood-forming cells in the bone marrow.

Chlorhexidine is a disinfectant that is used on its own or with antibiotics to clean wounds or to sterilize the skin.

Chloroform was one of the first general anaesthetics and, like ether, was in common use until the 1950s. Since then it has been gradually replaced by safer, less toxic drugs.

See also ANAESTHETICS.

Chlorophyll is the pigment in all green plants that absorbs light energy from the sun to convert carbon dioxide and water into carbohydrates. In high concentrations, it can destroy bacteria that produce odours. For this reason it is assumed that chlorophyll acts as a deodorant in toothpastes and aerosol sprays.

Chloroquine is a drug that is taken by people in malarious regions to prevent them from getting the disease. The standard preventive dose is 300mg weekly, but larger doses are required if a person actually gets malaria. In some parts of the world, however, the disease is resistant to the drug. Prolonged, high doses may cause permanent eye damage, and regular eye examinations are necessary. Chloroquine has also been used in the treatment of amoebiasis, lupus erythematosus, giardiasis, and rheumatoid arthritis.

Chlorpromazine is a tranquillizing drug that is used in the treatment of major psychotic states. It is also used as a sedative drug in anaesthesia, and in treating addiction to psychedelic and amphetamine drugs.

Choking (for EMERGENCY treatment, *see* First Aid p.526) is the inability to breathe following the obstruction of the larynx or windpipe (trachea) by food, mucus, or a foreign object that has been swallowed or inhaled.

Obstructions can usually be removed by striking the victim hard between the shoulder blades, or, in the case of a small child or baby, by holding the victim upside down. If the victim does not immediately start to breathe again, after the obstruction has been removed, artificial respiration must be given.

Cholagogue is any substance that increases the flow of the bile from the liver into the intestine. An example is the presence in the stomach of food containing fats.

Cholangiogram is an X-ray of the gall bladder and bile ducts, which are made visible by using a dye that blocks X-rays. The dye may be swallowed in solution or it may be injected into a vein; the X-ray is taken when the dye is excreted in the bile ducts. A gall bladder that is diseased (for example, from infection or stones) may not excrete the dye. A cholangiogram is also taken during an operation to remove the gall bladder (cholecystectomy), in order to ensure that there are no stones in the bile duct.

Cholangitis is inflammation of the bile ducts. It is usually caused by an obstruction of the bile ducts that link the liver with the gall bladder and duodenum. The obstruction may be caused by gallstones, parasitic worms, or a cancer, or it may occur following the removal of the gall bladder (cholecystectomy). Pain in the upper abdomen is accompanied by a high fever, often with vomiting, hot and cold sensations, and jaundice. Dark urine and pale faeces can be other symptoms.

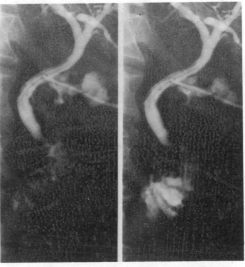

Cholangiogram is an X-ray of the bile duct taken after a radio-opaque dye is injected.

Cholecystectomy

Q: How is cholangitis treated?

A: Cholangitis may require hospital treatment consisting of antibiotic drugs and intravenous fluids, and an operation to remove the obstruction as soon as the patient is well enough.

Cholecystectomy is the surgical removal of the gall bladder.

Cholecystitis is an inflammation of the gall bladder. Acute cholecystitis is almost always caused by gallstones. Chronic cholecystitis commonly occurs in middle-aged persons, especially women, who are overweight and have gallstones.

Q: What are the symptoms of cholecystitis?

A: In acute cholecystitis, there is usually severe, sudden, or gradual pain in the right upper abdomen, with nausea, chills, vomiting, high fever, and sometimes referred pain in the back or the right shoulder. The symptoms of chronic cholecystitis are less severe, and include discomfort in the right upper abdomen, gas, belching, heartburn, or indigestion.

Q: How is cholecystitis treated?

A: Antibiotics and, if vomiting has been severe, hospitalization for intravenous fluids are preliminary treatments for acute cholecystitis. If there is no improvement, the gall bladder is removed (cholecystectomy). Sometimes it is necessary to drain the gall bladder (cholecystotomy) to allow the patient to become well enough for the gall bladder to be completely removed. For patients with chronic cholecystitis, weight loss and a low-fat diet are usually tried first.

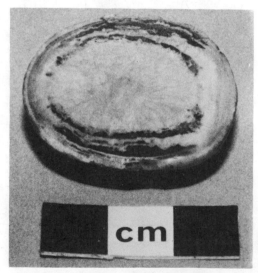

Cholelithiasis: picture shows cut surface of gallstone, about 3cm in diameter.

Cholelithiasis is the presence of gallstones in the gall bladder or bile ducts. Stones may form from precipitation of cholesterol, the bile pigment bilirubin, or a combination of both. This usually occurs when there is a high concentration of these substances in the bloodstream. This may happen in diabetes (high cholesterol) and haemolytic anaemia (high bilirubin). Other factors thought to be involved in the formation of gallstones include repeated infections of the bile ducts, some glandular or genetic factors, and a certain type of diet.

Q: What are the symptoms of cholelithiasis?

A: Many gallstones are "silent" (dormant) and produce no symptoms. Symptoms that can occur are pain in the right upper abdomen; wind; belching (made worse by eating foods containing fats); a spasm in the bile duct, causing severe pain, sweating, and vomiting, when a stone moves from the gall bladder (biliary colic); and jaundice, if a gallstone blocks the bile duct. Cholelithiasis increases the chances of infection in the pancreas and cancer of the gall bladder.

Q: Are some people more likely than others to get cholelithiasis?

A: Yes. Cholelithiasis occurs more often in middle-aged people (especially overweight women who have had children, and in some women taking the contraceptive pill). 10 per cent of people over the age of forty, and 20 per cent over the age of sixty, have gallstones. Gallstones often occur in patients with diabetes or haemolytic anaemia.

Q: How is cholelithiasis treated?

A: The usual treatment for gallstones that have produced symptoms is the removal of the gall bladder (CHOLECYSTECTOMY). In some cases, drugs that dissolve gallstones can be used if taken regularly over several months.

Cholera is an acute infectious disease caused by bacteria (*Vibrio cholerae,* or *comma*). Symptoms are severe diarrhoea and vomiting, with massive loss of body fluids, muscle cramps, and shock caused by dehydration. Cholera is transmitted by water, milk, or other foods, especially shellfish, that have been contaminated by the faeces of infected people. Cholera is mainly an epidemic tropical disease in Asia and Africa.

Q: How is cholera treated?

A: The patient requires replacement of fluids by drinking or by intravenous infusion to counteract the dehydration. Antibiotic drugs are also prescribed. During the recovery period, glucose and potassium tablets may be given.

Q: *How successful is the treatment of cholera?*

A: When proper treatment is available, it is usually effective and the patient recovers completely within two weeks. The death rate in adults is about five per cent, and in children ten per cent, but is much higher in regions where malnutrition and other diseases are widespread and facilities for treatment are inadequate.

Q: *Can cholera be prevented?*

A: People in epidemic areas are advised to avoid unsterilized water, fresh fruit, and shellfish. Cholera vaccinations provide some protection for at least three months. These consist of two injections given one to four weeks apart. International health regulations make vaccinations a condition of entry to certain countries in which cholera is endemic or of re-entry from such countries. Certificates of vaccination are valid for six months.

Cholesterol is a chemical that is found in the body's tissues and blood. The substance is manufactured in the liver as a by-product of the production of fats and fatty acids. Cholesterol is a normal constituent of bile. Many common foods contain cholesterol, but some foods contain more than others.

Q: *What may cause variations in the level of cholesterol in the body?*

A: Certain illnesses, such as diabetes and hypothyroidism, and excessive intake of food that contains cholesterol, result in increased levels of cholesterol in the blood. Although the relationship between cholesterol and good health is not fully understood, a high level of cholesterol appears to produce vascular disease (arteriosclerosis), and the likelihood of a stroke or coronary heart disease is increased. The tendency to have a high blood cholesterol level may be inherited. A high blood cholesterol level is usually accompanied by large amounts of other fatty substances in the blood.

Q: *Can a high cholesterol level be reduced?*

A: In all cases, treatment should be accompanied by a diet containing unsaturated vegetable fats instead of animal fats. These precautions may reduce the risk of strokes and heart disease. A doctor may prescribe the drug clofibrate (Atromid-S) to reduce a high cholesterol level in the blood. This is effective provided that a patient who is overweight loses weight.

Chondroma is a slow-growing, usually benign tumour of cartilage that may occur wherever cartilage is present in the body. It may or may not cause pain. Depending on its position, it may also increase the chance of breaking a bone. Chondroma occurs most commonly in adolescents and young adults.

Chondromalacia is the softening of cartilage in joints, especially that behind the kneecap (patella). It may cause pain and discomfort, but this usually improves with rest.

Chondrosarcoma is a malignant (cancerous) tumour that forms from cartilage cells. It may develop outside or inside a bone. *See* CANCER; TUMOUR.

Chordotomy. *See* CORDOTOMY.

Chorea is a disorder of the nervous system that is characterized by spasm of the facial muscles and involuntary contortions of the limbs. The two common forms of chorea are unrelated: Sydenham's chorea (St Vitus's dance) and Huntington's chorea.

Q: *What is Sydenham's chorea?*

A: Sydenham's chorea is a disorder in which the small arteries of the brain become inflamed. It is an allergic reaction to streptococcal infection. Sydenham's chorea commonly follows several months after an attack of rheumatic fever, and is most likely to occur in children between the ages of five and fifteen.

The symptoms of Sydenham's chorea include facial contortions, grunts, and occasionally difficulty in speaking. Sometimes, only one side of the body is affected.

Q: *How is Sydenham's chorea treated?*

A: The disorder is associated with rheumatic fever, and bed rest is essential. Sedative drugs help to control the involuntary contortions, and antibiotic drugs are usually prescribed to destroy infection.

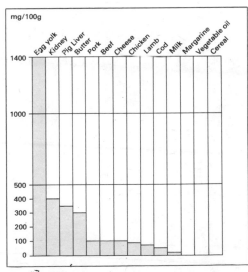

Cholesterol occurs in varying amounts in animal products, but not in vegetable foods.

Choriocarcinoma

The underlying disorder of the brain arteries is usually treated with regular high dosages of aspirin. Recovery may be complete within three or four months, but further attacks occur in about 30 per cent of cases.

Q: *What is Huntington's chorea?*

A: Huntington's chorea is a serious inherited disease of the central nervous system, which usually affects persons between the ages of thirty and fifty. The symptoms of Huntington's chorea are the gradual onset of involuntary jerky and contorting movements of the limbs. Mental deterioration and severe change of personality are associated symptoms, and the patient may eventually need institutional care.

Q: *Can Huntington's chorea be treated?*

A: No effective form of treatment has yet been found. Children of an affected parent have a 50 per cent risk of inheriting the disease. The usual medical advice to a person with the disorder is not to have children.

Choriocarcinoma is a malignant growth of the outer layer of the membrane (chorion) that surrounds a foetus in the womb. It is a rare condition that occurs in only one in 50,000 pregnancies. An obstetrician looks for signs of the disease in pregnant women in whom there has been degeneration of an ovum and the formation of a hydatidiform mole. Repeated blood tests are then made to determine the level of a certain hormone in the mother's bloodstream. If this level remains above normal, treatment with anticancer drugs (chemotherapy) is given, or the womb may be removed by an operation (hysterectomy).

Choroid is the middle coat of the eyeball that contains the dark colouring matter and blood vessels (*see* p.16). The term choroid plexus is applied to a small group of specialized blood vessels in the cavities (ventricles) of the brain, which produce CEREBROSPINAL FLUID.

Choroiditis is inflammation of the middle coat (choroid) of the eyeball. The symptoms of the disorder are a gradual blurring of vision, with flashes and bright circles of light. There is no pain, unless it is a sudden attack. Untreated, choroiditis may have serious complications.

Christmas disease, or haemophilia B, is an inherited defect in blood clotting which has the same symptoms as classic HAEMOPHILIA: prolonged bleeding from slight injuries and internal bleeding without any known cause. Treatment is transfusion of blood plasma containing the correct clotting factor. The condition gets its name from the patient in whom it was first discovered.

Chromosome is a thread-like structure in the nucleus of a cell. It is made up of many hundreds of genes, the messengers that carry the "instructions" that determine a person's hereditary make-up (*see* GENE). There are forty-six chromosomes (arranged as twenty-three pairs) in each human cell except the sex cells, which have only twenty-three chromosomes.

Q: *What happens to the chromosomes when a cell divides?*

A: The chromosomes divide at the same time as the cell, so that the two new cells, each with forty-six chromosomes, are identical to the parent cell. Exceptions are the cells that form sperm and ova, which divide to produce sex cells (gametes) with only twenty-three chromosomes each. This means that when a sperm joins an ovum at fertilization to form a new cell of forty-six chromosomes, it does so with half the genes from the mother and half from the father.

Q: *How do chromosomes decide the sex of an individual?*

A: The male chromosome is called Y. It is smaller, and contains fewer genes than the female chromosome. Each sperm contains either an X or a Y chromosome; each ovum contains a single X chromosome. When a sperm and an ovum combine to form a new individual, the fertilized ovum contains either two X chromosomes (XX) and is female, or it contains an X and a Y (XY) and is male.

Male chromosomes comprise 22 pairs, also found in females, plus one odd set (XY).

Chrysotherapy is the medical term for any treatment that employs gold or its compounds. *See* GOLD.

Chyme is the homogeneous pulp of partly digested food in the stomach. *See* DIGESTIVE SYSTEM.

Cicatrix is the medical name for a scar. *See* SCAR.

Cilia are the fine, hair-like projections of many cells of the body that sweep particles along. Microscopic cilia are found, for example, in the airways to the lungs (bronchi). Eyelashes are also sometimes known as cilia.

Circadian rhythm is the daily biological pattern in which sleep, hunger, and variation in body temperature occur. Moving to a distant time zone may disturb the rhythm, and the body may take ten days to adjust completely to the change.

Circulation, in medicine, usually means the flow of blood from the heart, through the arteries and capillaries, and back to the heart through the veins. The term may also be applied to the circulation of the cerebrospinal fluid around the brain and spinal cord, to the aqueous circulation of the eye, or to the lymphatic system.

Q: *Does all the blood go round one single circulation system?*

A: No. The systemic circulation is the passage of blood around the body. The pulmonary circulation is the passage of the blood through the lungs and back to the heart. In the foetal circulation, the blood by-passes the lungs from the pulmonary circulation into the systemic circulation through a special duct (ductus arteriosus). The placental circulation passes blood through the placenta of the foetus.

There are also the two portal circulation systems in which the blood flow starts and ends in the capillaries. One flows from the intestine to the liver (the hepatic portal system) and the other from the hypothalamus of the brain to the anterior lobe of the pituitary gland.

See also p.8.

A talk about Circumcision

Circumcision is the surgical removal of all or part of the FORESKIN (prepuce) of the penis. In infancy, it is usually carried out for social or cultural reasons. In later life it is less common, and usually performed for medical reasons.

Q: *How is circumcision carried out?*

A: There are two common methods. (1) A specially shaped piece of plastic is applied over the end (glans) of the penis and the foreskin is stitched over it before being cut off. (2) The foreskin is carefully cut and then stitched. An anaesthetic is not used for newborn babies, but is used for a child or an adult.

Q: *Are there any risks involved in the circumcision operation?*

A: Mistakes are extremely rare, but can occur. Too much skin, or not enough, may be removed, as may part of the glans itself. Damage may be caused to the urethra, or severe bleeding may occur.

Q: *What are the medical reasons for circumcision?*

A: In some rare instances, the foreskin is unusually long and the exit unusually narrow (phimosis) at birth. Or the glans, inside the foreskin, may become infected by bacteria (*see* BALANITIS) or from nappy rash. This causes the foreskin to become scarred and abnormally tight. Sometimes the foreskin stays retracted (paraphimosis). All of these conditions can be corrected by circumcision.

Q: *What are the social reasons for circumcision?*

A: These differ from culture to culture. Often circumcision forms part of a religious rite or an initiation into adulthood. Frequently, circumcision may seem desirable because it is in the tradition of the family or because the majority of boys in the neighbourhood are circumcised.

Q: *What possible advantages are there in not being circumcised?*

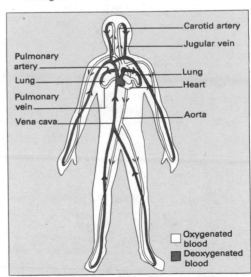

Circulation uses two main circuits, the systemic to the body, and the pulmonary to the lungs.

129

Cirrhosis

A: Ulceration of the glans is commoner in those who are circumcised than in those with a foreskin.

Q: *Does circumcision have any effect on the incidence of cancer of the penis or cancer of the cervix?*

A: There is some evidence, although it is not conclusive, that cancer of the penis is commoner in the uncircumcised and that circumcision reduces the possibility of cancer of the cervix (the internal opening to the womb) in the man's sexual partner.

Cirrhosis is a type of permanent and progressive liver damage. Any chronic liver disease, especially those caused by alcohol abuse or viral hepatitis, can lead to the formation of fibrous scars and nodules that connect to involve large areas of the liver. Once present, cirrhosis is permanent, but its progress can be stopped if the cause is removed. Untreated, it can be fatal.

Q: *What are the causes of cirrhosis?*

A: One of the commonest causes of cirrhosis is alcohol abuse. Other causes include infections, such as HEPATITIS and CHOLANGITIS; AUTOIMMUNE DISEASE; some rare inherited diseases (such as WILSON'S DISEASE and HAEMOCHROMATOSIS); and some drugs and chemicals, such as CARBON TETRACHLORIDE. In some parts of the world, virus infections or parasites are more common causes.

Q: *What are the symptoms of cirrhosis?*

A: Early symptoms can include weakness and a feeling of tiredness, loss of appetite, nausea and vomiting of blood, and constipation or diarrhoea. Symptoms of advanced cirrhosis include jaundice, broken blood vessels, a hard liver, a swollen abdomen, and swollen ankles. Some men suffering from the disorder experience an enlargement of their breasts, loss of pubic hair, and shrinking of the testicles (causing impotence).

Q: *How is cirrhosis treated?*

A: In cirrhosis caused by drinking alcohol, the only useful treatment is to stop drinking completely.

In cirrhosis caused by autoimmune disease, steroids and immunosuppressive drugs may be prescribed. Specialized care over a long period includes a high-protein diet with extra vitamins. Antibiotic drugs may be prescribed if there is infection (cholangitis). Occasionally the accompanying high blood pressure in the liver can be reduced by a surgical by-pass operation.

Q: *Can cirrhosis cause complications?*

A: Cirrhosis results in a kind of scar tissue that interferes with the flow of blood through the liver. This raises the blood pressure in the veins within the abdomen, especially at the lower end of the oesophagus, which becomes dilated and congested (oesophageal varices), and the rectum (haemorrhoids). If these veins burst, severe internal bleeding and vomiting of blood (haematemesis) can result.

Other complications of cirrhosis include jaundice, coma, bleeding disorders, peptic ulcers, and accumulation of fluid in the abdomen (ascites).

Claudication is the medical term for limping or lameness. Intermittent claudication is pain in the legs that is a symptom of arterial disease; the pain occurs only during exercise.

Claustrophobia is an abnormal fear of being in any confined area or enclosed space, such as a windowless room or lift. It is the opposite of AGORAPHOBIA.

Clavicle, or collar-bone, is one of two bones that connect the breastbone (sternum) with the shoulder blades (scapulas).

Claw hand is a deformity of the hand characterized by widely spread fingers, so that the hand resembles a claw. It is usually the result of a nerve injury.

Cleft palate is an abnormal fissure in the palate of the mouth that is present at birth. It is caused by faulty development of the facial structure of the foetus. Often, a cleft palate is accompanied by a similar division in the upper lip, called a hare-lip. In normal development, separate tissues fuse together to form the palate, upper lip, and upper jaw.

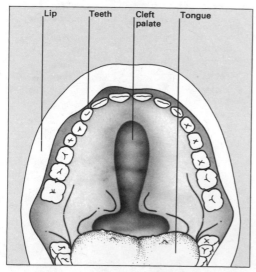

Lip Teeth Cleft palate Tongue

Cleft palate occurs because the roof of the mouth does not develop completely.

130

Q: *Does a cleft palate cause feeding problems for a baby?*

A: Yes. A cleft palate and hare-lip interfere with the natural sucking ability of a newborn baby, and the child must be fed with a bulb syringe or spoon, or with a special long nipple on a baby bottle.

Q: *Can a cleft palate be corrected?*

A: Most cases of cleft palate can be repaired by a series of operations during childhood. Plastic surgery is necessary to repair a hare-lip. If proper treatment is not started at a reasonably early age, the child may develop speech difficulties. Speech therapy may be necessary in any case for a person with a cleft palate.

Climacteric is the medical term for the time in a man's life when sexual activity naturally begins to decrease. In women, climacteric describes the changes that take place during the menopause (*see* MENOPAUSE).

Clitoris is a small, soft, sensitive area of tissue that is part of the female genitalia. It is situated below the pubic bone and is partially enclosed by the thin folds of the labia minora (*see* LABIUM). The clitoris plays an important part in the sexual stimulation of the female and, like the male penis, it becomes erect during sexual excitement.

Clonic refers to the alternate rapid contraction and relaxation of muscles.

Clostridium is a genus of spore-bearing, rod-shaped or spindle-shaped bacteria that are able to grow in the absence of oxygen. These bacteria are common in soil and in the intestines of animals. Some species are harmless to humans, but others produce toxins that are highly dangerous (*see* FOOD POISONING).

See also BOTULISM; TETANUS.

Clot is the jelly-like substance formed when a liquid coagulates. In medicine, the term is normally used to mean a blood or lymph clot (*see* BLOOD CLOT).

Clubbing is a condition of the ends of the fingers or toes, which become rounded and alter the shape of the nails. In most cases, clubbing is a sign of a serious underlying heart or lung disorder. It may also be a symptom of COELIAC DISEASE. If the cause is found and successfully treated, clubbing may disappear.

Clubfoot (known medically as talipes) is a deformity of the foot, present at birth. In the most usual form (talipes equinovarus), the sole of the foot is turned inward and the heel upward. It is more common in boys than in girls, and may affect both feet.

Treatment is most effective when started soon after birth. The foot is held in the correct position by a metal brace or a plaster of Paris cast. An orthopaedic surgeon may recommend an operation.

Coagulation is the formation of a clot in blood, lymph, or other liquid. It is a normal part of the healing process following an injury or surgery. Blood coagulation is a complicated process involving many factors to produce a BLOOD CLOT. If any of these factors is missing, coagulation occurs slowly or not at all. Haemophilia is a disease caused by a missing coagulation factor.

See also AGGLUTINATION.

Coarctation is a narrowing in a tube. The term usually refers to the narrowing of the aorta, the chief artery leading from the heart. This is usually a congenital defect (present at birth). Coarctation of the aorta prevents normal blood flow, causing high blood pressure in the head and arms, and low blood pressure in the rest of the body. It is treated by surgery, in which the narrowed section of the aorta is removed.

Cobalt bomb is a bomb-shaped lead casing that contains the radioactive isotope cobalt-60. The bomb is used to treat cancer by directing radiation from the cobalt-60 at a tumour.

Cocaine is a drug obtained from the leaves of the coca tree. The drug acts as a stimulant. Derivatives of cocaine are used as local anaesthetics in the treatment of minor conditions of the ears, eyes, nose, and throat. Cocaine is sometimes combined with opiate drugs in treating the painful, terminal stages of cancer. Large doses of cocaine cause hallucinations and trembling; in some patients, a marked sensitivity to cocaine can bring on these symptoms immediately.

Q: *Can a person become addicted to cocaine?*

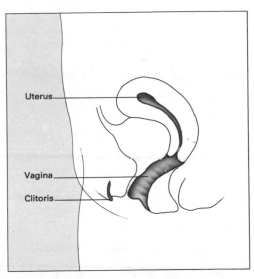

Clitoris, part of the female genitalia, is made of erectile tissue similar to the male penis.

Coccus

A: No, not in the physical sense, although some habitual users become psychologically dependent on cocaine to produce mental stimulation and excitement. Repeated use of cocaine leads to emaciation, memory loss, and mental deterioration. Because of the dangers of drug abuse, its prescription and use are tightly controlled by law.

See also DRUG ADDICTION.

Coccus is a spherical type of bacteria, which can be the cause of many infections. Streptococcus, pneumococcus, and gonococcus are examples of this group of bacteria.

Coccydynia is a severe pain in the region of the coccyx, at the base of the spine. It may occur after an injury or as a form of neuralgia. Treatment is generally with painkilling drugs or local anaesthetic. If this fails, the coccyx may be removed by surgery.

Coccyx is the final bone of the spine, usually formed from four small bones fused together and joined to the sacrum. The coccyx is sometimes called the tailbone.

Cochlea is a spiral-shaped organ in the inner ear. It contains the nerve endings that transmit sound to the brain, and is the most important organ of hearing. See p.16.

Codeine (known medically as methylmorphine) is a drug derived from opium. It is used as a painkiller, a cough suppressant, and a treatment for diarrhoea. Prolonged use of large quantities may produce mild addiction. Many painkilling preparations contain a small amount of codeine in addition to paracetamol or aspirin. Codeine by itself is available only by prescription.

Cod-liver oil is purified from the oil pressed from the fresh livers of codfish. The oil contains a high concentration of vitamins A and D, and was once used to supplement children's diets.

Coeliac disease is a disorder caused by sensitivity to the protein gluten, which is found in wheat, barley, and rye. The cells lining the small intestine are damaged and prevent the normal absorption of food, particularly fats. In adults, the disorder is also known as nontropical SPRUE.

Q: What are the symptoms of coeliac disease?
A: Babies and young children with the disease fail to gain weight normally, develop a swollen abdomen, and excrete loose, fatty stools. They may also suffer repeated respiratory infections, dry skin, and eventually, signs of anaemia, rickets, and other deficiency disorders. Adult patients suffer from tiredness, breathlessness, and muscle cramps. The abdomen is swollen, and the fingers may show clubbing.

Q: What is the treatment for coeliac disease?
A: Patients should be put permanently on a gluten-free diet, and treated for the anaemia or any deficiency disorder that is present. The diet should also be low in fats, with a high level of protein and vitamins to ensure adequate nourishment.

Coil is the common name for a type of intrauterine device (IUD) used in contraception. See CONTRACEPTION.

Coitus. See SEXUAL INTERCOURSE.

Colchicine is an alkaloid drug obtained from the roots of the autumn crocus. It is used to treat gout.

Cold. See COMMON COLD.

Cold abscess is an abscess that commonly accompanies tuberculosis. It develops so slowly that there is little inflammation, and becomes painful only when there is pressure on the surrounding area. A cold abscess may appear anywhere on the body, but is most commonly found on the spine, hips, lymph glands, or in the genitourinary organs.

See also ABSCESS.

Coldsore, or fever sore, is a small blister that appears, becomes an ulcer, and then heals with a scab. Coldsores usually occur around the lips and nose, but they are also common in the genital region, and tend to recur.

Coldsores, known medically as herpes simplex, are caused by the virus *Herpesvirus hominis*. This virus is present in many people and produces no symptoms when the person is in good health, but causes coldsores when another infection, such as the common cold, occurs.

Colectomy is an operation to remove part or all of the large intestine (COLON). It is usually performed to treat cancer of the colon or severe colitis. After a total colectomy or a partial colectomy close to the anus, an artificial opening is made in the wall of the abdomen (ileostomy or colostomy). When only a part of the colon is removed, the two ends are joined, but a temporary colostomy may be done to help healing.

Colic is acute pain in the abdominal cavity. The pain is usually localized in one of the ducts or hollow organs in the abdomen.

Q: What causes colic?
A: Colic in infants is usually related to diet, feeding methods, or emotional upset. An attack of infant colic is usually mild, although it may look severe and be accompanied by prolonged crying, abdominal distention, reddening of the face, and legs drawn toward the abdomen.

Colic in adults is in most cases severe. When its cause is an obstruction, such as a gallstone in the bile duct, the person may vomit and double up with pain. Colic may also accompany menstruation.

Q: How is colic diagnosed and treated?

A: Infant colic is usually diagnosed by observing the signs. The infant should be comforted until the pain subsides, and special attention paid to diet and feeding methods. Adult colic is usually diagnosed using special X-ray techniques and treated by eliminating the cause, such as removal of a gallstone.

Colitis is inflammation of the COLON. The commonest forms of the disorder are mucous colitis and ulcerative colitis.

Q: What is mucous colitis and how is it treated?

A: Mucous colitis is common and without signs of disease of the colon. It is thought to be brought about by psychological or emotional distress.

Diagnosis of mucous colitis is often made when a person under stress has symptoms, such as abdominal pain, insomnia, headache, fatigue, and diarrhoea, interspersed with constipation.

Treatment is primarily psychological, but the person's diet may need to be altered to correct irregular bowel movements, and sedatives may help the person to relax. In some severe cases, regular psychiatric help may be needed.

Q: What is ulcerative colitis?

A: Most cases of ulcerative colitis are severe and potentially life-threatening. The exact cause of the disorder is not known, but the commonest of its symptoms is explosive, and sometimes bloody, diarrhoea. Other symptoms may include severe abdominal pain, loss of weight, high fever, abdominal tenderness, toxaemia, and peritonitis.

Q: How is ulcerative colitis diagnosed and treated?

A: Examination of the rectum, with an instrument called a proctoscope, and X-rays of the colon usually detect this disorder. Treatment should be aimed at stopping the diarrhoea before dehydration and severe malnutrition occur. The attacks of diarrhoea must in any case be halted before a proctoscopic examination can be done or X-rays taken. When a positive diagnosis has been made, additional treatment may include admisson to hospital, corticosteroid drugs, intravenous fluids and blood transfusions, special diets, and sometimes, an operation.

See also DIARRHOEA; DYSENTERY.

Collapsed lung is a condition in which a section of lung contains no air. It may occur if there is an obstruction by a tumour or foreign body in the main bronchus (*see* ATELECTASIS), or if air enters the pleural cavity that surrounds the lung (pneumothorax), and compresses the lung.

Collar-bone. *See* CLAVICLE.

Colles' fracture is a fracture of the radius bone in the forearm, just above the wrist, in which part of the radius shifts and causes the wrist to be unnaturally positioned upward. A general anaesthetic is normally given while a surgeon restores the bone to its original position. The forearm is immobilized in a cast for about six weeks, after which physiotherapy is needed to restore normal movement to the wrist. A bad repair may leave the wrist permanently weak, and the tendons in the wrist may tear from rubbing against the fracture site.

Coloboma is a congenital eye defect that may appear as a white swelling or as a gap. Or it may appear as a groove or cleft in the iris, the lens, or the choroid. Sometimes the eyelid is also involved. Vision may be impaired, and there is no treatment for the condition.

Colon is the part of the large intestine that extends from the caecum to the rectum. ("Large" refers to diameter, not to length.) Sections of the colon have different names. For example, the ileum of the small intestine joins with the caecum of the colon. Where the colon extends upward, it is called the ascending colon; where it crosses the abdomen, it is called the transverse colon; and where it moves downward toward the pelvis, it is called the descending colon. The last part is the sigmoid colon, which meets the rectum.

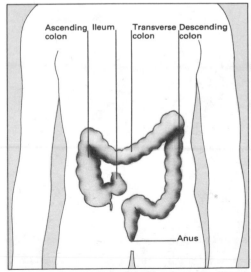

Ascending colon   Ileum   Transverse colon   Descending colon

Anus

Colon receives indigestible fibre from the ileum and passes it along to the anus by peristalsis.

Colonic irrigation

Q: What is the function of the colon?

A: Although most of the digestive process occurs in the small intestine, the colon absorbs excess water and salts to be taken into the blood. This function of conserving and recycling is an important one: without it, dehydration can take place. After the excess water and salts have been absorbed by the blood, the remaining contents of the colon take on the consistency of faeces, which are stored in the rectum until passed through the anus.

Colonic irrigation. *See* ENEMA.

Colostomy is an artificial connection between the large intestine (COLON) and the surface of the body on the abdominal wall, which is produced during an operation. A special bag over the opening in the abdominal wall is usually necessary to collect stools.

Q: Why might a patient need a colostomy?

A: A diseased area of colon may have to be removed (partial COLECTOMY). Then the two new ends each side of the removed portion may be brought to the surface. This type of colostomy may be temporary, until the two ends can themselves be joined surgically. But if the whole of the lower part of the colon is diseased and has to be removed, the upper end alone may be brought to the surface. This type of colostomy is permanent.

Q: What adjustments might a colostomy patient have to make?

A: Usually, a colostomy is no great inconvenience, once the patient has learned how to deal with it. The diet should be regulated to avoid constipation

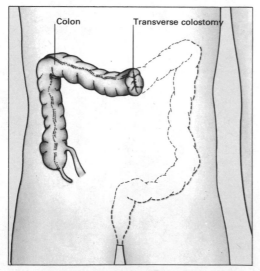

Colostomy performed on the transverse colon is managed post-operatively with a bag.

or diarrhoea. Some patients find that a morning ENEMA via the colostomy clears the colon for the day, and the bag may not be required.

The patient gains confidence from the emotional support of other colostomy patients. This can come from the many colostomy societies, which offer help and mutual advice.

Colostrum is the yellow fluid secreted by a woman's breasts for a few days before and after childbirth. It contains about twenty per cent protein, including the mother's antibodies to the diseases that she has had (*see* ANTIBODY). Colostrum has a higher concentration of salts but less fat and carbohydrates than normal breast milk.

Colour blindness is an inherited defect of vision resulting in a person's inability to distinguish between specific colours. Partial colour blindness is more common than total colour blindness, in which a person sees everything as shades of grey. The most common form of partial colour blindness leads to an inability to distinguish between red and green; rarely, the difficulty is between blue and yellow.

Colour vision depends on the stimulation of the 10 million cone cells in the light-sensitive membrane at the back of the eye (retina). The three colours distinguished by the eye – red, green, and blue – cause three different pigments in the cone cells to react. Absence of one or more of these pigments at birth results in defects of colour vision.

Q: How common is colour blindness?

A: The defect is genetically determined, and is passed on to about ten per cent of the male population. Only about one per cent of all women have some form of colour blindness. Total colour blindness is rare.

Q: How is colour blindness diagnosed?

A: ISHIHARA'S TEST is used. This is composed of a series of coloured cards on which numbers or lines of equal shade can be read by a person with normal colour vision but not by someone with defective colour vision.

Coma is a deep and sometimes prolonged unconsciousness state (for EMERGENCY, *see* First Aid, p.573). It may result from a head injury, stroke, reaction to drugs or alcohol, or an epileptic seizure. Or it may be caused by a disease such as diabetes or uraemia (retention in the blood of substances usually excreted by the kidneys).

Treatment is to place the patient in the recovery position and to keep the airway open (*see* p.544). Breathing and pulse rate should be monitored. The patient should be hospitalized at once.

Comedo. *See* BLACKHEAD.

Comminuted fracture is a bone fracture in which the bone is splintered.

Common cold, known medically as coryza and often called merely a cold, is a contagious virus disease of the respiratory tract. It is a droplet infection, that is, people catch a cold by inhaling airborne water droplets sneezed out by a patient with the disorder. Symptoms appear about forty-eight hours after exposure to the virus, which may be any one of more than forty different types.

Q: What are the typical symptoms of a cold?

A: Early symptoms of a cold include a runny nose, watering eyes, a headache, and a sore throat. Later, there may be a stuffy nose, a slight cough, and aching muscles. The patient may also have a chill and a slight fever.

Q: Can a cold be serious?

A: A cold, although extremely annoying, is seldom serious. But babies and young children and patients with asthma, bronchitis, a heart disorder, or kidney disease who have symptoms of a cold may be at risk and should have medical advice.

Q: Can a cold be cured?

A: There is no cure for a cold. Home treatment to relieve the symptoms includes regular doses of a mild painkiller such as aspirin or paracetamol, an antihistamine drug to help to dry up the nasal discharge, a cough medicine, and throat lozenges for the sore throat. Contrary to popular belief, antibiotics do not cure a cold (or any other virus infection). The patient should drink plenty of fluids, and avoid contact with others to prevent spreading the infection.

Communicable disease is one that is transmitted from one person or animal to another, either by indirect means or by direct contact (when it is said to be contagious). Sometimes the disease is transmitted by a CARRIER.

See also CONTAGIOUS DISEASES.

Complex is a psychological term, introduced by Carl Jung, for an idea or group of ideas repressed into the unconscious. It is because these ideas have a strong emotional charge that complexes may influence a person's behaviour. Examples of complexes include the Electra complex, the sexual love of a daughter for her father; Oedipus complex, the sexual love of a son for his mother; and inferiority complex, a state of mind in which a person feels inferior to others.

The term complex is often loosely used to mean an obsession. Complex also refers to the lines traced by an electrocardiograph that represent the beating of the heart. A collection of symptoms may also be called a complex, but such a collection is more usually termed a syndrome.

Compound fracture is a bone fracture in which the broken bone causes a surface wound. The bone may or may not be visible. A compound fracture is more serious than an ordinary fracture because of the risk of infection. For EMERGENCY, *see* First Aid, pp.546–553.

Compress is a pad of material by means of which heat or cold can be applied to the body.

Computerized axial tomography. *See* CAT SCANNER.

Conception is the moment in the reproduction cycle when a sperm fertilizes an ovum. This usually takes place in a woman's fallopian tube. The fertilized egg then passes into the womb (uterus), where it becomes implanted in the wall and develops first into an embryo and then into a foetus. *See* PREGNANCY AND CHILDBIRTH.

Concussion is an injury to a part of the body resulting from a blow or from violent shaking. Concussion usually refers to an injury to the brain. Brain concussion is commonly caused by a head injury, but it may also result from a fall on to the lower end of the spine.

Q: What are the symptoms of brain concussion?

A: The symptoms of brain concussion vary according to the site and extent of the injury. Brain concussion usually, but not always, produces unconsciousness. The

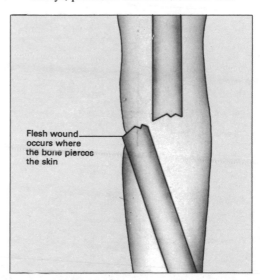

Flesh wound occurs where the bone pierces the skin

Compound fracture is susceptible to infection because the break creates an external wound.

135

Conditioned reflex

return to consciousness often occurs gradually. Following the initial injury, there may be headache; difficulty in concentrating; nausea; vomiting; difficulty in focusing; and a feeling of depression and irritability. Events immediately before the injury may be forgotten at first (retrograde amnesia), but the memory of them usually returns.

Q: *How is brain concussion treated?*

A: A doctor should be consulted in all cases of concussion because there may be more serious brain damage. Bed rest is essential for at least a day after the injury. Painkillers may be given to relieve the headache. Alcohol, sedatives, and tranquillizers may aggravate the symptoms. The patient should avoid sports and work requiring concentration or skill until he or she is completely recovered.

Conditioned reflex is either a modification of an inborn reflex or a completely new automatic response that is developed as a result of an individual's experience. Conditioned reflexes were first demonstrated by Ivan Pavlov in the 19th century. He taught a dog to salivate at the sound of a bell by first teaching the dog to associate the ringing of a bell with the appearance of food.

See also REFLEX.

Condom. *See* CONTRACEPTION.

Condyloma is an infectious wart-like growth on the genitals or near the anus. *See* SYPHILIS; WART.

Congenital refers to any characteristic or condition that is present at birth.

Approximate incidences of some congenital anomalies		
Defect	Ratio M:F	Incidence per 1,000
Congenital heart disease	1:1	
Pyloric stenosis	4:1	
Clubfoot	2:1	
Down's syndrome	1:1	
Spina bifida	1:1	
Hydrocephalus	1:1	
Anencephaly	1:2	
Congenital dislocated hip	1:6	
Harelip and cleft palate	2:1	
Klinefelter's syndrome	1:0	

Congenital anomalies are defects that occur in only a few of every 1,000 newborn children.

A talk about Congenital anomalies

Congenital anomalies are mental or physical abnormalities that are present at, and usually before, birth. Some anomalies may be medically insignificant and may not appear for some time. In other cases, the anomaly may pose a direct threat to life and require immediate attention. There are, however, some anomalies that cannot be treated.

Q: *What are examples of congenital anomalies?*

A: Congenital anomalies include BLINDNESS, BONE DISORDERS, CATARACT, CLEFT PALATE, CRETINISM, DEAFNESS, DOWN'S SYNDROME, ENDOCRINE GLAND disorders, CONGENITAL HEART DISEASE, HAEMOPHILIA, HYDRO-CEPHALUS, JOINT DISORDERS, PYLORIC STENOSIS, and SPINA BIFIDA.

Limbs or organs may be malformed, duplicated, or entirely absent. Organs may fail to move to the correct place, as in CRYPTORCHIDISM, fail to open correctly, as in IMPERFORATE ANUS, or fail to close at the correct time (*see* DUCTUS ARTERIOSUS). Congenital anomalies often occur together. For example, forty per cent of babies born with Down's syndrome also have heart disease.

Q: *What may cause the development of congenital anomalies?*

A: Congenital anomalies arise from the faulty development of a foetus, caused either by genetic disorders or other factors. Some anomalies arise from a combination of factors, and the underlying cause is far from clear in all cases.

Q: *How are genetic disorders responsible for congenital anomalies?*

A: Inherited congenital anomalies generally result from the presence of abnormal GENES or CHROMOSOMES. Heredity is determined by corresponding pairs of genes, called alleles. One of these paired genes is dominant and the other recessive, and it is the dominant gene that governs the transmitted trait or characteristic. Thus, if the abnormal gene of a pair is dominant, the abnormal or anomalous trait will be conveyed to the embryo. If the abnormal gene is recessive, then both genes in the pair have to be recessive for an abnormality to occur.

Some congenital anomalies, such as haemophilia, are linked to a defect of one of the sex chromosomes. Many genetic disorders, however, are neither wholly dominant, recessive, nor sex-linked, but may be caused by more than one abnormal pair of genes.

Congenital heart disease

Q: *What other factors may cause congenital anomalies?*

A: Infection in the mother is a common cause of abnormality in a baby. For example, an attack of GERMAN MEASLES during the first three months of pregnancy may cause her child to be born deaf or have cataracts, heart disease, jaundice, or other anomalies. Infectious HEPATITIS, MUMPS, and TOXOPLASMOSIS also cause congenital anomalies.

Certain drugs taken by a woman during pregnancy are often responsible for abnormalities in the child. For example, corticosteroid drugs may cause cleft palate, and drugs used in the treatment of thyroid disorders may result in GOITRE or cretinism in the baby. Other drugs may cause gross abnormalities, such as the defects arising from thalidomide.

Injury to a pregnant woman or to a foetus is another cause of congenital anomalies. For example, limbs may be malformed if an intrauterine device (IUD) is not removed early in the pregnancy. Smoking during pregnancy is implicated as one factor in the incidence of abnormally low birth weight in babies, and malnutrition seems to be related to a high incidence of congenital anomalies. The age of the woman at the time she conceives can also be a factor. For example, Down's syndrome occurs more frequently when conception occurs after the age of about forty.

Congenital anomalies have also been attributed to the effects of X-ray examination made early in a pregnancy.

Q: *It is possible to diagnose congenital anomalies in a foetus?*

A: Sometimes. The most reliable method of diagnosis is to examine a sample of fluid from the amniotic sac at about the fourteenth week of pregnancy. The sample is obtained by AMNIOCENTESIS, and microscopic examination of the cells in the fluid reveals possible abnormalities in the chromosomes. Congenital anomalies that can be diagnosed in this way include Down's syndrome, spina bifida, and anencephaly. Sometimes the diagnostic use of ultrasound can detect abnormalities of the skull or spine.

Q: *Can congenital anomalies be treated?*

A: Treatment depends entirely on the nature and severity of the condition. Many anomalies can be treated, but for some there is no treatment.

Q: *In what circumstances might abortion be considered?*

A: Abortion might be considered if serious foetal disorders are found early in a pregnancy. The decision to abort rests with the parents, and is taken after considering the advice of the doctor and specialists on the nature of the disorder and the consequences of abortion.

Q: *Are congenital anomalies more likely to occur in first-born babies?*

A: No. Statistics disprove this commonly held belief.

Q: *Does a congenital anomaly in a baby indicate that subsequent babies will be similarly affected?*

A: The branch of medicine that deals with such questions is GENETIC COUNSELLING. In many cases it is possible to state risks numerically. For example, a baby with congenital heart disease is likely to be followed by a similarly affected child in two per cent of pregnancies instead of the ordinary risk of one per cent. Spina bifida occurs in about one child in every 3,000 but if a previous child was born with the condition, there is about a one-in-forty chance that it will occur in a later child.

Congenital heart disease is any heart disorder that is present at birth, although the condition may not be diagnosed until later in life. The most common problems are due to failure of closure between the two sides of the heart ("hole in the heart"), or failure of closure of the DUCTUS ARTERIOSUS. In addition, narrowing of the opening of either of the main arteries is fairly common. Many defects are complex and some involve a hole

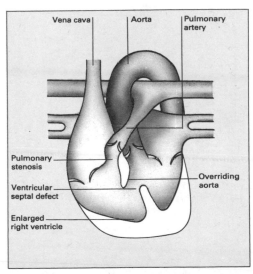

Vena cava | Aorta | Pulmonary artery

Pulmonary stenosis

Ventricular septal defect

Enlarged right ventricle

Overriding aorta

Congenital heart disease that affects four sites in the heart is known as Fallot's tetralogy.

Congestion

in the central portion of the heart, through which blood passes from one side to the other.

Q: *What are the symptoms of congenital heart disease?*

A: The symptoms, if present at all, depend on the nature of the disorder. For example, ventricular septal defect may be detected by a heart murmur. Breathing difficulty and a bluish colour to the skin may also be symptoms in a baby (*see* BLUE BABY; FALLOT'S TETRALOGY). An infant with congenital heart disease who survives is likely to have frequent respiratory infections.

Q: *What are the causes of congenital heart disease?*

A: Often the cause is unknown, although genetic factors are thought to be important. Some forms of congenital heart disease may be caused by a virus infection in the mother during the first three months of pregnancy.

Q: *How is congenital heart disease treated?*

A: Successful treatment depends on correct diagnosis. If possible, the appropriate type of heart surgery is then undertaken.

Q: *Are some babies more susceptible to congenital heart disease than others?*

A: Yes. Although less than one per cent of first-born babies have a congenital heart disease, the likelihood of it occurring in a subsequent baby is increased to one in fifty. There is a one in twenty-five chance that a baby born to parents who themselves have a congenital heart disorder will also have a heart problem.

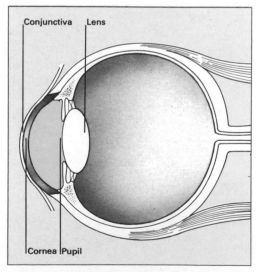

Conjunctiva lines the inside of the eyelids and covers the front portion of the eyeball.

Congestion is the swelling of body tissues due to the accumulation of blood or tissue fluid. It may be a reaction to infection or injury, or it may be caused by a blockage in veins returning blood to the heart.

Congestive heart failure is a condition in which the heart is unable to maintain the normal circulation of the blood. The blood in the veins increases in volume, and the veins become dilated. The lungs, liver, and intestines become congested with blood. There are various causes of congestive heart failure, including weakness of the heart muscle; high blood pressure; hardening of the arteries; and rheumatic or syphilitic disease of the heart valves. Untreated, the condition can be fatal.

Q: *What are the symptoms of congestive heart failure?*

A: The symptoms include breathlessness, swollen ankles (a form of oedema), and weakness.

Q: *How is congestive heart failure treated?*

A: A doctor may prescribe a diuretic drug, which helps to relieve any swelling (oedema) in the body tissues and reduces some strain on the heart. A salt-free diet is sometimes recommended, to help to prevent any further retention of fluids. In addition, Digoxin may be used to improve the strength of the heartbeat. Bed rest, with hospitalization if necessary, is advised for acute congestive heart failure. Oxygen may be required, and a source of oxygen should be kept available.

Conjunctiva is the thin, mucous membrane that lines the eyelid and covers the front of the eyeball.

Conjunctivitis (also called "pink eye") is inflammation of the membrane covering the eye (the conjunctiva). Acute conjunctivitis most commonly occurs during viral respiratory illnesses, such as the common cold or influenza. More severe attacks are usually caused by bacterial infections. Conjunctivitis that is not associated with respiratory disorders may be caused by irritants such as dust, cosmetics, or smoke, or by an allergic reaction to a specific substance, such as pollen. Conjunctivitis may also result from the tropical eye disorder trachoma, and from a number of other rare afflictions.

Q: *What are the symptoms of conjunctivitis?*

A: The eye tends to water profusely and the white of the eye is bloodshot or pink. The eye is painful when moved, and may be over-sensitive to bright light. Sometimes there is a discharge of pus from the eyelids.

Q: *How is conjunctivitis treated?*

A: A doctor usually prescribes an antibiotic drug and other treatments such as eye drops. Prolonged use of drops, however, may aggravate the inflammation. Conjunctivitis known to be caused by an allergy may be treated with corticosteroid drugs. Dark glasses give protection against bright light, but a patch over the eye may increase the inflammation. If the eye is painful, a mild painkiller such as aspirin gives relief. It is important not to rub the eye, because this may transmit the conjunctivitis to the other eye.

Connective tissue is any tissue that connects and supports other tissues or organs — for example, the fibrous tissue of ligaments. Dense connective tissue includes CARTILAGE and bone. Scars are formed from connective tissue.

A talk about Constipation

Constipation is the difficult or infrequent excretion of faeces. The frequency of bowel movements considered to be normal depends on the individual: "normal" may range from movements three times a day to three times a week. Greater intervals of time between movements than is customary for a particular person are a sign of constipation. The condition is not an illness in itself, but it may be a symptom of one, and a person should consult a doctor if it persists.

Q: What causes constipation?

A: Constipation is most often caused by insufficient bulk in the diet or the habit of ignoring the desire to defecate. This gradually makes the rectum tight as the faeces accumulate there, especially if a person's diet contains little vegetable fibre and a lot of highly processed food. Some effects of hormones produced during pregnancy may aggravate the problem. A marked change in diet, for example, as a weight-losing measure, may cause constipation. Painkilling drugs taken regularly are often a cause. A person taking drugs that are used as treatment for hypertension, rheumatic disorders, or depression may suffer from constipation.

Q: Why are babies often constipated?

A: Hot weather, insufficient fluid in the diet, or a fever may cause slight dehydration in babies. This means that most of the fluid in the colon is absorbed into the bloodstream, leaving the faeces hard and difficult to pass. If a baby is constipated from birth, it may be a sign of a developmental failure in the intestine called HIRSCHSPRUNG'S DISEASE.

Q: Are laxatives an effective treatment for constipation?

A: Laxatives are sometimes used for immediate relief from constipation, but they should be used sparingly and never taken if other symptoms indicate that the patient may have APPENDICITIS. The regular use of strong laxatives that contain chemicals and vegetable irritants (for example, senna or cascara), far from preventing constipation, actually maintains it.

Q: How else can constipation be treated?

A: Treatment must be aimed at removing the cause, such as depression. Non-irritant purgatives help to return the bowel to its normal rhythm; if the faeces are hard, special softening laxatives may be recommended. An attempt should be made to establish some regularity in bowel movements and eating habits. A diet containing vegetable fibre, bran, cellulose, or other bulk produces large soft faeces, which are easily passed.

Q: Does constipation affect certain groups of people more than others?

A: Constipation tends to affect twice as many women as men, and it occurs more frequently with advancing age. Those who spend many hours sitting down are more susceptible to constipation than those who are physically active.

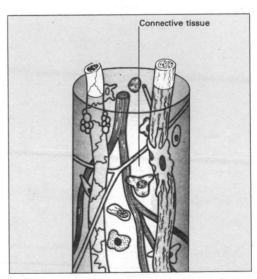

Connective tissue is a substance that supports cells and fibres in the body.

Consumption

Consumption. *See* TUBERCULOSIS.

Contact lens is a glass or plastic lens that fits over the cornea of the eye to correct a vision defect. Contact lenses adhere to the cornea and move with the eyeball, providing greater peripheral vision than conventional SPECTACLES. The modern soft, hydrophilic plastic lenses, which allow fluids to pass through, are more comfortable to wear than the older, harder types. And unlike hard lenses, soft lenses do not require a special salt solution to lubricate the cornea when they are put in.

Q: *What are the advantages and disadvantages of contact lenses?*

A: Apart from good general vision, contact lenses can provide the means of keeping medication in contact with the eyeball for persons with keratitis (inflammation of the cornea). They may also retard the progress of myopia.

But contact lenses may require skilful fitting, and be expensive. In the time needed for the eye to become used to a lens, conjunctivitis may occur: lenses must not be worn when the eye is inflamed, even with the mild conjunctivitis that occurs with a cold. The lenses must be removed and sterilized every night. They can also cause an allergic reaction.

Yet to many people they are more convenient than conventional glasses, when they have been worn for a time.

Contagious diseases are infectious diseases that are transmitted by direct physical contact (*see also* COMMUNICABLE DISEASE). The following is a list of contagious diseases, each of which has a separate entry in the A-Z section of this book.

BRONCHITIS	MONILIASIS
BRONCHOPNEUMONIA	(thrush)
CHICKENPOX	MUMPS
CHOLERA	PARATYPHOID
COMMON COLD	PLEURODYNIA
CONJUNCTIVITIS	PNEUMONIA
DIPHTHERIA	POLIOMYELITIS
GERMAN MEASLES	PUERPERAL FEVER
(rubella)	RINGWORM
GLANDERS	ROSEOLA
GLANDULAR FEVER	SCARLET FEVER
GONORRHOEA	SMALLPOX
HAND-FOOT-AND-	SYPHILIS
MOUTH DISEASE	TRACHOMA
INFLUENZA	TYPHOID FEVER
LEPROSY	VACCINIA
MEASLES	VENEREAL DISEASES
MENINGITIS	WHOOPING COUGH
MOLLUSCUM	(pertussis)
CONTAGIOSUM	YAWS

A talk about Contraception

Contraception, or birth control, is the prevention of pregnancy. There are various contraceptive methods. Some are designed to prevent the male sperm from fertilizing the female egg (ovum), and others to prevent the already fertilized egg from developing. The most suitable method is a matter of personal choice and medical advice, and often involves some experimentation. The failure rate of each method is expressed as the number of pregnancies per 100 that occur in women using the method each year.

Q: *What forms of contraception require no artificial aids?*

A: There are two common "natural" methods. (1) Coitus interruptus is the withdrawal of the penis from the vagina before ejaculation. It is probably still the most widely practised method, but is most unreliable, because some sperm nearly always escape before orgasm. The technique also induces stress during intercourse, and many couples find this method frustrating. The failure rate is about 30–40 per 100.

(2) In the rhythm method or safe period, intercourse is avoided on the days before and following ovulation, when an egg is released from an ovary and travels along a fallopian tube to the womb. These so-called "safe" days are calculated using the date of ovulation, with the knowledge that the egg survives for a maximum of one day and the sperm

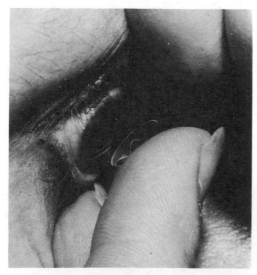

Contact lens is a cosmetic alternative to spectacles. It is shaped to fit over the cornea.

for not more than three days. Ovulation usually occurs between 12 and 16 days before a menstrual period is due. A woman can calculate her own ovulation time using either the calendar method or the temperature method, although neither method is totally reliable.

Q: What is the calendar method?

A: For this method, a record of menstruation must be kept for at least six months. The first "unsafe" day is found by subtracting 19 from the shortest recorded cycle, and the last by subtracting 10 from the longest cycle. Thus, if a woman's shortest cycle was 27 days and her longest 32, she must avoid intercourse from days 8 to 22, counting the first day of menstruation as day 1.

Q: How does the temperature method work?

A: Each month a woman's body temperature rises slightly at the time of ovulation. She can record this rise if she takes her temperature every morning before (and not after) getting out of bed. The "safe" period is usually from three days after until five days before the next rise in temperature. The failure rate is about 20–30 per 100.

Q: What are the artificial aids to contraception?

A: Two methods use simple physical barriers between the sperm and the egg. (1) The condom, worn by the man, is a sheath of thin rubber or plastic, and often has a small teat at the end to collect the ejaculated sperm. The condom is rolled on to the erect penis just before intercourse. After orgasm the penis must be withdrawn from the vagina before it becomes flaccid, or the condom may fall off in the vagina. For added protection the woman should use a spermicide.

The condom is probably the most widely used form of artificial contraceptive, and has a failure rate of about 10–20 per 100.

(2) The diaphragm, or Dutch cap, is a dome-shaped piece of rubber or plastic attached to a flexible wire ring. It is placed across the upper end of the vagina covering the cervix to prevent sperm from entering the womb.

Q: How does a woman choose the correct size of diaphragm?

A: The first fitting must be made by a gynaecologist. After an examination, a woman is given the correct size of diaphragm and taught how to fit it herself. She should fit it each night as a matter of habit, whether or not she has intercourse. For maximum effectiveness, the diaphragm should be used with a spermicide and left in place for at least six hours after intercourse. The failure rate is about 5 per 100, but is higher if the diaphragm does not fit well.

Q: How do spermicides work?

A: Spermicides are chemicals available as jellies, foams, or pessaries that kill sperm in the vagina. They are inserted high into the vagina at least five minutes before intercourse and must be reapplied before further intercourse. Spermicides should never be used alone.

Q: How does an IUD work?

A: The intrauterine device (IUD) is a small, flexible piece of plastic that is inserted into the womb through the vagina. It is usually shaped as a coil, loop, or ring, and may contain copper, zinc, or progesterone. The copper, zinc, or progesterone is believed to increase the effectiveness of the plastic by its poisonous effect on the fertilized egg.

An IUD should be changed every two years.

Some forms of IUD, such as the loop and the coil, are best suited to women who have borne children. Also, women who suffer particularly heavy periods are advised against using an IUD, since it tends to increase the menstrual flow.

Q: How is an IUD fitted?

A: A woman must consult a gynaecologist, who first examines her carefully for infection or pregnancy. A thin plunger containing the IUD is then inserted through the cervix into the womb, where

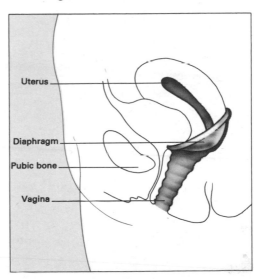

Diaphragm has a springy outer rim that holds it in position over the entrance to the womb.

Contraception

it is released. Insertion is easiest during a period, when the cervix expands a little.

Q: *What are the side effects of an IUD?*

A: After insertion there may be intermittent bleeding and some abdominal cramp, as the womb tries to expel the IUD, but these symptoms should disappear after a few weeks. Another side effect is that the first few periods may be heavier and cause more backache than usual.

Q: *What happens if the side effects of the IUD persist?*

A: A woman should consult her gynaecologist, in case she is not suited to an IUD. If side effects are accompanied by irritation and a heavy vaginal discharge, they may be caused by an infection. This infection can spread from the womb to the fallopian tubes and may lead to infertility if left untreated.

    Any woman with an IUD should have regular gynaecological check-ups.

Q: *Is the IUD a safe and effective contraceptive?*

A: Yes. Although about ten per cent of users expel the device, serious complications are unusual and fewer than those from the contraceptive pill. An IUD does not need a spermicide and is less bother than a condom or a diaphragm. The failure rate is about 2 in 100.

Q: *What is the birth control pill?*

A: Oral contraceptives, or the pill, were introduced in the 1950s as hormone preparations used to prevent pregnancy. The pill must be prescribed by a doctor. It is by far the most reliable

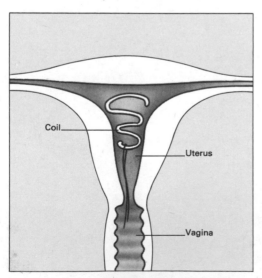

Coil is thought to work as a contraceptive by preventing the implantation of a fertilized egg.

contraceptive, and possible side effects are its only drawback. Recently, side effects have been greatly reduced by using the lowest dosage of hormone capable of preventing pregnancy.

Q: *How does the pill work?*

A: There are many different types of birth control pills, but they all contain synthetic preparations of one or both of the hormones known as oestrogen and progesterone. The oestrogen works by preventing ovulation each month in the same way as the natural hormones do during pregnancy. As a result, there is no egg to be fertilized by the sperm. The progesterone has three functions: (1) it helps to prevent ovulation; (2) it thickens the cervical mucus, thus presenting a barrier to the sperm; and (3) it affects the lining of the womb, making it unreceptive to a fertilized egg.

Q: *What is the combined pill?*

A: This pill has both oestrogen and progesterone hormones. One pill is taken each day for three weeks in the menstrual cycle, thus allowing menstruation to occur in the fourth week, when no pills are taken. The withdrawal of hormones usually produces a lighter and shorter period. The first course of pills is started on the fifth day after menstruation starts, but additional contraceptive precautions must be taken for at least two weeks during the first course. The failure rate is about 0.025 in 100.

Q: *How does the progesterone-only pill work?*

A: This so-called "minipill" relies solely on the effects of progesterone. The dosage is continual and low, and menstruation occurs irregularly, sometimes with breakthrough bleeding between periods. It is essential that the pill be taken each day, preferably at the same time. If two consecutive pills are missed, the woman must use an additional means of contraception until her next period. Even when used correctly, the minipill incurs a higher risk of pregnancy than the combined pill. The failure rate is about 1 in 100.

Q: *What are the side effects of the pill?*

A: Common side effects of the pill are: (1) occasional nausea and weight gain, which may occur in the early weeks of use; (2) an increase in tenderness of the breasts and in vaginal discharge; (3) variable effect on the skin, with either an improvement in, or worsening of, acne, and occasionally a brownish discoloration of the face (chloasma); (4) slight fatigue or weariness in muscles, loss of sexual drive, and mild depression; (5) increase or decrease in headaches and migraine; and (6) spotting and breakthrough bleeding. (Spotting is slight blood loss from the womb, and the pill should be continued for the rest of the cycle. Breakthrough bleeding is like normal menstruation, and the pill should be stopped and a new cycle started after a week.)

If adverse symptoms persist for more than two or three months, a gynaecologist should be consulted, because a different preparation may be needed.

Q: *What are the more serious complications associated with the pill?*

A: (1) A woman's fertility may be affected temporarily after she stops taking the pill and before the return of normal menstruation. This happens more often to women whose periods have previously been irregular. (2) Although diabetes is not caused by the pill, mild diabetes may be made worse by it. (3) Hypertension may occur in some women, particularly in those who have had high blood pressure in pregnancy. (4) Recent studies have shown that thrombosis has slightly increased in women taking a pill containing oestrogen. The risk of thrombosis increases in those over the age of thirty-five, but the risk is much less than that associated with pregnancy and childbirth.

Q: *Is it true that the pill can cause cancer?*

A: Research is still continuing, but there is no conclusive evidence yet that the pill causes cancer of the breast or the womb.

Q: *Can any woman take the pill?*

A: The pill should be prescribed only after a gynaecologist has made a thorough examination and selected the type of pill most suited to the woman. Any woman using the pill should have regular pelvic examinations and cervical smear (Pap) tests.

Q: *Is there a surgical form of contraception?*

A: Yes. Surgical sterilization may be performed on men or women to make them infertile. It is a minor operation for either, but one that is difficult to reverse. Sterilization of men is known as vasectomy; sterilization of women is known as tubal ligation.

Q: *How should a woman decide which contraceptive to use?*

A: In a younger woman, the combined pill is the safest and most convenient form of contraception, unless there are reasons why she cannot use it. Women often express anxieties about continuing it for possibly fifteen or twenty years. In this case, they may use the IUD, which offers

convenience and safety, provided it does not cause side effects. If an IUD is uncomfortable, a woman may try the diaphragm or return to the pill.

The increasing awareness of the hazards of pregnancy after the age of forty leads many women at this age to choose sterilization. It is important that, before selecting a contraceptive, a woman consult her doctor, consult the nearest branch of the Family Planning Association, and talk to other women friends to learn about each method.

Contrecoup injury is an injury to one side of the brain as a result of a blow to the head on the opposite side. For example, a blow on the back of the head can cause the front parts of the brain to be rotated and bruised.

Contusion is a superficial injury in which the skin is not broken, often producing a bruise. There may be pain, swelling, and a discoloration of the skin.

Convalescence is the period of recovery from the end of an acute stage of an illness or operation to the return of a normal level of health and activity. During this period, a person may be weak and in need of both physical and psychological help.

Q: *What practical measures should be provided during convalescence?*

A: Most of the specific measures provided during convalescence are, of course, determined by the person's doctor.

There are, however, some general measures that are applicable to

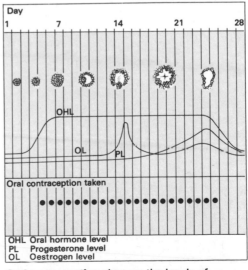

Oral contraception taken

OHL	Oral hormone level
PL	Progesterone level
OL	Oestrogen level

Oral contraception changes the levels of hormones in the blood and stops ovulation.

most people during convalescence. For example, conditions favouring rest should be provided. Meals should be small in quantity but more frequent than normal to help encourage the return of a healthy appetite. As the person's strength returns, regular exercise such as walking should be encouraged to help restore normal muscle tone. The person's morale will benefit from companionship, especially during a long convalescence.

Convulsion (for EMERGENCY treatment, *see* First Aid, p.528) is a series of sudden muscular spasms, activated by the brain and involving contortions as muscles alternately contract and relax. Loss of consciousness is also usual. A convulsion (also called a seizure or fit) may occur as a symptom of various disorders: epilepsy; infection in the brain (for example, encephalitis or meningitis); drug withdrawal; diabetes; high fever, particularly in children; brain tumour; arteriosclerosis (in elderly people); toxaemia of pregnancy; and poisoning.

Q: *What immediate treatment should be given?*

A: The first priority is that the patient should be protected against injury. An unconscious patient should be put in the recovery position and the airway should be kept open to prevent choking. A convulsion in a feverish child can be treated by sponging with cool or tepid water, so that heat is lost by evaporation. A diabetic should be given sweets or sugar because the convulsions may be caused by excess insulin.

Extra sugar is not harmful to a diabetic in such circumstances.

Cooley's anaemia. *See* THALASSAEMIA.

Cordotomy is an operation to cut some of the nerves in the spinal cord. It is a method of relieving chronic severe pain.

Corn is the thickening of the skin on or between the toes. It is usually produced by friction or pressure caused by tight or ill-fitting shoes. If present on exposed surfaces, a corn is hard; if it occurs between the toes, it is soft and may become inflamed.

See also First Aid, p.579.

Cornea is the clear transparent layer on the front of the eyeball. Its curvature is greater than that of the other layers of the eyeball, and so it acts (with the lens) to refract light rays and focus them on to the retina at the back of the eye.

Corneal graft is a form of eye surgery in which a damaged cornea is replaced by a healthy cornea. A cornea removed from the eye of a deceased donor within six hours of death can be preserved in special frozen solutions before it is needed for a corneal graft.

Q: *How might the cornea be damaged?*

A: Scarring of the cornea from injury or disease often renders it useless. If the damage is severe, a graft may not be possible. In such cases it may be possible to replace the cornea with one made from plastic.

Coronary generally refers to the heart. The term "coronary" is also sometimes used to mean a HEART ATTACK, in which case it is actually an abbreviation of "coronary thrombosis".

See also CORONARY HEART DISEASE.

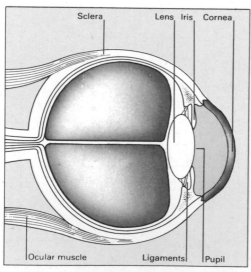

Cornea is the transparent front portion of the sclera, the fibrous coat that surrounds the eye.

Sclera   Lens Iris   Cornea

Ocular muscle   Ligaments   Pupil

A talk about Coronary heart disease

Coronary heart disease is any damage to the heart muscle resulting from reduced blood supply from the two coronary arteries, which encircle the heart. Normal blood supply is reduced by the narrowing of any section of an artery. ARTERIOSCLEROSIS, a build-up of fatty deposits in the arterial walls, is the most common cause, and the artery most commonly affected is the first descending branch of the left coronary artery.

Q: *What are the symptoms of coronary artery disorders?*

A: Sometimes a pain in the centre of the chest (angina pectoris) occurs during exercise. Such pain goes when the exercise ceases. Often there are no symptoms at all until thrombosis (occlusion) completely stops the blood supply. This causes death of part of the heart muscle, a condition known medically as myocardial infarction. In popular usage it is called a "coronary", "heart attack", "infarct", or "thrombosis". For EMER-GENCY, *see* First Aid pp.554–557.

See also HEART DISEASE.

Q: *What are the symptoms of a heart attack?*

A: The patient usually complains of severe, tight, constricting pain in the chest. This may extend to the shoulders, arms, hands, into the neck and jaw, and some-times down into the upper abdomen. The pain may be accompanied by shortness of breath, nausea, and sweating. A patient with these symptoms should be taken to hospital as soon as possible. It is also possible to have a "silent" heart attack, with no symptoms, which may only be discovered much later on an electrocardiogram (ECG).

Q: *How long does the pain last?*

A: The pain may last from a few minutes to several hours, after which the patient is exhausted.

Q: *Does the heart stop beating?*

A: Sometimes if the condition is severe, the heart may stop beating, which causes death if the heartbeat is not restored. About 70 per cent of patients survive a heart attack; about 20 per cent die before reaching the hospital; and the remaining 10 per cent die within a month of the infarct.

Q: *How is a heart attack diagnosed?*

A: The diagnosis of a heart attack is made from several facts: (1) by studying the patient's history of pain; (2) by observing characteristic changes in the electro-cardiogram; (3) by detecting the presence of various enzymes in the blood.

Q: *What is the treatment for a heart attack?*

A: The patient may be admitted to a coronary care unit, where electro-cardiographic monitoring is done to detect any irregularities in the pulse. Such irregularities may indicate that the heart is weak and may be about to stop. Pulse irregularities can be treated with drugs. Injections of painkilling drugs can be given if needed. Patients under about the age of 60 may be given anticoagulant drugs (for example, heparin or warfarin) to prevent further thrombosis. After two to three days, the most dangerous period is over and the patient is usually allowed out of bed. This reduces the chance of deep vein thrombosis in the legs.

Q: *For how long may a coronary heart disease patient stay in hospital?*

A: It depends on the size of the heart muscle

that has died (infarcted), whether the whole thickness of the heart wall is involved, and any complications. But a patient may be in hospital for about ten days to three weeks.

Q: *What advice can be given about con-valescence?*

A: The patient should live a quiet and relaxed life, without stress, and take increasing amounts of exercise. The taking of anticoagulant drugs may be continued at home for several weeks. Sexual intercourse may be resumed after the first month. Heavy lifting and strains should be avoided for two months following the attack. After six weeks, the dead muscle in the heart will have been replaced by scar tissue. To strengthen the heart, the doctor may recommend exercise in a coronary rehabilitation unit.

Q: *Does a heart attack alter the life style of a patient?*

A: There are a number of precautions that a patient must observe for life. Most doctors advise physical exercise for 10–15 minutes a day. Initially, exercises may be taught at a coronary rehabilitation centre, where monitoring equipment shows up any signs of heart strain in the patient.

A person who has had a heart attack must never smoke, but can drink alcohol in reasonable quantities if it does not interfere with a weight-reducing, low cholesterol diet. If the patient suffers from hypertension (high blood pressure), this must be treated and kept well under control.

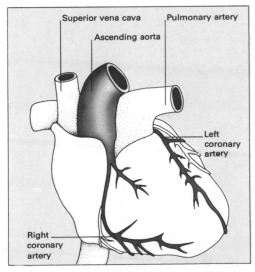

Coronary heart disease is caused by reduced blood supply in the two coronary arteries.

Coroner

Q: *What are the complications of coronary heart disease?*

A: Damage to the electrical conducting mechanism of the heart may cause atrial FIBRILLATION, with the symptom of an irregular, rapid pulse. Congestive heart failure (due to inadequate pumping by the heart) may occur at times, and if the heart muscle has been damaged, ANGINA PECTORIS may be a complication.

Q: *Are certain groups more prone to coronary heart disease than others?*

A: Four times as many men as women have coronary heart disease; also it tends to affect more men earlier in life than women. Coronary heart disease is more common in women after the menopause. There is a high incidence of the disorder in the following groups: smokers; those with hypertension; the overweight; those with high blood cholesterol levels; those with physically inactive jobs; and those with anxious or aggressive dispositions. The possibility of a heart attack is greatly increased in those who have had one already, those who have a family history of them, and those who are diabetic.

Coroner is an official – usually a doctor – appointed by the Home Office to preside over a court that investigates the circumstances of any death possibly not due to natural causes (an inquest). The medical facts of death are examined, including the result of any autopsy, together with the surround-

ing circumstances. Witnesses and pathological experts may be called, and there is sometimes a jury. The verdict reached concerns the deceased's manner of death only; the medical facts stated are merely evidence.

Corpuscle is the medical term for any small, rounded body. It is usually applied to blood cells: red blood corpuscles (erythrocytes) and white blood corpuscles (leucocytes).

Corpus luteum is a small, yellow hormone-producing structure that develops in an ovary at the site of a released egg (ovum). In addition to the hormone called oestrogen, also being produced by the ovaries and the adrenal glands, the corpus luteum produces progesterone. These hormones prepare the lining of the womb (endometrium) for the implantation of a fertilized ovum. If conception takes place, and an ovum becomes fertilized, the corpus luteum remains; if not, it degenerates and shrinks when menstruation starts.

Cortex is the outer layer of an organ, as distinct from the inner portion (medulla).

Corticosteroid drugs are synthetic derivatives of CORTICOSTEROIDS used to treat Addison's disease, allergies, rheumatic disorders, and inflammation. They must be used with particular care in the presence of infection.

Corticosteroids (corticoids) are various steroid hormones produced in the outer layer (cortex) of the adrenal glands. The term is also used for a number of synthetic derivatives (corticosteroid drugs) that have similar properties to the natural hormones.

There are three main groups of naturally-occurring corticosteroids: (1) ALDOSTERONE, which regulates the excretion of sodium and potassium salts through the kidney; (2) CORTISOL (hydrocortisone), which promotes the synthesis and storage of glucose and regulates fat distribution within the body; and (3) sex hormones, which have only a minor effect on the body of an adult. Aldosterone and cortisol are essential to life, and they affect many chemical processes within the body. They work together to maintain a constant internal environment, despite the fact that the body is continually subjected to changes.

Corticotropin. *See* ACTH.

Cortisol (hydrocortisone) is the most important naturally occurring of the CORTICOSTEROIDS. It controls the level of glucose, fats, and water in the body. Several synthetic cortisol drugs are available. They all work by preventing the body's normal reaction to disease or damage. This effect can be useful in treating such conditions as allergy or inflammation, but cortisol must never be used if infection is present.

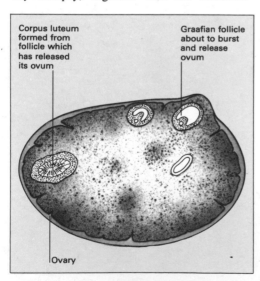

Corpus luteum formed from follicle which has released its ovum

Graafian follicle about to burst and release ovum

Ovary

Corpus luteum is a structure that develops in an ovary and secretes progesterone.

Q: *What are the medical uses of cortisol?*

A: It is given in small daily doses to treat
ADDISON'S DISEASE, in which there is a lack
of natural cortisol. In tablet form it is
used to treat some types of asthma,
muscle pains, acute allergies, and some
forms of cancer. As an injection it is used
to treat some rheumatic conditions (for
example, rheumatoid arthritis) and shock.
Cortisol is also available in cream, lotion,
and ointment forms, which are used to
treat localized inflammation of the skin
and eyes. A recent use of cortisol is in the
suppression of organ rejection following
transplant operations.

Q: *Can cortisol produce any adverse effects?*

A: Yes. Although the level of naturally-
produced cortisol is carefully regulated by
the body, excessive use of cortisol as a
drug may cause diabetes, calcium loss
from bones (osteoporosis), weight
increase, and muscle weakness. Wounds
heal slowly and the onset of infections
and internal abscesses may be
overlooked, because cortisol prevents the
body from reacting normally. Prolonged
use of cortisol may cause acne and red
stripes on the skin because of changes in
metabolism; the adrenal glands may also
stop working. This may cause problems
when trying to reduce the dosage, which
must be done gradually to allow the
adrenal glands to recover.

People taking cortisol and similar
synthetic drugs should carry a card
stating they do so, in case they are
involved in a traffic accident or other
emergency.

Cortisone is one of the CORTICOSTEROID hormones. It is inactive until changed into
CORTISOL by the liver.

Coryza. *See* COMMON COLD.

A talk about Cosmetic surgery

Cosmetic surgery is a form of surgery done to
improve a person's appearance. It is a branch
of PLASTIC SURGERY.

Q: *Why do people have cosmetic surgery?*

A: Usually because they are distressed or
dissatisfied by their natural face or figure,
or because they have been involved in a
disfiguring accident. Skilful surgery can
alleviate mental as well as physical
anguish, giving or restoring confidence to
those who would otherwise avoid normal
contacts.

Q: *What kinds of cosmetic repairs can be
made?*

A: Almost any kind that is required. A cleft

lip may be closed; a hand made immobile
by scars can be restored to function;
injuries to the face, from car accidents or
industrial accidents, can be repaired by
sculpting and realigning the delicate
bones. In such cases, wires and splints are
used to reconstruct facial features, and
flaps of muscle fill the vacant spaces left
by bone that has been destroyed or
removed. Bone grafts may also be used.

Women who are dissatisfied with the
shape or size of their breasts can have
them altered by MAMMOPLASTY. This
technique is safe, but not all women are
satisfied with the results.

Q: *What other methods of cosmetic surgery
are there?*

A: Skin GRAFTS are sometimes made to cover
large raw areas, as in severe burns, and to
serve as an efficient dressing to protect
the raw area from infection and loss of
body fluid. A thin layer of skin is
surgically removed from one part of the
body and laid over the injured area,
where the skin cells are soon nourished
by the tiny blood vessels of the injured
area.

Pitting of the skin, caused by acne or
smallpox for example, may be treated by
a surgeon with surgical planing, often
called dermabrasion. In this method, a
general anaesthetic is given, and the
doctor uses a rapidly rotating wire brush
to remove the pitted surface of the skin.
Healing takes place beneath a
scab in a little more than a week. The
new skin that forms is usually a great

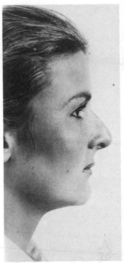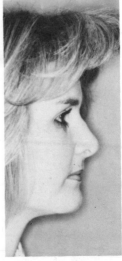

Cosmetic surgery performed on the nose (left)
results in a smaller nose with a better shape.

improvement over the scarred and pitted one. Wrinkles, if they are not deep, may also be removed or made less conspicuous in this way.

Another method used is chemical peeling, in which the skin is painted with a chemical. This produces peeling of old, scarred, or wrinkled skin.

Q: Can scars result from cosmetic surgery operations?

A: Every surgical operation leaves a scar, but its size depends partly on the skill of the surgeon and partly on the healing properties of the individual.

Cot death. *See* SIDS.

Cough is an action that clears an irritated area of the lungs or throat. It is a common symptom of a number of disorders, such as a common cold, influenza, or a minor respiratory illness. It may also accompany a respiratory tract disorder or heart disease.

Any cough that lasts for more than a few days should be discussed with a doctor.

Q: Should medicine be taken to stop a cough?

A: Coughing is a useful and protective mechanism, and treatment that completely suppresses it could do more harm than good. When a person coughs, a deep breath is taken in, the vocal cords close, and pressure builds up within the lungs. When the cords open, a violent expulsion of air takes place as the body attempts to expel any foreign material in the throat or lower respiratory tract.

Cough syrups that help the person to bring up phlegm are called EXPECTORANTS, and many kinds are available without prescription from a chemist. Other preparations containing ANTIHISTAMINES may help to dry up secretions. A cough suppressant, sometimes prescribed by a doctor, contains a drug such as codeine or dextromethorphan.

Q: Apart from infection, what else can cause a cough?

A: Smoking can produce a cough, especially in the morning, because in people who smoke the lining of the air passages to the lungs (the bronchi) is damaged and the lungs fail to empty themselves naturally during the night.

Q: What can be done for a dry cough?

A: Eating something dry, such as a dry biscuit or cake, may help to stop the irritating tickle. In a dry, overheated room, a vaporizer can relieve congestion of the nose and throat membranes.

Sometimes a dry cough, especially in a child, can be exhausting and debilitating, as in WHOOPING COUGH (pertussis) or some of the virus illnesses that commonly occur during the winter months. In such cases, a medicine that suppresses the cough to some extent is helpful, but should be used only on medical advice.

Cowpox, medical name vaccinia, is an infection of cattle that can cause a mild illness in human beings. It is the virus originally used by Edward Jenner in 1796 for vaccinating human beings against SMALLPOX. In the milk cow, the udder and teats are affected by a slight eruption. Similar, pus-filled blisters appear on the skin of human beings who have either been inoculated with cowpox vaccine or been in contact with infected cows.

Coxalgia is the medical name for pain in the hip.

Coxa vara is a deformity of the thigh-bone (femur). The angle of the neck of the bone, where it joins the part leading to the hip joint, is reduced.

Coxa vara is much more common than the associated condition coxa valga, in which the bone angle is increased.

There are various possible reasons for coxa vara: it may be congenital; caused by a fracture; or caused by a softening of the bone from rickets, osteomalacia, or parathyroid disease. The condition may also result from any injury during childhood that causes the head of the thigh-bone to slip or move out of position. The patient has a limp because one of the legs acts as if it were shorter than the other. There is often pain in the hip (coxalgia).

Treatment depends upon the cause, which

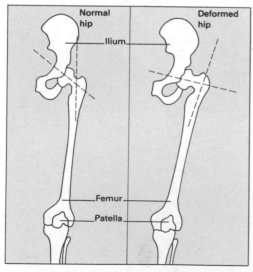

Coxa vara is a deformity of the hip that may occur as a result of injury, or rickets.

should be diagnosed by a bone specialist.

Coxsackie infection is caused by a family of viruses that can produce a number of serious disorders, including a severe, influenza-like illness (Bornholm disease) and a virus form of meningitis. It is named after a city in New York State where it was first isolated in 1948. Diagnosis is usually made by means of blood tests after the patient has recovered, and treatment is with painkilling drugs and rest. *See* PLEURODYNIA, EPIDEMIC.

Cramp is a sudden, involuntary, and often painful contraction of a muscle or a group of muscles. The affected muscles may become hard and knotted. Cramp in the intestine is called colic, and cramp in the leg may occur during the night (night cramps). Cramp may occur after prolonged exercise, such as swimming; at night, especially in the elderly and usually affecting the leg muscles; or at the start of menstruation. The causes of cramp are not fully understood, but in some cases cramp may be caused by salt loss from excessive sweating or diarrhoea, or from poor blood circulation.

Q: How can cramp be treated?

A: Because the causes of cramp are so little understood, there is no single treatment for all types of cramp. Stretching and warming the affected muscle may help. Drinking water to which salt has been added may relieve cramp caused by salt loss. If cramp occurs frequently, especially in the calf muscles after walking (intermittent claudication), a doctor should be consulted because there may be a more serious underlying cause, such as a disorder of the blood circulation.

Craniotomy is an operation to make an opening in the skull, as a preliminary to brain surgery.

Cranium is the anatomical name for the skull. It usually refers to the part that surrounds the brain, but excludes the bones of the face and the jaw.

Cretinism is a condition of stunted body growth and impaired mental development. The symptoms, which appear during early infancy, are the gradual development of a characteristic coarse, dry skin, a slightly swollen face and tongue, and an open mouth that drools. The baby is usually listless, slow moving, constipated, and a slow feeder. Cretinism is the result of a congenital deficiency in the secretion of the hormone thyroxine from the thyroid gland. In some cases this is thought to be caused by an insufficient amount of iodine in the diet of the child's mother during pregnancy.

Q: How is cretinism treated?

A: After the condition has been diagnosed with the help of blood tests, treatment with thyroid hormone promotes normal physical and mental development. It is essential that treatment be started during the first six weeks of life, or irreversible changes may take place.

Crohn's disease (regional ileitis or regional enteritis) is a chronic inflammatory condition of the intestine. There is no known cause for the disease, although it may be hereditary. It is usually confined to the lower end of the small intestine (ileum), but may involve the large intestine (colon). The symptoms of Crohn's disease include intermittent attacks of diarrhoea and abdominal pain, weight loss, and fever. Rarely, the intestine may burst (causing PERITONITIS) or become blocked, or ulcerate into adjacent areas. Treatment involves a nutritious diet, painkilling drugs, antibiotics, and sometimes corticosteroids. If complications occur, the doctor usually recommends surgery to remove the diseased section of intestine.

Cross-eye. *See* STRABISMUS.

Cross infection is the infection of one patient by another. This is a serious problem in hospitals, especially if the disease-producing organism is resistant to most antibiotics.

Croup is an acute breathing disorder, most often occurring in young children. The mucous membrane of the larynx, trachea, and bronchial tubes becomes inflamed and swollen, and produces excessive mucus.

Q: What causes croup?

A: Respiratory infections caused by various kinds of bacteria can often result in

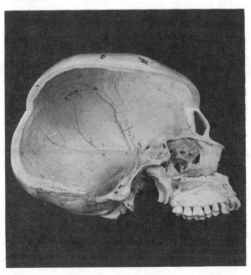

Cranium is that portion of the skull that encloses the brain.

Crush syndrome

croup. The condition is usually mild but is capable of being serious, and it may develop rapidly.

Q: *What are the symptoms of croup?*

A: For most cases of croup, there is loss of appetite, fever, noisy breathing, and a barking cough that ends with a whistle upon inhalation. Only in the most severe cases of croup do certain other symptoms occur, such as cyanosis (blue-tinged skin) due to insufficient oxygen. This condition is a medical emergency.

Q: *How are most cases of croup treated?*

A: Generally, croup is treated with antibiotics, which help destroy bacteria causing the infection. Antihistamines may also be prescribed, along with the use of a steamy atmosphere, to aid breathing.

Crush syndrome is the failure of the kidneys and liver to function after severe injuries, especially a crushed leg. It occurs because large amounts of proteins from damaged muscles have been released into the circulation system, and the kidneys cannot cope with them; shock is another factor. Treatment of this very serious condition requires hospitalization. KIDNEY DIALYSIS may be necessary until the kidneys recover.

Cryosurgery is a surgical technique in which tissues are exposed to extreme cold, usually below−20°C (−4°F). It is used to remove cataracts and malignant tumours. Cryosurgery is also used in brain surgery, in the treatment of cervical erosion and warts, and to reduce bleeding.

Cryptorchidism (cryptorchism), commonly

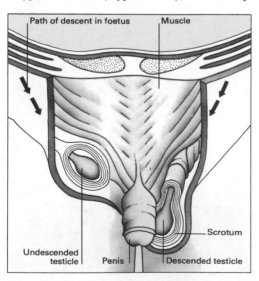

Cryptorchidism is the failure of a testis to descend from the abdomen to the scrotum.

known as undescended testicles, is the condition in which one or both of the testicles have not descended into the scrotum. It is often accompanied by a hernia in the groin.

Q: *Why does cryptorchidism occur?*

A: The reason is not known. The testicles develop in the abdomen of a foetus, and before birth they descend through the abdominal wall into the scrotum. If this fails to happen, cryptorchidism results. In many boy babies the testicles appear to be absent, because the attached muscles pull them up to the abdominal wall. This is perfectly normal and should not be confused with cryptorchidism.

Q: *How is cryptorchidism treated?*

A: If the testicle can be located outside the abdomen an operation may be performed to fix the testicle in the scrotum. If the testicle is in the abdomen, major surgery is involved. It may still not be possible to find the testicle. An alternative, but less certain, method is the administration of human chorionic gonadotrophic hormone, which may stimulate the testicle to descend.

Curare is the general name for a wide variety of poisonous extracts from several South American trees. Curare causes rapid paralysis of the muscles throughout the body and was originally used on poisonous arrows by the South American Indians. A refined preparation of curare called d-tubocurarine may be used as a muscle relaxant drug during anaesthesia.

Curettage is the scraping clean of the interior of a body cavity with a spoon-shaped instrument called a curette. See D AND C.

Cushing's syndrome is a rare glandular disorder in which there is excessive production of cortisol and similar corticosteroids by the adrenal glands. Cushing's syndrome may occur spontaneously or it may be caused by a tumour of the adrenal glands, or a tumour of the pituitary gland, causing an excessive amount of corticotropin to be produced and overstimulation of the adrenal glands. Cushing's syndrome may also result after prolonged medication with large doses of corticosteroid drugs.

Q: *What are the symptoms of Cushing's syndrome?*

A: The symptoms of Cushing's syndrome include fatty swellings on the back of the neck; a characteristic "moon face"; fatigue; weakness; obesity of the trunk, while the limbs remain thin; and skin discoloration with pink streaks. There may also be excessive hair growth, reduced sex drive in men, and the cessation of menstruation in women. In

150

cases where the cause is cancer, Cushing's syndrome may be fatal.

Q: How can Cushing's syndrome be treated?

A: There are drugs available that may temporarily control the symptoms, but surgical removal of either the tumour or the overproductive tissue is the most common treatment. Radiation therapy is also sometimes used. If an adrenal gland is surgically removed, there will be a lack of the hormones that it normally produces. Such a lack may be compensated for by taking corticosteroid drugs.

Cut. For treatment of cuts, *see* First Aid, p.582.

See also HAEMORRHAGE.

Cutaneous refers to the skin. For example, cutaneous nerves are sensory nerves that are situated in the skin.

Cuticle is a layer covering the free surface of epithelial cells. It may be horny or calcified, as in tooth enamel. The term is also used for the thin outer layer of the skin, often that adjacent to a fingernail.

Cyanosis is a bluish discoloration of the skin, most easily seen in the lips. It is caused by a lack of oxygen in the blood. This, in turn, may be caused by sluggish surface circulation in cold environments, failure of the lungs to oxygenate the blood fully, pneumonia, heart failure, asphyxiation, or overdose of certain drugs. It also occurs in children with some forms of congenital heart disease (*see* BLUE BABY). Treatment depends on the cause.

Cyclamate is any salt of cyclamic acid. Today cyclamates are available only on prescription, because they were implicated as cancer-forming agents (carcinogens) in experiments on animals.

Cyclopropane is a colourless gas that is used as a general anaesthetic. *See* ANAESTHETICS.

Cyst is an abnormal swelling or sac that usually contains fluid. Cysts can occur in almost any body tissue, but they are most frequently found in the skin and ovaries, where they may grow to a large size. There are several kinds of cysts: (1) nonmalignant tumours with cells producing liquids that cannot escape; (2) cysts containing cells of tissues that are normally found elsewhere in the body (for example, a DERMOID CYST may contain elements of skin and hair); (3) cysts caused by parasitic infection (for example, *see* HYDATID CYST); and (4) ordinary glands that have become blocked (for example, a sebaceous gland in the skin blocked by a plug of fat forms a sebaceous cyst). Treatment, if any, depends on the type of cyst.

See also TUMOUR.

Cysticercosis is a disorder caused by infection with the pork tapeworm (*Taenia solium*).

The tapeworm embryos penetrate the intestinal wall and spread throughout the body, causing small cysts in the muscles, eye, heart, liver, or tissue of the central nervous system. During the first weeks of infestation, there may be no symptoms, but later fever, headache, and aching muscles usually occur. Other symptoms may take many years to appear: epilepsy, heart disease, nerve damage, or even personality changes. A doctor may diagnose cysticercosis by means of X-rays, blood tests, and biopsy. The treatment is the removal of any cyst that causes specific problems, or the drug mepacrine.

See also TAPEWORMS.

Cystic fibrosis is a noncontagious, inherited disorder in which mucous secretions from several parts of the body become thick and sticky and interfere with normal functioning. Commonly involved are the lungs, liver, and pancreas. Mucus in the lungs can block the bronchi, making breathing difficult. Thick mucus can also block the ducts of the liver and the pancreas, causing improper digestion.

Q: What are the symptoms of cystic fibrosis?

A: Persons with cystic fibrosis seem to be born healthy, but begin showing signs of this disorder between infancy and adolescence. Such signs may include greasy, foul-smelling stool; chronic cough; persistent wheezing; and recurrent respiratory problems.

Q: How is cystic fibrosis diagnosed?

A: Along with observation of symptoms common to this disorder, special tests often help in the diagnosis. It seems that the sweat glands are also affected by

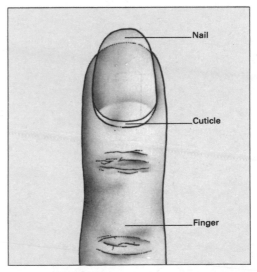

Cuticle is the hard skin at the base of a nail. If it is injured, a hangnail may form.

Cystitis

this disorder and produce excessive amounts of salt, which can be detected by testing the sweat.

Q: *How is cystic fibrosis treated?*

A: There is no known cure for this disorder, which can be fatal during childhood. Treatment usually involves alleviating symptoms. For example, antibiotics against infections and special diets for malnutrition may be prescribed. Sometimes digestion can be improved by taking preparations of missing digestive enzymes. Inhalation of water mist helps to thin mucus in the lungs.

A talk about Cystitis

Cystitis is the acute or chronic inflammation of the bladder. It causes frequent, painful, cloudy urination. Milder symptoms may be only a slight increase in the frequency of urination, which is accompanied by a burning sensation. Fever, blood in the urine, and backache may occur, particularly if infection has spread to the kidneys (pyelonephritis). The pain during urination may be so severe that children refuse to pass urine.

Q: *What causes cystitis?*

A: Cystitis is usually caused by infection of the bladder, usually from the urethra. Causes other than infection may be the after-effects of radiotherapy for bladder tumours.

Q: *Can other disorders increase the chances of getting cystitis?*

A: Yes. The presence of any abnormality

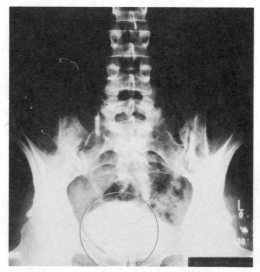

Cystogram is an X-ray of the bladder after a radiopaque dye has been injected into it.

that affects the bladder may make cystitis more likely: an obstruction that affects the normal flow of urine (for example, an enlarged prostate gland); pouches in the bladder resulting from a birth defect; the presence in the bladder of stones or a tumour; or, in tropical countries, schistosomiasis. A distended womb during pregnancy may obstruct the normal flow of urine and cause cystitis.

Q: *How is cystitis diagnosed and treated?*

A: Cystitis is usually diagnosed by testing a urine sample for the presence of infection. The disorder can be treated effectively by simple methods. Large quantities of fluids (at least one glass of water every hour) should be drunk. Potassium citrate mixture, an old-fashioned remedy, often brings relief from the burning pain that accompanies urination. A short course of an antibiotic drug may be prescribed by a doctor. After an attack of cystitis, a doctor may test a urine specimen again to make sure that the infection has disappeared.

Q: *Does treatment differ if another attack of cystitis occurs?*

A: No, but the disorder should be more fully investigated. This may involve blood tests; examination of the prostate gland; and X-rays with intravenous pyelography (IVP) and a cystogram. Sometimes the doctor examines the bladder with a special instrument (cystoscope), to make sure that stones or other abnormalities are not present. Urine specimens may have to be examined on several occasions to make sure that a low-grade infection is not present all the time, and to rule out the rare possibility of tuberculosis. Recurrent (chronic) cystitis commonly affects women.

Q: *Why is chronic cystitis a common problem in women?*

A: In women, the urethra is short, and this makes it easy for bacteria to reach the bladder. Sexual intercourse may move external bacteria into the urethra (honey-moon cystitis).

Q: *What precautions might prevent honey-moon cystitis?*

A: Simple measures such as emptying the bladder immediately after intercourse remove any bacteria that may have passed up the urethra. Hygiene is important, and the anus should be wiped from front to back to prevent intestinal bacteria from entering the vaginal area. Washing from the groin to the anus should take place twice a day. If these simple measures are not successful, an antiseptic cream should be applied around the vaginal entrance and urinary exit before intercourse. A doctor may prescribe a single dose of an antibiotic to be taken after intercourse, so that the first urine that enters the bladder kills the infection before it has time to grow. Most attacks of honeymoon cystitis improve spontaneously with these measures. Sometimes, however, a CYSTOSCOPY is done to make certain there is no anatomical reason for the cystitis.

Cystogram is a special X-ray taken after a radiopaque dye has been placed in the urinary bladder, usually after the bladder has been emptied by means of a catheter. X-rays can be taken before and during urination to detect the presence of stones in the bladder.

See also CALCULUS.

Cystoscopy is the examination of the inside of the bladder using a special instrument that is equipped with a lens (cystoscope) and a light. The cystoscope is introduced through the urethra, the tube that carries urine from the bladder to the outside of the body. Long, thin instruments can be passed into the bladder to take a biopsy of a tumour, to crush stones, or to treat the bladder tissue.

Cytology is the study of the structure, function, and formation of cells. It is now widely used, for example, in the early diagnosis of cancer, especially cancer of the cervix. *See* CERVICAL SMEAR.

Cytotoxic drugs are drugs that destroy cells or prevent their multiplication. They are mainly used in the treatment of cancer, but are occasionally used to treat other disorders, such as psoriasis. The administration of cytotoxic drugs must be carefully controlled, because excessive doses may cause serious blood disorders, hair loss (alopecia), and reduced resistance to infection.

D

Dacryocystitis is inflammation of the tear duct, caused by a blockage of the duct or by infection from the nose. The symptoms are pain, swelling, and tenderness in the corner of the eye, with the discharge of pus, and tears that cannot drain normally. To treat the condition, a doctor may syringe the duct with an antibiotic solution, prescribe antibiotic tablets, or resort to surgery.

D and C is the abbreviation commonly used for dilation and curettage. Specifically the expression refers to dilation (stretching) of the cervix, the neck of the uterus, and curettage (scraping with an instrument called a curette) of the inside of the uterus. D and C is a surgical procedure, performed while the patient is under anaesthetic. The technique is valuable for the diagnosis of gynaecological disorders. It is also used to remove any placental tissue remaining after an abortion or after childbirth, to clean the inside of the uterus, or as a method of producing an abortion or removing polyps.

Dandruff is a minor condition in which the scalp is dry and scaling, and may represent an inherited variation of a normal skin pattern. Dandruff tends to get worse when it occurs with seborrhoea (a disorder of the sebaceous glands) or atopic eczema. To treat dandruff the hair should be washed well two or three times a week. A doctor may prescribe a preparation containing corticosteroid hormones to be applied at night.

Dangerous drugs. In the United Kingdom, the prescribing of certain drugs is carefully controlled by legal regulations under the Misuse of Drugs Act 1973. The drugs concerned fall into three categories: the strong pain-relieving drugs such as heroin and morphia, pethidine and similar preparations; stimulant drugs such as cocaine and the amphetamines; and certain addictive sedative drugs such as methaqualone. It is possible that other drugs such as barbiturates may in the future be added to this list.

On the prescription, the doctor must write, in handwriting, the patient's name and address and the exact details of the drug,

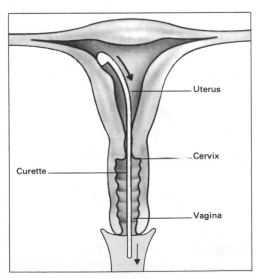

D and C is done under general anaesthetic. A curette is used to scrape the uterus lining.

Dapsone

all in a particular way. The pharmacist must recognize the handwriting before dispensing the prescription, and may even telephone the doctor to check.

Such prescriptions cannot be used to obtain drugs more than once: the patient may not regard them as "repeat prescriptions". For more drugs, the doctor has to write another prescription.

The drugs are known as Dangerous Drugs after being listed in the earlier Dangerous Drugs Act.

Dapsone is a drug that is used to treat LEPROSY. It is taken by mouth in increasing doses to a maximum of 300 mg a week for three or four years. Side effects may include anaemia, fever, and dermatitis.

DDT is a common abbreviation of dichloro-diphenyltrichloroethane, now known also as chlorophenothane. DDT was once an extremely effective odourless insecticide, but many pests have now developed an immunity to it. DDT is no longer used when substitutes are available because its presence in food-stuffs is thought to be harmful to animals and human beings. DDT taken through the mouth causes acute poisoning.

Deaf and dumb describes a person who can neither hear nor speak. The condition exists in a person who is born deaf, or who becomes severely deaf in early life, and who is unable to imitate the sounds of speech. Using specialized methods, it is possible to teach severely deaf people how to speak, and those who cannot learn to speak may learn instead to lip-read and to communicate by finger spelling and sign language.

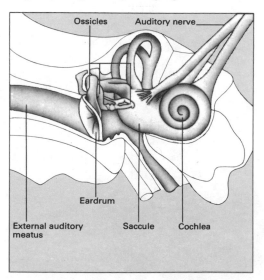

Labels: Ossicles, Auditory nerve, Eardrum, External auditory meatus, Saccule, Cochlea

Deafness may be conductive as in otosclerosis when a growth of bone stiffens an ossicle.

Deafness is the inability to hear. It may affect both ears or only one, either totally or only partially. Deafness may be present at birth (congenital deafness) or it may occur at any age, suddenly or gradually.

Q: Are there any obvious signs that a person may be deaf?

A: Yes. Deafness may be suspected if a person fails to react to sounds at various levels or speaks more loudly than is necessary. A child who is partially deaf may give the impression of being bored or disinterested and will have difficulty in learning to speak. Such a child may not progress well at school, and it is often a teacher's report that first leads a parent to suspect that the child may have impaired hearing. Deafness in an older person can lead to a sense of isolation and make the person bad-tempered. The degree of hearing loss, however, depends on the kind of deafness involved.

Q: What different kinds of deafness are there?

A: It is usual to categorize deafness as being either conductive deafness or perceptive deafness. Some persons, however, suffer from a combination of the two.

Q: What is conductive deafness?

A: Conductive deafness is hearing loss resulting from interference with the transmission of sound waves through either the outer or the middle ear. Conductive deafness may be either a temporary or a permanent condition.

Q: What causes conductive deafness?

A: Conductive deafness can have many causes, perhaps the most common of which is earwax (cerumen) that obstructs the ear canal and prevents sound waves from reaching the inner ear. Another common cause of conductive deafness is infection of the middle ear (otitis media), which often arises from various childhood diseases, particularly those involving the upper respiratory tract. Infections of the upper respiratory tract often cause swelling in or around a Eustachian tube. This tube connects the middle ear with the nasopharynx and helps equalize air pressure on both sides of the eardrum. When the pressures are unequal, as often happens during upper respiratory tract infections, deafness can result. Flying in aircraft, or deep-sea diving, can also change pressure within the ear and cause conductive deafness. *See* BAROTRAUMA.

Q: How is conductive deafness diagnosed?

A: In addition to direct observation of the signs, otologists and audiologists (specialists in problems of the ears and of hearing) use various tests to diagnose this kind of hearing impairment. One such test involves the use of a tuning fork. If the sound of a vibrating tuning fork is heard more clearly when the fork is placed against the skull than when it is placed close to the ear, the deafness is likely to be conductive. Specialists may then use an audiometer to determine the degree of deafness and X-ray photographs of the skull to pinpoint obstructions that may be causing the deafness.

Q: *How is conductive deafness treated?*

A: Treatment depends on the cause. For example, if earwax is the cause, removal of the wax often restores hearing. This removal should be done only by a trained person, however, because an untrained person may force the wax deeper into the ear or puncture the eardrum.

Other forms of treatment for conductive deafness may also include antibiotics, as in the case of otitis media; draining the fluid build-up from the middle ear; and surgery, in the case of a punctured eardrum or an immobile stapes. Surgery in cases of otosclerosis is a common procedure.

Q: *What is perceptive deafness?*

A: Perceptive, or nerve, deafness arises from the inability of nerve impulses to reach the auditory centre of the brain because of nerve damage either to the inner ear or to the brain. For example, nerve damage to the cochlea, which contains the sense organ for hearing (the organ of Corti), can result in perceptive deafness, as can damage to the ear's auditory nerve and nerve damage to the cerebral cortex of the brain.

Q: *What causes perceptive deafness?*

A: Diseases are a common cause of perceptive deafness. The diseases include ANAEMIA, ARTERIOSCLEROSIS, INFLUENZA, LEUKAEMIA, MÉNIÈRE'S DISEASE, MENINGITIS, MUMPS, RH DISEASE, and SYPHILIS.

Many children born with perceptive deafness have mothers who contracted GERMAN MEASLES (rubella) during the first three months of pregnancy. Such a child is called DEAF AND DUMB.

Other causes of perceptive deafness include tumours of the brain or the middle ear, severe head injury, blows to the ear, and exposure to repeated loud sounds. The toxic effects of certain drugs may also cause perceptive deafness.

Q: *How is perceptive deafness diagnosed and treated?*

A: Together with observation of the obvious

signs of deafness, audiologists and otologists use electronic equipment to detect and diagnose perceptive deafness. Such equipment, which includes various types of audiometer, can also help specialists to determine if tumours or other problems are involved. Perceptive deafness is usually irreversible and cannot be treated.

Q: *Can hearing aids help all deaf persons?*

A: No. Hearing aids amplify sound, but such devices are helpful only to persons who retain some nerve hearing.

A talk about Death

Death occurs when all activity of the brain ceases and life is completely extinct (*see* DYING). It may come at the end of a long illness, or be sudden and unexpected as the result of an accident or a heart attack. But in every case, everyone can spare his or her family a great deal of unnecessary anguish by giving clear instructions, in advance, concerning all the details and instructions surrounding arrangements for his or her own death. The funeral will have to be organized; the family must be comforted and cared for; and any other special circumstances, such as a part of the body left for medical research or transplant surgery, must be considered.

Q: *What is the first thing to think about when death has occurred?*

A: A death certificate will be issued and signed by a doctor familiar with the deceased or the doctor who was in

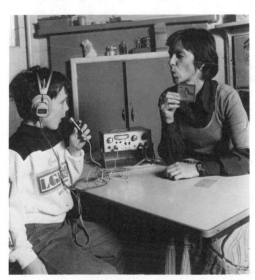

Deafness is a handicap that many children can overcome with the help of specialized training.

Debility

attendance at the time of death. When a person dies in hospital, the certificate will be signed by an attending doctor and is obtained from the hospital office along with any personal effects belonging to the deceased. Receipt of these is usually acknowledged by signature. Copies of the certificate are made available from the Registrar's office. In the event of an accidental or unexplained death, the certificate will be issued by the coroner, who may not be able to state the cause of death without performing a post-mortem examination.

Q: *Isn't a post-mortem examination too distressing for the relatives to bear?*

A: It is as distasteful to the hospital staff as it is to the bereaved to have to face the decision to perform a post-mortem examination. But so much has been learned from post-mortem studies that the request should never be resented.

Q: *How are the arrangements made for the funeral?*

A: The services of a good undertaker can considerably ease the administrative burden of the funeral arrangements. Following instructions from the family, the funeral director obtains permission to remove the body to the undertaker's chapel, and, in consultation with a responsible relative, helps to make the necessary arrangements concerning the coffin, the type of funeral service, the hours of visiting for people to pay their last respects, and so on. The director may also take care of the press notices.

Q: *Who takes care of medical bequests by the deceased?*

A: If the deceased has left his or her body to a medical school, the undertaker will usually convey the body there for a small fee. In cases of sudden, accidental death in young, fit people, thought must be given to kidney, heart, and liver donation, if facilities are available. If the deceased has bequeathed his or her corneas for transplant or experimental use, the local eye bank or hospital will send a technician immediately upon notification. Speed is essential, and it is important to know about such bequests ahead of time.

Q: *What is the best way to help the bereaved relatives?*

A: Somebody must take charge of affairs, and most families look to one or two members to do this. Often it will be the eldest child of the deceased, or an old and trusted friend who may be executor of the estate. It is usually better that the individual concerned be able to be fairly detached, in order to take the burden off the closest relative (usually the deceased's spouse), especially in the choice of an undertaker. The telephone will be in frequent use for a time, and it is advisable that the family member who is in charge use a phone nearby, leaving the home phone clear for calls of sympathy and help from other relatives and friends. The family solicitor should be told immediately, particularly if the deceased had left any special instructions. The family priest, minister, or rabbi should also be informed at the earliest opportunity.

Death is a test of a family's strength: it can bring out the best or the worst in family and friends. Perhaps the best guide to conduct is to try to act in a manner that would have been approved of by the deceased.

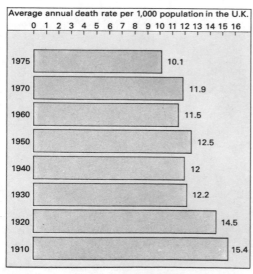

Average annual death rate per 1,000 population in the U.K.

Year	Rate
1975	10.1
1970	11.9
1960	11.5
1950	12.5
1940	12
1930	12.2
1920	14.5
1910	15.4

Death rate in the U.K. is decreasing because of better nutrition and medical care.

Debility. See WEAKNESS.

Débridement is the cleansing of a wound by the surgical removal of foreign matter and dead or damaged tissue or bone.

Decalcification is the loss of calcium salts from the bones. This condition may occur in persons who are confined to bed for long periods of time, and in persons who are subjected to long periods of weightlessness. Decalcification may result from various disorders: overactive parathyroid glands, causing osteitis fibrosa; rickets and osteomalacia, caused by vitamin D deficiency; and osteoporosis. Local decalcification may be caused by bone tumours (osteosarcomas), or the spread of cancer from other parts of the body. Decalcification may lead to the formation of stones in the kidneys and bladder (*see* CALCULUS).

Deciduous teeth. *See* MILK TEETH.

Decompression sickness. *See* BENDS.

Decongestant is a drug or other agent that reduces any congestion of mucus produced by various mucous membranes, particularly those in the nose. Decongestants should be used strictly according to the prescribed dosage, and for no longer than two or three weeks, or the chemical effects of the drugs may further irritate the mucous membranes and prolong the presence of mucus.

Decubitus ulcer. *See* BEDSORE.

Defecate is the medical term for having a bowel movement. It also applies to the release of faeces from an artificial opening that has been made in the intestines, such as a colostomy or an ileostomy.

Defibrillation is the term used for stopping the trembling, or fibrillation, of the heart muscle by means of drugs or an electric shock. In certain conditions, for example, coronary heart disease, the heart may stop beating while the heart muscle continues to fibrillate. Sometimes, normal heart contractions can be restored by electric shocks from a machine called a cardiac defibrillator.

Deficiency diseases are disorders that are caused by a lack or deficiency of a substance that is essential to the proper functioning of the body, such as various vitamins, minerals, and proteins. Deficiency diseases often result from an inadequate diet, but they can also be caused by metabolic disorders such as pernicious anaemia (which is caused by inadequate absorption of vitamin B_{12}); intestinal disorders; over-excretion of the substance in the urine, faeces, or by vomiting; the presence of a parasite; or by a prolonged illness.

Q: What are the most common deficiency diseases?

A: The most common deficiency diseases are those caused by a lack of vitamins or minerals. They include anaemia (lack of iron); scurvy (lack of vitamin C); beriberi (lack of vitamin B_1); night blindness (lack of vitamin A); rickets and osteomalacia (lack of vitamin D); and goitre (lack of iodine).

Q: How are deficiency diseases treated?

A: In most cases the disorder is treated by a special diet that is rich in foods that restore the deficient substance. The diet is sometimes supplemented with vitamin tablets or specific drugs.

See also VITAMINS.

Dehydration is the excessive loss of water from the body. In normal conditions an adult needs about 2.4 litres (5 pints) of water each day to replace that lost by breathing, sweating, urinating, and defecating. If this fluid loss is not replaced, dehydration results.

The major symptom of dehydration in adults is thirst, and muscle cramps may occur if dehydration is combined with fatigue. Dehydration is potentially serious, especially in babies and young children. Danger signs are drowsiness, constipation, wrinkled skin, and a depressed "soft spot" (fontanelle) in a young baby's skull. The major causes of dehydration include diarrhoea, vomiting, excessive water loss through sweating caused by fever or high air temperatures, illness such as diabetes, and a reaction following surgery.

Q: How is dehydration treated?

A: A seriously dehydrated baby should be hospitalized immediately. A lesser degree of dehydration can be treated with small and frequent drinks of water or milk and water. In adults, dehydration can usually be treated with water to which a little salt has been added. If the cause is a disorder such as cholera or diabetes, hospital treatment is required.

Delhi boil. *See* LEISHMANIASIS.

Delirium is a state of mental confusion and extreme excitement, commonly accompanied by hallucinations and continual but aimless physical activity. Delirium is the immediate result of a disturbance in brain function, but the disturbance itself can be caused by any, or by a combination of several, generally serious, conditions. High fever, particularly

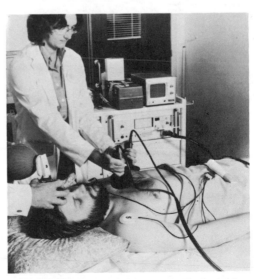

Defibrillation is used either to stop the heart for surgery, or to restart it beating.

Delirium tremens

from pneumonia, may cause delirium, as may malaria, meningitis, encephalitis, or heart failure. Another cause is alcoholism, which can lead to DELIRIUM TREMENS, a dangerous psychiatric disorder that involves both visual and auditory hallucinations. Drug overdoses and some mental disorders, such as schizophrenia, may also cause delirium.

Delirium may be reduced with sedatives or tranquillizers, but hospital treatment is generally necessary for treatment of the underlying serious condition.

Delirium tremens (DTs) is a form of DELIRIUM that occurs in severe ALCOHOLISM and in opium addiction. It is a potentially fatal condition, and hospitalization is urgently necessary. Delirium tremens may be accompanied by epilepsy, pneumonia, and heart and liver failure.

Q: *What are the symptoms of delirium tremens?*

A: The symptoms of delirium tremens include sleeplessness, anxiety, and nausea, and there is often an aversion to food. Persons with delirium tremens may suffer delusions and hallucinations and become extremely agitated. For example, such persons may experience strange skin sensations, see monstrous creatures, and make wild gestures with the hands.

Q: *What is the treatment for delirium tremens?*

A: Treatment usually consists, initially, of bed rest, sedation, and a controlled diet. Long-term treatment aims at helping patients to overcome their addiction to alcohol or opium.

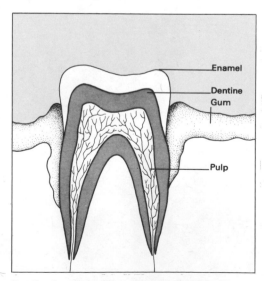

Dentine is a bone-like substance surrounding the tooth pulp and protected by enamel.

Delivery is the final stage of childbirth. The term also includes the expulsion of the placenta. *See* PREGNANCY AND CHILDBIRTH.

Delusion is a false and unshakable belief that is inconsistent with reality. There is no clear distinction between mild, harmless delusions and simple mistakes. Such delusions are thought to be part of a person's normal defence mechanisms, and help to maintain an individual's self-image. But in a serious mental disorder, such as SCHIZOPHRENIA, a person's delusions may be both extreme and harmful. Delusions in such cases are often an integral part of the person's loss of contact with reality. For example, persistent delusions of persecution and grandeur are characteristic of PARANOIA.

Q: *How are serious delusions treated?*

A: Serious delusions are often difficult to treat because they are usually part of a mental disorder that affects many aspects of the personality. Treatment of the underlying disorder may overcome the delusions, and such treatment may include regular psychiatric consultations and some form of drug therapy. Hospitalization may be necessary if patients are a danger to themselves or to others.

Dementia is a form of mental deterioration that is often associated with loss of physical control of the body. The progress of dementia is gradual, and it often begins with memory loss, particularly of recent events. This forgetfulness may be accompanied by childish and unreasonable behaviour. As deterioration progresses, there may be disturbances of the patient's speech, which may become disconnected and incomprehensible. In the final stages, the patient may be incontinent, unable to perform simple tasks, and unresponsive to his or her surroundings.

There are various causes of dementia, including old age (senile dementia); Alzheimer's disease (presenile dementia); general paralysis of the insane (GPI), a form of syphilis; arteriosclerosis of the arteries serving the brain; alcoholism; schizophrenia; and, rarely, brain tumour.

Dementia praecox. *See* SCHIZOPHRENIA.

Dengue (also known as breakbone fever) is an acute tropical disease, caused by a virus infection transmitted by the mosquito *Aedes aegypti.* The disease is rarely fatal. Symptoms include fever, vomiting, skin rash, headache, and severe pains in the muscles and joints. The symptoms often subside after the fifth or sixth day, but then return for another three or four days.

There is no specific treatment, although painkilling drugs and plenty of fluids may ease the symptoms. An attack of dengue is often followed by a period of depression and severe debility before normal health returns.

Dental caries. *See* TOOTH DECAY.

Dental disorders. The following table lists some common disorders of the teeth and gums. These disorders come within the competence of a dentist or an orthodontist. Each disorder has a separate article in the A-Z section of this book.

Symptom	Possible disorder
Teeth	
Decay	PLAQUE (saliva and food sugar containing harmful bacterial enzymes)
Sharp pain	ABSCESS
	TOOTH DECAY affecting the dentine
Temperature sensitive	TOOTH DECAY affecting the enamel and dentine
Dull, throbbing pain	ABSCESS
	TOOTH DECAY affecting the tooth pulp (soft inner part of tooth containing nerves and blood vessels)
	IMPACTED or emerging tooth
Acute pain	ABSCESS at base of tooth
Loose tooth	Infected GINGIVITIS
	MILK TEETH (in young children only)
	PLAQUE (saliva and food sugar containing harmful bacterial enzymes)
Overcrowded teeth	MALOCCLUSION
Speckled enamel	Excessive FLUORIDE
Gums	
Irritation	PLAQUE (saliva and food sugar containing harmful bacterial enzymes)
An open sore	MOUTH ULCER (ulceration of the mouth or lips)
	Badly fitting DENTURES
Pus-filled swelling	ABSCESS due to badly fitting DENTURES
	PYORRHOEA

Dentifrice. *See* TOOTHPASTE.

Dentine is the hard substance that makes up a tooth. It surrounds the central pulp, and is itself covered by harder external enamel.

Dentures are artificial teeth. The term may refer to any number of teeth attached to a plastic or metal appliance (plate), which is fitted to the upper or lower jaw. The appliance may be removable or permanently fixed. Dentures should be cleaned at least once a day.

Deodorants are agents used to destroy or disguise odours of the body or the breath. Most body odours arise from the decomposition of bacteria in a mixture of dead skin cells and sweat, usually because a person does not wash often enough (*see* BROMHIDROSIS). Most commercial skin deodorants contain an antiperspirant, such as aluminium chloride; usually perfumes are also added. However, care should be taken in the use of deodorants because some can cause skin reactions in those people who are allergic to them.

Bad breath is often caused by food decomposing between the teeth (*see* BAD BREATH). Commercial mouthwashes and deodorants disguise the smell of bad breath but do not treat the cause.

Deoxyribonucleic acid. *See* DNA.

Depersonalization is a term used in psychiatry to describe a loss of personal identity. An individual may seem to ignore or forget about the body, be unaware of pain, or be concerned about a non-existent disfigurement. Depersonalization is usually associated with mental illness.

Depilatory is a substance or device that removes hair. Chemical depilatories are alkaline creams that remove the hair painlessly without damaging the root. ELECTROLYSIS is a method of removing hair permanently. It destroys each hair root by an electric current. Electrolysis is particularly useful on sensitive areas of the body, but it is impractical for areas of dense hair growth, and may cause inflammation and pain.

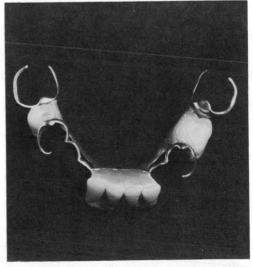

Dentures shown above contain replacement front teeth and molars in a metal clip.

Depression

A talk about Depression

Depression is a mental state that is characterized by feelings of guilt, lack of hope, melancholy, dejection, and the general feeling that life is not worth living. There may also be an impairment of mental and physical functions, such as appetite, sleep, work, and libido.

Q: *What are the signs and symptoms of depression?*

A: Boredom, overeating, quietness, inhibitedness, insomnia, pessimism, irritability, an inability to concentrate, and general listlessness may all indicate mild, or normal, depression.

When these signs and symptoms become persistent, however, a more serious type of depression should be suspected. Other indications of serious depression include loss of appetite, loss of weight, constant fatigue, chest pains, and headaches that may become chronic. The abuse of alcohol or other drugs may also indicate a serious depression, and there may be a tendency for seriously depressed persons to offer violence to others or even to harm themselves.

Q: *Can depression be normal?*

A: Yes, to some degree. Many women, for example, feel depressed prior to menstruation (*see* PREMENSTRUAL TENSION), and the onset of middle age might cause an ordinarily healthy person to feel depressed.

Almost everyone suffers from periods

of sadness, grief, loneliness, or discouragement under certain circumstances. It is normal for a person to be depressed by the terminal illness or death of a relative or friend, for example. But this type of depression is generally soon overcome and does not usually cause the person to lose touch with reality.

Q: *What is endogenous depression?*

A: Endogenous depression is a mental disorder that stems from factors within the person. The depression may affect the victim's personality, and may be so immobilizing that hospitalization is necessary. There are two main types of endogenous depression: manic-depressive psychosis and involutional melancholia.

Manic-depressive psychosis is characterized by alternating periods of high elation (the manic phase) and periods of severe depression with feelings of persecution and a distorted sense of bodily appearance (the depressive phase).

Involutional melancholia is more common and occurs in late middle age and is characterized by despondency, possibly suicidal tendencies, and often feelings of personal unworthiness.

Q: *What causes depression?*

A: The precise underlying causes of depression are not known. Almost anybody can become depressed if subjected to enough emotional stress, but some persons seem to become depressed more easily than others. A personal trauma or stressful event may trigger a depressive episode, and depression frequently occurs with withdrawal from drugs or following a surgical operation. Some types of depression, such as PREMENSTRUAL TENSION and MENOPAUSAL DEPRESSION, are apparently related to a person's metabolism and age.

Many psychiatrists believe that depression may have its roots in the experiences of a person's childhood, and studies undertaken by researchers indicate that some types of depression may run in families. For example, hereditary origins of depression may be suspected in persons who persistently become depressed for no apparent reason. Such persons display many of the common signs of depression for weeks or even months at a time, and then appear to make a gradual and complete recovery, but their depression usually recurs.

Q: *What are the dangers of depression?*

A: In all types of depression, the main danger is that of suicide. The risk

The number of men and women admitted to hospital in the U.K. in 1976 for depressive psychoses		
Age group (in years)	Men	Women
Under 15	4	3
15 to 24	240	364
25 to 34	683	1266
35 to 44	811	1908
45 to 54	1142	2733
55 to 64	1163	2839
65 to 74	920	2662
75 and over	281	1031

Depression is a mental condition experienced by more women than men.

of suicide is always present and cannot be judged by the apparent depth of the depression. Making light of a person's depression, or trying to cheer the person up, is likely to increase the feeling of isolation.

Q: *How is depression treated?*

A: Treatment for depression depends on the type of depression and its severity. For example, the so-called normal depression that stems from the death of a relative or friend usually needs no medical treatment. But both persistent mild depression and endogenous depression usually require medical intervention.

Medical treatment for such cases may include psychiatric counselling; drug therapy (such as tranquillizers, sedatives, and antidepressants); and hospital confinement. Hospitalization is imperative for suicidal patients.

In persons who are so ill that their condition constitutes an emergency, electroconvulsive therapy may be necessary (*see* ELECTROCONVULSIVE THERAPY). How this method works is not fully understood, but it has proved useful in a number of patients.

Above all, persons suffering from depression should be treated with care and consideration, and every effort should be made to re-establish their sense of personal worth.

Dermatitis is inflammation of the skin. In the past, dermatitis referred to external causes of inflammation, but it is now used as another name for eczema, and the terms are interchangeable.

Treatment depends on the diagnosis by a dermatologist. Most forms of dermatitis respond to skin preparations containing corticosteroid drugs. If infection is present, the doctor may also prescribe antibiotics and, sometimes, antifungal agents.

See also ECZEMA.

Dermatographia is a form of urticaria (hives). It is a sensitive condition of the skin, in which scratching or rubbing produces raised red areas. The term literally means "skin writing," and gentle drawing of a blunt point over the skin causes visible lines to appear and remain for a time. Usually, dermatographia is not a serious condition and does not require medical treatment. But it may be a symptom of a reaction to a drug. If this is suspected, a doctor must be consulted.

Dermatology is the branch of medical science concerned with diseases of the skin and the treatment of skin disorders.

Dermoid cyst is a nonmalignant CYST formed from surface skin cells. The cyst may contain elements of skin, hair, sweat glands, and bone, and forms a small, hard swelling in the body. A dermoid cyst is caused by a fault in the folding of tissues during embryonic development or by a wound that forces surface skin cells under the skin. The usual treatment is surgical removal of the cyst.

Desensitization is a method of treating an ALLERGY. Tests on the patient identify the substance causing an allergy. Sensitivity is reduced by regular injections of the specific allergen in solutions of increasing strength.

Detached retina is the separation of the retina in the eye from its pigmented base on the choroid. It causes partial loss of vision. The symptoms include "floating" specks and transient flashes of light, followed later by mistiness in front of the eye.

Q: *How is detachment caused?*

A: Detachment results from a hole in the retina that allows fluid to leak through and separate the retina from its base. The hole is usually a result of degenerative changes in the retina, most common in nearsighted people, or from a blow on the eye. Detachment may also be caused by a tumour or disease in the eye.

Q: *What is the treatment?*

A: Various surgical techniques are used to reseal the retina to the choroid. Treatment must be prompt, before vision loss becomes permanent.

Deviated nasal septum is a condition in which the partition in the nose (the septum) is bent, so that it partly blocks one or both nasal

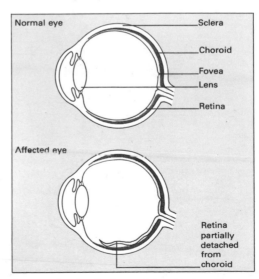

Detached retina is the partial or total separation of the retina from the choroid of the eye.

Devil's grip

passages. Deviation is caused by a broken nose, but it may be congenital, or occur for no obvious reason. One nostril may be smaller than the other, with symptoms of snoring, difficulty in breathing, mucus, and recurrent sinusitis.

When a deviated septum causes chronic or acute symptoms, a doctor may recommend an operation called a submucosal resection. The deformed part of the septum is removed, and the nose firmly filled with gauze for 24 hours while it heals. Or, an operation called a septoplasty may be required, to rebuild the septum.

Devil's grip is another name for pleurodynia, a sharp pain in the muscles of the chest wall. *See* PLEURODYNIA.

Dextrans are forms of carbohydrate that are soluble in water. With the addition of salt they can be made into sterile solutions that may be used in the emergency treatment of severe bleeding, shock, or burns, if a blood transfusion is not available or while blood is being grouped and crossed-matched to ensure that it is safe to use in the patient.

Dextrans are safe and seldom cause allergic reactions. They are rapidly destroyed by the body and excreted in the urine.

Dextrocardia is a congenital abnormality in which the heart is located in the right side of the chest instead of the left. Dextrocardia is often associated with reverse positioning of all the organs, known as situs inversus. In the absence of other associated abnormalities, this condition produces no real problems, although it may cause some confusion in diagnosis of other conditions.

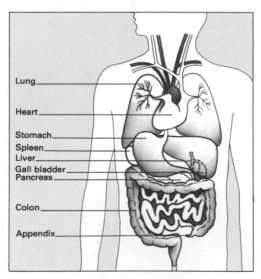

Lung
Heart
Stomach
Spleen
Liver
Gall bladder
Pancreas
Colon
Appendix

Dextrocardia may be part of a condition in which organs are located abnormally.

Dhobie itch is the common name for any groin irritation of the skin, especially those caused by the fungal infection tinea cruris. Originally, dhobie itch was a form of dermatitis in the groin caused by an allergic reaction to the dye used for laundry-marking the washing of Europeans in India.

Diabetes is the name of several metabolic disorders that are generally serious. Usually, however, the term by itself represents an abbreviation of DIABETES MELLITUS, which is one of the two major forms; the other is DIABETES INSIPIDUS.

Diabetes insipidus is a disorder that arises from a hormonal imbalance that makes the kidneys overactive or renders them unable to reabsorb the water passed to them from the blood. A person who has the disorder urinates excessively (polyuria) and has a raging thirst (polydipsia) and an increased appetite (polyphagia). These are symptoms also of DIABETES MELLITUS, but the two disorders are otherwise unrelated.

Q: *What are the causes of diabetes insipidus?*

A: Diabetes insipidus generally occurs because of a lack of vasopressin, an antidiuretic hormone (ADH) that controls the body's urine output. The hormone is produced in the hypothalamus (a part of the brain) and is stored in and secreted by the pituitary gland. The normal secretion of vasopressin can be disturbed by any disease or injury to either the pituitary gland or the hypothalamus. Other causes of diabetes insipidus include diseases such as encephalitis, meningitis, and syphilis. In extremely rare cases, the cause may be the impaired ability of the kidneys themselves to hold water.

Q: *How is diabetes insipidus treated?*

A: Following diagnosis by skull X-rays and special tests, a doctor may advise an injection of ADH to correct the hormone deficiency. Recent treatment involves synthetic ADH used as a nasal spray. If the cause of the disease is a kidney disorder, treatment with a diuretic is sometimes effective. Diabetes insipidus cannot be cured, but treatment greatly improves a patient's condition.

A talk about Diabetes mellitus

Diabetes mellitus, or sugar diabetes, is a disorder in the way the body regulates sugar concentrations in the bloodstream. A key element in sugar-level regulation is the hormone insulin, which is secreted by special cells (beta cells) in an area of the pancreas known as the islets of Langerhans. Diabetes results from either a lack of insulin or an inability of tissues to use the insulin properly, but the cause of diabetes is often not known. Damage to the pancreas arising from viral diseases such as measles or mumps may be a cause, and such persons may inherit a tendency toward diabetes. Alcoholism and gall bladder disease may also be factors in the onset of diabetes.

There are two forms of diabetes mellitus, juvenile-type and adult-type diabetes. They are so named because one is usually found in persons under age twenty; the other, in persons over thirty-five.

Diabetes is a serious, sometimes fatal disorder. The British Diabetic Association has calculated that approximately two per cent of the total population of the U.K. are diabetic. There are approximately 600,000 diagnosed cases of diabetes in the U.K., of which approximately 30,000 are children under the age of sixteen. There are at least another 600,000 cases of diabetes that have not been diagnosed.

Q: *What causes the imbalance in blood-sugar levels?*

A: Normally, food digested in the intestine releases a form of sugar called glucose into the blood. This increase in blood-sugar level causes beta cells in the islets of Langerhans to release insulin, which aids in transporting glucose from the blood to storage in such tissues as the liver and muscle.

In victims of juvenile-type diabetes, the pancreas is unable to produce insulin. In adult-type diabetes, the pancreas produces some insulin, but the tissues do not respond to it properly. As a result, in both cases, high concentrations of sugar build up in the blood after eating (hyperglycaemia). A vicious circle then begins.

The fatty acids released from tissue throughout the body are converted by the liver into biochemicals called ketone bodies. These also pour into the bloodstream, causing a condition in which the blood becomes dangerously acidic (ketoacidosis). This can lead to a diabetic coma and, if untreated, to death.

Q: *What are the symptoms of diabetes?*

A: Rarely, juvenile-type diabetes develops so rapidly that a victim lapses into a coma before any other noticeable symptoms develop. The general symptoms of diabetes include increased frequency of urination and persistent thirst. In juvenile-type diabetes these symptoms are often accompanied by weakness and loss of appetite.

A doctor can diagnose diabetes by testing for sugar in the urine and blood. A GLUCOSE TOLERANCE TEST determines how well the body uses and stores sugar.

Q: *What is the treatment for diabetes mellitus?*

A: Any diabetic who has lapsed into a coma requires immediate emergency medical attention and must be hospitalized.

Juvenile-type diabetics need daily injections of insulin. A doctor determines the correct dosage, and patients are taught how to prepare and administer the insulin themselves. The technique is simple, even for children. Most diabetics also test their urine daily for sugar.

A strict diet is important in controlling juvenile-type diabetes to keep the levels of insulin and sugar in the blood from fluctuating too widely. Careful regulation of activity, food intake, and insulin is also necessary to prevent insulin shock (hypoglycaemia), in which the insulin level rises too high and blood sugar drops too low.

The first signs of insulin shock are mild hunger, dizziness, sweating, and heart palpitations; then follows mental confusion and coma. Diabetics can stop insulin shock by consuming some substance high in sugar, and should always carry sugar or sweets. It is advisable for diabetics to have an identification card, tag, or bracelet so that they will receive emergency care.

Adult-type diabetes is much easier to control. Some cases are treated with

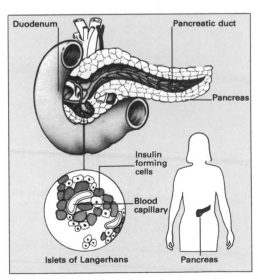

Insulin is made in the islets of Langerhans, located in the pancreas.

Diagnosis

sugar-restricted diet alone, others with diet plus oral antidiabetic drugs. Some cases are treated with insulin.

Most adult-type diabetes can be controlled with diet alone, at least at the onset of the illness, if the patient maintains proper body weight. Ninety per cent of all adult-type diabetics are overweight.

Q: *What complications arise from diabetes mellitus?*

A: If the body cannot use up sugar, it burns fat instead. This causes an increase in the blood of cholesterol and fatty substances (lipids). The increase in turn leads to a much greater incidence in such patients of arteriosclerosis, and therefore coronary heart disease, strokes and blockage of the leg arteries that may result in gangrene of the feet. Elderly diabetics are particularly liable to arterial complications, and it is most important that they should pay special attention to the cleanliness of the skin on their legs and feet to prevent infection occurring.

Another complication of diabetes is the degeneration of small blood vessels. In the kidney, this leads to kidney disease and failure. In the eyes, it results in a form of tissue degeneration (diabetic retinitis) that may eventually result in blindness.

A similar disorder of the arteries to the nerves causes a gradual degeneration producing muscle weakness and loss of skin sensation.

In general, the longer the diabetes has lasted, the more likely the patient is to suffer from these complicatons. The better the control of the diabetes, the less likely the complications are to develop.

Q: *Is it safe for a diabetic woman to have a baby?*

A: Although there is some risk involved, most diabetic women who have not suffered from the disease for a long period of time have perfectly healthy children, but there is definitely a need for special care during pregnancy, childbirth, and just after. During pregnancy, a diabetic woman's blood sugar level may vary widely, which means that if she needs insulin, her insulin requirement will vary also. Usually, the doctor takes regular blood-sugar tests and instructs the woman about testing her urine to be sure she has the proper insulin dosage.

The foetus carried by a diabetic woman is usually larger than normal. The newborn infant of a diabetic mother may be particularly prone to respiratory disorders for the first twenty-four hours of life, and lose a considerable amount of weight for the first week. After that time, however, the progress of the baby should be the same as that of other children.

Most medical experts recommend that diabetic women have no more than two pregnancies, because pregnancy tends to aggravate the disease.

Q: *Can diabetes be prevented?*

A: Maintaining proper body weight is the best precaution for an individual with a family history of adult-type diabetes, especially if a glucose tolerance test reveals that the person's sugar-processing mechanism is not normal.

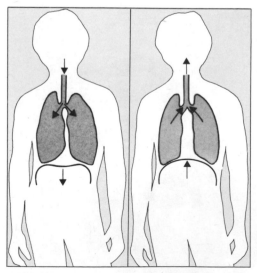

Diaphragm contracts and flattens during inhalation, then relaxes during exhalation.

Diagnosis is the process by which a doctor identifies a disease or disorder from its symptoms, causes, and signs. In order to get information for making a diagnosis, the doctor may ask the patient to undergo an X-ray examination or various medical tests.

Dialysis is a method of separating microscopic particles in a solution, using a special membrane as a filter. It is this method that is used for purifying blood in an artificial kidney: blood from an artery is passed into a dialysis machine, which filters out unwanted substances, and is then passed back into one of the patient's veins. *See* KIDNEY DIALYSIS.

Diamorphine, or diacetylmorphine, is the medical term for HEROIN.

Diaphoretic is a substance that increases sweating, for example, aspirin.

See also PERSPIRATION.

Diaphragm is any thin tissue that separates one structure from another. The term is most commonly applied to the large sheet of muscle between the abdominal cavity and the chest cavity. Diaphragm is also the name of a device used in CONTRACEPTION.

Diarrhoea is a condition characterized by frequent bowel movements and faeces that are soft or watery, and that may contain blood, pus, or mucus. The condition can prevent the body from absorbing necessary water and salts into the bloodstream, which may lead to DEHYDRATION. Diarrhoea can be acute or chronic.

Q: *What can cause acute diarrhoea?*

A: Attacks of mild acute diarrhoea can often be traced to a simple dietary cause, such as eating rich food, or to an emotional upset. But serious acute diarrhoea may be caused by CHOLERA, DYSENTERY, FOOD POISONING, or OTITIS MEDIA. Among other causes of serious acute diarrhoea are chemical poisoning and certain respiratory infections.

Q: *How is acute diarrhoea treated?*

A: All persons with acute diarrhoea should drink plenty of fluids, to prevent dehydration. Most people with mild acute diarrhoea benefit from a diet of bland foods, such as boiled or poached eggs, biscuits, custards, gelatins, and rice. In some cases doctors may prescribe antidiarrhoeal or antispasm preparations to help ease the symptoms.

Persons with serious acute diarrhoea usually need immediate medical help, because of the high risk of dehydration. Signs that dehydration is taking place include a decrease in urine output, dark or light brown urine, sunken eyeballs, rapid pulse rate, vomiting, constant thirst, and drowsiness or even unconsciousness. Dehydration is a serious condition that may prove fatal, especially to infants and young children.

Q: *What can cause chronic diarrhoea?*

A: Chronic diarrhoea may be a symptom of various serious disorders. Among such disorders are infections of the colon, colitis, intestinal cancer, sprue, and infestation of the intestines with worms.

Q: *How is chronic diarrhoea treated?*

A: All persons with chronic diarrhoea should drink plenty of fluids, to avoid dehydration. Treatment for chronic diarrhoea depends partly on the cause, which may be determined by diagnosis of the symptoms and by the results of certain tests. These tests may include sigmoidoscopy, barium enema, and stool-sample examination.

Diastole is the normal period of relaxation of the heart muscle; it alternates with the period of contraction (SYSTOLE). During the diastole, the heart cavities fill with blood; the diastole of the atria (upper chambers) occurs momentarily before that of the ventricles. The diastolic blood pressure is the point of least pressure in the arteries, because blood is not being pumped by the heart during this phase

See also p.8.

Diathermy is the painless production of heat within the body tissues by means of a high-frequency electric current. Physiotherapists use shortwave diathermy to relieve the symptoms of inflammation and stiff, painful joints and muscles. Surgical diathermy is a method of sealing blood vessels using an electrically heated probe.

See also CAUTERY.

Diathesis is a constitutional or hereditary tendency to develop a particular disease or disorder. With some disorders that apparently run in families, it is the diathesis that is inherited, not the actual disorder. It may be possible to avoid developing such a disorder by taking appropriate preventive measures.

Diazepam is the active chemical in several tranquillizing drugs.

A talk about Diet

Diet refers to the types of food a person eats regularly. Diet also refers to the deliberate effort to control the types and amounts of food eaten because of health problems.

A normal diet should provide the body

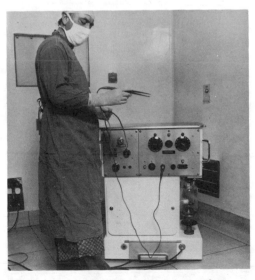

Diathermy machine is used in an operating theatre as an aid to surgery.

Diet

with all the substances necessary to maintain growth, keep in good health, and repair damaged tissues. These substances come from a balanced diet that contains proteins, fats, carbohydrates, vitamins, minerals, and water. A normal diet should also contain the exact amount of food to satisfy the body's energy needs and no more. When a body takes in more food than it can use for energy, the excess may be stored as fat (*see* WEIGHT PROBLEMS).

Q: How is the energy content of foods measured?

A: Foods are measured for their heat energy value in metric units called calories. One calorie is the energy needed to raise the temperature of one gram of water one degree centigrade. Nutritionists use the kilocalorie (1,000 calories), properly written Calorie (with a capital C), to express the energy content of foods. But by convention, in this context, the kilocalorie is written calorie.

The daily number of calories needed depends on a person's age, size, and occupation. Generally, men need more calories than women, and youngsters more than older persons.

Carbohydrates and fats are the chief source of calories in a balanced diet.

Q: What foods make up a balanced diet?

A: Nutritionists classify foods for a balanced diet in various categories. One such system uses seven basic food groups.

Meat, poultry, fish, eggs, beans, peas, and nuts make up the first group. They are rich sources of protein, vitamin B,

iron, niacin, phosphorus, and some carbohydrates. A balanced diet requires one or two servings of these foods a day.

Leafy, green, and yellow vegetables provide folic acid, vitamin A, the B vitamins, vitamin C, calcium, iron, and non-nutritive fibre. A person should have at least one serving from this group each day.

Citrus fruits, green vegetables and tomatoes supply vitamins A and C, calcium, and iron. At least one daily serving is recommended.

Potatoes, other vegetables, and non-citrus fruits provide carbohydrates, minerals, and small amounts of most vitamins. One potato and another food from this group is recommended in the daily diet.

Whole-grain bread, breakfast cereal, and enriched flour are rich sources of carbohydrates, vitamins, and minerals. Some, such as bran, also supply fibre. Nutritionists recommend at least four daily servings.

Butter and fortified margarine supply vitamin A and fats.

Milk and such milk products as ice cream and cheese provide vitamin A, vitamin B_2, calcium, protein, and fats.

Q: Why are proteins important?

A: Proteins are body-building foods. They are essential for growth and maintenance of tissue. Skin, hair, muscle, blood, and other parts of the body are made up largely of proteins. *See* PROTEINS.

Q: Why are carbohydrates important?

A: Carbohydrates are starches and sugars. They are the main source of energy in the diet. Before the body can use carbohydrates as fuel, the food has to be broken down by the digestive system into the simple sugar, glucose. In a well-balanced diet, carbohydrates make up about 45 per cent of the calorie intake. A diet too high in carbohydrates, however, leads to overweight. *See* CARBOHYDRATES.

Q: Why are fats important?

A: Fats are another major source of body energy. They provide about twice as much energy as does an equal weight of carbohydrate or protein. Fats make up about 40 per cent of the calories in a balanced diet. Because fats give off a great deal of heat when they are "burned" by the body, a person needs more fat in the diet during winter and less during summer. Fats are also needed by body cells and to transport fat-soluble vitamins. High intakes of saturated fats, derived mainly from animals, have been

Percentage composition of some common foods						
Food	Fat	Protein	Carbo-hydrate	Vitamins and minerals	Water	Fibre
Bread	3	13.5	70	2	10	1.5
Chicken	16	20	0	1	63	0
Meat	17	18	0	1	64	0
White fish	0.25	17.5	0	1.25	81	0
Egg	12	12	1	1	74	0
Milk	4	3.5	4.5	1	87	0
Cheese	29	25	2	4	40	0
Tomato	0	0.5	3	0.5	95	1
Potato	0	2	17	0.5	80	0.5
Apple	0.25	0.50	13	0.25	84	2

Diet can be controlled so that a person can achieve a well-balanced food intake.

correlated with coronary heart disease. Therefore, most doctors believe that unsaturated fats, derived mainly from vegetables, pose less of a risk. *See* FATS.

Q: *What roles do vitamins play?*

A: The body cannot make most vitamins, and some it makes in only small quantities. Therefore, the body must get vitamins from food. Vitamins are not a source of energy, but they are indispensable to good health and the effective functioning of the body. Scientists have identified about twenty-five vitamins.

Vitamin A is essential for healthy skin, eyes, teeth, and bones.

Vitamin B (thiamin) aids the body in releasing energy from sugars and starches.

Vitamin B_2 (riboflavin) helps cells to use oxygen and aids in tissue repair.

Vitamin B_6 is necessary for healthy blood vessels and nerves.

Vitamin B_{12} and folic acid are needed by red blood cells and nerves.

Niacin, or nicotinic acid, is necessary for healthy skin, cell metabolism, and the absorption of carbohydrates.

Vitamin C (ascorbic acid) maintains supportive tissue, such as ligaments and tendons, and is needed for healthy gums and bones.

Vitamin D aids the body's use of calcium and phosphorus.

Vitamin E is needed by the heart and skeletal muscles.

Vitamin K is essential for proper blood clotting.

See also VITAMINS.

Q: *What are the roles of minerals?*

A: Minerals, like vitamins, do not provide energy but are needed for the growth and maintenance of body structure.

Important minerals include iron, which is essential for red blood cells; iodine, which is used by the thyroid gland; and calcium, magnesium, and phosphorus, which are necessary for healthy teeth and bones. Potassium, sodium, sulphur and other minerals are essential components of digestive juices and body fluids in and around cells.

Q: *Why is fibre important in the diet?*

A: The indigestible fibre found in fruits, vegetables, and cereals aids in eliminating solid waste from the body. Adequate fibre in the diet helps to prevent constipation, and may reduce the likelihood of haemorrhoids or diverticular disease.

See also DIGESTIVE SYSTEM.

Q: *Can eating the wrong foods cause illness?*

A: Good nutrition is definitely essential for general good health. But lack of specific elements in the diet can cause serious diseases. *See* DEFICIENCY DISEASES.

Too much of a certain type of food can also contribute to disease.

Digestive system is the series of organs that process and convert food into simpler substances that the body uses for nourishment. Starch and complex sugars are digested to simple sugars; fats to fatty acids and glycerine; and proteins to amino acids. These simpler substances consist of small molecules that can then pass through the intestinal wall and into the bloodstream for distribution to all parts of the body. The digestive system consists of the alimentary canal – mouth, pharynx, oesophagus, stomach, and small and large intestines – aided by secretions from the liver and pancreas.

Q: *What happens to food in the mouth?*

A: The teeth break up food by chopping and grinding it into fine particles. Glands in the mouth lubricate and moisten food with saliva, which also contains a digestive enzyme. The tongue conveys food to the throat, and the pharynx muscles push it down the oesophagus (gullet), a muscular tube about 25cm (10 inches) long that leads to the stomach.

Q: *What happens to food in the stomach?*

A: The stomach both stores and helps to digest food. The stomach of an average adult can hold about 0.9 litres (1 quart). The muscular stomach churns food around and mixes it with gastric juice,

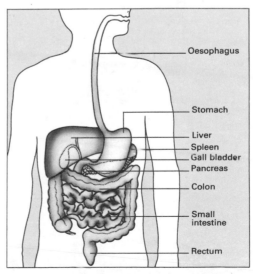

Digestive system processes food by means of many individual organs, from mouth to anus.

Digitalis

which includes hydrochloric acid to sterilize the food particles and the enzyme pepsin to break down protein. The partly digested food (chyme) passes from the stomach to the small intestine, usually after two to five hours.

Q: *How does the small intestine function?*

A: The digestive process is completed in the small intestine, a narrow muscular tube about 6 metres (20 feet) long. Enzymes from the pancreas mix with enzymes from the duodenum. Bile, made by the liver and stored in the gall bladder, also enters the small intestine. Bile helps in the digestion of fats.

The digested food particles are then absorbed by lymph or blood vessels in the intestinal wall. Tiny finger-like projections (villi) on the walls of the small intestine increase the surface area that can absorb the food. The digested particles are then carried by the bloodstream to the liver, which converts them into substances needed by the body.

Q: *What is the role of the large intestine?*

A: Eaten material that cannot be digested as food, such as plant fibre, passes into the large intestine, which is about 1.5 metres (five feet) long. There water is removed from the liquid waste and bacteria convert it to its final form, faeces. The waste material is excreted from the body through the end of the large intestine (rectum).

Q: *How does food move through the digestive system?*

A: Food is propelled along by wavelike contractions of muscles in the stomach and intestines. This is called peristalsis. The food moves in one direction only. Sphincters, circular muscles that close tightly, prevent the food from moving backward. There are sphincters at the lower end of the oesophagus, at the exit from the stomach, at the lower end of the small intestine, and at the exit from the rectum.

Q: *What are common diseases or disorders of the digestive system?*

A: One fairly common disorder is ulcers of the stomach or duodenum, the first part of the small intestine. If bile stagnates in the gall bladder because of a blocked bile duct, gallstones can form and must be removed surgically. Disorders of the intestinal tract include colitis, diverticular disease, and enteritis.

Digitalis is a drug made from the dried leaves of the foxglove (*Digitalis purpurea*). Prescribed as tablets, capsules, or liquid, digitalis is important in the treatment of congestive heart failure, and some forms of heart palpitation. Treatment is normally continued for some time after the heart failure has been corrected.

Digitalis makes a failing heart more efficient by strengthening the contractions of the tired muscle, and making the heart beat more slowly. Digitalis indirectly reduces blood congestion in veins and the accumulation of fluids in the body, as well as increasing urine production by the kidneys. Great care has to be taken when prescribing digitalis, particularly in the elderly, or in those suffering from vomiting and diarrhoea, as excessive dosage may cause nausea, vomiting, heart irregularities, and, occasionally, death. The drug is eliminated from the body so slowly that doses may accumulate with correspondingly harmful effects.

Digitoxin is a heart stimulant drug prepared from the plant *Digitalis purpurea*. Its effects are similar to those of the related drugs DIGITALIS and DIGOXIN.

Digoxin is a heart stimulant drug prepared from the plant *Digitalis lanata*. Its effects are similar to those of the related drugs DIGITALIS and DIGITOXIN.

Digoxin makes the heart beat more strongly and more effectively, and slows a rapidly beating heart. It is administered orally or by injection, and its use is preferred to digitalis because it acts more quickly and dosages can be more accurately controlled.

Dilation and curettage. *See* D AND C.

Dimercaprol is a drug that is usually injected intramuscularly in the treatment of poisoning by certain metals, such as arsenic

Action of the digestive system			
Site	Secretion	Food affected	Action
Mouth	Saliva, alkaline	Starch	Water to aid lubrication of food
Stomach	Gastric juice, acid	Proteins	Provides acid medium for pepsin and kills most bacteria. Absorbs only alcohol
Duodenum	Duodenal/ pancreatic secretions, bile	Fats Starch Proteins	Breaks down food for absorption
Ileum	Succus entericus	Fats Starch Proteins	Most absorption of food occurs here
Colon			Absorption of water

Digestive system breaks down food into elements that can be absorbed by the body.

and mercury, antimony and gold. It is also used in the treatment of a rare congenital disorder in which copper is retained in the body eventually causing serious symptoms. *See* CHELATING AGENTS.

Dioptre is the unit of measurement of the focusing power of a lens. *See* SPECTACLES.

Diphtheria is an acute infectious disease caused by the bacillus *Corynebacterium diphtheriae*. This bacterium usually grows on the membranes of the nose and throat, but can infect other mucous membranes and occasionally infects the skin. Diphtheria is now a rare disease, because of widespread vaccination against it. It occurs most frequently in children under the age of ten.

Q: How is diphtheria spread?

A: The disease is usually spread in minute airborne droplets that are breathed out by an infected person. As a result, it can spread extremely rapidly.

The diphtheria bacillus can be transmitted by a carrier, a person who is immune to the disease, who does not exhibit any symptoms, and who may be unaware of the infection.

Q: What are the symptoms of diphtheria?

A: Before any symptoms become apparent, there is an incubation period of up to five days; this period varies and symptoms may appear after only one day. There is a sudden onset of a sore throat and fever, accompanied by rapidly increasing feelings of ill health and weakness. A typical sign is a thick, white, crustlike membrane at the back of the throat. The inflamed tissues are painful, and the lymph nodes in the neck often become swollen, but the infection rarely spreads any further.

Q: Are there any complications associated with diphtheria?

A: Yes, although the complications are not permanent and complete recovery can be expected. The thick membrane overlying the swollen and congested throat commonly leads to obstruction of breathing, and an urgent operation to make an opening in the windpipe (a tracheostomy) may be necessary. The toxin produced by the infection may also cause weakness of the heart muscle (myocarditis). Nerve damage may also occur, causing further difficulty in swallowing; occasionally this neuritis involves nerves to the eyes and limbs, causing areas of localized weakness and possible double vision (diplopia).

Q: How may diphtheria be treated?

A: A patient with diphtheria requires hospital treatment in isolation. This usually involves the administration of diphtheria antitoxin and antibiotics. The antitoxin counteracts the effects of the toxin, and the antibiotics kill the bacteria. Complete bed rest is essential during the acute stage of the disease, with a gradual return to normal activity afterward.

Q: Can diphtheria be prevented?

A: Yes. Diphtheria immunization is usually carried out in the first year of life. A SCHICK TEST determines whether or not a person is susceptible to diphtheria. If an individual is susceptible, he or she can be immunized with specially-treated toxin (toxoid). In practice, however, the Schick test is not often used today.

Diphyllobothrium latum is the largest of the parasitic tapeworms that infest human beings. The adult worm lives in the intestine, and may grow to about 9 metres (30 feet) long. Most cases of infestation arise from eating raw or undercooked fish. The first sign of infestation is often worm segments in the faeces. Treatment is usually with drugs that kill the worm.

Diplegia is paralysis of like parts on both sides of the body, for example, both arms or both legs. *See* PARALYSIS.

Diplopia. *See* DOUBLE VISION.

Dipsomania. *See* ALCOHOLISM.

Disarticulation is an amputation through a joint. *See* AMPUTATION.

Disc is any flat, round, platelike structure. In medicine, the term commonly has two meanings. The optic disc is the point at which the optic nerve enters the back of the eye. An intervertebral disc is a fibroelastic ring with a

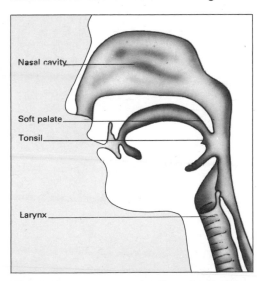

Nasal cavity

Soft palate

Tonsil

Larynx

Diphtheria most commonly affects the mucous membranes of the nose, mouth and throat.

Discharge

soft, gelatinous centre, which lies between each pair of vertebrae of the backbone. The intervertebral discs act as shock absorbers and enable the backbone to flex. Occasionally an intervertebral disc ruptures, causing the condition known as SLIPPED DISC.

Discharge is the loss of a substance through a body opening. It may be the result of a normal body process, for example, urination, or it may be abnormal, for example, bloody pus from the ear.

Disinfectant is a substance that destroys infection-causing organisms. The term is generally applied to chemicals used for treating such things as surgical instruments and sickroom floors.

See also ANTISEPTICS.

Disinfestation is the process by which lice, fleas, and parasites that live on the skin are exterminated and cleared away. Drugs given to do this are generally applied as a solution, but may also be used in the form of a powder. *See* SCABICIDE.

Dislocation (luxation) is the displacement of a structure from its normal position in the body. In most joints, dislocations of bones are rare, except as a complication of a fracture or as a result of weakened joint ligaments. Dislocations most commonly occur in the shoulder, where there may be a congenital weakness of the surrounding ligaments. A dislocation always causes torn ligaments, and it may take several weeks for the tears to heal. Various surgical operations have been devised to strengthen or replace weak ligaments, and so overcome the problem. Occasionally, one or both hips may be dislo-

cated from birth (congenital hip dislocation), and early diagnosis and treatment are required to prevent permanent disability.

Disorientation is a loss of normal awareness of place or time. Such mental confusion may occur in serious physical illnesses, with fever, as a result of certain drug treatments, or as a symptom of a mental illness.

Dissection is the surgical cutting of tissue, usually using instruments such as a scalpel and forceps, to expose an area for examination or to effect a surgical removal.

Disseminated sclerosis. *See* MULTIPLE SCLEROSIS.

Diuretics are drugs that act on the kidneys to increase the output of urine. This is accompanied by a loss of sodium or, more commonly, potassium salts. Alcohol, tea, and coffee are mild, but nonmedical, diuretics.

Q: Which disorders may diuretics be used to treat?

A: Diuretics are used to treat virtually any disorder in which there is an excessive build-up of fluid in the body (oedema). These include disorders of the heart, liver, and kidneys. Some weak diuretics are used to decrease excessive fluid pressure within the eyeball (glaucoma). Diuretics are used to treat certain lung disorders in which fluid accumulates in the lung tissue (pulmonary oedema). They may also be used to decrease high blood pressure (hypertension) and to treat overdosage of certain drugs.

Q: Can diuretics produce any adverse effects?

A: Yes. The adverse effects of diuretics vary according to the specific drug used. The commonly prescribed diuretics may cause nausea, weakness, skin rashes, and allergic reactions. All diuretics should be used with care by diabetics and by those with impaired liver or kidney function.

Diverticulitis and diverticulosis (diverticular disease) are common, related diseases of the colon, the main part of the large intestine. Diverticulitis develops from diverticulosis, which involves the formation of pouches (diverticula) on the outside of the colon. Diverticulitis results if one of these diverticula becomes inflamed. Bacteria may then infect the outside of the colon. If the infection spreads to the lining of the abdominal cavity (peritoneum), this can cause a potentially fatal illness (peritonitis). Sometimes inflamed diverticula can cause narrowing of the bowel, leading to an obstruction. Also, the affected part of the colon could adhere to the bladder or other organ in the pelvic area. These diverticular disorders most often affect middle-aged and elderly persons.

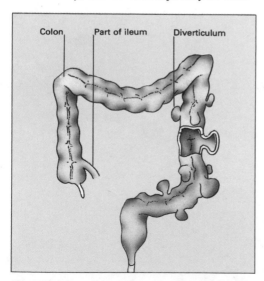

Colon   Part of ileum   Diverticulum

Diverticulitis occurs when a small pocket in the bowel becomes inflamed.

Q: *What are the symptoms of diverticular disease?*

A: Usually there are no symptoms accompanying diverticulosis. However, if diverticulitis develops, some patients experience abdominal pain and rectal bleeding. This occurs when an ulcer on a diverticulum erodes a blood vessel. A barium enema X-ray examination reveals the presence of diverticula.

The symptoms of diverticulitis include localized abdominal pain and tenderness, loose bowel movements, and fever. A blood test shows an increased number of white blood cells.

Q: *What is the treatment for diverticular disease?*

A: Persons with diverticulosis are put on a high-fibre diet, which aids in passing waste through the colon and thus reduces intestinal pressure. This could help to prevent diverticulitis from developing. However, in cases of severe bleeding, surgery is necessary.

An acute attack of diverticulitis is usually treated with antibiotics. When the infection has been controlled, patients suffering from such an attack are also placed on a high-fibre diet. However, recurring acute attacks or complications, such as peritonitis, require surgical treatment.

See also DIET; DIGESTIVE SYSTEM.

Diverticulum (plural: diverticula) is a small, finger-like pouch, most often found in the intestinal wall but also occurring in other parts of the body. Diverticula may occur normally or they may result from a rupture of intestinal mucous membrane. MECKEL'S DIVERTICULUM, however, is present at birth. It is a pouch that protrudes from the ileum, and represents the yolk stalk of the embryo. In most persons, the stalk structure disappears at birth, but Meckel's diverticulum is fairly common, and does not require treatment.

See also DIVERTICULITIS AND DIVERTICULOSIS.

Dizziness is a sensation of unsteadiness or lightheadedness; the term is synonymous with giddiness. Dizziness should not be confused with vertigo, which is a feeling of movement, either of the external world rotating about the person, or of the person spinning.

See also BALANCE.

DNA (deoxyribonucleic acid) is the chemical found in the nucleus of every living cell. It is the carrier of the basic genetic information used in reproduction, and thus structures the GENE, groups of which form the CHROMOSOMES.

Dominant is a term used in the study of HEREDITY to describe a gene that affects the physical characteristics (phenotype) of an individual in preference to another gene of the same type. For example, the gene for brown eyes is dominant over the gene for blue eyes (which is said to be RECESSIVE).

The term dominant is also used by psychiatrists to describe persons with strong, overpowering personalities.

Dorsal means relating to the back (dorsum) of a structure or the body.

Double vision (known medically as diplopia) is when a single object is seen as two, which may or may not overlap. (People with squints do not have double vision because they have the ability unconsciously to ignore the vision from one eye.)

Q: *What causes double vision?*

A: Double vision is a common and generally insignificant symptom in people who are tired, who have had too much alcohol to drink, or who have suffered minor head injuries resulting in mild concussion. But double vision may also be a symptom of more serious disorders that affect the power of the eye muscles. It most commonly follows serious head injuries or strokes, but other neurological conditions (such as multiple sclerosis and diabetic neuritis, or the muscle disorder myasthenia gravis) may be the cause too.

Sometimes, blurred vision may be described as double vision by a patient.

Brief, non-recurrent double vision should be of no concern; a remaining or recurring symptom should be diagnosed by a doctor.

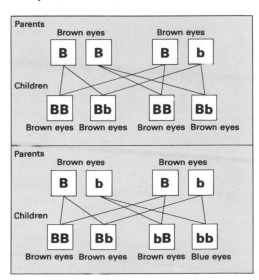

The dominant gene for brown eyes (B) prevails unless two recessive genes (bb) coincide.

Douche

Douche is a stream of vapour, water, or antiseptic fluid directed against a part of the body. It may be used either for personal hygiene or to treat a local disorder. The term is usually used to describe the washing of the vagina. The vagina cleanses itself naturally and is also cleansed in the normal bathing process, so there is little reason for a healthy woman to use a vaginal douche. Despite popular belief, there is no evidence that a vaginal douche following sexual intercourse is an effective method of contraception.

A talk about Down's syndrome

Down's syndrome, or Trisomy 21, is the medical name for mongolism, a congenital defect of mental and physical development. It is caused by an extra chromosome. There are forty-seven chromosomes instead of the normal forty-six. The defect is usually caused by an extra number twenty-one chromosome. The syndrome is associated with increasing age of the mother, and not with the number of pregnancies. A mother between the age of thirty-five and thirty-nine has a 0.4 per cent chance of having a mongoloid child; a woman over the age of forty has a 1–2 per cent chance of having a mongol. The physical characteristics include a flat, round head, which is also smaller than normal; small, low-set ears; a flattened nose; skin folds over the inner corner of the eyes; a large tongue that protrudes from a small mouth; and a typical pattern of creases on the palm. However, the most important feature is mental retardation; an affected child may have an intelligence quotient (IQ) of fifty or lower.

Q: Are there any other abnormalities associated with Down's syndrome?

A: Yes. Down's syndrome is often associated with other congenital disorders, such as heart disease, umbilical hernia, and Hirschsprung's disease (a bowel disorder that causes constipation). Leukaemia may develop in childhood or later.

Q: What can be done to help children with Down's syndrome?

A: There is no medical treatment that can cure Down's syndrome. However, with specialized education, most affected children can learn to look after themselves and to lead useful lives. Parents of a child with Down's syndrome should discuss education with their doctor and a specialist who has a special interest in the disorder.

Q: After the birth of one affected child, what is the likelihood of subsequent children having Down's syndrome?

A: Because Down's syndrome is rarely inherited, there is an excellent chance that any subsequent children will be normal, unless the mother is over age 40. Rarely, however, Down's syndrome is inherited. In either event, it is advisable to seek expert medical advice, for example, to obtain GENETIC COUNSELLING before starting another pregnancy.

Q: Can Down's syndrome be detected during pregnancy?

A: Yes. By testing a sample of the fluid from around the foetus in the womb (amniocentesis), a geneticist can discover whether a baby will be born with Down's syndrome, while there is still time to consider an abortion.

DPT vaccine is a combination of diphtheria, pertussis (whooping cough), and tetanus vaccines, used in immunizing infants.

Dracunculiasis is infestation with the parasitic guinea worm. *See* GUINEA WORM.

Dreams are thoughts, emotions, and experiences that occur during sleep. Any of the senses may contribute to a dream, but most dreams are visual and are accompanied by rapid eye movements (REM). Everybody dreams, although not everybody can remember dreaming.

The purpose of dreams is not known. But persons who are deliberately deprived of dream sleep become irritable and restless. Dream deprivation may also cause emotional problems. Many psychiatrists believe that the events within dreams relate to the

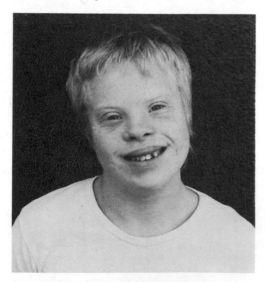

Down's syndrome is a congenital anomaly that produces typical facial characteristics.

dreamer's life and that by studying a patient's dreams they can find clues to the underlying causes of the dreamer's problems.

See also NIGHTMARE; SLEEP.

Drop foot. *See* FOOT DROP.

Dropsy is an obsolete term for excessive fluid retention in the body; it is now called OEDEMA.

Drop wrist. *See* WRIST DROP.

Drowning is death caused by smothering in liquid. *See* First Aid p.532.

A talk about Drug addiction

Drug addiction, or drug dependence, is the uncontrollable craving for a drug. Such craving may occur periodically or continuously, and is usually accompanied by an overwhelming compulsion to obtain the drug. The addict becomes preoccupied with thoughts about the anticipated effects of the drug.

The uncontrollable craving for a drug may be of physical origin, psychological origin, or both, and with some drugs the craving may develop in as short a time as twenty-four hours. In a person who is physically addicted to a drug, the body's chemical processes are altered so that the drug becomes essential for some of the normal metabolic functions. Psychological dependence on a drug does not involve a modification of the body's chemistry, but the addicted person believes that the drug is necessary in order to function normally.

Q: *Why do people take drugs for nonmedical reasons?*

A: There are many reasons for the nonmedical use of drugs. For example, some people with difficult problems, such as unemployment or large debts, become anxious, frustrated, and depressed. They feel trapped by problems that seem to have no solution and seek a release from reality in the effects of drugs.

Other people may take drugs out of boredom or curiosity, and some because their friends do and they feel the need to conform. This need to conform with friends is, perhaps, strongest among teenagers.

Q: *Are some people more likely than others to become dependent on drugs?*

A: Yes. In general, the likelihood of a person becoming dependent on a drug involves three interrelated factors; an individual's personality, the social environment, and the type of drug involved.

Some people are more sensitive than others to the effects of drugs and may feel euphoric states more intensely. This may result in a relatively rapid attraction to and dependence on drugs. In others, feelings of tension or depression may be more acute, and the relief provided by drugs correspondingly greater, and so the dependence more probable.

A person's environment affects the likelihood of drug dependence in many ways. For example, poor housing and unemployment are known to cause depression and anxiety, two states that are common causes of drug addiction. It is also likely that dependence on a drug will be greater in a person who has to steal to get money for the drug than it will in a person who does not. There is for some people a special attraction in doing something illegal or merely antisocial, and this attraction may put people in danger of becoming drug dependent.

In some cases, the nature of the drug taken affects the likelihood of dependency. For example, a person taking heroin is more likely to become drug dependent than a person taking barbiturates.

Q: *Which drugs may cause dependency?*

A: There are many drugs on which people can become dependent. These drugs can be categorized as those that depress the central nervous system; those that stimulate the central nervous system; and those that produce hallucinations, and also affect the central nervous system. The main group of drugs that depress the central nervous system are the narcotics, such as codeine, heroin, methadone, morphine and pethidine. Other drugs in this category include alcohol, barbiturates, nicotine, tranquillizers, and some sleeping pills.

Drugs that stimulate the central nervous system include cocaine and the amphetamines, such as dexamphetamine.

Drugs that produce hallucinations are known as hallucinogens or psychedelics. Some of the more common hallucinogens are DMT, DOM, LSD, MDA, psilocybin, mescaline, and THC.

Marijuana is classified as a mild hallucinogen, but it is much less powerful than other drugs in this category.

Q: *What effects do depressants produce?*

A: Depressants slow down the activities of the central nervous system. If this system slows down too much, the body's vital functions may stop, which could be fatal. Dependence on depressants usually takes

Drug addiction

the form of both physical and psychological dependence. The narcotic depressants can cause dependence much more quickly than other depressants.

The short-term effects of depressants include euphoria; relief of pain; and prevention of withdrawal symptoms. The long-term effects include depression; malnutrition; and constipation. The addict may also become infected with hepatitis or tetanus by using infected needles. If the drug is stopped, the addict will suffer withdrawal symptoms.

Q: *What symptoms may be caused by withdrawal from a depressant?*

A: The symptoms of depressant withdrawal vary according to the drug involved, but are often extremely severe, and may be fatal. For example, within about eighteen hours of the sudden withdrawal of alcohol from an alcoholic there may be convulsions and delirium (delirium tremens). Delirium tremens (DTs) may also occur when an addict stops taking sleeping pills.

Other symptoms of depressant withdrawal include weakness; high blood pressure and pulse rate; profuse sweating; gooseflesh; diarrhoea; vomiting; severe abdominal cramps; and, sometimes, cardiovascular collapse. The diarrhoea and vomiting may cause dehydration.

Q: *What effects do stimulants produce?*

A: The short-term effects of stimulants include excitation; sleeplessness; hyperactivity; and euphoria. In the long-term, some heavy users of stimulants may also experience hallucinations, delusions, and toxic psychosis.

Dependence on stimulants is mainly psychological, although some degree of physical dependence may also develop. Amphetamines are perhaps the most dangerous of the stimulant drugs and many amphetamine addicts develop a high tolerance as part of their dependence on the drug. Tolerance usually occurs rapidly and the addict has to take larger dosages to achieve the desired effects. The larger amounts may cause the amphetamine addict to stay awake for several days, during which the addict may hallucinate, become disoriented, and suffer from paranoia. Following this ordeal the amphetamine addict may sleep for a day or more. On waking, the addict usually feels severely depressed and often takes another dose of the drug to relieve the depression, which begins the cycle all over again.

Q: *What symptoms may be caused by withdrawal from a stimulant?*

A: The symptoms of stimulant withdrawal include severe depression; muscle pains; apathy; and a strong desire to take more stimulants. These symptoms are felt most keenly by amphetamine addicts. Generally, however, the symptoms of stimulant withdrawal are milder because stimulants are less physically addictive than depressants.

Q: *What effects do hallucinogens produce?*

A: The effects of hallucinogens vary widely,

Deaths recorded as due to drugs: 1974–1977				
Nature of substance	1974	1975	1976	1977
Opiates and synthetic analogues (including heroin and morphine)	20	25	36	41
Analgesics (pain-relieving drugs) and antipyretics (fever-reducing drugs)	376	458	471	583
Barbiturates (sedative drugs derived from barbituric acid)	1261	1121	966	809
Barbiturates and alcohol	255	223	173	176
Other sedative and hypnotic drugs	132	121	143	121
Psychotherapeutic drugs (including tranquillizers and antidepressants)	347	349	342	390
Toxic effect of alcohol	75	79	88	94
Other drug and medical agents alone or with alcohol	446	461	544	612
Other chemical substances of non-medicinal source	721	651	729	849
Total	3633	3488	3492	3675

Drug addiction and abuse of drugs cause a significant number of deaths.

Despite improved facilities for care and rehabilitation, drug addiction is increasing.

both between individuals and even in the same individual on different occasions. The main effects include exhilaration, sensory distortion, and illusions. But in some cases there may be feelings of paranoia and panic. Occasionally, "flashbacks" may occur. These are brief recurrences of a previous hall-ucinatory state that may occur weeks or months later without the person having taken a hallucinogen.

The hallucinogens do not seem to produce physical dependence, but they may produce psychological dependence. The long-term effects of these drugs are not known. But scientists are trying to determine whether long-term usage of hallucinogens can cause chromosome damage or genetic mutation.

Q: *Are babies of drug-dependent women born drug dependent?*

A: Yes, although the symptoms of drug dependence in babies vary according to the drug involved. For example, the newborn child of a heroin-addicted mother may be of small size and generally poor health. The baby may display withdrawal symptoms in the form of irritability, high-pitched crying, trembling, sweating, vomiting, and diarrhoea. The withdrawal symptoms usually occur within about three days of birth, but withdrawal from barbiturate dependence usually takes longer. Methadone-dependent babies may exhibit breathing distress, convulsions, and fever.

Q: *What is the clinical treatment for drug dependence?*

A: The first stage of treatment is withdrawal of the drug (detoxification). In cases of physical dependence this usually involves a gradual reduction of the addict's intake over a period of about ten days. Sometimes a less harmful substitute with similar effects is administered, for example, methadone instead of heroin. The treatment of alcoholism may also include vitamin supplements and the administration of a deterrent drug, such as Antabuse. This drug produces nausea whenever alcohol is drunk. Withdrawal may be delayed if the person is in poor health.

In addition to withdrawal, treatment may also include a programme of mental and social rehabilitation, which may involve psychiatric counselling. The treatment of drug dependence is often not completely successful, although the success rate varies from drug to drug.

The rehabilitation programmes, such as therapeutic communities and Alcoholics Anonymous, greatly increase the chances of success.

See also ALCOHOLISM.

Drugs. The following table lists the major types of drugs and their medical usage. Each type of drug has a separate article in the A–Z section of this book.

Drug	Medical usage
AMPHETAMINES	To treat narcolepsy and depression
ANAESTHETICS	To reduce pain
ANORECTICS	To reduce appetite
ANTACIDS	To counteract excess stomach acidity
ANTHELMINTICS	To destroy worms
ANTIBIOTICS	To treat micro-organismal infections
ANTICOAGULANTS	To treat thrombosis
ANTICONVULSANTS	To prevent convulsions
ANTIDEPRESSANTS	To treat depression
ANTIHISTAMINES	To treat allergies
ANTINAUSEANTS	To treat nausea
ANTIPRURITICS	To relieve itching
ANTIPYRETICS	To reduce fever
ANTISPASMODICS	To prevent or relieve muscular spasm
ANTITUSSIVES	To relieve coughing
ANTIVENINS	To treat poisonous bites or stings
BARBITURATES	To treat insomnia
BRONCHIAL DILATORS	To treat bronchial asthma
CHELATING AGENTS	To treat poisoning by heavy metals
CONTRACEPTIVES	To prevent conception (*see* CONTRACEPTION)
DIURETICS	To treat oedema and high blood pressure
HYPNOTICS	To induce sleep
INSULIN	To treat diabetes
MUSCLE RELAXANTS	To relax muscles
RESPIRATORY STIMULANTS	To treat breathing stoppage
SCABICIDES	To destroy mites
SEDATIVES	To treat insomnia
THYROID PREPARATIONS	To treat goitre, hypothyroidism, hyperthyroidism, and thyroiditis
TRANQUILLIZERS	To treat anxiety and mental disorders
URICOSURIC AGENTS	To treat gout
URINARY ACIDIFIERS	To increase the effectiveness or elimination of certain drugs

Drunkenness. *See* ALCOHOLISM; INTOXICATION.

DTs

DTs. *See* DELIRIUM TREMENS.

Duct is any narrow tube in the body that carries secretions or fluids from one part of the body to another.

Ductless gland is another name for ENDOCRINE GLAND.

Ductus arteriosus is a blood vessel that joins the main artery leading to the lungs (the pulmonary artery) with the main artery that leads from the heart (the aorta). This link is present in a foetus so that the blood supply bypasses the lungs, which do not function until after birth. The ductus arteriosus closes off soon after birth. Failure to close is a common type of congenital heart disorder; the condition is corrected by tying off the vessel in a surgical operation.

Dumb. *See* MUTE.

Dumping syndrome is a digestive disorder that occurs in a patient who has had an operation removing or bypassing a large part of the stomach. Symptoms of sweating, dizziness, and weakness may be accompanied by pain and headache. The cause of dumping syndrome is not fully understood, but what happens is that the stomach "dumps" its contents too quickly into the small intestine. The symptoms can be reduced by eating several small meals instead of one or two large ones, and by drinking fluids separately.

Duodenal ulcer. *See* PEPTIC ULCER.

Duodenum is the first part of the small intestine, surrounding the head of the pancreas. It is about 25cm (10 inches) long, and receives partially digested food from the stomach. The digestive process is continued in the duodenum by the enzyme-containing fluids

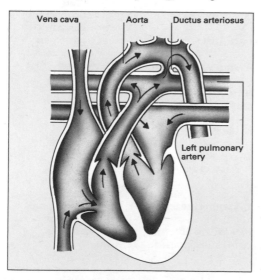

Ductus arteriosus is the blood vessel that bypasses the foetal lung; it closes after birth.

from the pancreas and the glands lining the duodenal wall, and the action of bile from the liver and gall bladder. When the digestive processes have been completed in the duodenum, the food passes into the jejunum.

Dupuytren's contracture is the inability to straighten the little and ring fingers, due to a thickening of the fibrous tissue lining the palm. Occasionally Dupuytren's contracture can involve the soles of the feet as well. The cause is not known, but it may be inherited. Treatment involves a surgical operation to remove the thickened fibrous tissue and release the tendons.

Dutch cap is a rubber diaphragm that is used with sperm-killing creams as a form of contraception. The woman inserts it into the vagina to cover the cervix (neck of the womb) before intercourse takes place. *See* CONTRACEPTION.

Dwarfism is the physical condition of being abnormally undersized. A dwarf may have normal body formations that are proportionally smaller throughout, or the condition may involve disproportionate stunting (achondroplasia). Dwarfism may be caused by abnormal foetal development (congenital), malnutrition, and other environmental factors, or hormone deficiency. Treatment of dwarfism depends on the cause.

Q: Which types of dwarfism are congenital?

A: The most common congenital disorder is achondroplasia, the form of dwarfism in which growth of the long bones is retarded. An achondroplastic dwarf has a normal sized head and trunk, but relatively disproportionally short arms and legs. If one parent has this condition, there is a 50 per cent chance with each pregnancy of having an affected child. There are other rare congenital disorders associated with dwarfism.

Q: What environmental factors may result in dwarfism?

A: Poor nutrition deprives the body of the food and vitamins that are needed for normal growth. This can be seen in poor families with a low standard of living, and in Third World countries where disorders such as kwashiorkor may occur. An improvement in diet, provided it is started soon enough, will produce rapid and eventually normal growth.

Chronic illnesses, such as those caused by coeliac disease or congenital heart disease, cause slow growth and undersized children. If the condition is treated, normal growth usually returns.

The treatment of some illnesses with corticosteroid drugs by mouth may, if continued for a long period of time, seriously interfere with normal growth and produce apparent dwarfism.

It has also been shown that the normal rate of growth may be affected by emotional deprivation, especially if the warm supportive environment that children need is lacking and replaced by hate and violence (*see* BATTERED BABY SYNDROME).

Q: How do hormonal deficiencies cause dwarfism?

A: Growth hormone is produced by the pituitary gland at the base of the brain. If for any reason the pituitary gland of a child is underactive, dwarfism results. The body of a child with this deficiency remains small but is correctly proportioned. There is no mental impairment.

See also CRETINISM.

A talk about Dying

Dying is a natural process involving the progressive degeneration of those body functions essential to maintain life. To be dying of old age is the best example of this: the body's organs are worn out and eventually they cease to function. Drug treatment and other applications of medical knowledge have made it possible to postpone the dying process.

Q: Should a dying patient be made aware of the situation?

A: Many patients prefer to know if they are to die from their illness and press the doctor for a frank opinion. If direct questions are asked, it is generally because the patient wants honest answers. Close associates of the patient sometimes prefer that their friend or relative be spared the anguish of knowing, but the wishes of the patient must be the primary consideration. In other cases, the patient suspects the prognosis but prefers not to have it confirmed. It is unlikely that a doctor will offer the information unless directly requested.

Q: How strong does fear seem to be in people who are dying?

A: It seems that most people dread that time in the future when they will know that death is imminent. However, people who are dying and know it usually manage to come to terms with the fact. It seems clear from experienced witnesses such as doctors and nurses that the dying process is not frightening in itself: as death

draws near, the patient tends to become peaceful and accepting of a death which may well be desired by the final stages.

Q: What is it about a drawn-out death that people think will be frightening?

A: The fear of pain and suffering is probably the most common fear for those who contemplate their dying. This is why people often say that they would prefer to die instantaneously (for example, from accident or heart attack). Another fear is that approaching death will bring remorse or terrifying revelations.

Q: What type of requests might a dying person make?

A: It is natural for the patient to wish to be with close friends; such companions are of most comfort during this time and their understanding and concern may reduce the loneliness of the ordeal. The patient may feel the need to speak in confidence with certain people who are trusted, sympathetic, or admired. During such intimacies, it is likely that death will be discussed freely, and this can be a type of therapy. If other people can allay his or her alarm and fear, the dying person may more readily embrace what is natural and inevitable. Some patients cope with the thought of death by making sure that affairs consequent upon their death will cause as little inconvenience as possible to those who must attend to them. Matters of the will may be settled, funeral arrangements decided, and the patient may wish to participate in discussions about what everyday

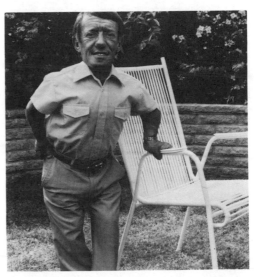

Dwarfism of the achondroplastic variety affects the growth of the long bones.

Dysarthria

adjustments may have to be made both short-term and long-term.

Q: *What practical care should be given the patient?*

A: The patient needs the regular, thorough care of home nursing. This requires patience in overcoming the initial difficulties of bed-bathing, feeding someone who has little or no appetite, and learning how to deal with possible involuntary urination and defecation. Prescribed medicines have to be administered regularly and drugs have to be given as needed according to the advice of the doctor. Measures to ensure greatest comfort for the patient should be taken such as propping up the pillows, regulating the amount of light entering the room, changing the bed linen, and ensuring adequate entertainment.

Q: *How can the family help?*

A: People who live in the patient's home cope best with the nursing requirements if the small everyday chores are shared. Intensive care of the patient means that regular daily activities may have to be curtailed. It is good to remember that in time of crisis, neighbours or friends are only too willing to be of assistance; if help is needed, there should be no hesitation in seeking it.

Q: *Might a person be conscious immediately before death?*

A: Yes. Sometimes a patient remains weak but alert until the moment of death. The presence of the family at this time is always a comfort. Often when a

patient appears to be unconscious, the sense of hearing still remains; this should be considered at all times when discussing the illness in the presence of the patient.

Q: *Is it always obvious when a patient dies?*

A: No. Although a pallor and stillness typically occur with death, the exact moment of death is difficult to define even for doctors and nurses. Breathing prior to death may follow a cycle of being alternately shallow and deep for any length of time before death finally occurs during a shallow period (*see* CHEYNE-STOKES BREATHING). Within a few minutes of the event, the eyes become staring and the muscles of the face sag.

See also DEATH.

Dysarthria is the inability to speak clearly. The causes of the disorder include emotional stress, paralysis, and lack of co-ordination of the tongue and facial muscles, and of those supplying the voice box. Disease of the muscles or nerve disorders may also be causative factors.

Dysentery is an infectious disease characterized by severe diarrhoea, with blood and mucus in the stools. It is accompanied by pain in the abdomen and, sometimes, contracting spasms of the anus with a persistent desire to empty the bowels (tenesmus).

There are two forms of dysentery: bacillary dysentery, caused by bacteria (*Shigella*); and amoebic dysentery, caused by an amoeba (*Entameba histolytica*). Both forms are transmitted by contaminated water or food. Dysentery is particularly common in tropical countries where standards of hygiene are poor.

Q: *What are the symptoms of bacillary dysentery?*

A: There are several forms of *Shigella* infection, which cause dysentery of varying severity. The symptoms start after about 48 hours with the acute onset of vomiting, diarrhoea, and abdominal pains. A high fever may occur, and diarrhoea continues for several days with blood and mucus in the stools. In babies and young children, life-threatening DEHYDRATION may occur rapidly.

Q: *What is the treatment for bacillary dysentery?*

A: It is most important to ensure that the patient drinks plenty of fluids. A doctor may prescribe antispasmodic and antidiarrhoeal drugs to control the worst of the symptoms until the condition improves naturally. This may take up to ten days, although the patient is often

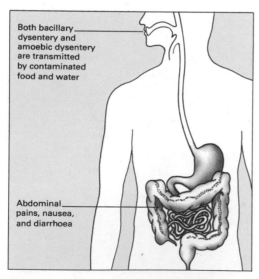

Both bacillary dysentery and amoebic dysentery are transmitted by contaminated food and water

Abdominal pains, nausea, and diarrhoea

Dysentery is an intestinal disorder caused by bacteria or by the ingestion of amoebae.

better within 48 hours. Babies and children may have to be admitted to a hospital for intravenous infusion, if serious dehydration occurs. Antibiotics are used only in the severest cases.

Q: *What are the complications of bacillary dysentery?*

A: Sometimes a patient develops an eye inflammation, such as conjunctivitis or iritis. Because the stools may remain infectious for some weeks, it is necessary for the patient to take great care with personal hygiene, washing the hands thoroughly after each bowel movement. The doctor may culture the patient's faeces on several occasions to check whether the infective organism has disappeared.

Q: *In what way does amoebic dysentery differ from bacillary dysentery?*

A: Amoebic dysentery may take some time to appear. Often some other minor intestinal disorder causes it to flare up, resulting in recurring attacks. The attacks are accompanied by colicky abdominal pain and, sometimes, fever. Intermittent attacks may already have gone on for several months, causing the patient to feel vaguely unwell, before a major attack necessitates consulting a doctor.

Q: *How is amoebic dysentery diagnosed?*

A: A doctor diagnoses amoebic dysentery by examining the faeces for the infective organism, and by examining the inside of the colon with a lighted tube (sigmoidoscope). The doctor can often see small ulcers in the colon; specimens from these ulcers contain the infection.

Q: *How is amoebic dysentery treated?*

A: It can be treated with a variety of drugs. The drug metronidazole is usually effective in uncomplicated cases.

Q: *What are the complications of amoebic dysentery?*

A: The infection may form a palpable mass inside the intestine or infect the liver, forming a liver abscess. It may also extend into the lung to produce a lung abscess. Both are serious conditions, and require specialized treatment.

Q: *What precautions can a person take to prevent catching dysentery?*

A: Because dysentery is more common in tropical countries, it is important in such localities to avoid eating uncooked foods and to ensure that all foods are prepared in the most hygienic way. It is essential not to drink unboiled water, because this may carry the infection. All foods must be kept covered to prevent flies from contaminating them with the disease.

Dyslexia is an imprecise term used to describe a variety of reading and writing disorders. It may be a disturbed understanding of what is read, ranging from a minor disability to a complete and permanent inability to read, which is inconsistent with the individual's intelligence. It is usually accompanied by an inability to spell correctly. The specific causes of dyslexia are disputed, but it may be due to congenital or acquired brain damage, probably affecting the speech centres. Dyslexia is not a sign of low intelligence, and some affected individuals may benefit from special teaching.

Dysmenorrhoea is pain associated with menstruation. Primary dysmenorrhoea occurs for no apparent cause. Secondary dysmenorrhoea, usually happening later in life, has an underlying cause.

Q: *What are the symptoms of primary dysmenorrhoea?*

A: The pain begins just before or at the onset of menstruation, and is centred in the lower abdomen. It may be cramplike, and lasts for the first day or two of the menstrual period. The abdominal pain is often accompanied by backache and, sometimes, vomiting.

Q: *How is primary dysmenorrhoea treated?*

A: Painkilling and antispasmodic drugs may be prescribed. They should be started just before menstruation, and continued for the first two or three days of the period. The drugs should be taken regularly, not just when pain reappears. If these measures fail to control the symptoms, certain hormonal drugs, such as birth

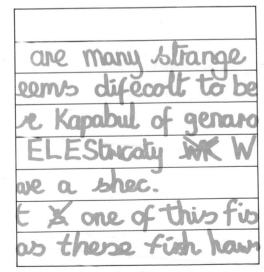

Dyslexia may be a cause of poor spelling but does not indicate lack of intelligence.

Dyspareunia

control pills, will prevent ovulation and stop the pain. Sometimes it is necessary to lie down with a heated pad over the lower abdominal area.

Q: *Are the symptoms of secondary dysmenorrhoea different from those of primary dysmenorrhoea?*

A: Yes. The pain usually starts after the onset of menstruation, causing a dull ache deep in the pelvis, and it often continues throughout the period.

Q: *What are the causes of secondary dysmenorrhoea?*

A: Secondary dysmenorrhoea is usually caused by some gynaecological disorder, such as inflammation of the womb (endometritis) or of the fallopian tubes (salpingitis), or by the spread of intestinal inflammation. In some cases the cause may be ENDOMETRIOSIS, in which tissue resembling womb lining occurs in other parts of the pelvic cavity.

Q: *How can secondary dysmenorrhoea be treated?*

A: The treatment must be directed at the cause. If there is infection, prolonged treatment with antibiotics may be necessary, as well as deep heat treatment given by a physiotherapist. Occasionally a cause has to be dealt with surgically.

Q: *Are there any other reasons for a woman to experience dysmenorrhoea?*

A: Yes. It is common for menstruation to be accompanied by mild abdominal discomfort, a feeling of pressure in the pelvis, headache, and slight nausea.

These symptoms may be much worse if the woman is overtired or has been under emotional stress. Psychological factors, such as depression, may aggravate these symptoms enough for the woman to complain about them.

Dyspareunia is painful sexual intercourse. There are two forms of the condition, primary dyspareunia and secondary dyspareunia.

Q: *What causes primary dyspareunia, and how is it treated?*

A: The cause of primary dyspareunia is involuntary contraction of the muscle around the vagina, which makes sexual intercourse difficult, and sometimes impossible. The reason for the involuntary muscular contraction is usually psychological, for example, an excessive anxiety about the act of sexual intercourse or perhaps the fear of an unwanted pregnancy. Treatment for this form of dyspareunia is to remove the person's sexual fears and anxieties.

Q: *What causes secondary dyspareunia, and how is it treated?*

A: In secondary dyspareunia the pain arises from some other disorder, such as inflammation or a structural defect. It is the only form of dyspareunia experienced by men, the most common cause being inflammation of the foreskin. In women the causes of secondary dyspareunia include inflammation or infection of the vagina (vaginitis), the fallopian tubes (salpingitis), or the womb (endometriosis), or an unusually rigid hymen.

The pain can be expected to disappear after the underlying cause has been treated.

Dyspepsia. *See* INDIGESTION.

Dysphagia is difficulty in swallowing.

Dysphasia is the lack of co-ordination of speech and failure to arrange words in a comprehensible way. It is a less severe form of APHASIA. Dysphasia commonly follows brain damage caused by a stroke or injury involving the side of the brain that controls SPEECH. There is a tendency for the condition to improve naturally, and careful speech therapy can teach the patient how to talk, even though this may take many months.

Dyspnea is the medical term for breathlessness. The essential characteristic of dyspnea is that shortness of breath may occur without undue physical exertion. This is often a symptom of a disorder. *See* BREATHLESSNESS.

Dystrophy is a wasting condition.

Dysuria is painful or difficult urination. It is a symptom of various disorders, including

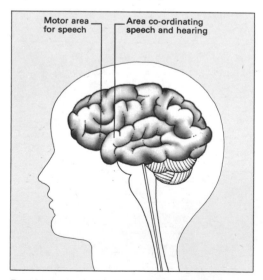

Motor area for speech   Area co-ordinating speech and hearing

Dysphasia a speech defect, is caused by a disorder of the left hemisphere of the brain.

cystitis, prostatitis, and urethritis. Rarely, it is caused by cancer of the cervix in women or pelvic peritonitis. Any person with dysuria should consult a doctor, so that the precise cause can be diagnosed and treated.

See also BLADDER DISORDERS.

E

Ear is the organ of hearing and balance. It consists of a series of sensitive structures that detect sounds and create impulses in the auditory nerve leading to the hearing centre in the brain. There are three sections in the ear: (1) the outer ear; (2) the middle ear; and (3) the inner ear.

Q: What is the function of the outer ear?

A: The outer ear has two main parts: the visible flap, called the auricle or pinna, and the auditory canal. The funnel-shaped auricle picks up sound waves and passes them along the auditory canal to the middle ear. In the outer third of its length the auditory canal has a lining of fine hairs and a number of glands that secrete wax (cerumen). The hairs and the cerumen protect the ear's delicate structures by collecting dust that enters the canal.

Q: How does the middle ear function?

A: The middle ear is separated from the outer ear by the eardrum, or tympanic membrane. As sound waves vibrate the eardrum, they set up vibrations in three tiny bones (ossicles) in the middle ear; the bones are called the hammer (malleus), anvil (incus), and stirrup (stapes). The auditory ossicles intensify and pass on the vibrations to a membrane of the inner ear called the oval window.

Pressure in the middle ear is kept the same as atmospheric pressure, allowing the eardrum to vibrate, by means of the Eustachian tube, which connects the middle ear with the back of the throat (pharynx). Two small muscles join the ossicles to the surrounding bone. These muscles contract in reaction to loud noises, and protect the inner ear by limiting its vibration.

Q: How does the inner ear function as an organ of hearing?

A: The inner ear, or cochlea, is a tube that is coiled like a snail's shell and is filled with fluid. It contains the organ of Corti. Vibrations of the oval window activate the nerve endings within the organ of Corti causing impulses to pass along the auditory nerve to the hearing centre in the brain, where sound is registered.

Q: How does the ear act as an organ of balance?

A: The inner ear also contains three fluid-filled loops, called semicircular canals, set at right angles to each other. Any movement of the head affects the fluid in one or more of them. The ends of the canals contain receptor cells that register movements of the fluid and pass the information to the brain. The whole system of canals and cavities in the inner ear is called the labyrinth.

Another organ in the inner ear contains sensitive cells with fine hairs that include small "stones" (otoliths) of calcium carbonate. When the head is held upright, the otoliths press on certain receptors. If the head is tilted, the otoliths press on other receptors. In this way, receptors register any position of the head, and pass this information also to the brain. The sense of balance comes from a combination of movement and position of the head (*see* BALANCE).

See also EAR DISORDERS; p.17.

A talk about Earache

Earache is a variable and often intense throbbing pain deep inside the ear. Normally, atmospheric air pressure inside the middle ear is maintained by a channel (Eustachian tube) that connects with the back of the throat. If this tube becomes blocked during a

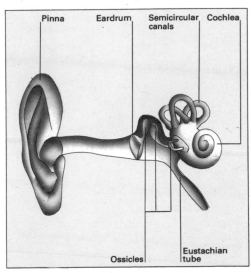

Ear has complex parts, some of which are used for hearing, and others for sensing balance.

Ear disorders

respiratory infection, a build-up of pressure in the middle ear affects the sensitive eardrum and causes pain. Sudden changes in atmospheric pressure (for example, when flying or diving) may cause a similar condition in the middle ear (*see* BAROTRAUMA).

Inflammation in the outer ear (for example, a boil) also causes pain because the lining adheres tightly to the underlying bone.

Pain may be referred to the ear from disorders elsewhere in the body, for example the neck, the pharynx, or the sinuses.

Q: *Can infection spread to the ear from other parts of the body and cause earache?*

A: Yes. Infection can spread from the throat along the Eustachian tube to the middle ear. The eardrum becomes inflamed from the inside, and pus forms. The pressure of the pus may be enough to burst the eardrum, in which case there is a discharge from the outer ear. The infection may also spread to the mastoid bone just behind the outer ear or, in the most serious cases, through the bone to the brain.

Q: *What conditions affecting the outer ear can cause earache?*

A: Wax, secreted by the glands in the outer ear, may irritate the auditory canal and cause earache. If particles lodge in the outer ear, interference with the auditory canal may cause pain. Skin infections such as boils, inflammations resulting from swimming, cuts, or bruises sometimes cause earache.

Q: *How is earache treated?*

A: Because of potential damage to the ear, a doctor should be consulted. Until the cause is determined, little can be done other than to take painkilling drugs. Middle ear disorders are treated with antibiotics, decongestant nasal drops, or antihistamines. Infections in the outer ear are treated with antibiotic eardrops. Any foreign object or lump of hardened wax in the outer ear should be removed by a doctor.

Ear disorders. The following table lists some of the disorders that affect the ear and the basic characteristics of each disorder. Each disorder has a separate article in the A-Z section of this book.

Disorder	Basic characteristics
BOIL (inside and outside the ear)	Abscesses, causing pain and diminished hearing
CAULIFLOWER EAR	Deformed ear
DEAFNESS	Nearly complete or total loss of hearing
LABYRINTHITIS	Inflammation of inner ear, resulting in noises in ear and dizziness
MASTOIDITIS	Inflammation of the mastoid process
MÉNIÈRE'S DISEASE	Deafness, noises in the ear, and vertigo
MYRINGITIS	Inflammation of eardrum
OTITIS externa, media, or interna	Inflammation of external, middle, or inner ear
OTOMYCOSIS	Fungus infection of outer ear and/or auditory canal
OTORRHOEA	Discharge from the ear
OTOSCLEROSIS	Bone growths in inner ear, resulting in hearing loss
TINNITUS	Buzzing in ears
TUMOUR (in auditory canal, middle ear, or acoustic nerve)	Impaired hearing, deafness
WAX	Impaired hearing

The following table lists some general health disorders that may cause ear problems grouped according to symptom. The symptoms listed may also indicate other clinical disorders. A good medical history and physical examination by a doctor are essential for adequate diagnosis of a problem.

Each disorder has a separate article in the A-Z section of this book.

Symptom	Disorder
Auditory hallucinations	DRUG ADDICTION SCHIZOPHRENIA (and other mental disturbances)
Earache	COMMON COLD GUMBOIL

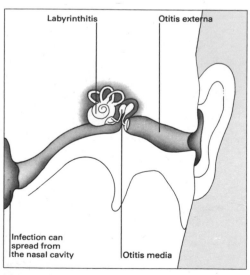

Labyrinthitis
Otitis externa
Infection can spread from the nasal cavity
Otitis media

Ear disorders that cause inflammation can affect the outer, middle, or inner ears.

Symptom	Disorder
Earache	INFLUENZA
	MENINGITIS
	OCCUPATIONAL INJURIES AND DISORDERS
	PHARYNGITIS
	PIMPLE or foreign body in the outer ear
	SINUSITIS
	TONSILLITIS
Impaired hearing/deafness	GERMAN MEASLES (in pregnant mother)
	HAEMORRHAGE (into inner ear)
	INFLUENZA
	MUMPS
	OCCUPATIONAL INJURIES AND DISORDERS
	SCARLET FEVER
Outer ear skin problems	Aural IMPETIGO
	DERMATITIS
	ECZEMA
	PIMPLE
	RODENT ULCER
	Sebaceous CYST

Eardrum, known medically as the tympanic membrane, is a layer of skin, fibrous tissue, and mucous membrane at the end of the auditory canal that separates the outer ear from the middle ear.

See also EAR; EAR DISORDERS.

ECG. *See* ELECTROCARDIOGRAM.

Echinococcus is a small TAPEWORM that may cause hydatid disease. *See* HYDATID CYST.

Echocardiogram is a record of the echo produced when ultrasonic sound waves are reflected from the heart. Analysis of the echo pattern can aid diagnosis of heart disorders. *See* SONOGRAPHY.

Echogram is a record of the echo produced when ultrasonic sound waves are reflected from various body tissues. *See* SONOGRAPHY.

Eclampsia is the serious form of TOXAEMIA of pregnancy. It can occur in women during the final three months of pregnancy or after the delivery of the baby.

Eclampsia is an extremely grave, but rare, condition, characterized by convulsions, high blood pressure (hypertension), and finally coma that may be fatal. The cause of eclampsia is not known, but usually the condition follows pre-eclampsia.

See PRE-ECLAMPSIA.

Q: *What is the treatment for eclampsia?*
A: Urgent hospitalization is essential. Treatment varies but commonly sedatives are used to prevent further convulsions, and other drugs are given to reduce blood pressure. If treatment appears to be failing, labour is induced immediately or a Caesarian section is performed.

ECT. *See* ELECTROCONVULSIVE THERAPY.

Ecthyma is an ulcerative form of the skin infection impetigo in adults. *See* IMPETIGO.

Ectopic pregnancy occurs when a fertilized ovum, instead of passing along the fallopian tube from the ovary and implanting in the lining of the womb, implants in the tube or, rarely, on the ovary. Such as pregnancy seldom lasts more than two months; usually, the fallopian tube then bursts. Occasionally the embryo dies and is absorbed, although there have been cases in which a foetus has survived long enough to be born by Caesarean section. Ectopic pregnancy may be caused by infection of the fallopian tube.

Q: *What are the symptoms of ectopic pregnancy?*
A: In its early stages it may be impossible to distinguish between a normal and an ectopic pregnancy. Later there may be a sudden onset of vaginal bleeding with severe abdominal pain caused by bursting of the fallopian tube. This internal bleeding causes shock and collapse.

Q: *How is an ectopic pregnancy treated?*
A: If the embryo is detected before the tube ruptures, it may be removed surgically. When the fallopian tube ruptures, urgent hospitalization is necessary and the entire tube has to be removed.

Q: *Can a woman conceive after having had an ectopic pregnancy?*
A: Yes, further pregnancies are usually possible if one healthy fallopian tube remains. Expert gynaecological advice should be sought.

See also PREGNANCY AND CHILDBIRTH.

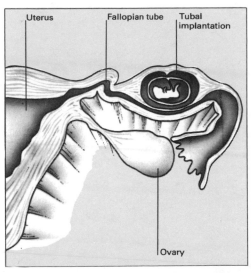

Ectopic pregnancy can occur anywhere outside the uterus – a common site is in the tube itself.

Ectropion

Ectropion is the turning inside out of an edge, commonly the edge of the eyelid. It may be caused by a relaxation of the skin or, rarely, by damage to the facial nerve. The condition may also result from an infection of the eyelid. Ectropion is common among elderly persons.

Q: Can an ectropion be treated?

A: Yes, in most cases. The condition can be corrected either by a special surgical technique using a cautery needle, or by plastic surgery.

Q: Can ectropions affect any other parts of the body?

A: Yes. If the womb has been lacerated, during childbirth, for example, the edges of the neck-like exit (cervix) may turn inside out.

See also ENTROPION.

Eczema is a red, itching, slightly discharging inflammation of the skin. Like DERMATITIS, it is a descriptive term without an indication of its cause; eczema and dermatitis are used as interchangeable words. Eczema is often called atopic eczema as it is an inherited condition associated with other allergic conditions, such as hay fever or asthma, that may affect other members of the family.

Q: When may atopic eczema first appear?

A: Usually between the ages of two and six months, areas of redness and scaling on the skin commonly appear on the scalp and face and spread to the limbs and body. The condition varies greatly in babies. If it is mild it typically involves the bends in the elbows and behind the knees; if it is severe, it will cause itching and sleeplessness.

Q: What is the progress of atopic eczema?

A: The condition tends to improve naturally. The milder form may disappear by the age of three or four, and the more severe form by adolescence. Many children with eczema eventually develop asthma or hay fever.

The condition may be made worse by extremes of heat or cold, changes in the diet, or minor illnesses, such as the common cold. Constant scratching may cause infection, such as impetigo.

Q: How is atopic eczema treated?

A: In infancy it is essential to protect the affected areas, and babies often have to wear gloves to stop them scratching. Certain items of food, such as cow's milk and egg white may aggravate the condition. These may be temporarily excluded from the diet to see if there is an improvement.

The skin should be cleaned with special creams, not with soap. Cotton, not wool, should be worn next to the skin.

Antihistamine drugs, to reduce itching, and careful use of corticosteroid creams are an essential part of the treatment prescribed by a doctor.

EEG. *See* ELECTROENCEPHALOGRAM.

Effort syndrome, or neurocirculatory asthenia, is a nervous condition brought about by anxiety. Characteristics of the syndrome include chest pain around the heart, breathlessness, palpitations, irregular pulse, dizziness, fatigue and sweating. Treatment is to remove the patient from the stressful situation. Tranquillizing drugs may help; a doctor may also recommend psychotherapy.

Effusion is the accumulation of fluid in a body space. The cause of effusion is generally inflammation or congestion.

Ejaculation is the emission of semen from the penis at the climax of sexual excitement (orgasm). Emission of semen before the sexual partner has achieved satisfactory excitement is known as premature ejaculation (*see* SEXUAL PROBLEMS).

Elbow is a hinge joint between the lower end of the upper arm bone (humerus) and the two bones of the lower arm (radius and ulna). Two muscles in the upper arm, the biceps and the triceps, control the action of the elbow. When the biceps contracts, the arm bends; when the triceps contracts, the arm straightens. The funny bone is not a bone, but a nerve that lies on the inner side of the tip of the elbow, near the humerus.

Elbow injuries produce symptoms that differ from those due to ARTHRITIS. The most common injuries are fractures, of which there

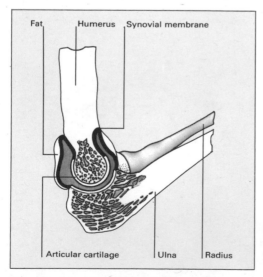

Fat Humerus Synovial membrane

Articular cartilage Ulna Radius

Elbow is a hinge joint that articulates with the larger of the two forearm bones, the ulna.

are many types. The elbow may be dislocated, especially following a fall on an outstretched hand. Like other joints, the elbow is vulnerable to sprains, twists, and torn ligaments.

For EMERGENCY treatment, *see* First Aid, pp.546, 592.

Q: *What complications might result from a fracture?*

A: The chief risk with an elbow fracture is that the main artery supplying the forearm and hand may become blocked by pressure from the broken bone. This quickly causes death to the muscles the artery supplies. For this reason the pulse should always be checked at the wrist immediately after the accident. If the pulse is absent, urgent hospital attention is needed. Temporary paralysis may result if there is pressure on nerves.

If a fracture sets badly, friction of the ulnar nerve on the back of the bones of the elbow may cause tingling in the forearm and in the fourth (ring) and fifth (little) fingers of the hand. Muscles in the hand may also become weak. If the symptoms are severe, surgical repositioning of the nerve to the front of the elbow is necessary.

Q: *What is a "pulled elbow"?*

A: The bones of the elbow or surrounding muscle fibres may join together, resulting in a stiffening of the joint. This condition is known medically as ANKYLOSIS. "Pulled elbow" may occur after infection or inflammation of the tissues surrounding the elbow joint. It is a difficult condition to treat. Mobility in the joint is often restored by heat therapy, exercise, and manipulation.

Q: *Why does an elbow become inflamed?*

A: Inflammation of the elbow is a form of BURSITIS, in which the fluid-filled sac (bursa) surrounding the joint becomes swollen. This may be the result of injury, or it may be a symptom of such conditions as gout or rheumatoid arthritis. "Students' elbow" (olecranon bursitis) is inflammation of the bursa at the elbow caused by constant rubbing on a flat surface such as a desk or table. If the bursa becomes infected, a doctor may prescribe antibiotic drugs.

See also TENNIS ELBOW.

Electric shock. For EMERGENCY treatment, *see* First Aid, p.538.

Electrocardiogram (ECG) is a record of the electric currents that occur in the heart muscle during every heartbeat. The electric currents are monitored by a highly sensitive machine known as an electrocardiograph.

Q: *How is an electrocardiogram obtained?*

A: Electrodes (metal strips) are attached to the skin on the patient's wrists and legs, and a fifth electrode can be placed on the chest over the heart. A combination of different impulses picked up by the electrodes produces the electrocardiogram.

Q: *What is the purpose of an electrocardiogram?*

A: A study of the recording assists a doctor in the diagnosis of heart disorders. *See* HEART ATTACK; HEART DISEASE.

Electroconvulsive therapy (ECT), sometimes called shock therapy or electroshock therapy (EST), is the passage of an electric current through the brain to induce alterations in the brain's electrical activity. It is used in treating certain mental disorders, such as depression or schizophrenia, but ECT is increasingly being replaced by drug therapy.

Electroencephalogram (EEG) is a record of the electric currents that occur in the brain. It takes the form of an irregular line traced on a moving strip of paper. The instrument that monitors the brain's electrical activity is known as an electroencephalograph.

Q: *How is an electroencephalogram obtained?*

A: Electrodes are attached to the patient's scalp, and the difference in electrical potential between two sites on the skull is monitored. Changes in the usual brain rhythms are recorded during rest, sleep, and during mental concentration. It is a painless procedure.

Q: *What is the purpose of an electroencephalogram?*

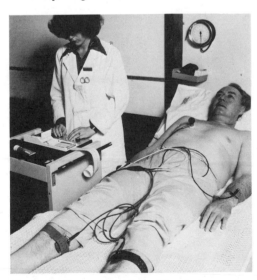

Electrocardiogram is obtained by placing electrodes on the outside of the body.

Electrolysis

A: The test assists doctors in the diagnosis of epilepsy and in the identification of sites of tumours or lesions in the brain. An EEG is also used in the definition of clinical death when a patient has been kept alive by artificial means. When no electrical activity is recorded, brain death is said to have occurred.

Electrolysis, in medicine, is the decomposition of certain body tissue by the passage of an electric current through it. It is possible to destroy hair follicles by this method, and electrolysis is often used to remove unwanted hair.

See also DEPILATORY.

Electrolyte, in medicine, is a term used to describe many varieties of salt solution that may be administered intravenously.

Electromyogram (EMG) is a record of the electrical impulses produced by the muscles. A doctor uses an electromyogram in the diagnosis of muscle or nerve disorders.

Elephantiasis is a condition characterized by gross swelling of the skin and underlying tissues. Arms, legs, and feet are most commonly affected. In males, the genitals may also be affected; in females, the breasts. The first symptoms are attacks of dermatitis, before the affected part begins to swell, accompanied by fever; the skin surface may become ulcerated and discoloured.

Q: *What causes elephantiasis?*

A: Elephantiasis, which occurs most commonly in tropical countries, is caused by an infestation of the lymph channels by the filarial worm *Wuchereria bancrofti*. The worm enters the body through the bite of an infected mosquito (*see* FILARIASIS).

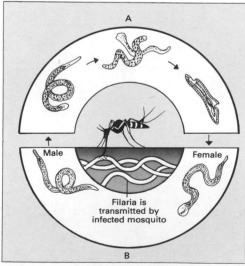

Elephantiasis is caused by worms from a mosquito (A), which infest humans (B).

Eventually, the lymph vessels that normally drain fluid away from tissues become obstructed, and swollen.

Q: *Is there any treatment for elephantiasis?*

A: Drugs poisonous to the filarial worm are available, but may have uncomfortable side effects. Treatment for swelling of the lymph vessels (lymphoedema) depends on severity.

Mild cases of elephantiasis in the legs may require only rest with the legs raised, an elastic stocking, and scrupulous foot care to prevent further infections. But elephantiasis of other parts of the body may require surgery.

Emaciation is the state of being extremely thin, as can happen after prolonged starvation, or physical or mental illness. When the body's store of energy-giving carbohydrate becomes depleted, fat under the skin and elsewhere is used for energy. Once the store of fat is exhausted, the body uses protein from the muscles. The nervous system and the heart are never used for energy, but the rest of the body can lose up to half its weight before death occurs, usually from infection due to lowered resistance.

Embolism is a blockage of an artery, or less commonly a vein, by material that has been brought to it in the bloodstream. The material is called an embolus, and may be a blood clot (thrombus); a clump of cancer cells; infected tissue from an abscess; or air bubbles that have entered the circulation. Occasionally, a small piece of calcified lining of an artery breaks free.

If an embolus starts in a vein, it will be carried in the venous circulation through the heart and into the lung, producing a pulmonary embolus. If the embolus starts in the heart, it may pass to any part of the body, including the brain (where it causes a stroke), the leg (where it may cause gangrene), or the kidney, where it produces kidney infarction and haematuria.

Q: *What are the symptoms of embolism?*

A: If an embolus is small there are often no symptoms. A larger embolus will usually cause death of the tissue supplied by the artery, causing a stroke or gangrene of the intestine, the leg, or even the kidney.

An embolus in the lung (pulmonary embolism) may produce few or no symptoms if it is small, but a large one may cause death or symptoms similar to those of coronary thrombosis with severe chest pain, shock, and collapse followed by a cough with bloodstained sputum (haemoptysis).

Q: *What is the treatment for embolism?*

A: Recurrent small emboli are difficult to diagnose, and may require special investigations and tests. A large pulmonary embolism requires immediate admission to hospital for treatment with oxygen. Rarely, an embolectomy, an operation to remove the clot from a leg or lung, can be performed.

A patient in whom an embolism has occurred is usually given blood thinning agents (anticoagulants) for some weeks.

Q: Can embolism be prevented?

A: The chances of an embolus forming can be reduced by the use of anticoagulants before an operation. All patients who are kept in bed for long periods of time must be encouraged to do breathing and leg exercises.

Embryo is an offspring from the moment of fertilization (conception) to the end of the third month of pregnancy.

See also PREGNANCY AND CHILDBIRTH.

Emetic is a substance that induces vomiting. Emetics are of two kinds. One type works by irritating the stomach, for example, common salt and ipecac (ipecacuanha). The other type stimulates a reflex centre in the brain, for example, the drug apomorphine.

EMG. *See* ELECTROMYOGRAM.

EMI scanner. *See* CAT SCANNER.

Emphysema is air in the body tissues. Pulmonary emphysema is a chronic lung disease in which the normal lung structure breaks down, allowing air into areas from which it is normally excluded. Surgical emphysema is air introduced into tissues as a result of injury or a surgical procedure. The air is gradually absorbed; usually, surgical emphysema requires no treatment, and no permanent damage is caused.

Q: What are the symptoms of pulmonary emphysema?

A: There is gradually increasing breathlessness during exercise, and the chest moves less easily than normal, producing a constricted feeling. There may also be frequent bouts of coughing, and production of sputum. The patient feels generally unwell.

Q: What causes pulmonary emphysema?

A: Emphysema is often seen at an advanced stage of chronic bronchitis. It is also associated with other factors such as smoking, asthma, and various respiratory and occupational diseases. Heavily polluted air aggravates lung disorders that lead to emphysema. Frequent coughing causes the alveoli to rupture and they join together to form larger sacs (*see* ALVEOLUS).This decreases the surface area of the lungs available for the exchange of the gases oxygen and carbon dioxide, and makes the lungs less elastic.

Q: How is pulmonary emphysema treated?

A: The only effective way of dealing with the condition is to treat the preceding disease before emphysema develops. If emphysema is already present, treatment is directed toward preventing further lung damage. Affected persons should stop smoking, make sure that all respiratory infections receive medical treatment immediately, and perform breathing exercises to clear any mucus from the lungs. People with severe emphysema may require oxygen before any physical exertion or sleep.

See also BRONCHITIS.

Empyema is the accumulation of pus in a body cavity, usually the pleural cavity between the lung and the chest wall. It generally occurs because of a secondary bacterial infection that accompanies a lung disorder, for example, pneumonia or pleurisy. Infection may also come from the outside, for example, as the result of a stab wound. The symptoms of empyema include fever and sweating, other serious illness, chest pain, and cough.

Q: How is empyema treated?

A: The pus must be removed. This can be done either by sucking it out through a hollow needle (aspiration), or by a surgical operation to remove part of a rib and drain the pus away through a tube. Antibiotic drugs are prescribed to combat the infection, and the underlying cause is treated at the same time.

Enamel. *See* TEETH.

Encephalitis is inflammation of the brain. It

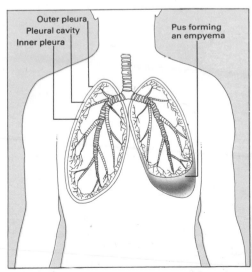

Empyema is a collection of pus in the cavity between the pleura and the lung tissue.

Encephalitis lethargica

is a serious disorder, usually caused by one of several viruses, but it can occasionally be caused by bacteria. Encephalitis viruses may be transmitted by various carriers such as ticks and mosquitoes. This form of the disease is more common in tropical countries. Rarely, encephalitis occurs as a complication of virus infections such as mumps, measles, cold sores (herpes simplex), shingles (herpes zoster), chickenpox, and some of the Coxsackie viruses. A smallpox or antirabies vaccination may lead to encephalitis.

Q: *What are the symptoms of encephalitis?*

A: Headache, high fever, vomiting, and stiffness of the neck are early symptoms. The patient's mental state varies from irritability and lethargy to confusion, delirium, convulsions, and coma in severe cases. The severity of the symptoms depends on the type of virus infection.

Q: *How is encephalitis treated?*

A: There is no specific treatment for encephalitis caused by a virus, but if the condition is traced to bacterial infection, antibiotic drugs are effective. Particular attention is paid to supportive care: an operation to make a hole in the windpipe (tracheotomy) may be performed if the patient has difficulty in breathing due to coma; fluids are given intravenously if the patient is unable to drink. If encephalitis is the result of a tumour or abscess in the brain, surgery is necessary to treat it.

Encephalitis lethargica is a particular form of brain inflammation. It is sometimes called sleeping sickness.

See also ENCEPHALITIS; PARKINSON'S DISEASE.

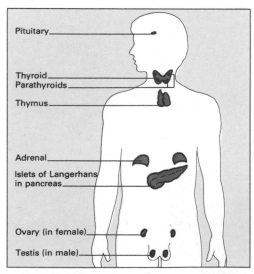

Endocrine glands secrete hormones directly into the bloodstream.

Encephalopathy is any irritation of the brain substance. It is similar to ENCEPHALITIS, but may be caused by poisons such as lead or other industrial chemicals.

Endemic refers to any disease that is always present in a region or population.

See also EPIDEMIC; PANDEMIC.

Endocarditis is inflammation of the endocardium, the inner lining membrane of the heart. The area most commonly affected is the lining of the heart valves, and sometimes the membrane lining the heart's chambers. The cause of the inflammation is usually microorganisms in the bloodstream that lodge in a deformed heart valve.

Q: *How does infection enter the bloodstream?*

A: The most common point of entry for bacteria is following minor surgery, or the extraction of an infected tooth. Bacteria may also be released into the bloodstream following a tonsillectomy, or via the womb of a woman shortly after delivery of a baby. People with a history of rheumatic or congenital heart disease should take antibiotic drugs several hours before visiting a dentist or before any surgical procedure, and the dentist or surgeon should be informed. A course of antibiotics may be prescribed afterward.

Q: *What are the symptoms of endocarditis?*

A: Symptoms begin gradually with fatigue, chills, and intermittent fever. If the condition is not diagnosed at this stage, increasing pallor due to progressive anaemia and loss of appetite follow. Small blood spots may appear on the skin and under the nails, caused by infected clots (emboli) that have broken away from the site of the heart infection.

Q: *How is endocarditis treated?*

A: If endocarditis is suspected, hospitalization is necessary, and treatment with large doses of antibiotics is continued for at least six weeks. Penicillin is the antibiotic most commonly used, until a more specific one is selected after tests. Bed rest is an essential part of treatment. The patient may be given a blood transfusion if anaemia is severe. Medical care should continue for several years.

Endocrine gland, also called a ductless gland, is a gland that produces chemicals (hormones) and secretes them directly into the blood for circulation to all parts of the body. Many endocrine glands do not act independently of each other: the balance of the body's hormones is maintained by a "feedback" system between the stimulus to produce a hormone and the ability of the hormone to regulate the strength of that stimulus.

Q: *What are the main endocrine glands?*

A: The main endocrine glands are: (1)
PITUITARY GLAND; (2) THYROID GLAND; (3)
PARATHYROID GLANDS; and (4) ADRENAL
GLANDS (adrenal cortex and adrenal
medulla).

These glands are purely endocrine. But
(5) the GONADS (ovaries and testes) also
have an endocrine function, producing
sex hormones. Similarly, (6) the PANCREAS
secretes insulin directly into the blood (an
endocrine function) and conveys digestive
juices along a duct to the duodenum.

See also HORMONE DISORDERS.

Endocrinology is the study of the endocrine
glands. *See* ENDOCRINE GLAND.

Endometriosis is the presence of fragments of
the lining of the womb (endometrium) in
other places, such as the muscle of the womb
or in the ovaries. The causes of this condition
are not known.

Q: *What are the symptoms of endometriosis?*

A: Often there are no definite symptoms and
the condition is found only during a
surgical operation for some other
disorder. When present, symptoms
include heavy periods, often more
frequent than usual, accompanied by pain
(dysmenorrhoea); pain during sexual
intercourse (dyspareunia); and sometimes
pain on defecation during a period.

The abnormally placed fragments of
endometrium pass through the same
monthly cycle as does the normal
endometrium: they swell before a period
and then bleed. Because there is no
outlet for the blood, cysts form. These
occasionally rupture, causing severe
abdominal pain. The symptoms disappear
during pregnancy, which may cure the
condition, and after the menopause.

Q: *How is endometriosis treated?*

A: In mild cases, painkilling drugs may
lessen the symptoms. Rarely, the fragments of endometrium can be found and
removed surgically. All of the symptoms
are relieved by artificially inducing
menopause by irradiation or surgical
removal of the ovaries, so that the womb
and the abnormal tissue cease to be
stimulated by ovarian hormones. The
hormone pills used for contraception may
also help, and these work without
sterilizing the patient. A woman with the
symptoms should consult a gynaecologist.

Endometritis is inflammation of the lining of
the womb (endometrium) caused by bacterial
infection, which may spread to the rest of the
womb and other tissues. The infection most
commonly follows an abortion (miscarriage)
or a full pregnancy; it may also follow

gonorrhoea, infection of the cervix, or some
gynaecological operations.

Q: *What are the symptoms of endometritis?*

A: The symptoms include fever, low
backache, abdominal pain, foul-smelling
vaginal discharge, and painful periods
(dysmenorrhoea).

Q: *How is endometritis treated?*

A: The usual treatment is with antibiotic
drugs to combat the infection.

Endometrium is the mucous membrane that
lines the inner surface of the womb. The
endometrium is under hormonal influence
and undergoes various changes during the
menstrual cycle. During the cycle the
endometrium becomes thicker and develops
a copious blood supply. If an egg is fertilized,
it implants in the endometrium, part of which
develops into the placenta. If fertilization
does not occur, the endometrium is shed each
month, causing the menstrual flow.

See also MENSTRUATION.

Endoscopy is the examination of the interior
of the body using a lighted and pliable
fibrous glass tube, usually with a system of
lenses. A surgeon can pass instruments down
a straight endoscope to take a small sample
of tissue for analysis (biopsy).

Endotracheal tube is a tube that is passed
down the throat and into the windpipe
(trachea). It is used to provide an airway and
to prevent the inhalation of foreign material
during a surgical procedure.

Enema is the introduction of a liquid into the
rectum and colon through the anus. Soap and
water is used to wash out constipated faeces;
oil to lubricate the large intestine. A barium

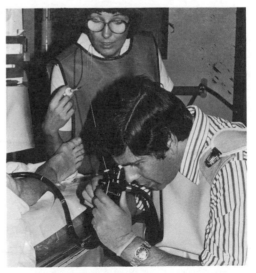

Endoscopy enables a doctor to examine the
internal organs without the need for surgery.

enema (a suspension of barium sulphate in water) is used in X-ray examinations to diagnose disorders of the large intestine such as diverticulitis, ulcerative colitis, and cancer.

Q: *Are there any dangers from the regular use of enemas?*

A: Constant home use of enemas as a treatment for chronic constipation is dangerous, because (1) the bowels' natural ability to expel faeces is weakened; and (2) there is a possibility that an underlying disorder of the intestine is masked. Enemas should be given only under medical guidance.

See also COLONIC IRRIGATION.

ENT is an abbreviation for ear, nose, and throat, the medical specialty called OTO-RHINOLARYNGOLOGY.

Entameba histolytica is a species of amoeba that infects the intestine of human beings. It is the cause of amoebic dysentery and amoebic abscess. *See* DYSENTERY.

Enteric fevers are intestinal infections of the typhoid and paratyphoid group. *See* PARA-TYPHOID; TYPHOID FEVER.

Enteritis is inflammation of the intestine, particularly the small intestine. If the stomach is also inflamed, the condition is known as GASTROENTERITIS; if the colon is involved, it is called COLITIS.

Enteritis may be due to infection by a virus or bacteria; food poisoning; or chemical irritation. Symptoms of the condition are diarrhoea, abdominal pain, and vomiting. Treatment is directed at the cause, and antispasmodic drugs may also be prescribed.

See also CROHN'S DISEASE.

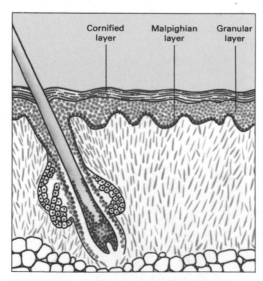

Cornified layer   Malpighian layer   Granular layer

Epidermis is continuously renewed with cells from the Malpighian layer.

Enterobiasis is infestation of the intestines by the parasitic worm *Enterobius vermicularis*. It is commonly known as the pinworm or threadworm. *See* WORMS.

Enterostomy is a surgical opening in the abdominal wall to form an artificial anus. The term is also used to describe an artificial opening between two parts of the intestine.

See also COLOSTOMY; ILEOSTOMY.

Entropion is the turning inward of an edge or margin. It occurs most commonly on the edge of the lower eyelid following infection or as a condition of old age. An entropion can be treated by a special method of cautery or by plastic surgery.

See also ECTROPION.

Enuresis is involuntary urination. Nocturnal enuresis, or BED-WETTING, is common in children.

See also INCONTINENCE.

Enzymes are chemical substances, produced by living cells, that act as catalysts and speed up the rates of chemical changes in other substances. All enzymes are complicated proteins.

Q: *What kinds of enzymes are there?*

A: Enzymes that bring about the breakdown of complex substances into simpler compounds are found particularly in the digestive juices. Sucrase is one of the enzymes responsible for the digestion of carbohydrates: ordinary table sugar, sucrose, is broken down into smaller compounds (fructose and glucose), which the body can digest. Other digestive enzymes break down proteins into amino acids, and fats into fatty acids.

Some enzymes have an assimilating action on body substances. Carbonic anhydrase, an enzyme in red blood cells, converts the gaseous waste product carbon dioxide into soluble carbonic acid, which is then carried to the lungs dissolved in the blood.

Q: *Can deficiency of an enzyme cause disease?*

A: Yes. The absence of a particular enzyme is often inherited. The disorder known as PHENYLKETONURIA is caused by the absence of an enzyme that normally prevents the build-up of the amino acid phenylalamine by converting it to tyrosine.

Epidemic is an outbreak of an infectious disease or condition that afflicts many persons at the same time and in the same geographical area.

See also ENDEMIC; IMMUNIZATION; PANDEMIC; QUARANTINE.

Epidermis is the surface layer of the SKIN.

Epididymis is an oblong structure at the side

of the testicle (testis), consisting of a tightly coiled tube five and a half to six metres (eighteen to twenty feet) long. Connected with the epididymis are about twenty small tubes through which the sperm flow from the testis. The sperm gradually mature in the epididymis, before travelling along the spermatic cord to the seminal vesicles.

Epididymitis is inflammation of the EPIDIDYMIS. The inflammation causes the epididymis to become swollen and painful. The person may need to urinate more frequently, and urination may be painful. In some cases fever may occur.

The condition may be caused by the spread of the bladder infection cystitis or urethritis, or it may be a complication of gonorrhoea, prostate disorders, or tuberculosis. Epididymitis can be effectively treated with antibiotic drugs and bed rest with support for the scrotum. Painkilling drugs may be prescribed until the pain subsides.

Epidural anaesthetic is a local anaesthetic injected into the space in the dura mater of the meninges, the tough fibrous membrane that covers the spinal cord.

See also ANAESTHETICS.

Epiglottis is a leaf-shaped structure in the throat that lies in front of the base of the tongue and over the opening of the larynx and windpipe (trachea) that prevents food and liquids from passing into the trachea.

A talk about Epilepsy

Epilepsy (for EMERGENCY treatment, *see* First Aid p.528) is a symptom of brain dysfunction characterized by periodic, recurrent seizures. Seizures occur in various forms, ranging from brief periods of impaired awareness to severe convulsions with loss of consciousness. Some people with epilepsy experience an aura, a physical sensation such as a smell, at the beginning of a seizure.

Seizures used to be described as grand mal, petit mal, psychomotor, and focal. But the new International Seizure Classification groups and describes seizures according to the area of the brain involved. The two major classes are partial seizures, which involve only a portion of the brain, and generalized seizures, which involve all of the brain.

Q: What are partial seizures?

A: Partial seizures involve only a part of the brain. Therefore only a specific area of the body or a particular level of consciousness is affected. Partial seizures with simple symptoms (traditionally called focal seizures) produce brief twitching movements of specific muscle

groups, such as those controlling an arm or leg. If the area of the brain affected controls sight, hearing, or another of the senses, brief visual, auditory, or other hallucinations are experienced. The patient usually retains consciousness with simple partial seizures. Partial seizures with complex symptoms (traditionally called psychomotor seizures) involve impairment of consciousness and involuntary complicated acts. During a typical complex partial seizure, the individual appears to be conscious but is unresponsive, or inappropriately responsive, to his or her surroundings. The patient may perform purposeless activities, such as lip-smacking, picking at his or her clothing, or aimless wandering. This type of seizure may be brief, last for several hours, or progress to a generalized seizure.

Q: What are generalized seizures?

A: Generalized seizures affect all of the brain. The two most common forms are absence seizures (traditionally called petit mal), and tonic-clonic seizures (traditionally called grand mal). Absence seizures consist of brief lapses of consciousness lasting usually five to thirty seconds. The person may stare blankly and appear to be daydreaming or experience slight movements of the facial muscles, head, or arms. When the seizure ends, the person resumes his or her previous activity and has no awareness of the seizure. Absence seizures commonly begin in childhood and may be as frequent as 50 to 100 a

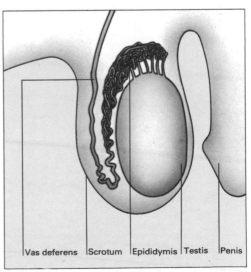

| Vas deferens | Scrotum | Epididymis | Testis | Penis |

Epididymis is a twisted tube about 6 metres (20 ft) long leading from testis to vas deferens.

Epilepsy

day or may occur only a few times a month.

Generalized tonic-clonic seizures are what most people think of as epilepsy. The seizure begins with a sudden loss of consciousness. The patient falls and the muscles become rigid (the tonic phase). The patient may also give a sharp cry, which is caused by the sudden contraction of the abdominal muscles forcing air from the lungs through the larynx. Because there is a brief cessation of breathing, the skin may turn blue. The clonic phase then follows, consisting of jerking contractual movements of the major muscle groups. Breathing resumes but is heavy and irregular, causing frothing of saliva. The patient may bite his or her tongue or lose bladder control. Following the seizure, the patient may have a headache, be confused, and want to sleep. Generalized tonic-clonic seizures usually last from three to five minutes.

Q: What are some of the rarer forms of epilepsy?

A: Rare forms of epilepsy include Jacksonian seizures in which motor activity begins in the distant part of a limb, such as a toe or thumb, and "marches" or progresses up the limb to involve major portions of the whole body. Autonomic seizures are partial seizures involving the part of the brain that controls the autonomic nervous system. Seizure activity includes headaches, stomachaches, nausea, vomiting, fever, or similar symptoms that recur without apparent cause. In

atonic seizures, the patient experiences a loss of muscle tone and falls with no convulsive activity. In myoclonic seizures, the individual experiences brief muscle jerks, sometimes violent enough to throw him or her to the ground. In unilateral seizures, only one hemisphere, or half, of the brain is involved and consequently seizure activity is limited to one side of the body.

Q: What are the causes of epilepsy?

A: Seizures are caused by the uncontrolled discharge of electrical energy by brain cells. An electroencephalograph (EEG) is used to record the electrical activity of the brain to help in the diagnosis of epilepsy. In about half of epilepsy patients, no cause can be found for the uncontrolled electrical activity, and in these patients, epilepsy is termed idiopathic. For the remaining 50 per cent, an underlying cause can be identified and the epilepsy is called symptomatic.

Anyone can experience an injury to the brain or central nervous system which can result in epilepsy. Some of the more common causes are antenatal damage, injury during birth, brain tumours, head injury, cerebrovascular disease, and serious infections during childhood.

Q: Can epilepsy be an inherited condition?

A: A number of genetic disorders, usually rare, include recurrent seizures among their symptoms. In such cases, it is the genetic disorder and not a tendency toward seizures which is inherited.

In a low percentage of cases, an abnormal EEG pattern may be inherited. Such a condition may increase the chances that epilepsy may develop.

Q: Does epilepsy develop only in childhood?

A: No. Epilepsy may develop at any age, but because most cases are diagnosed in patients younger than aged eighteen, epilepsy is often mistakenly regarded as a childhood condition. People over the age of 55, because of the increased incidence of cerebrovascular disease, are the second most susceptible age group. Because epilepsy is not cured, but controlled by currently available treatment, it is usually a lifelong disorder.

Q: Are there other disorders with symptoms similar to epilepsy?

A: Yes. Breath-holding spells in children may resemble convulsive seizures. Fainting in adults may be mistaken for epilepsy. Heart disease causing rapid changes in the pulse rate may cause symptoms similar to those of epilepsy. High fever in young children can cause

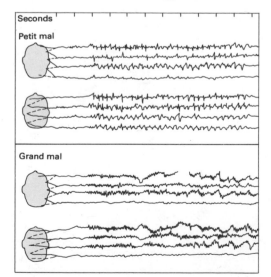

Epilepsy produces changes in the brain patterns picked up by electrodes on the head.

convulsions called febrile seizures. In otherwise normal children, febrile seizures do not usually have any serious consequences, but a doctor should be consulted. In children with a family history of epilepsy or other neurological disorders, an increased chance of developing epilepsy may be present and preventive treatment may be necessary.

Q: *How is epilepsy treated?*

A: There are a number of anticonvulsant or antiepileptic drugs approved for use. Not all are effective for every type of seizure. A doctor will begin by prescribing a single drug and increase the dosage until seizures are controlled. If side effects appear, the dosage will be reduced until a balance between a minimum of side effects and a maximum of satisfactory control is achieved. If a single drug is not satisfactory, a second drug is usually added.

A large percentage of epileptic patients experience several different types of seizures. Sometimes the type of seizure experienced by a person may change as he or she grows older. Epileptic patients should be regularly checked by their doctors.

Because the patient's body chemistry causes him or her to absorb anticonvulsant drugs in an individual way, the doctor periodically takes blood samples to determine the level of drug present in the patient's system. Blood level monitoring allows the doctor to accurately adjust the drug dosage to each patient to achieve maximum seizure control with a minimum of drug side effects. Some of the most commonly used antiepileptic drugs are phenobarbitone and phenytoin for generalized tonic-clonic seizures; paramethodione, valproic acid, or ethosuximide for absence seizures; and primidone or carbamazepine for complex partial seizures.

Surgery may be used to treat epilepsy when the cause can be traced to such things as a scar on the brain or a tumour. But even in these cases, drug treatment will be used unless it can be determined that the scar or tumour is located where it can be safely treated surgically.

Other forms of treatment are currently being assessed. Biofeedback can teach some patients to control the brain's electrical activity. This may in the future help patients to prevent seizures. Another experimental technique involves the permanent implanting of electrodes in an epileptic patient's brain.

These electrodes can be periodically activated. The hope is that this periodic electrical activity will help to stabilize the brain's uncontrolled electrical activity and thus prevent seizures. However, it must be emphasized that both techniques are only experimental and will require more research before they can be evaluated.

Q: *What complications can result from seizures?*

A: Sometimes one seizure will immediately follow another and result in continuous seizure activity. This condition (called status epilepticus) can be life-threatening in the case of generalized tonic-clonic seizures and requires emergency medical treatment to prevent cardiac arrest or respiratory failure.

In generalized tonic-clonic, myoclonic, and atonic seizures, the person may injure himself or herself by falling against hard or sharp objects. In other seizure forms, such as absence or complex partial seizures, status epilepticus results in prolonged periods of impaired consciousness which prevent the person from behaving normally.

Untreated seizures prevent the patient from carrying out a normal life. With current treatment, more than 50 per cent of persons with epilepsy can achieve complete seizure control and lead a normal life. Another 30 per cent can achieve partial control over their seizures and engage in most activities.

Q: *Is epilepsy a permanent condition?*

A: In most cases, epilepsy is chronic.

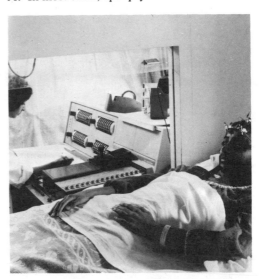

Electroencephalograph: brainwave recordings are made with complex electronic machinery.

Episiotomy

However, with consistent treatment, seizures may decrease in frequency after a number of years, and drugs can be gradually reduced or withdrawn. Doctors will usually begin reduction if a patient remains seizure-free for several years, but seizures often recur. A patient should never reduce medication without the advice of a doctor. Abrupt withdrawal of antiepileptic drugs may result in an increase in the number and severity of seizures. Such withdrawal has also been known to trigger incidents of status epilepticus.

Q: What precautions should a person with epilepsy take?

A: People with epilepsy whose seizures are controlled can lead normal lives. However, they should be aware that excessive use of alcohol, poor eating habits, and lack of rest may precipitate seizures. Most countries permit a person with epilepsy to drive if he or she has been seizure-free for a specific period. The person whose seizures are less well controlled or are triggered by a specific stimulus should limit activities accordingly so as not to endanger himself or herself. The epileptic patient should always take his or her drugs exactly as prescribed and report any changes in seizure activity or drug side effects to a doctor so that dosage can be adjusted.

Q: Should a woman with epilepsy consider bearing a child?

A: A woman with epilepsy should consult a doctor before becoming pregnant.

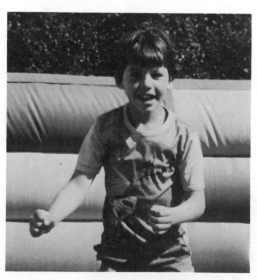

Epilepsy can be medically controlled and need not stop a child from enjoying life.

Pregnancy has been known to increase both the number and severity of seizures. Further, some anticonvulsant drugs have been shown to have a relationship to an increase in the incidence of certain birth defects, primarily cleft palate.

Episiotomy is a cut that is made into the edge of the birth canal, at the ending of the second stage of labour. It may be made to prevent tearing or to help the delivery. *See* PREGNANCY AND CHILDBIRTH.

Epithelium is the layer of cells that covers the internal and external surfaces of the body: for example, the skin, trachea, bladder, intestines and blood vessels. Hair, tooth enamel and the nails are a modified form of epithelium. General functions of epithelium are protection, secretion and absorption; there are also specialized functions such as sensory reception and the moving of substances through ducts in the body.

Epsom salts. *See* MAGNESIUM SULPHATE.

Epulis is any swelling or growth on the gums caused by infection or irritation. *See* GINGIVITIS; GUMBOIL.

Erection, in males from puberty onwards, is a state of enlargement and stiffness of the penis that results from sexual stimulation, physical or mental. Blood flowing into the penis is prevented from flowing out again by the contraction of special muscles around the veins. The spongy tissue of the penis swells and causes the penis to become erect, a prerequisite for sexual intercourse. Failure to produce an erection is one type of IMPOTENCE; it may be caused by damage to the penis, damage to the nerves that supply the veins, the use of certain drugs, or by psychological factors.

Ergosterol is a steroid substance that is now obtained mainly from yeast, but was originally obtained from ERGOT. Ergosterol is exposed to ultraviolet rays to yield vitamin D_2, which is sometimes used in the treatment of rickets. *See* RICKETS.

Ergot is a fungus (*Claviceps purpurea*) that grows as a parasite on rye. It is extremely poisonous, but its alkaloid chemicals are the source of many drugs.

Ergot poisoning can occur by eating rye bread made from contaminated grain or by taking an overdose of an ergot drug. The poison causes blood vessels to contract. This gives rise to symptoms such as vomiting, diarrhoea, tingling in the limbs, and, occasionally, convulsions. The victim needs emergency medical attention. If the patient survives, cataracts and gangrene may develop as secondary complications.

Two of the many drugs derived from ergot are ergometrine and ergotamine. Ergometrine causes the womb to contract, and may be prescribed after childbirth to stop bleeding. Ergotamine acts on the blood vessels in the head, and is used to treat migraine.

See also ERGOSTEROL.

Erosion is the breaking down of the body tissues. *See* CERVICAL EROSION.

Erysipelas is an acute, streptococcal skin infection. It tends to spread rapidly causing inflammation, fever, nausea, vomiting, and, occasionally, red lines stretching along the limbs. Erysipelas is treated with penicillin and sulphonamide drugs. A doctor should be consulted if erysipelas is suspected.

Erysipeloid is an unusual bacterial skin infection resembling erysipelas. Erysipeloid produces red swellings on the skin, with tingling and itching. It is usually confined to the hands and seldom makes the patient ill. The symptoms last for several days before spontaneous recovery occurs, leaving a brown stain on the skin. Erysipeloid is generally acquired by handling fish or meat products, and it is more common in the summer. Although no treatment is necessary, antibiotics can shorten the time taken for recovery.

Erythema nodosum is a condition in which red, oval nodules appear on the skin. Over a period of several weeks, the nodules change from red to a brown colour. Erythema nodosum often occurs on the shins and may be accompanied by fever, aches, and fatigue. It usually follows a streptococcal throat infection. In children, the condition can be associated with rheumatic fever. In adults, it may occur with sarcoidosis, tuberculosis, or ulcerative colitis. Certain drugs, such as the sulphonamides, may also produce erythema nodosum.

The treatment consists of bed rest and aspirin until the condition improves. If the cause of the condition is a streptococcal infection, penicillin is prescribed.

Erythroedema. *See* PINK DISEASE.

Erythroblastosis foetalis. *See* HAEMOLYTIC DISEASE OF THE NEWBORN.

Erythrocyte. *See* RED BLOOD CELL.

ESR is an abbreviation of erythrocyte sedimentation rate, the rate at which red blood cells settle when an anticoagulant is added to them. *See* SEDIMENTATION RATE.

Ether is the general name for a class of organic chemical compounds derived from alcohols. Ether is used as a cleansing agent, and was once widely used as an anaesthetic (*see* ANAESTHETICS).

Eugenics is the science that deals with physical and mental improvement by means of genetic control. It was founded in the nineteenth century by the British scientist Francis Galton, whose main proposition was the improvement in inherited characteristics through the careful selection of parents.

Although at one time the subject of a social movement, eugenics was discredited early in the twentieth century because of its association with racist views.

See also GENETIC COUNSELLING.

Eunuch is a male who has had both testicles removed. The resulting absence of the male sex hormones produces certain symptoms: weight gain, especially around the hips; loss of facial hair; and sometimes slight development of breasts.

If castration occurs before puberty, the voice remains unbroken. Adult men who have had their testicles removed, possibly because of disease or injury, retain their adult voice. They may also be given regular injections of male hormones so that other masculine characteristics are preserved.

Euphoria is a feeling of elation and wellbeing. In psychiatry, it may be one of the symptoms of the manic phase of manic-depressive illness, since it may have no obvious cause. Certain drugs, such as heroin and cocaine, can also produce a temporary feeling of euphoria.

Eustachian tube is the narrow tube about 4cm (1.5 inches) long that connects the back of the nasal passages with the cavity of the middle ear. The Eustachian tube has two functions: it allows the natural secretions from the ear to drain into the throat; and it equalizes the pressures on each side of the eardrum. During swallowing, the lower end

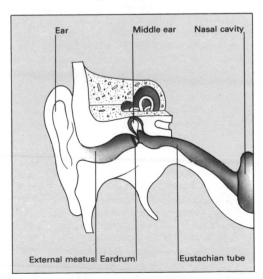

Eustachian tube connects with the nasal cavity and equalizes air pressure in the middle ear.

Exanthem

of the Eustachian tube closes momentarily. Blockage of the Eustachian tube, with mucus or infection (otitis media), can lead to temporary deafness. If the tube is blocked and sudden pressure changes occur, as may happen during flying or diving, there may be pain and the eardrum may rupture (see BAROTRAUMA).

See also EAR; EARACHE.

Euthanasia is the act of painlessly terminating a patient's life in order to relieve suffering from pain or an incurable illness. The term does not refer to the practice of deliberately withholding drugs or other treatment that might prolong a patient's life. The legal issues involved in euthanasia have not been clarified; suicide is not a criminal offence in the U.K., but aiding a person to take his or her own life still is.

Exanthem. *See* RASH.

Exhaustion is a state of extreme fatigue, often accompanied by a reduced ability to respond to external stimuli.

See also FATIGUE; HEATSTROKE.

Exophthalmos is abnormal protrusion of the eyeballs. It is usually a symptom of HYPERTHYROIDISM, but may have other causes, such as a tumour behind the eye. A doctor should be consulted so that the underlying cause can be treated.

Expectorant is a substance that helps the loosening and the discharge of phlegm.

Exploratory operation is a surgical procedure that is performed to aid the precise diagnosis of a disorder; when the urgency is such that there is no time for conventional diagnostic testing; or when conventional diagnostic methods have failed to reveal a disorder.

Exposure is a debilitated body state that results from being subjected to extremes of hot, cold, or windy weather without adequate protection. Lack of treatment may lead to loss of consciousness and further complications. Prolonged exposure may lead to death.

Exposure to extreme heat can lead to the gradual or sudden onset of HEATSTROKE. Headache, weakness, and nausea may occur in the early stages. The body ceases to sweat, the skin becomes hot and dry, and the body temperature rises rapidly. Finally, there may be mental confusion, shock, and convulsions, which can lead to coma and sometimes death. *See* First Aid, p.567.

Exposure to extreme cold, especially in wet and windy weather conditions, can lead to HYPOTHERMIA. The onset is gradual, with symptoms of mental confusion and poor physical coordination. The body's ability to produce heat by shivering is reduced, and its temperature drops. In severe cases, hypothermia can lead to unconsciousness,

coma, and death. *See* First Aid, p.558.

Extradural haematoma is bleeding between the dura mater (the tough fibrous membrane that covers the brain) and the skull. The blood comes from a ruptured artery that supplies the internal surface of the skull. Extradural haematoma usually follows a head injury involving a skull fracture.

Q: What are the symptoms of an extradural haematoma?

A: The first sign may be a temporary loss of consciousness, followed by a period of apparently normal behaviour. Other symptoms may begin hours or sometimes days after the injury. The patient's speech becomes slurred, and he or she walks unsteadily. The patient may suffer a headache, followed by unconsciousness caused by the pressure of the clotted blood on the brain.

Q: How is an extradural haematoma treated?

A: The patient needs urgent hospitalization. Special X-rays are taken to diagnose the condition. A surgeon then performs an operation to remove the clot.

Extrasystole is a disturbance of the natural rhythm of the heart. An extra heartbeat occurs, as a premature and weak beat. When the next heartbeat is due, the heart muscle is still recovering from the extrasystole and may not respond: the heart may miss a beat.

The sensation of a missed beat is usually felt in the chest, or throat, and may cause anxiety, but in an otherwise normal heart extrasystoles are no cause for alarm. They are common in many healthy persons while resting, especially in those who smoke or who drink a lot of coffee. If the extrasystoles disappear on taking exercise, they can safely be ignored. But if extrasystoles continue after exercise or occur with some regularity, a doctor should be consulted.

Extrauterine pregnancy is another name for ectopic pregnancy. *See* ECTOPIC PREGNANCY.

Extravasation is the escape of a body fluid from its normal containing vessel into the surrounding tissue.

Extrovert is a psychological term that describes a person whose interests centre on external objects and actions.

See also INTROVERT.

Exudate is a fluid that penetrates the walls of blood vessels and seeps into adjoining tissues. The process happens as a body defence mechanism associated with inflammation caused by infection: blood vessels dilate and become more permeable, so allowing a fluid rich in serum protein containing antibodies and white blood cells to escape. Pus and nasal mucus are also termed exudates.

See also TRANSUDATE.

A talk about the Eye

Eye is the organ of sight. It is an almost perfect sphere about 2.5cm (one inch) in diameter. The eye is filled with jelly-like fluid (*see* HUMOUR) that helps to maintain its shape. The front of the eye is covered with the CONJUNCTIVA. The eye muscles are between the orbit and the SCLERA.

The eye's outer surface is covered with the sclera, except for a transparent area in the front, the CORNEA. Lining the sclera is the CHOROID. The front edge of the choroid is called the ciliary body. The IRIS is the coloured disc in front of the LENS. The RETINA is a layer of millions of light-sensitive nerve cells that overlies the choroid. There are two types of nerve cells in the retina: rods and cones. The individual nerve fibres from these cells join to form the optic nerve.

Q: How is the amount of light entering the eye controlled?

A: This is controlled by the iris, which contains circular muscles and radial muscles. When the circular muscles contract, the pupil gets smaller. When the radial muscles contract, the pupil gets larger. These muscles are controlled by the AUTONOMIC NERVOUS SYSTEM.

Q: How is light focused on the retina?

A: Light is focused by the cornea and the lens. The cornea is the major focusing component; the lens performs fine focusing. The lens can change its shape so that near and far objects can be focused; this is called ACCOMMODATION.

Q: What happens when light hits the retina?

A: Light is focused mainly on one area of the retina called the MACULA. In the centre of the macula is the FOVEA, the region that gives the greatest visual acuity. Visual acuity depends upon the number and density of the rods and cones, since each cell can record only the presence of light and, in cones, its colour. There are about ten million cones and one hundred million rods in each eye.

When light falls on a rod or cone, the cell sends impulses along the optic nerve to the brain, which interprets them into a representation of the image.

Q: How do cones detect colour?

A: The mechanism of colour vision is not fully understood, but some specialists claim that there are three types of cone cell. Each type of cone cell is sensitive to either red, green, or blue light. These colours stimulate particular cone cells so that colour is perceived.

Eye disorders. The following table lists some of the disorders that affect the eye and the basic characteristics of each condition. Sometimes an eye disorder is symptomatic of some other disorder (for example, diabetes, nephritis, or stroke). Each disorder has a separate article in the A-Z section of this book. For eye injuries, *see* First Aid, p.552.

See also BLINDNESS.

Disorder	Basic characteristics
ADENOMA (of pituitary gland)	Loss of vision due to pressure on optic nerve by a tumour
AMAUROSIS	Progressive loss of sight, leading to blindness
AMBLYOPIA	Dimness of vision
APHAKIA	Absence of the lens of the eye, causing blurred vision
ASTIGMATISM	Distorted and blurred vision
BLEPHARITIS	Inflammation of the eyelid
CATARACT	Blurred vision and loss of sight
CHALAZION	Lump on the eyelid
COLOBOMA	Cleft in the iris, the choroid, or other part of the eye
COLOUR BLINDNESS	Inability to identify one or more primary colours
DACRYOCYSTITIS	Inflammation of tear duct
DETACHED RETINA	Flashes of light, followed later by sensation of curtain drawn over the eye

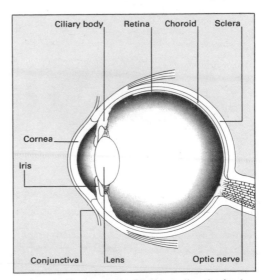

Eye is the organ of sight that supplies the body with thirty per cent of sensory perception.

Eyeglasses

Disorder	Basic characteristics
DIABETES	Dimness of vision, loss of sight
ECTROPION	Inside of eyelid is turned outwards
ENTROPION	Edge of eyelid is turned inwards
EXOPHTHALMOS	Bulging eye or eyes
GLAUCOMA	Increased pressure within eye, resulting in gradual loss of vision
GLIOMA (optic)	Tumour of optic nerve, with loss of vision
HEMIANOPIA	Defective vision or blindness in half the visual field
HYPERTENSION	Degeneration of retina as result of high blood pressure
IRITIS	Inflammation of iris
KERATITIS	Inflammation of cornea
LONGSIGHTEDNESS	Hyperopia, diminished ability to see things at close range
MIGRAINE	Blurred vision and flashes of light followed by intense headache
NEPHRITIS (chronic)	Degeneration of retina as result of kidney disease
NIGHT BLINDNESS	Absence of or defective vision in the dark
OPTHTHALMIA	Inflammation of the eye or the conjunctiva
PAPILLOEDEMA	Swelling of the optic nerve where it enters the back of the eye

Disorder	Basic characteristics
PRESBYOPIA	Longsightedness, due to ageing
RETINITIS	Inflammation of retina
RETINITIS PIGMENTOSA	Degeneration of retina; may lead to blindness
RETROBULBAR NEURITIS	Inflammation of optic nerve and sudden blindness
SCOTOMA	A blind or partly blind area in the visual field, surrounded by area of normal vision
SHORTSIGHTEDNESS	Myopia, objects can be seen distinctly only when close to eyes
STROKE	Blind spots, actual blindness, or temporary loss of vision due to interruption of blood supply to the brain
STYE	Infection of one or more of the small glands of the eyelid
TAY-SACHS DISEASE	Impairment of sight, resulting in blindness

Eyeglasses. *See* SPECTACLES.

Eyelid is one of two movable folds of skin that protect the front of each eyeball. When closed, the eyelids cover the visible area of the eye. The upper lid is larger and capable of more movement than is the lower one. It contains a fibrous plate of tissue that gives additional protection to the eyeball. Each eyelid has on its undersurface a mucous membrane, called the conjunctiva. The conjunctiva is lubricated by tears produced by the lacrimal apparatus.

Q: Which disorders affect the eyelids?

A: Eyelid disorders include BLACK EYE, BLEPHARITIS, CHALAZION, CONJUNCTIVITIS, ECTROPION, ENTROPION, PTOSIS, and STYE. The eyelids are also susceptible to general skin disorders such as ECZEMA and RODENT ULCER.

    See also EPICANTHUS; EYE.

F

Face-lift. *See* COSMETIC SURGERY.

Face presentation describes a baby emerging face first from the vagina. *See* PREGNANCY AND CHILDBIRTH.

Facial paralysis is weakness of the muscles of the face, caused by damage to, or infection of, the nerve that supplies them.

    See also BELL'S PALSY.

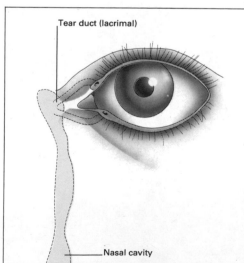

Tear duct (lacrimal)

Nasal cavity

Dacryocystitis is inflammation of the lacrimal duct and sac, causing swelling.

Faecal analysis is the medical examination of a patient's faeces to aid in the diagnosis of various disorders. *See* FAECES.

Faeces are the waste or end products of digestion that accumulate in the bowel (large intestine) and are expelled through the anus during defecation. The expelled product is commonly called a stool or a bowel movement. Faeces are composed of: undigested or indigestible food, especially vegetable fibre such as cellulose; water; mucus and other secretions from the glands that supply the intestinal tract; bacteria; enzymes that have assisted digestion; inorganic salts; and, occasionally, foreign substances.

Q: What is the normal appearance of faeces?

A: Faeces are normally brown or dark brown in colour, soft, and firm. Bile pigments give faeces their characteristic colour. The typical odour is caused by nitrogen compounds that are produced by the action of bacteria. Medical examination of the faeces for abnormalities is important in the diagnosis of disorders of the intestinal tract.

Q: What disorders affect the colour of faeces?

A: Black faeces may result from taking drugs, such as iron tablets, or drinking red wine. The presence of blood in the faeces may make them either black or bright red in colour. This can occur because of infection; ulceration of the intestines; diverticular disease; malignant or non-malignant tumours; abrasive foreign bodies; or haemorrhoids. Pale yellow or white faeces suggest a disorder of bile production, usually an obstruction of the bile ducts. In children, greenish faeces indicate that food has passed quickly through the digestive tract.

Q: What disorders affect the consistency of faeces?

A: Hard, nodular faeces are associated with constipation, which may be a symptom of some other disorder. Diarrhoea produces excessively watery faeces. Faeces that are flat and ribbon-like may be caused by spasm or an obstruction in the rectum. With jaundice, the faeces may be pale.

Q: What disorders can be revealed by an analysis of faeces?

A: Worms are detected by inspecting the patient's faeces. Chemical and microscopic analysis of a stool may show up abnormal amounts of fats, proteins, or sugars, which may indicate a disorder of digestion or malabsorption of food.

Fahrenheit is a temperature scale on which the freezing point of water is 32° and the boiling point of water is 212°.

See also CENTIGRADE.

Fainting, or syncope, is a momentary loss of consciousness. It is caused by a temporary deficiency in the blood supply to the brain, usually following a sudden drop in blood pressure. *See* First Aid, p.544.

Fallopian tube (oviduct) is a muscular tube that extends from the womb (uterus) to an ovary. It is about 10cm (four inches) long. There are two fallopian tubes, one for each ovary.

After ovulation, the egg (ovum) passes from an ovary along the fallopian tube to the womb. Finger-like tissue at the end of the tube nearest the ovary helps to direct the egg into the tube, and hair-like cells inside the tube propel the egg along it. Sperm swim up the tube from the womb and meet the egg. If the egg becomes fertilized, fertilization usually takes place while the egg is in the fallopian tube. If for any reason the fertilized egg then moves too slowly, it may implant in the fallopian tube instead of in the lining of the womb, resulting in an ectopic pregnancy. *See* ECTOPIC PREGNANCY.

See also PREGNANCY AND CHILDBIRTH.

Q: Can a disorder of the fallopian tubes cause sterility?

A: Yes. After inflammation (salpingitis), any scar that remains may block the tube, or damage the finger-like tissue at its opening, or damage the hair-like cells. If the inflammation and scarring occur in both tubes, the woman is in danger of being unable to conceive. (*See* SALPINGITIS.)

Q: Does artificial sterilization of a woman involve the fallopian tubes?

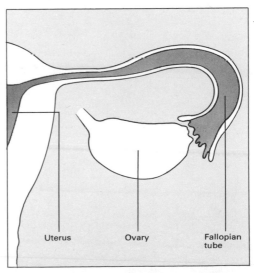

| Uterus | Ovary | Fallopian tube |

Fallopian tube extends from the ovary to the uterus and is lined with mucous membrane.

Fallot's tetralogy

A: Yes. The surgical cutting and tying of both fallopian tubes is the usual method of sterilization.

See also STERILIZATION.

Fallot's tetralogy is a congenital heart malformation that comprises four separate problems. These are: (1) a hole in the wall between the left and right ventricles; (2) narrowing of the artery that leads to the lungs (pulmonary artery); (3) blood reaching the aorta from the right ventricle as well as from the left ventricle; and (4) an increase in the thickness of the muscle of the right ventricle.

Q: What are the symptoms of Fallot's tetralogy?

A: The main symptom is a bluish tinge to the skin (cyanosis), caused by the presence in the arteries of blood that has not been properly oxygenated. Fainting sometimes occurs and a child with the disorder is often breathless.

Q: How is the condition treated?

A: Cardiac surgery during childhood may correct the condition.

False labour pains are abdominal pains that make a pregnant woman think that labour is beginning when in fact it is not. The womb contracts and relaxes slightly throughout pregnancy. A contraction may be strong enough to cause mild cramp-like pain.

See also PREGNANCY AND CHILDBIRTH.

False pregnancy (pseudocyesis) is a condition in which a patient shows most of the outward, physical signs and symptoms of pregnancy, but is not pregnant. Among these signs are an enlarged abdomen, absence of menstruation, morning sickness, and weight gain. False pregnancy is thought to have an emotional origin, which causes the pituitary gland to be affected in the same way as during a real pregnancy. It occurs in women with a strong desire to have a child or in those who are anxious not to conceive. The condition has also been reported in men.

Q: Is there any treatment for a false pregnancy?

A: Psychiatric help may be useful. When the patient is asleep or under hypnosis, the enlargement of the abdomen disappears.

False teeth. *See* DENTURES.

Family planning is the control by couples of when they have children, and how many. It is achieved by practising some form of birth control and then stopping the practice when conception is desired. *See* CONTRACEPTION.

Farsightedness (hyperopia, or hypermetropia). *See* LONGSIGHTEDNESS.

Fascia is a sheet of tough fibrous tissue that covers, supports, and separates muscles, or unites skin with the tissues beneath it.

Fasting is deliberate abstinence from food over a period of time. It is a medical requirement for some X-ray examinations (for example, a barium meal test), blood tests (for example, a glucose tolerance test), and before a general anaesthetic.

Fasting is a requirement in some religious rites; it is also used as a means of political or social protest. Some people fast as a means of losing weight rapidly, but this method is not recommended.

Q: What happens to the body's metabolism during fasting?

A: In the absence of food, the body's energy requirements are supplied first by the body's sugar, then by reserves of fat. The "burning up" of fat is incomplete, resulting in mild KETOSIS, due to the production of by-products of fat metabolism.

Pangs of hunger occur during the first few days of a fast, but then become less noticeable.

Q: What precautions should be taken by a person who is fasting?

A: A person who intends to fast for more than two days should seek the advice of a doctor. Vitamin supplements are recommended. When a fast is broken, a normal diet should be resumed gradually, beginning with light, easily digested foods.

See also WEIGHT PROBLEMS.

Fat embolus is a globule of oil, fat, or bone marrow that obstructs an artery. Such an obstruction can occur after the fracture of a large bone or after some forms of orthopaedic surgery. *See* EMBOLISM.

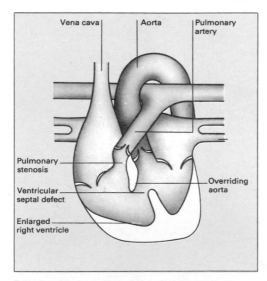

Fallot's tetralogy is a congenital heart disease that affects four sites in the heart.

Fatigue is a feeling of tiredness or weariness. Fatigue may be caused by many factors. Physical exertion, inadequate sleep, mental strain, boredom, or poor posture may all cause fatigue. Chronic (persistent) fatigue often occurs as a symptom of infection, deficient diet, anxiety depression, or an underlying disorder such as anaemia, diabetes, tuberculosis, or cancer.

Q: Does fatigue require medical treatment?

A: Persistent fatigue should be brought to the attention of a doctor. The cause of the condition may not be medical, in the true sense, at all, but even if the root of the problem is the patient's mental or physical over-exertion at work, proper investigation by a doctor is worth while.

Occasional fatigue is best treated by rest. A balanced diet is a good preventive for fatigue. "Pep pills", coffee, and other stimulants should be avoided: their effects are shortlived, and the feeling of fatigue may recur more strongly.

A talk about Fats

Fats are one of the three kinds of energy-giving foods in the diet. They are an extremely rich source of energy, with a calorie content of about 255 calories per ounce (9 calories per gram). This is twice as much as provided by the other foods (proteins and carbohydrates). The most common fat-containing foods are butter, cream, eggs, fat meats, margarine, oily fish, and vegetable oils. Fats are acted on by bile salts, which change them into soluble forms that can be absorbed from the intestines.

Q: What are the functions of fats in the body's metabolism?

A: Most fats are burned up (oxidized) to produce energy (in addition to carbon dioxide and water). Other fats become an essential part of cells. Fats that are not required immediately as a source of energy are stored in layers of fatty (adipose) tissue under the skin. They are available as fuel for energy at any time. The stored fats surround and protect internal organs such as the kidneys, and act as insulation that prevents heat loss. Fats also provide an environment in which vitamins A, D, E and K can be stored. Some fat is stored in the liver.

Q: What is the difference between saturated and unsaturated fats?

A: Saturated and unsaturated fats differ chemically in the way their carbon and hydrogen atoms are arranged. Basically, unsaturated fats can absorb hydrogen,

whereas saturated fats cannot. Most animal fats are saturated fats; saturated vegetable fats include coconut oil. Unsaturated fats include cottonseed oil, corn oil (polyunsaturated fats that may be constituents of margarine), and olive oil.

Q: What is the significance of this distinction?

A: Research suggests that large amounts of saturated fats in the diet may be associated with vascular disease (arteriosclerosis). Surveys have shown that countries with high living standards, such as the U.K., have a high incidence of arteriosclerosis. But whether or not this is directly caused by staple "rich man's food" such as meat, eggs, cream, and so on (the saturated fats) is still under investigation.

Q: Can fats be eliminated from the diet?

A: A fat-free diet must be extremely bulky to provide enough calories because proteins and carbohydrates are only half as rich in calories as fats. Dieticians usually advise that about thirty to forty per cent of a normal diet should consist of fats – preferably unsaturated.

Fatty degeneration is a disorder involving the accumulation of fat in cells, especially of the liver and the heart. It occurs because the cells are deprived of oxygen or certain foods that make the disposal of fat possible. Poor circulation, anaemia, or poisoning by alcohol or industrial chemicals, such as dry cleaning fluids, may cause fatty degeneration.

Favism is a form of acute haemolytic anaemia

Type of fat content in some foods	
Food	Type of fat
Beef	
Pork	
Chicken	
Lamb	
Eggs	
Milk/butter	
Margarine	
Emulsified	
Non-emuls	
Vegetable oils	
Corn	
Soya bean	
Olive	

▨ Saturated fat   ■ Polyunsaturated fat
■ Monounsaturated fat   ☐ Glycerol

Fats of the saturated variety are high in animal meat, and are linked with some disorders.

Favus

caused by inhaling or swallowing fava pollen or the fava bean. It is caused by an inherited metabolic sensitivity of the red blood cells. The symptoms are fever, vomiting, diarrhoea, and sometimes coma. Favism is common in the eastern Mediterranean.

Favus is a form of ringworm affecting the scalp, caused by a fungus (*Trichophyton schoenleinlii*). *See* RINGWORM.

Febrile. *See* FEVER.

Feet. *See* FOOT.

Felon is an infection of the fingertip. *See* PARONYCHIA.

Femur is the thighbone, the bone that extends from the hip to the knee. It is the longest and strongest bone in the body; some of the most powerful muscles in the body are attached to the femur.

Fenestration is an operation in which an artificial opening is made into the labyrinth of the inner ear. It was once a standard operation in the treatment of deafness due to advanced OTOSCLEROSIS. More reliable, less drastic operations, such as a STAPEDECTOMY, are now preferred.

> *See also* DEAFNESS.

Fertility is the ability to reproduce. In a woman, fertility is the capability of an egg (ovum) to be fertilized. In a man, it is the capability of sperm to fertilize an ovum.

Fertilization is the union of an egg (ovum) and a sperm to produce a single cell (zygote) that then develops into an embryo. Fertilization usually takes place in a fallopian tube. *See* PREGNANCY AND CHILDBIRTH.

Fester is to become inflamed and produce pus. *See* INFLAMMATION; PUS.

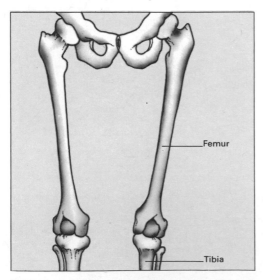

Femur is the longest bone in the body, and can bear more weight than any other bone.

Fetish is a person's finding sexual significance in an object rather than a person. It can be involved in normal sexual stimulation, but in isolation it requires psychiatric consultation.

A talk about Fever

Fever is an abnormally high body temperature. In adults the normal temperature, taken orally, is up to 37°C (98.6°F). When the temperature is taken under the armpit, it is about 1°F lower than the oral temperature. The rectal temperature is about 1°F higher than the oral temperature. Children have a greater range of body temperature than adults so a moderate temperature increase in children is of less significance than the same increase in an adult. For practical purposes, fever may be defined as a temperature that is at least 0.5°F above normal on two recordings taken at least two hours apart.

Q: Are there different types of fever?

A: Yes. Most febrile illnesses are accompanied by a temperature that is lowest in the morning, that rises during the day to reach a peak in the evening, and that falls during the night. In other illnesses, the temperature may fluctuate widely without returning to normal.

With a relapsing fever, there are periods of normal temperature that may last for two or three days, separated by bouts of fever. A fever in which the temperature remains high with little variation is known as a sustained fever.

Q: What are the symptoms that commonly accompany a fever?

A: The accompanying symptoms depend on the underlying cause of the fever. They may include loss of appetite, headache, thirst, and aching throughout the body.

Q: What causes a fever?

A: Fever is usually caused by infection, but may also occur with certain blood disorders, increased metabolism with overactivity of thyroid gland (hyperthyroidism) and, sometimes, cancer.

Q: How does an illness cause a fever?

A: Usually, the microbes of the invading infection produce poisons that disturb the normal functioning of the heat-regulating centre of the brain, the hypothalamus. Such disturbance to the hypothalamus can also be produced by tissue damage, as may occur in coronary thrombosis or severe bruising; by poisoning; by drug overdose; by dehydration; by certain diseases, such as cancer; or by direct damage to the hypothalamus.

When the hypothalamus is disturbed

in this way, it stimulates the body to produce more heat: the blood vessels near the skin surface constrict and the muscles undergo rapid contractions (shivering). The patient at first may feel cold, but once the temperature has been raised, may perspire in an attempt to reduce the temperature.

Q: *When is a fever considered to be serious?*

A: Any fever that is accompanied by mental confusion or disorientation is serious and requires expert medical attention. If the temperature rises above 39.4°C (103°F); if a continued fever has no obvious cause; or if a fever is accompanied by vomiting or diarrhoea, consult a doctor.

Q: *Can a fever produce complications?*

A: In young children, a high fever can cause convulsions. This is not a sign of epilepsy. However, fever may trigger convulsions in an epileptic child. If convulsions do occur in a young child, a doctor should be consulted at once, for they may recur if the temperature is not lowered.

A fever may also produce cold sores, due to the herpes simplex virus.

Q: *How is a fever treated?*

A: For EMERGENCY treatment, *see* First Aid, p.584.

A doctor should be consulted so that the underlying cause can be determined and treated. Aspirin given at four-hourly intervals may help to reduce the temperature. Antibiotics should not be given unless they have been prescribed by the doctor.

A person with fever should stay in bed in a warm, well ventilated room and should be given plenty to drink. Anyone with a fever may well be infectious: visitors should not be allowed until a definite diagnosis has been made.

Fever sore, or fever blister, is a sore that occurs on the lips, often during a fever. *See* COLD SORE.

Fibrescope is a flexible instrument used for inspecting the body's internal organs and tissues (see ENDOSCOPY). A fibrescope is made of glass or plastic fibres that conduct light.

Fibrillation is rapid, irregular twitching of muscle fibres. Any muscle can fibrillate, and the fibrillation sometimes accompanies degenerative disorders such as motor neuron disease. It may also occur in skeletal muscle that has recently been deprived of its nerve supply. But the most serious site of fibrillation is the heart, in which the condition affects either of the two pairs of chambers, the atria (auricles) or the ventricles.

Q: *What is atrial fibrillation?*

A: Atrial (or auricular) fibrillation is extremely rapid twitching of the muscle of the upper chambers of each half of the heart (atria). The atria no longer contract rhythmically, causing inefficient pumping of the blood. The pulse at the wrist is irregular because the main chambers (ventricles) of the heart are not receiving a regular stimulus from the atria.

Atrial fibrillation may be caused by any kind of heart disease, such as coronary artery disease due to arteriosclerosis, following rheumatic fever with valve disease, or as a result of hyperactivity of the thyroid gland (thyrotoxicosis). In some cases, however, the cause cannot be identified.

Q: *What is ventricular fibrillation?*

A: This condition resembles atrial fibrillation in its action but affects the lower chambers in each half of the heart (ventricles). The disorder is rapidly fatal, because the weak, rapid heartbeats pump little or no blood into the circulation. Ventricular fibrillation may be caused by coronary thrombosis, the effect of drugs such as digitalis or chloroform, or an electric shock.

Q: *How is fibrillation in the heart treated?*

A: Atrial fibrillation is effectively treated either with digoxin or with other drugs used to bring the rhythm of the heart under control. All such drugs are used under medical supervision. If the cause of atrial fibrillation is known it must also be treated.

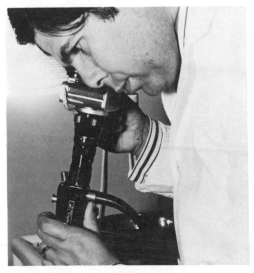

Fibrescope is used to study internal organs, and can be used to photograph them.

Fibrin

Ventricular fibrillation is an emergency treated as a cardiac arrest, and regular heart rhythm is restored using a special machine that causes defibrillation.

Fibrin is an insoluble web of protein that forms the framework of a blood clot. Synthetic fibrin, made from gelatin (fibrin foam), is sometimes used as a surgical dressing to stop a haemorrhage.

See also FIBRINOGEN.

Fibrinogen is a soluble protein in the blood plasma. It is essential for the clotting of blood: through the action of the enzyme thrombin, fibrinogen is converted into the insoluble protein FIBRIN.

Fibroadenosis is a condition that occurs in the breasts of women: the many milk-secreting ducts become enlarged and are surrounded by fibrous tissue, and the breast feels tender and lumpy to the touch, usually due to hormonal changes.

Fibrocystic disease. *See* CYSTIC FIBROSIS.

A talk about Fibroids

Fibroid is a common, benign (non-cancerous) tumour that consists mainly of fibrous and muscle tissue. It forms in the muscle of the womb (uterus), and is also known medically as leiomyoma uteri. One or several fibroids may be present. They are of various shapes, firm, and slow-growing. They may range in size from less than 2.5cm (one inch) to more than 30cm (one foot) across.

Q: What are the symptoms of a fibroid?

A: Often a fibroid produces no symptoms

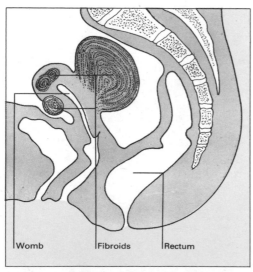

Fibroids may grow comparatively large, but generally produce no symptoms at all.

and is discovered only in a gynaecological examination. Possible symptoms include heavy menstrual bleeding (menorrhagia), occasionally with pain (dysmenorrhoea); if a fibroid causes pressure on the bladder, urination is more frequent. A large fibroid can sometimes be felt through the abdominal wall.

Q: What causes a fibroid?

A: Each month the womb increases in size, in response to the sex hormones, and then decreases at the time of menstruation. It is likely that an area of muscle in the womb fails to shrink with the rest of the womb. Each month, the area grows slightly larger under the stimulus of hormones and, as the bulk increases, a fibroid is formed. After menopause, fibroids decrease in size as the womb becomes smaller.

Q: Can fibroids affect fertility?

A: Sometimes fibroids cause STERILITY. They may also be a factor in producing a miscarriage.

Q: How are fibroids treated?

A: Fibroids need treatment only if they produce symptoms.

They are treated surgically either by removal of the fibroid from the womb (myomectomy) or by complete removal of the womb (hysterectomy).

Fibroma is a benign (noncancerous) tumour of connective tissue. It may occur anywhere in the body, for example, in the fibrous covering of bone (periosteum) or nerve. It has a firm consistency, is irregular in shape, and grows slowly. A fibroma is not painful unless it causes pressure.

Fibrosarcoma is a rare malignant tumour formed from fibroblasts, the cells of connective fibrous tissue. A fibrosarcoma is treated by surgical removal.

See also TUMOUR.

Fibrosis is the formation of fibrous scar tissue. It is a normal reaction to infection or injury, and may occur in the lungs, following pneumonia, or form adhesions in the peritoneum following peritonitis.

Fibrositis is a popular term used imprecisely for pain experienced in the muscles. Often, tender nodules can be felt in the affected muscle. These are caused by small areas of muscle spasm, and can usually be relieved by heat and massage. However, if the pain is extremely severe, an injection of local anaesthetic may be necessary.

Fibrous tissue is tissue containing or composed of fibres that holds organs and other structures in place.

Fibula is the long, slender bone on the outside of the lower leg, extending from just below the knee to the ankle. Its lower end forms the outer side of the ankle joint. Unlike the shinbone (tibia), the fibula does not bear weight but serves as an attachment for some of the leg muscles.

Filariasis is a general term for infection by any of several tropical WORMS of the family Filarioidea. *See* ELEPHANTIASIS; LOIASIS; ONCHOCERCIASIS.

Filling, in dentistry, is the process of repairing a tooth cavity.

Finger is any of the digits of the hand. A finger consists of three bones (phalanges), except for the thumb, which has only two. The phalanges are connected by hinge joints. Tendons along the upper and lower surfaces of the fingers move the joints. These are controlled by muscles in the forearm. Other muscles in the hand help with fine finger movements. *See* DUPUYTREN'S CONTRACTURE; FROSTBITE; HEBERDEN'S NODE; RAYNAUD'S PHENOMENON.

Fingernail. *See* NAIL.

First Aid is assistance administered in an emergency to a person who has been injured or otherwise suddenly disabled. *See* First Aid, pp.503–597.

Fissure is a medical term for a crack or groove. It can be a natural division in a structure such as the brain, liver, and spinal cord, or it can refer to a crack-like sore. An anal fissure (fissure-in-ano), the most common example, is a tear in the skin of the anus. It is usually caused by passing hard, constipated faeces. Pain from the fissure is sharp and there may be bleeding during defecation. In small children, the pain may prevent defecation.

Q: How is an anal fissure treated?

A: Anal fissures often heal on their own after several days or when the constipation ceases (*see* CONSTIPATION). An anaesthetic ointment may be applied to the area to prevent pain. If the condition does not improve, the anus may have to be stretched surgically under general anaesthetic, to provide a wider opening.

Fistula is an abnormal channel from a hollow body cavity to the surface (for example, from the rectum to the skin), or between two cavities (for example, from the vagina to the bladder). A fistula may be congenital (for example, bladder to navel), the result of a penetrating wound (for example, skin to lung), or formed from an ulcer or abscess (for example, appendix abscess to vagina or tooth socket to sinus). Fistulas arise from an abscess or wound that is unable to heal because it receives the fluid contents of some body cavity. A fistula-in-ano, for example, begins with the infection of the mucous lining of the rectum, perhaps by tuberculosis, Crohn's disease, or ulcerative colitis. The area becomes an abscess as it is constantly reinfected by the faeces, and eventually a fistula breaks through to the skin near the anus.

Q: How is a fistula treated?

A: A fistula from a wound kept free from infection, normally closes spontaneously. If a fistula is allowed to develop beyond the early stages, an operation to close it is the usual treatment.

    See also COLOSTOMY.

Fit. *See* CONVULSION.

Flatfoot is a common disorder in which the entire sole of the foot, instead of being arched, is in contact with the ground when the person stands. Normally, the bones of the foot form three arches to raise the sole; support is provided by strong ligaments in the sole and by the muscles, especially those of the big toe. Flatfoot occurs when the larger, inner arch of the bone collapses.

All children have flat feet for at least two years after they start walking. A slight outward twist of the foot (called a valgus deformity) can cause flatfoot to become a permanent condition, because it forces the inner arch of the foot downwards. If the arch appears when a person with flatfoot stands on tiptoe, it is an indication that the foot is still supple enough to form a normal arch with corrective treatment.

Q: Are there any other causes of flatfoot?

A: Occasionally, flatfoot may be associated with muscular disorders or paralysis.

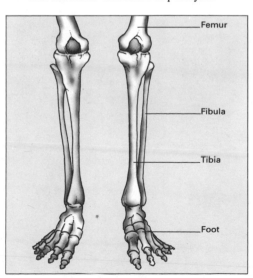

Femur

Fibula

Tibia

Foot

Fibula is a thin, long bone extending from the knee downwards to the ankle.

Flatulence

Q: *What is the treatment for flatfoot?*

A: For a child, a chiropodist may suggest wedging the heels of the shoes on the inner side of the foot, and remedial exercises. But for an adult, there is no medical need to correct flat feet unless they disturb the patient.

Flatulence results from excessive gas in the stomach and intestines. A person may belch, and pass "wind" (flatus). Some wind is normally produced from fermentation in the large intestine. Flatulence often accompanies indigestion; it may also result from the nervous habit of swallowing air (aerophagia). Commercial products for the relief of indigestion help to reduce flatulence. When the condition is caused by aerophagia, it may be best treated after discussion with a doctor or psychotherapist.

Flatus is gas in the intestines. Excess flatus causes FLATULENCE.

Fleas are wingless, jumping, bloodsucking insects that belong to the order *Siphonaptera.* Most fleas are parasitic on one specific species of animal, including human beings. *Pulex irritans* injects its saliva into the skin of human beings as an irritating bite.

Q: *Can animal fleas afflict people as well?*

A: Yes. Fleas from cats and dogs (*Ctenocephalides felis* and *C. canis*) may bite human beings, but this is unusual. One of the rat fleas, *Xenopsylla cheopis*, carries bubonic plague if the rat itself was infected. This flea can pass on the disease in its bite. The same rat flea may carry a form of typhus.

See also LICE.

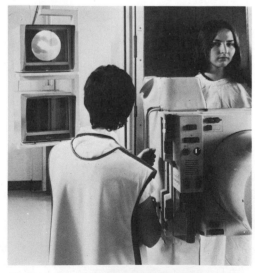

Fluoroscope is a type of X-ray device that projects the image onto a screen instead of film.

Flexibilitas cerea is a condition in which the limbs remain in any position in which they are placed. It is a rare symptom of catalepsy, a phase of schizophrenia.

Flies are winged insects that belong to the order *Diptera*. The housefly, like other flies, feeds on decomposing organic matter and can pick up disease germs on its feet and legs. A fly that settles on food contaminates it by shedding germs from its feet, in its droppings, and through its mouth while it is feeding. Illnesses that may be spread by flies include bacillary dysentery and other intestinal disorders, cholera, conjunctivitis, poliomyelitis, sandfly fever, and typhoid.

Flooding is excessive bleeding during menstruation, often occurring with clots of blood. *See* MENORRHAGIA; MENSTRUAL PROBLEMS.

Flu. *See* INFLUENZA.

Flukes are flatworms of the class *Trematoda*. They can cause various parasitic infections in human beings. The life cycle of a fluke is complex: a small organism (miracidium) hatches from an egg, invades a snail, and develops there. When it changes into a small cyst-like structure (cercaria), it is excreted by the snail and finds its home in plants, crabs, or fish. If human beings drink or come into contact with water containing the cysts, flukes that evolve from the cysts invade the tissues and produce clinical symptoms.

See also WORMS; SCHISTOSOMIASIS.

Fluorescein is a dye that is used to detect damage to the cornea of the eye, either from foreign bodies or from lesions.

Fluoridation is the addition of fluoride to the water supply. Many water supplies naturally contain an adequate amount of fluoride, and the addition of more is controversial.

Fluoride is a chemical compound of fluorine. Fluoride, in the form of calcium fluoride, occurs naturally in the soil, and in the water supply in some regions. It helps in the formation of bones and teeth. Fluoride helps to prevent tooth decay in children, but authorities are not agreed on whether or not it has the same effect in adults.

A prolonged deficiency of fluoride may lead to osteoporosis, a disorder in which the bones become softer. A prolonged high intake of fluoride in adults may cause yellowing of the teeth; weakening of the tooth enamel; and, rarely, bone disorders, such as osteosclerosis.

Fluoroscope is a machine that aids in diagnosis. It projects onto a screen X-ray pictures of what is happening inside a person's body. The screen, which looks like a television screen, is activated when X-rays strike it. By using a fluoroscope, a doctor can study the movements of internal organs.

Flush is sudden redness of the skin, particularly of the face and neck. The cheeks may be flushed with a fever, or flushing may be part of such illnesses as chronic pulmonary tuberculosis. A hot flush is accompanied by a sudden feeling of heat caused by an oversensitivity of the surface blood vessels to minor changes of temperature or emotion. This often occurs in women at time of menopause. A hot flush is also sometimes symptomatic of various neuroses.

Flutter is a state of extremely rapid, regular, vibration or pulsations. It usually occurs in the upper chambers (atria) of the heart, where the number of contractions can rise to between 200 and 400 per minute. The lower chambers (ventricles) cannot contract at such a rapid speed; instead they contract on every third or fourth atrial beat, causing irregular pulsations.

Atrial flutter may be caused by heart disease, particularly rheumatic valve disease, or by the effects of an overactive thyroid gland (THYROTOXICOSIS). Sometimes no cause can be found.

See also FIBRILLATION.

Foetus is an unborn baby from three months after conception to the time of birth.

See also EMBRYO; PREGNANCY AND CHILDBIRTH.

Folic acid is a vitamin of the B group. *See* VITAMINS.

Folk medicine is any nonorthodox but traditional way of treating illnesses and injuries. It may use herbal mixtures, physical manipulations, religious rituals, or a combination of these. It differs from orthodox medicine in that the treatments are not the products of scientific medical research, but some old remedies have now been incorporated into standard medical practice because their benefit has been scientifically proven.

Many folk remedies that do not work are useless rather than harmful. But harm might occur indirectly if a person uses such remedies instead of consulting a doctor.

Follicle is a small, roughly spherical cavity or a small secretory gland.

Follicle-stimulating hormone (FSH) is a hormone that stimulates the growth of an ovarian follicle in the first half of each menstrual cycle. It also affects sperm formation in men. The hormone is produced by the front part of the pituitary gland. When the ovarian follicle has matured, the membrane surrounding it bursts, and a single egg cell (ovum) is released. *See* OVULATION.

Folliculitis is an inflammation of the hair follicles on the skin. It first appears as scattered pimples that later dry out and form crusts around the follicles. The affected area is itchy and nearby lymph glands may become swollen. In most cases, folliculitis is caused by streptococcus or staphylococcus bacteria. Sycosis barbae on the face and neck of males is a form of folliculitis.

Q: How is folliculitis treated?

A: The application of antiseptic creams or lotions to the infected area reduces the infection. A doctor may prescribe antibiotic drugs.

Fomentation. *See* POULTICE.

Fontanelle (or fontanel) is a gap between the bones of the skull of a newborn baby. At birth there are six fontanelles in a baby's skull. The two main ones lie along the centre-line of the scalp; one towards the front of the skull just above the forehead, and the other at the back of the skull near the nape of the neck. The bones of a baby's skull are still unjoined at birth. The fontanelles allow the bones to overlap and the skull to change shape during birth to fit the birth canal.

Q: Is it possible to see any of the fontanelles on a baby's head?

A: Yes. The fontanelle at the front of the skull, sometimes known as the "soft spot," can usually be seen and felt. It bulges when the baby cries, and may form a hollow if the baby needs fluids.

Q: Is it possible to harm the fontanelle?

A: No, not through normal handling. A tough membrane covers the gap and protects the brain. It can be touched and washed without harming the baby.

Q: When does the fontanelle disappear?

A: It is usually completely closed when the child is eighteen months old.

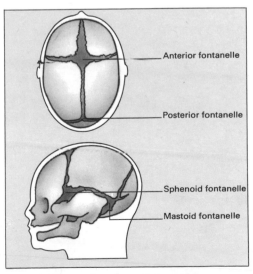

Fontanelles are the spaces between the unjoined bones of the baby's skull.

Food poisoning

A talk about Food poisoning

Food poisoning (for EMERGENCY treatment, *see* First Aid, p.562), is an acute illness caused by eating contaminated or poisonous food. The usual symptoms are vomiting, diarrhoea, and sharp abdominal pain. Cramps, headache, and sweating may be additional symptoms. The patient may collapse with weakness and exhaustion. Food poisoning is rarely fatal and recovery usually takes place after about six hours.

Q: *What are the causes of food poisoning?*

A: There are several possible causes of food poisoning, the most common of which involve bacteria. (1) Bacteria in contaminated food may grow in the food and produce their own toxin. The germs usually enter the food from a staphylococcal infection (such as a boil, abscess, or other skin infection) in a person who has handled the food during processing. Although cooking kills the germs, it does not destroy the toxin that has been produced. Poisoning from the toxin takes place within two hours of eating contaminated food. Toxins produced in foods from other kinds of bacteria are rare, but BOTULISM (from the bacteria *Clostridium botulinum*) is one example.

(2) Another type of poisoning occurs when bacteria contained in food develop in the intestines of the patient (for example, salmonella or typhoid fever). Salmonella bacteria are found in many animals and the foods most likely to contain them are meats (especially chicken and processed frozen meat) and duck's eggs. The bacteria need time to grow in the intestines, and so symptoms may not appear for one or two days.

(3) Water and foods such as unwashed fruit and vegetables may be contaminated by chemicals such as pesticides, or by other poisons.

(4) Many plants and some animals are naturally poisonous to human beings. These include some types of fungi and some shellfish. Food poisoning results with varying severity if these substances are eaten.

(5) Certain foods that are wholesome to most people may cause food poisoning as an allergic reaction in others.

Q: *What is ptomaine poisoning?*

A: Ptomaines are evil-smelling products of bacteria present in putrefying food. They were once believed to cause food poisoning, but it is now known that so-called ptomaine poisoning is bacterial infection of the intestines.

Q: *How is food poisoning treated?*

A: A doctor normally concentrates on treating the symptoms by giving anti-nauseant drugs. The doctor may also treat any water and salt deficiency, the consequence of the vomiting and diarrhoea.

Q: *What measures can be taken to avoid food poisoning?*

A: Persons involved in the processing or preparation of food should be checked for skin and intestinal infections. All fresh fruit and raw vegetables should be washed thoroughly before being eaten. Cooked food should be covered, cooled quickly, and stored in a refrigerator to prevent the growth of bacteria. Food that is reheated should be eaten at once and not kept warm, because this encourages the growth of bacteria.

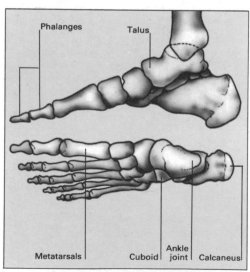

Foot is formed from twenty-six bones and a complex set of muscles that balance the body.

Foot is joined at the ankle to the lower end of the leg. The calcaneus, which is the largest bone in the foot, forms the HEEL. Above the calcaneus, and resting on the front part of it, is the talus bone, leading to several tarsal bones, and then to the elongated metatarsals and TOES. The cuboid bone is also in front of the calcaneus, and from it the fourth and fifth metatarsal bones connect with the fourth and fifth toes. The arch of the foot is raised higher on the instep because the talus projects farther forward than does the cuboid bone. The weight of the body is taken by the calcaneus and transmitted to the heads of the metatarsal bones.

See also FLATFOOT.

Foot disorders. The following table lists some of the disorders that affect the feet, and the basic characteristics of each condition. Each disorder has a separate article in the A-Z section of this book.

Disorder	Basic characteristics
ATHLETE'S FOOT	Skin eruptions, usually between the toes
BLISTER	Collection of fluid under the skin causing top layer to puff out
BUNION	Thickening of the skin over the joint at the base of the big toe and inflammation
BURSITIS	Inflammation of the bursa
CALLUS	Hard, thickened areas of skin on the foot
CELLULITIS	Inflammation of cellular tissue
CHILBLAIN	Itching, swelling, and painful reddening of skin
CLUBFOOT (talipes)	Forepart of the foot is twisted out of shape
CORN	Hard, cone-shaped, thickened areas of the skin on the toes
FLATFOOT	Arch of foot sinks down and the inner edge of the foot rests upon ground
FOOT DROP	Inability to lift front part of foot
FROSTBITE	Reddened or whitened skin with swelling, blistering, and numbness
GANGLION	Cystic tumour near a tendon or joint
GANGRENE	Dead tissue
GOUT	Inflammation of joint of big toe usually, but also of instep or heel
HALLUX VALGUS	Outwards deviation of the great toe from the mid-line
HAMMER TOE	First joint of toe bent downwards and tending to form corns
IMMERSION FOOT	Blueness of skin
INGROWING TOENAIL	Edges of nail overgrown with tissue, causing pain and possible infection
MADURA FOOT	Swollen feet with ulcers
METATARSALGIA	Pain in the metatarsal region

Disorder	Basic characteristics
OSTEOARTHRITIS	Inflammation and degeneration of bone and cartilage that form joints
PES CAVUS	Abnormally high arch
POLYDACTYLISM	Extra toes
RHEUMATOID ARTHRITIS	Inflammation and degeneration of joints
SYNDACTYLY	Webbed toes
TOE, CLAW	Toes abnormally curved
WART, PLANTAR	Epidermal tumour on sole of foot

Foot drop is a condition in which the toes drag and the foot hangs, caused by weakness or paralysis of the muscles on the side of the shin-bone. It may occur as a result of damage to the nerves supplying the muscles, poliomyelitis, polyneuritis, or a muscle disorder such as myasthenia gravis or one of the muscular dystrophies.

The treatment of foot drop depends on the underlying cause. If foot drop remains after the treatment, the patient may wear a special splint or a spring on the shoe to prevent stumbling. Sometimes an operation may be performed to fix the foot (arthrodesis) at right angles, or one to move a tendon from one side of the leg to the other, thereby strengthening the weak side.

Forceps are pincers that are used in surgery for holding, seizing, or extracting.

Foreign body is an alien particle or small object that has lodged in the skin, in surface organs (for example, the eyes, ears, or nose), or internally.

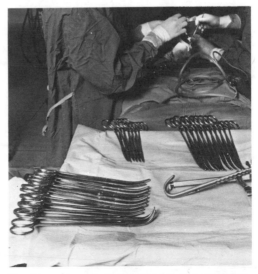

Forceps are used, during an operation, to splice blood vessels, and expose tissues and organs.

Forensic medicine

Forensic medicine is the branch of medical science that is related to the law and legal processes. It applies medical knowledge to legal (especially criminal) problems.

Foreskin (or prepuce) is the fold of skin that covers the end of the penis (glans penis). Before the age of eighteen months, it is held down by fine strands of tissue; after this age, it can be pulled back. Because the foreskin is subject to irritation and inflammation (balanitis), it should be pulled back and the penis washed regularly as a standard part of male hygiene.

See also CIRCUMCISION.

Formaldehyde is a pungent, poisonous gas. It is a component of formalin, a solution used in medicine as a disinfectant and preservative.

See also FORMALIN.

Formalin is a watery (aqueous) solution of the organic chemical formaldehyde, with some added methanol (methyl alcohol). It is used in medicine as a disinfectant and preservative. As a disinfectant, formalin is a component of soaps for hospital use. Clothing and towels, and samples of faeces and sputum, may be sterilized in formalin. Body tissues soaked in formalin become hard, and the solution is used to preserve biological specimens for examination by a pathologist. Formalin is also sometimes used in the treatment of warts.

Formic acid (or methanoic acid) is an organic chemical. It is probably the cause of the pain from certain insect bites and nettle stings. It is a clear, pungent liquid that is chemically related to formaldehyde and methanol (methyl alcohol). Formic acid is occasionally used in medicine for the relief of deep-seated inflammation.

Formication is the sensation of insects crawling over the skin. It is a form of paraesthesia (an abnormal sensation without cause). Formication is sometimes a symptom of DELIRIUM TREMENS, and it is a common side effect of alcohol and cocaine withdrawal.

Fovea is any small cup-shaped depression that occurs naturally on many structures of the body; an example is the pit in the head of the thigh bone (femur). The term most commonly refers to the fovea centralis retinae, the depression on the retina of the EYE onto which light is naturally focused, and which contains only cones and no blood vessels.

A talk about Fractures

Fractures are broken bones. (For EMERGENCY treatment, *see* First Aid, pp.546–553.) Any bone in the body can accidentally be broken (fractured). But some bones, because of their awkward shapes or vulnerable positions (for example, the long bones of the arms and legs), tend to fracture more often than others. Chunky bones such as the carpals in the wrist and the tarsals in the ankle are less liable to fracture.

Q: What can cause a bone fracture?

A: Most fractures occur as the result of injury or accident. Sometimes a bone breaks following repeated minor strains. Some bones have a tendency to fracture easily because they are weak from disease.

Q: Do bones always fracture in the same way?

A: No. Doctors recognize five main kinds of fractures. (1) A transverse fracture is a straight break in a bone from side to side. (2) An oblique fracture is an angled break in a bone (for example, diagonally). (3) A spiral fracture is one in which the bone breaks as a result of a twisting action. (4) A comminuted fracture is one in which the bone is broken and splintered into more than two pieces at the fracture site. (5) A greenstick fracture usually occurs in children: because the bones are pliable, a break occurs on one side of a bone and the other side bends but, like a green twig, remains intact.

Q: Can fractures damage tissues other than bone?

A: Yes. A medical description usually classifies a fracture in terms of the effect that it has on surrounding tissues. (1) A simple (or closed) fracture does not pierce the surface of the skin. (2) A

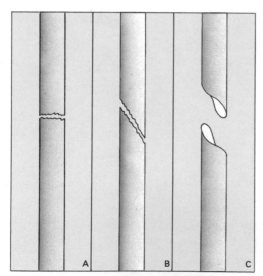

Fractures of bones are known medically as (A) transverse; (B) oblique; or (C) spiral planes.

compound fracture causes a surface wound, either leading to the site of the fracture, or caused by a broken bone piercing the skin. (3) A complicated fracture is one that damages a nearby structure such as a blood vessel, nerve, or body organ. (4) An impacted fracture is a type of fracture in which one end of the broken bone becomes wedged or compressed into another bone.

Q: *What is the standard treatment for fractures?*

A: The basis of treatment for all fractures is to reposition the bone in its normal anatomical position and to hold it there until new bone has had time to heal the break.

Q: *How are unstable fractures treated?*

A: Unstable fractures may be held together by an operation that employs various fixers, such as screws, metal plates, thick pins (for the hip), or wires.

Q: *How is a complicated fracture treated?*

A: A complicated fracture is treated in the same way as other fractures except that repair of the internal damage is given priority.

Q: *Is a fractured bone always displaced?*

A: No. With some fractures, particularly those of the hand, foot, or skull, the bone breaks but may not change position.

Q: *How long does a fracture take to heal?*

A: In general, an arm fracture is kept immobilized for about six weeks, but it takes at least three months for a leg fracture to heal sufficiently for the patient to be able to walk unaided.

Q: *Are there complications that can prolong the healing time?*

A: Fractures in elderly people often take a long time to heal (called delayed union), especially when there is an underlying bone disease.

Sometimes not enough blood reaches the site of the fracture, and the bone fails to heal (non-union); this is common in fractures of the neck of the femur (thigh-bone) in old people.

Q: *Are there any other possible complications of fractures?*

A: Yes. If the bone has not been set in its correct position, shortening of the limb may result. A poor joining of the fractured bone (called mal-union) results if one end is allowed to rotate slightly so that its contour does not lock smoothly with the other piece of bone. This problem is most common with multiple fractures, in which it is not always possible to set all the bones in their exact, original positions. If infection occurs, it is usually associated with a compound fracture, but it may also occur with simple fractures as a post-operative complication.

Q: *Can nearby muscles be exercised while the bone is healing?*

A: Yes. It is essential that the patient exercises the muscles while a limb is in a cast. Physiotherapists teach muscle contraction exercises that can be done while the limb is immobile (isometric exercises). After the cast or splint has been removed, the nearby joint is usually stiff and therapy is necessary to restore the full range of movement. Swimming is an excellent means of restoring muscle power. A high protein diet with additional vitamins is another measure that helps the return of normal use to a fractured bone.

Fragilitas ossium is a congenital condition in which the bones are abnormally brittle. *See* OSTEOGENESIS IMPERFECTA.

Framboesia. *See* YAWS.

Fraternal twins are twin babies that result from two separate eggs (ova) that were fertilized at the same time. Unlike identical twins, fraternal twins are not necessarily of the same sex. *See* TWINS.

Freckles are small brown or yellowish-brown patches of pigment in the skin. They appear in response to sunlight: the body's cells produce more of the dark pigment MELANIN as a protection against further harmful action by sunlight's ultraviolet rays. These collections

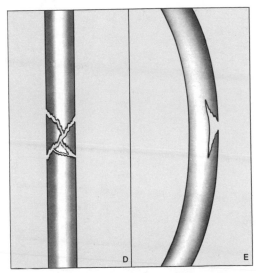

Fractures: comminuted (D), and greenstick (E), when bone is broken on one side only.

Friar's balsam

of pigment tend to fade in the absence of sunlight.

Friar's balsam is an alcoholic solution of the resins from trees growing in Thailand and Sumatra which is mixed with aloes and storax. It is used as an antiseptic solution for the treatment of cold sores, minor wounds, and as a surgical dressing. It can be diluted in hot water as an inhalation for bronchitis and laryngitis.

Friedreich's ataxia is a serious, rare, inherited disorder of the central nervous system. It is caused by the imperfect development of some nerve fibres in the spinal cord. The first symptom of Friedreich's ataxia is poor co-ordination of muscles in the legs, usually beginning in childhood or early adolescence. The feet later become deformed (claw feet), the gait becomes shambling, and muscular unco-ordination spreads throughout the body. Commonly, the spine curves to one side, and the patient becomes increasingly bent. Sputtering, hesitating speech is another symptom.

Q: *What are the complications of Friedreich's ataxia?*

A: Friedreich's ataxia is a cause of para-plegia in children and young people. If the heart becomes involved, heart failure may occur. Diabetes is a frequent complication, and the patient is also more liable to get pneumonia.

Q: *How is Friedreich's ataxia treated?*

A: No effective treatment is known. But attempts can be made with physiotherapy to slow down the stiffening of the muscles. Death usually occurs within ten

to twenty years, although this results from secondary infection.

Frigidity is the lack of sexual desire, and a consequent inability to reach orgasm, in a sexually mature person in good health. Frigidity is usually attributed to women only. The cause of frigidity is almost always psychological: for example, it may be a fear of becoming pregnant. Emotional problems may prevent vaginal secretions during sexual arousal, resulting in a dry genital area and painful intercourse (DYSPAREUNIA). A doctor or psychiatrist can usually determine the reasons for a woman's frigidity once her sexual history is known; appropriate treatment can then begin. Sympathetic and careful counselling is necessary.

Fröhlich's syndrome is a rare glandular disorder of childhood, more common in boys than in girls. It is caused by a disturbance in the hypothalamus, the part of the brain that regulates the supply of hormones from the pituitary gland. Essential pituitary hormones are not produced, so that the sex organs remain underdeveloped. Excess fatty tissue is distributed in areas normal for the female build: thighs, hips, and breasts. If the condition begins in early childhood the patient may be a dwarf; if it occurs just before puberty, the child is fat and sluggish. The skin of an adult man with Fröhlich's syndrome remains soft, and he has effeminate features due to the distribution of fat throughout the body. Fröhlich's syndrome in a girl causes extreme obesity.

Q: *What is the treatment for Fröhlich's syndrome?*

A: Provided treatment is started early enough, Fröhlich's syndrome can be most effectively treated with modern hormone therapy. *See* HYPOPITUITARISM.

Frostbite is an acute skin reaction to extreme cold. Particularly vulnerable areas of the body include the toes, fingers, ears, and the tip of the nose.

Q: *What are the symptoms of frostbite?*

A: The affected area turns unnaturally white. The victim is unaware of the condition because there is no sensation of pain at this stage. Within a few hours blood seeps back into the tissues turning them purple or black. The area becomes red, swollen, and painful. The skin may blister, and the blisters break down into ulcers. In severe cases the circulation does not return on warming, and the damage leads to gangrene.

Q: *What causes frostbite?*

A: In extreme weather conditions of cold and wind, the blood and tissue moisture in the affected area freezes. In severe

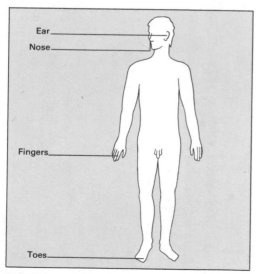

Ear

Nose

Fingers

Toes

Frostbite is more likely to effect a person's fingers, toes, nose and ears.

cases, the blood vessels supplying the arca shut down, preventing normal circulation even when gently warmed.

Q: How is frostbite treated?

A: The affected area must be warmed very gradually, preferably at the same time as the rest of the body, and constrictive clothing should be removed. Rubbing increases the damage to the already injured tissues. If the area remains white after warming, a doctor must be consulted immediately. If gangrene sets in, amputation may be necessary.

Q: How can a person avoid frostbite?

A: During extremely cold weather, clothing must be well-fitting, warm, and wind-resistant. Tight shoes, socks, or gloves cut down the circulation and endanger the specific area. People with diabetes or any form of circulatory disorder are more likely to develop frostbite.

Frozen section is a technique in which an area of tissue (from a biopsy) is frozen and a thin slice cut off for examination under a microscope. The technique is useful for the immediate detection of cancer.

See also CRYOSURGERY.

Frozen shoulder is pain and stiffness in the shoulder. It is caused by inflammation of the joint capsule. This usually follows a minor injury or strain, although sometimes the cause may not be known. The inflammation restricts normal movement in the shoulder. Usually the stiffness and pain become gradually worse over a period of weeks. The pain then disappears, but the stiffness remains, with slow improvement over the next six to twelve months.

Q: What is the treatment for frozen shoulder?

A: At first the arm must be kept in a sling and only those movements that do not cause pain should be allowed. Painkilling and anti-rheumatic drugs may be prescribed; pain may also be relieved by applying ice-packs to the affected shoulder. Sometimes, injections of corticosteroid drugs produce an improvement but, in severe cases, radiotherapy or manipulation of the affected shoulder while the patient is under general anaesthetic may be necessary, followed by physiotherapy.

FSH. *See* FOLLICLE-STIMULATING HORMONE.

Fugue is a temporary disturbance of consciousness in which a person nevertheless behaves as though conscious. On "waking" from a state of fugue, a person suddenly realizes that he or she cannot account for, nor remember in any way, the time during which the fugue lasted. Because the condition usually represents a hysterical state of repressed emotions concerning some unfaceable crisis, a person in a fugue state commonly acts a completely different role in society (*see* HYSTERIA). The condition may also be associated with epilepsy or concussion.

A fugue differs from AMNESIA, in which state a person acts consciously but without memory of previous events.

Fulguration is the destruction of living tissue using an electric current. It is sometimes used to treat skin tumours.

See also DIATHERMY.

Fumigation is a method of disinfecting an area using poisonous fumes.

Functional describes a disorder in which the workings of an organ are affected, but no organic or structural cause is evident.

Fungal disorders may be caused by microscopic fungi or their spores. Many of these disorders are difficult to treat because the fungi resist most bactericidal agents. The following table lists some of the common fungal disorders and the basic characteristics of each condition. Each disorder has a separate entry in the A-Z section of this book.

Disorder	Basic characteristics
ACTINOMYCOSIS	Fibrous masses about the mouth or tongue that burst and become sinuses or ulcers; also abscesses in the lungs
ASPERGILLOSIS	Lumps in the skin, ears, sinuses and, especially, the lungs
ATHLETE'S FOOT	Skin eruptions on the foot, usually between the toes

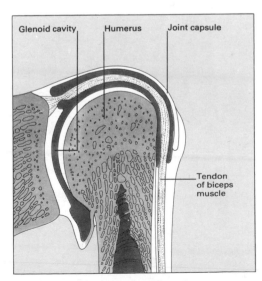

Frozen shoulder is inflammation of the shoulder joint capsule that causes stiffness.

Funny bone

Disorder	Basic characteristics
BLASTOMYCOSIS	Lesions all over the body but, especially, infection of the lungs
HISTOPLASMOSIS	Infection of the lungs, ulcers in the gastro-intestinal tract
MADURA FOOT	Swollen feet with ulcers
MONILIASIS (thrush)	White patches inside the mouth that later become shallow ulcers; also in the vagina
RINGWORM	Raised, round sores of the skin, scalp, or nails
TINEA VERSICOLOR	Patches on the shoulders and upper arms

Funny bone is at the inner, lower end of the HUMERUS (upper arm bone). The ulnar nerve lies over this section of the humerus, close to the surface of the skin at the back of the ELBOW. A blow on the ulnar nerve is painful, and often accompanied by tingling or numbness in the fingers of the affected hand.

Furred tongue is a condition in which the tongue is coated with a furry substance. It occurs during most fevers, but is an inconclusive diagnostic aid, because thirst or reduced appetite may also cause a furred tongue.

Q: What causes furring of the tongue?

A: Dead cells from the tongue are constantly being shed, and are normally removed with the saliva. When the flow of saliva is reduced, this debris, together with food particles and dried mucus, accumulates on the surface of the tongue.

A furred tongue is also a symptom of chronic indigestion, poor oral hygiene,

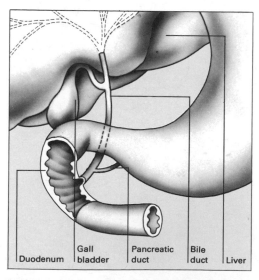

Gall bladder, situated underneath the right lobe of the liver, secretes bile into the duodenum.

or a throat infection such as tonsillitis.

Heavy smoking stains the tongue dark brown, and this is sometimes mistakenly thought to be a furred tongue.

Furuncle (or furunculus). *See* BOILS.

G

Gall is another name for bile. *See* BILE.

Gall bladder is a pear-shaped organ beneath the right side of the liver. It is about 7.6–10.2cm (three to four inches) long, and about 2.5cm (one inch) wide. The function of the gall bladder is to store BILE, a digestive liquid continually secreted by the liver. The bile emulsifies fats and neutralizes acids in partly digested food. A muscular valve in the common bile duct opens and the bile flows from the gall bladder into the cystic duct, along the common bile duct, and into the duodenum (part of the small intestine).

See also CHOLANGITIS; JAUNDICE.

Gallstone is a mass of concentrated bile, resembling a stone, that forms in the gall bladder, or sometimes in the common bile duct. Medically, it is a type of CALCULUS. A gallstone is usually a mixture of cholesterol, bilirubin (a bile pigment), and protein. The size of a gallstone can vary from a tiny crystal to a lump the size of a small egg. Usually, more than one gallstone is formed.

See also CHOLELITHIASIS.

Gamma globulin is a plasma protein, a component of blood serum that contains antibodies (*see* ANTIBODY). It can be extracted from the blood of a person who is immune to a certain infection and injected into another person who has been exposed to the disease (hyperimmune globulin). These extracts can provide temporary immunity to infectious hepatitis, measles (rubeola), poliomyelitis, tetanus, yellow fever, or smallpox (*see* IMMUNIZATION). Gamma globulin injections do not seem to be of benefit against mumps or German measles (rubella).

Q: Are gamma globulin extracts used to give immunity to any other conditions?

A: Yes. A special preparation of gamma globulin, RhO (D) immune globulin, is given to a mother who has Rh— (Rhesus negative) blood after she has given birth. *See* HAEMOLYTIC DISEASE OF THE NEWBORN.

Q: How important is an adequate amount of gamma globulin in the blood?

A: There is a serious risk of infection if a person has a low level of gamma globulin. For example, in a rare inherited disorder called AGAMMAGLOBULINAEMIA, there is almost no gamma globulin in the blood. Infections of all kinds occur more often, and are more serious. Decreased gamma globulin levels sometimes result from the treatment of leukaemia or cancer by chemotherapy. The only treatment in such circumstances is regular doses of gamma globulin.

Ganglion is an anatomical term for a bundle of nerves within the nervous system that act as a relay station outside the brain and spinal cord. A basal ganglion, however, is located within the brain and spinal cord. Ganglions are present throughout the autonomic nervous system.

As a surgical term, a ganglion is a cystlike tumour that appears on tendons.

Gangrene is the decay and death of tissue caused by a lack of blood supply to an area. It is a complication of external or internal injury, or of damage to an artery. External causes include infected bedsores; crushing injuries; deep burns; frostbite; boils; and chemical damage of the skin. Internal causes include blood clotting (thrombosis) in a diseased artery; an embolus; severe arteriosclerosis; diabetes; a strangulated hernia; torsion of the testes; Buerger's disease (a rare disorder of the arteries); and Raynaud's phenomenon (spasm-like contraction of the arteries in the fingers and toes).

Medically, gangrene is considered either "dry" or "moist."

Q: What is dry gangrene?

A: Dry gangrene is the withering and drying out of tissue, without infection by bacteria. This process may continue unnoticed for weeks or months, especially in elderly people. Dry gangrene is most often a complication of advanced diabetes or arteriosclerosis.

Q: What is moist gangrene?

A: Moist gangrene occurs usually in the toes, feet, or legs after a crushing injury or some other factor that causes a sudden stoppage of blood. The gangrene spreads rapidly as invading bacteria thrive and multiply unchecked by the defences normally carried in the blood.

See also GAS GANGRENE.

Q: What are the symptoms of gangrene?

A: Areas of both dry and moist gangrene are conspicuous by a red line on the skin that often marks the border of the gangrenous tissue. Dry gangrene causes some pain in the early stages. The area becomes cold, and the skin changes in colour to brown, then black. Moist gangrene begins with swollen skin that may be blistered, red, and hot. The area then becomes cold as the tissues begin to die, and the skin

appears bruised. The putrefactive bacteria produce an offensive odour.

Q: Which parts of the body are susceptible to gangrene?

A: The limbs, especially the ends of the toes and fingers, are most commonly affected. The intestine may become gangrenous if an artery supplying it is twisted (volvulus), obstructed by a hernia, or diseased by arteriosclerosis. Bone gangrene is also possible.

Q: What is the treatment for gangrene?

A: The only treatment is surgical removal, with large doses of antibiotics.

Q: Can any measures be taken to guard against gangrene?

A: Patients who have severe arteriosclerosis, or diabetes, should take particular care of their feet and hands, especially the nails, because the risk of infection even from a minor injury, for example, one caused by a ragged nail, is increased. This is because the narrowed blood vessels in their fingers and toes cannot carry sufficient blood to combat infection. Any abrasion or infection should be treated immediately.

Gas gangrene is a type of moist GANGRENE that is usually a complication of crushing injuries. The infection is caused by the bacteria *Clostridium welchii* (*see* CLOSTRIDIUM) that thrive without oxygen and release a foul-smelling gas as well as a poisonous toxin. The bacteria breed in the damaged tissue and spread rapidly to healthy tissue. Symptoms include a high fever, putrid-smelling pus, and the formation of gas bubbles under the skin.

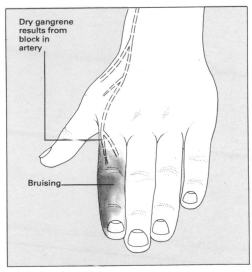

Dry gangrene results from block in artery

Bruising

Gangrene occurs when the blood supply is disrupted, causing gradual death of tissues.

Gas poisoning

Urgent hospitalization is necessary. Death occurs within about two days if the condition is not treated.

Gas poisoning (for EMERGENCY treatment, *see* First Aid, p.562). Many poisonous gases are released when solids and liquids such as mineral acids, ammonia, cyanides, and mercury are heated. Others are specially manufactured as war gases. Poisonous gases affect the body in various ways, and many are potentially fatal.

Q: *What are some examples of the effects of poisonous gases?*

A: Carbon monoxide and mixtures that contain it prevent the blood from carrying oxygen to tissues; hydrogen sulphide causes respiratory paralysis; carbon tetrachloride damages the liver and kidneys; carbon disulphide ultimately causes paralysis and psychoses; tear gases, such as xylyl bromide, severely irritate the eyes, nose, and throat; the various nerve gases prevent the proper functioning of nerve impulses; lung irritant gases, such as chlorine and phosgene, attack the eyes, nose, throat, and lungs; vesicant gases, such as mustard gas and lewisite gas (containing arsenic), cause blisters and ulcers on the skin; nauseant gases, such as chloropicrin, induce vomiting; nose irritant gases, such as diphenylchlorarsine, cause pain, sneezing, depression, and sometimes vomiting.

Q: *How can people come in contact with such gases?*

A: Carbon monoxide is the most poisonous

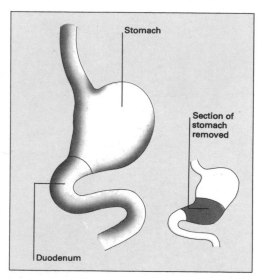

Gastrectomy of the partial type may reduce the capacity of the stomach by as much as half.

gas likely to be present in domestic surroundings. For example, it is present in a closed garage when a car engine has been left running. Carbon tetrachloride is used in dry cleaning. Hydrogen sulphide is a poisonous gas produced in some chemical processes. Tear gases are used by police and military personnel. Carbon disulphide is used in the rubber industry, and in making rayon.

Gastrectomy is the surgical removal of part or all of the stomach. The operation is performed to remove a perforated or bleeding stomach ulcer (partial gastrectomy), to remove scarred tissue that obstructs the passage of food, or to remove a cancerous growth. A partial gastrectomy is also one method of treatment for a peptic ulcer in the duodenum.

Q: *How is the digestive process affected after a gastrectomy?*

A: The small intestine is capable of maintaining the preliminary breakdown of proteins that normally takes place in the stomach. After the total removal of the stomach, however, a patient may have to make some dietary adjustments.

Q: *What dietary adjustments may have to be made?*

A: Supplements of vitamins and iron may be necessary. The absorption of vitamin B_{12} depends on the presence of gastric (stomach) juices; after a total gastrectomy, injections of this vitamin have to be given. Iron supplements reduce the risk of ANAEMIA if a gastrectomy interferes with the amount of iron normally absorbed during digestion. After a partial gastrectomy, the patient has to adopt a routine of eating smaller amounts of food, more often.

Gastric flu is a common term for gastroenteritis caused by a virus. *See* GASTROENTERITIS.

Gastric ulcer is the ulceration of an area of the stomach lining. *See* PEPTIC ULCER.

Gastrin is a hormone that is released into the blood from cells in the lower part of the stomach after a meal.

Gastrin and the parasympathetic vagus nerve stimulate the secretion of acid from the upper part of the stomach, and help produce secretions from the gall bladder, the pancreas, and the small intestine.

Gastritis is inflammation of the stomach lining. The inflammation may be caused by viral infection, alcohol, smoking, certain drugs, or highly spiced or poisoned food. Gastritis may be acute or chronic.

Q: *What are the symptoms of gastritis?*

A: Acute gastritis causes vomiting, furred tongue, thirst, severe stomach pain, and mild fever. Chronic gastritis usually produces few symptoms although in some cases a person may experience one or more of the following discomforts: mild indigestion; slight nausea; a bloated feeling after a small meal; a bad taste in the mouth; and vague stomach pain.

Q: *How is gastritis treated?*

A: Acute gastritis improves of its own accord, so treatment is directed at the symptoms; antacid preparations and anti-nauseant drugs are often prescribed. Chronic gastritis can be treated only by eliminating the causative factor, for example, alcohol, smoking, or highly spiced or other foods that are difficult to digest. Sometimes antacid drugs are recommended for the relief of indigestion.

Gastroenteritis is any inflammation of the lining of the stomach and intestinal tract. The inflammation is usually caused by a viral infection. If it occurs in infants, there is severe liquid loss, and the patient may require hospital treatment. But gastroenteritis can also be caused by alcohol, certain drugs, food allergies, contaminated food, and certain bacterial and viral infections. The symptoms of gastroenteritis are vomiting, abdominal cramps, diarrhoea, and, in severe cases, exhaustion.

Q: *How is gastroenteritis treated?*

A: The symptoms are treated, not the cause. The patient must stop drinking alcohol and must replace essential nutrients, especially liquids, that are lost through vomiting or diarrhoea. A bland diet is often prescribed. A doctor may prescribe antinauseant drugs for vomiting; anti-spasmodic drugs for cramps; antihist-amine drugs for food allergies; or antibiotic drugs, such as penicillin or ampicillin, for bacterial infection.
See also GASTRITIS.

Gastroenterostomy is an artificial opening that is made between the stomach and the small intestine. The operation (gastroenter-ostomy) is necessary if the muscle that surrounds the stomach opening is scarred and unable to pass food normally from the stomach. It is sometimes done as alternative surgical treatment for a duodenal ulcer (*see* ULCER). When removing part of the stomach (partial gastrectomy), a surgeon may perform a gastroenterostomy to connect the remaining part of the stomach to the small intestine. The lower opening is made into the jejunum beyond the duodenum.

Gastroscopy is the examination of the internal surface of the stomach through a special instrument (gastroscope) that is passed through the mouth and down the oesophagus. The gastroscope may be either a straight tube or flexible FIBRESCOPE. Gastro-scopy is a branch of ENDOSCOPY.

Gastrostomy is an opening that is made from the outside surface of the abdomen into the stomach. The operation (called a gastros-tomy) may be performed if there is some obstruction in, or damage to, the oesophagus that prevents foods from passing down it (for example, cancer, or severe scarring following acid poisoning at the lower end). A gastro-stomy allows the patient to be fed through the opening directly into the stomach. Gastrostomies are often performed as a tem-porary measure after major gastrointestinal surgery to allow stomach and abdominal tissue to heal completely.

Gaucher's disease is a rare inherited disorder caused by the absence of an enzyme that is necessary for the processing by the body of a particular group of fatty acids. The age of onset varies greatly. There is no treatment for this disease. Children generally die of the disease within one to two years of its onset, but death in adults usually results from a complication such as pneumonia.

Gene is the basic unit of HEREDITY that car-ries "instructions" for a particular charac-teristic. Within the nucleus of nearly all human cells there are twenty-three pairs of CHROMOSOMES, which contain an unknown number of genes. Exceptions are sex cells (eggs and sperm), which contain only twenty-three single chromosomes each. When an egg and a sperm fuse at fertilization, the resultant embryo carries genes from each parent cell.

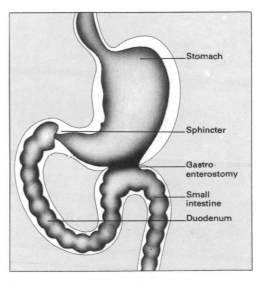

Gastroenterostomy connects stomach and small intestine to by-pass the duodenum.

Stomach

Sphincter

Gastro-enterostomy

Small intestine

Duodenum

Genetic abnormality

Genetic abnormality is a disorder caused by an abnormality of a GENE, or by an incorrect number of chromosomes.

Q: What genetic abnormalities commonly occur?

A: Conditions such as ACHONDROPLASIA, HAEMOLYTIC DISEASE OF THE NEWBORN, SICKLE CELL ANAEMIA, DOWN'S SYNDROME, and CLEFT PALATE are among the commonest genetic abnormalities. There are more than 2,000 genetic disorders, some of which are extremely rare, such as PHENYLKETONURIA, an inherited metabolic disorder.

Q: Are all genetic abnormalities immediately apparent?

A: No. Some genetic abnormalities, such as TAY-SACHS DISEASE, affect the metabolism in subtle ways and may not become apparent until several months after birth. Others, such as HUNTINGTON'S CHOREA, may not appear until the individual reaches middle age.

Q: Can normal parents have children with genetic abnormalities?

A: Yes. The effects of an abnormal gene may be masked by a normal gene in either one or both of the parents. In such a case, the parents will appear to be completely normal, but their children may be affected. HAEMOPHILIA is an example of a condition in which this situation could occur. Genetic abnormalities in children with normal parents may also occur if there is a spontaneous mutation, or change, of the parental genes, or if there is a

fault in the process of egg or sperm production.

Q: Can genetic abnormalities be treated?

A: Although most genetic abnormalities are untreatable, there are a few that can be treated. Those suffering from phenylketonuria can be given a phenyl-alanine-free diet during the first few years of life while the nervous system is developing, after which they can lead a normal life. Those with COELIAC DISEASE can prevent the occurrence of any symptoms by having a gluten-free diet throughout their lives. Cleft palate and SPINA BIFIDA may be treated surgically, although with spina bifida, the success of the treatment depends upon the initial severity of the condition.

See also GENETIC COUNSELLING.

Genetic counselling is a branch of medicine that provides and interprets information about human genetics. The main object of genetic counselling is to prevent the occurrence of congenital anomalies.

Q: What information will a genetic counsellor require?

A: A counsellor will need to know the ages of the couple; whether either of the couple, or any of their close relatives, has a congenital abnormality; and whether either has had children with an inherited disorder. A counsellor will need as complete a family health history as possible, perhaps going back for several generations. A counsellor may also perform certain tests to determine whether either of the couple has an inherited disorder.

Q: Are there any disorders that do not affect the parents but which may occur in their children?

A: Yes. If both parents have one recessive gene for the same disorder, neither will exhibit any abnormality. However, if a child inherits both recessive genes, one from each parent, then the disorder will appear. In such a situation, there is a 25 per cent chance that the child will inherit both genes.

Q: What information does a genetic counsellor give?

A: A counsellor explains about dominant and recessive genes; the kinds of chromosomal abnormalities that may occur; and why certain conditions appear. If the couple has a child with a genetic disorder, a counsellor explains the chances of a second child suffering from the same disorder. Similarly, if one or both parents has an inherited disorder, a counsellor tells them about the chances of

Down's syndrome occurs when an extra chromosome appears in the cell make-up.

a child inheriting the same disorder.

A genetic counsellor's task is to provide as much information as possible. It is not for the counsellor to advise on whether to have a baby or not. That decision rests with the couple. But many couples have found the decision easier to make when they have been made aware of the facts.

Q: *Can anything be done to warn a pregnant woman of an abnormal foetus?*

A: Yes. In the fourth month of pregnancy AMNIOCENTESIS, the sampling of fluid from the bag around the foetus, may be performed. If an abnormality is detected, the pregnancy may be terminated if the parents wish it.

Q: *How can genetic counselling be obtained?*

A: If a couple want genetic counselling, they should consult their family doctor or an obstetrician, who will refer them to a genetic counsellor.

See also GENETIC ABNORMALITY; PREGNANCY AND CHILDBIRTH.

Genitourinary. *See* UROGENITAL.

Genu valgum. *See* KNOCK-KNEE.

Genu varum. *See* BOW-LEGS.

Germ is any microorganism, especially one that causes disease, such as a specific bacterium, virus, fungus, or protozoan. The term also describes rudimentary living matter that has the capacity to develop into an organ, part, or organism. Germ cell is another name for a single egg (ovum) or sperm.

German measles, or rubella, is an infectious viral disease that produces a rash. The incubation period varies between two and three weeks. The patient can transmit the virus during a period from one week before the appearance of the rash to one week after it first appears. Quarantine is three weeks.

Q: *What are the symptoms of German measles?*

A: Initial symptoms include drowsiness, headache, fever, and a sore throat. There may be swelling of the lymph glands behind the ears and down the side of the neck.

The eruption of an itchy rash of small pink and red spots follows, and the patient's temperature rises to about 38°C (101°F). The rash spreads from the face down the whole body, and usually lasts between two and four days.

Q: *How is German measles treated?*

A: There is no cure for German measles. Treatment is directed towards alleviating the symptoms, with aspirin for fever and for pain in the joints.

Q: *What complications may occur with German measles?*

A: Rarely, a form of ENCEPHALITIS (inflammation of the brain) may develop, and a mild temporary form of arthritis. German measles is particularly dangerous to an unborn child if the mother is in the first three months of pregnancy because it may cause CONGENITAL ANOMALIES. If this occurs, the pregnancy can be terminated (by an abortion) if the parents wish it.

Q: *What should a pregnant woman do if she is exposed to German measles?*

A: She should consult a doctor immediately. The doctor may test her blood for rubella antibodies which, if present, will prevent infection. If the blood is low in antibodies, further tests are needed to see whether infection has occurred.

Q: *Can German measles be prevented?*

A: Yes. German measles vaccine is given to girls at puberty, usually at the age of eleven, by school medical authorities, and may give lifetime immunity.

Gigantism is an adolescent condition of abnormal height resulting from excessive growth hormone secretion from the pituitary gland. *See* ACROMEGALY.

Gingivitis is inflammation of the gums accompanied by pain, swelling, and a tendency to bleed. If the inflammation is left untreated the teeth may become loose or fall out. The most common cause of gingivitis is poor dental hygiene. Gingivitis may also be caused by ill-fitting dentures; vitamin C deficiency disease, known as scurvy; generalized inflammation of the mouth (stomatitis); or as a complication of diabetes, leukaemia, or pregnancy. In severe cases of gingivitis,

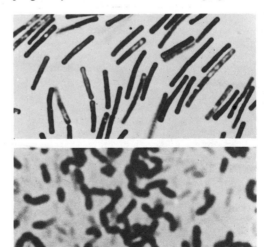

Germs of the anthrax (above) and streptococcal (below) varieties, highly magnified.

Gland

some of the inflamed gum may be removed.

See also DENTAL DISORDERS.

Gland is a body organ made up of specialized tissue that secretes a fluid. There are two types of glands: an exocrine gland secretes fluid into a duct or tube, and an ENDOCRINE GLAND secretes directly into the bloodstream. *See* ADRENAL GLANDS; BARTHOLIN'S GLAND; CORPUS LUTEUM; ISLETS OF LANGERHANS; OVARY; PANCREAS; PARATHYROID GLANDS; PITUITARY GLAND; PROSTATE GLAND; SALIVARY GLANDS; TESTIS; THYROID GLAND.

See also LACRIMATION; LACTATION.

Glandular fever, also called mononucleosis and infectious mononucleosis, is an infectious illness caused by a herpes virus (Epstein-Barr virus). Most common in people aged between fifteen and twenty-five, glandular fever is spread by saliva and nasal secretions. It is only mildly infectious.

Q: What are the symptoms of glandular fever?

A: About a month after contracting the disease, the patient has a period of in- creasing fatigue, lethargy, and a slight fever that lasts for seven to ten days. This is followed by a sore throat, similar to tonsillitis, with a high fever and general- ized enlargement of the lymph glands in the neck. There may be a faint pink rash over the body. The acute phase of the illness lasts for seven to ten days, and the fever then subsides slowly.

There is no cure for glandular fever. It should be treated, as for fever, with ample bed rest, painkilling drugs, and mouthwashes for the sore throat. Anti- biotics are of little help, unless a secondary bacterial infection occurs.

The acute phase of the illness is followed by several weeks of lethargy and vague discomfort. During this time a relapse may occur.

Q: How is glandular fever diagnosed and treated?

A: An examination of the white blood cells and a special blood test (the Paul-Bunnell test) confirm the diagnosis and eliminate other conditions with similar symptoms.

Glaucoma is a group of eye diseases charac- terized by the build-up of fluid pressure within the eyeball. The pressure severely affects the eye lens and optic nerve, resulting eventually in blindness.

Primary glaucoma usually occurs without known cause. A high incidence of glaucoma in certain families suggests that it may be an inherited tendency.

Secondary glaucoma is a complication of other eye disorders, such as inflammation of the iris (iritis). Diabetics seem more likely to develop this condition.

Q: What are the symptoms of glaucoma?

A: Acute glaucoma usually occurs suddenly with pain and a dramatic blurring of vision. The patient begins to notice rainbow-coloured halos around lights and bright objects, and a loss of vision at the sides of the field of view (tunnel vision). Eyesight deteriorates, and blindness results if treatment is not obtained promptly. It is more common in long- sighted people.

Chronic glaucoma occurs slowly and without pain, so that an individual is usually unaware of the disorder until it is well advanced.

Q: How does glaucoma cause loss of vision?

A: The pressure of the fluid (aqueous humour) in the front of the lens increases the pressure in the fluid (vitreous humour) behind the lens. The resulting pressure on the optic nerve damages its blood supply and results in field defects which the patient may not notice until they are quite advanced.

Q: How is glaucoma treated?

A: If the condition is detected early, drug treatment prevents later damage to sight. Various eye drops can be used at regular intervals to reduce pressure within the eyeball. An ophthalmologist may prescribe pilocarpine, which increases the size of the opening through which the aqueous humour drains. Many other drops can also decrease the secretion of the aqueous fluid. A common one is timolol maleate. These drugs reduce the pressure in the eyeball. Diuretic drugs, such as acetazolamide, not only increase the loss of water from the body but also reduce the secretion of aqueous fluid.

If drug treatment fails, surgery is necessary. An ophthalmic surgeon makes a new drainage channel for the aqueous fluid so that it can escape more easily. The pressure within the eye is thus permanently reduced.

Glioma is a malignant (cancerous) tumour in the web-like tissue that supports nerves and the brain. A glioma may develop slowly, or grow rapidly. It is treated either by surgical removal or with RADIOTHERAPY.

Globulin is one of a group of simple proteins in the blood plasma. Its main subgroups are alpha, beta, and gamma globulin. The blood clotting agent, fibrinogen, is a globulin.

Globus hystericus is the feeling of a lump in the throat at times of anxiety or emotion. It is also a symptom of HYSTERIA. The "lump" is caused by the throat muscles remaining under greater tension than usual.

Glucose

Glomerulonephritis is a form of NEPHRITIS that involves the glomeruli, clusters of tiny blood vessels that filter the blood to extract urine in the kidneys. Glomerulonephritis may be either acute or chronic.

Q: What are the symptoms of acute glomerulonephritis?

A: Acute glomerulonephritis often follows a sore throat caused by a streptococcal infection. It is more common in children than in adults. About two weeks after the onset of infection, the patient may suddenly suffer from headaches, and backache. The face swells, and the patient passes bloodstained, "smoky", or brown urine. These symptoms last for several days and the condition gradually improves within a few weeks.

Q: What causes acute glomerulonephritis?

A: In most cases, it results from a reaction to one of the types of streptococcal bacteria that cause sore throats or skin infections. The reaction damages the glomeruli, and leads to the retention of salt, water, and nitrogenous waste substances in the bloodstream, and haematuria (blood in the urine). In many cases, the cause of glomerulonephritis is not known.

Q: How is acute glomerulonephritis treated?

A: In most cases, the disease is mild enough to be treated by a restriction of salt and fluid intake, with total bed rest. If a bacterial infection is present, a doctor usually prescribes antibiotic drugs.

Q: What are the symptoms of chronic glomerulonephritis?

A: The symptoms develop slowly over a period of several months, and the condition may not be detected until it is in its final stages. The symptoms include nausea, vomiting, and kidney failure. There is also high blood pressure, and the risk of heart failure. Usually, chronic glomerulonephritis is detected during a routine examination, when protein and small amounts of blood are found in the urine.

Q: How is chronic glomerulonephritis treated?

A: Treatment involves a strict diet, with restriction of salt and protein intake, and drugs to reduce high blood pressure. In severe cases, kidney dialysis and kidney transplantation may be necessary.

Glomus tumour is the painful but benign (noncancerous) enlargement of the glomus, a collection of tiny arteries with nerve endings found in the nailbeds and the pads of the fingers, toes, ears, hands, and feet. Usually located beneath a fingernail, a glomus tumour causes purplish-red discoloration with slight swelling, extreme tender-

ness, and sometimes shooting pain. Treatment is surgical removal.

Glossitis is inflammation of the tongue. Acute glossitis is often associated with other mouth disorders, such as GINGIVITIS or generalized STOMATITIS. Symptoms of acute glossitis include a painful, sometimes ulcerated, tongue, thick and sticky saliva, and difficulty in swallowing. The patient may also complain of unpleasant taste and odour.

Chronic glossitis is associated with chronic ill health, DYSPEPSIA, and septic teeth. Other causes include gastritis, smoking, alcohol consumption, and sometimes the use of antibiotic drugs.

Q: How is glossitis treated?

A: Acute glossitis is treated with antiseptic mouthwashes and an anaesthetic solution to reduce pain. Chronic glossitis is treated by improving the general health of the patient.

Glucagon is a hormone secreted by the pancreas. It stimulates the conversion in the liver of GLYCOGEN into GLUCOSE, and the release of glucose into the bloodstream.

Glucose is a simple sugar that is essential to body cells for energy. It is the intermediate product in the breakdown of carbohydrates in food (sugars and starches). Glucose passes into the bloodstream from the intestines and is stored, as GLYCOGEN, in the liver. The amount of glucose in the blood is called the blood sugar content. This is carefully regulated by the pancreatic hormone INSULIN and, to a lesser extent, by other hormones such as glucagon, cortisol, thyroxine, and adrenaline. Insufficient insulin produces

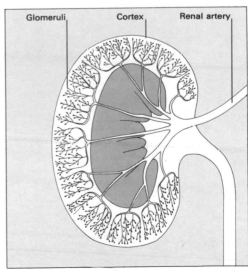

Glomerulonephritis occurs when the glomeruli within the kidney become inflamed or infected.

221

Glucose tolerance test

high blood sugar. *See* DIABETES MELLITUS.

Q: *What other disorders are associated with abnormal blood sugar levels?*

A: High blood sugar, or HYPERGLYCAEMIA, is associated with acromegaly, haemochromatosis, hyperthyroidism, and hyperadrenalism. Low blood sugar, or HYPOGLYCAEMIA, is associated with Addison's disease, insulin shock, hypopituitarism, and myxoedema. *See* GLUCOSE TOLERANCE TEST.

Glucose tolerance test is a procedure that a doctor carries out to determine whether a patient is able to use and store GLUCOSE normally. The test is most commonly carried out to diagnose DIABETES MELLITUS, but is also used to assess the functioning of the liver and the thyroid gland.

After a period of fasting, the patient's blood and urine are tested for glucose. Then, a measured quantity of glucose is administered as a drink or by injection. Further blood and urine samples are taken at regular intervals for two to four hours. A normal result shows a maximum level of glucose in the blood about an hour after the dose, followed by a gradual return to the normal level during the second hour. An abnormal result reveals an unusually high rise in the blood sugar level, an extremely slow return to normal, and sugar in the urine (glycosuria).

Glue ear is an accumulation of sticky glue-like mucus in the middle ear. It occurs most often in children aged five to eight, and usually after acute otitis media has been treated with antibiotics. It is treated by decongestant medicines and by the insertion of small tubes (grommets) to drain out the mucus.

Gluten is the insoluble protein component of cereal grains such as barley, oats, and wheat. It is also found in certain vegetables.

See also COELIAC DISEASE.

Glycogen is the form of carbohydrate in which GLUCOSE is stored in the liver and muscles. It acts as an energy reserve for the body, and can quickly be changed into glucose.

Glycosuria is the medical term for glucose in the urine. *See* GLUCOSE TOLERANCE TEST.

Goitre is an enlargement of the THYROID GLAND. The resulting bulge on the neck may become extremely large, but most simple goitres are brought under control before this happens. Occasionally a simple goitre may cause some difficulty in breathing and swallowing. An overactive thyroid gland, known as HYPERTHYROIDISM, may also produce a goitre.

Q: *What causes a goitre?*

A: Iodine is the principal component of thyroxine, the thyroid gland's main hormone. If there is not enough iodine in the diet, there is insufficient thyroxine, and the pituitary gland responds by releasing more thyroid-stimulating hormone. This causes enlargement of the thyroid gland.

However, a goitre may also be caused by overactivity of the pituitary gland or by overactivity of the thyroid gland itself. Other causes include reduced activity of the thyroid gland because of inflammation (thyroiditis), so that the gland swells in order to produce more thyroxine.

Q: *How is a simple goitre treated?*

A: Iodized salt added to the diet is an effective treatment, as well as a preventative measure. The best drug for treating goitre caused by hypothyroidism (underactivity of the thyroid gland) is thyroxine. Such treatment prevents the pituitary gland from secreting too much thyroid-stimulating hormone. Lumps or nodules on the thyroid gland are removed surgically in case they are cancerous. Inflammation (thyroiditis) may be part of a general illness, and the goitre improves when the patient recovers. Goitres resulting from the hormone requirements of adolescence or pregnancy disappear when the demand for thyroxine is reduced naturally.

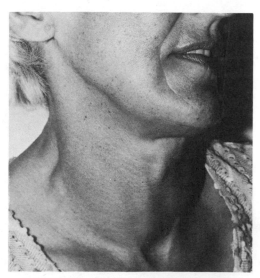

Goitre is an enlargement of the thyroid gland caused by a number of different disorders.

A talk about Gonorrhoea

Gonorrhoea is a highly contagious venereal (sexually transmitted) disease. It is common throughout the world and is widespread in the U.K. If left untreated it can lead to sterility. In babies infected by their mother, it can be a cause of blindness.

Most cases of gonorrhoea can be treated successfully with antibiotics, if reported to a doctor in time, although no immunity is given against reinfection. Any person who has a discharge from the genitals should report it to a doctor at once. This consultation is important because it increases the chances of successful treatment.

Q: *What are the symptoms of gonorrhoea?*

A: In a male, a thick, yellow discharge from the penis occurs within two to ten days after infection. Inflammation and pain in the urethra (the tube through which urine is passed) are common, and urination becomes slow and difficult. If left untreated, the discharge becomes clear and sticky for several months before symptoms of fever and swollen lymph glands in the groin appear. A small number of males may develop no symptoms at all, though they are still capable of spreading the infection to a sexual partner.

In a female, the infection may not produce symptoms and so she is unaware that she may be infecting the person, or people with whom she comes into sexual contact. Occasionally, however, symptoms do develop slowly. These include vaginal discharge, painful or frequent urination, or pain in the lower abdomen. Gonorrhoea in the rectum causes anal discharge and pain; in the throat the condition causes a sore throat.

Q: *What causes gonorrhoea?*

A: Gonorrhoea is caused by the gonococcus bacterium, *Neisseria gonorrhoeae*. In most cases, the bacteria cause inflammation of the mucous membranes of the urogenital tract, but they may also affect the membranes of the mouth, the conjunctiva, or the rectum.

Q: *How is gonorrhoea diagnosed?*

A: For a male, a test (Gram's stain) of the urethral discharge produces a reliable diagnosis. In a female, diagnosis is not as reliable; however, the organism can often be cultured.

Q: *How is gonorrhoea treated?*

A: All cases of gonorrhoea, even if only suspected, must be treated by a doctor. The patient's partner must also see the doctor. There is no home cure for the disease, nor will it disappear if left alone. Antibiotic treatment with penicillin is usually successful. Some strains of the bacteria are resistant to penicillin,

however, and these can be treated with other antibiotics.

Q: *What are the possible complications of gonorrhoea?*

A: Neglected cases of gonorrhoea become chronic. In a male, infection spreads from the mucous membranes into deep tissues, such as the bladder, prostate gland, and epididymis. Sometimes the urethra becomes scarred, which makes urination slow and difficult, and in some cases sterility may result.

In a female, the chronic infection may spread to the womb, fallopian tubes, and ovaries, and cause sterility. A pregnant woman with untreated gonorrhoea infects her baby's eyes during birth as the baby passes through the birth canal.

Q: *How can a person avoid catching gonorrhoea?*

A: A person can avoid catching gonorrhoea by avoiding sexual contact with an infected person. Use of the condom (sheath) offers some protection against catching the disease.

See also VENEREAL DISEASES.

Gout is a metabolic disorder characterized by inflammation and pain in affected joints. It is caused by an excess of URIC ACID in the blood and tissues. Crystals of the acid form under the skin and in the joints, causing local pain. In normal circumstances, uric acid above a certain low concentration is excreted in the urine. Gout occurs either when too little uric acid is excreted, or when there is too much of

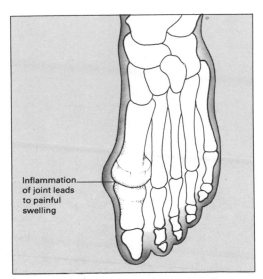

Inflammation of joint leads to painful swelling

Gout is caused by the formation of uric acid crystals that cause joint inflammation.

Graafian follicle

the acid for the kidneys to excrete. Contrary to popular belief, gout has little to do with diet, or alcohol intake.

Q: *What are the symptoms of gout?*

A: An attack begins suddenly with severe pain and swelling in a joint, often in the big toe. The overlying skin becomes red and shiny. A severe attack may cause fever and nausea. Untreated, an attack of gout lasts between three and seven days. Even when the symptoms disappear, further attacks are likely.

Q: *What brings on an attack of gout?*

A: In general, the causes of acute attacks of gout are not known, but some drugs, for example, diuretics, and minor injuries or excessive drinking and eating can bring on an attack.

Q: *How is gout diagnosed?*

A: A doctor has to make sure that the inflamed joint is not the result of infection, osteoarthritis, or acute rheumatoid arthritis. A diagnosis of gout is made after a blood test reveals an abnormally high level of uric acid in the blood. Sometimes the fluid from an inflamed joint is examined for crystals.

Q: *How is gout treated?*

A: In an acute attack, the joint is rested until the pain subsides. The drug colchicine can bring relief within a few hours, but possible side effects often make it unsuitable. Other drugs prescribed include phenylbutazone and indomethacin. Allopinurol is taken daily to prevent attacks of gout.

Q: *Does gout have any complications?*

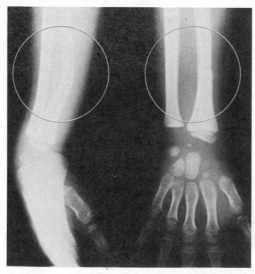

Greenstick fracture occurs when the bone splits and bends, without breaking cleanly.

A: Yes. If gout is not treated in its early stages, the condition may become chronic. Chronic gout results in deposits of uric acid (tophi) in the joints. These deposits may cause permanent arthritis. The most serious danger is that crystals may be deposited in the kidneys.

Graafian follicle is the mature follicle in an ovary that contains the ovum before OVULATION. When the follicle ruptures under the influence of luteinizing hormone (LH) the ovum is released. The CORPUS LUTEUM develops within the ruptured follicle.

Graft is healthy tissue that is transferred surgically from one place to another. Skin is the tissue most commonly grafted, although bones, tendons, and nerves can also be grafted. A cornea from the eye of a recently dead donor can be grafted to a patient's damaged cornea. The technique of skin grafting is invaluable for the treatment of deep burns and similar injuries. Healing time is reduced and the grafted skin is stronger and less disfiguring than the scarred tissue that would otherwise form.

Grand mal. *See* EPILEPSY.

Granuloma inguinale is a venereal (sexually transmitted) disease caused by the bacterium *Donovania granulomatis*. The first symptom is a small, painless lump in the genital area. If neglected, this rapidly breaks down and forms a deep ulcer that spreads slowly. New ulcers may develop and cover the entire genital area, buttocks, and abdomen. Effective treatment can be given with antibiotic drugs.

Graves' disease. *See* THYROTOXICOSIS.

Greenstick fracture is a type of bone fracture common among children. The fractured bone cracks only half across its width; the remaining half merely bends. *See* FRACTURES.

Grief is a normal emotion of intense sorrow expressed in response to a great loss, such as the death of a friend or relative.

Q: *How may somebody be helped in the initial stages of grief?*

A: There are many ways to help a grieving person. Give practical help with the domestic tasks. Give emotional support by listening to the grieving person as he or she talks about the loss. The person may also be helped by talking to a clergyman. Encourage the person to have a rest during the day to maintain physical strength. Sedatives, prescribed by a doctor, may help to restore a normal sleep pattern, and the doctor may also prescribe tranquillizers for times of acute stress, such as a funeral.

Q: *How may a grieving person be helped after the initial stages?*

A: The grieving person should be continually

invited to join in family and social events, even if the invitations are always refused.

Despite the good will and efforts of family and friends, some people seem to cling morbidly to grief. This prolonged grief is sometimes a sign of underlying guilt and remorse and the person may require psychiatric help.

Gripes. *See* ABDOMINAL PAIN; COLIC.

Grippe. *See* INFLUENZA.

Gristle. *See* CARTILAGE.

Group therapy is psychiatric treatment based on discussions among a group of people who have similar problems. *See* PSYCHOTHERAPY

Growing pains is a vague term for muscle pains in children. These pains usually have no obvious cause; they are not caused by an injury, and they are not related to rapid growth. Reassurance that nothing is seriously wrong and gentle massage of the affected limb is usually the only treatment necessary.

Guinea worm is a long, thin worm (*Dracunculus medinensis*) that is common in parts of Africa, India, Turkey, thé West Indies, and South America. People who drink water containing larvae of the worm become infected. The larvae develop in the human body into worms that in turn bore toward the surface to discharge their larvae. Local swelling and pain are often accompanied by an itching rash, vomiting, and diarrhoea. Drug treatment usually cures the condition.

Gullet is a common term for the oesophagus. *See* OESOPHAGUS.

Gum, in medicine, is the dense fibrous tissue that surrounds the necks of the teeth. The gums are covered by a mucous membrane. It is important to keep the gums healthy by massaging them when cleaning the teeth, and by keeping the teeth free of tartar and food particles.

Fairly common gum disorders include GINGIVITIS, GUMBOIL, MOUTH ULCER, PERIODONTITIS, and VINCENT'S ANGINA. Spongy, ulcerated gums may be a symptom of DIABETES MELLITUS, LEUKAEMIA, TUBERCULOSIS, STOMATITIS, and digestive disorders. Gums that bleed easily usually indicate gingivitis, but such a condition may also be caused by SCURVY or inflammatory illnesses such as PYORRHOEA or TRENCH MOUTH.

See also DENTAL DISORDERS.

Gumboil is a swelling on the gum. It is a type of abscess, usually caused by local infection at the root of a tooth. The affected area of gum is typically red, swollen, extremely tender, and painful.

Q: How is a gumboil treated?

A: Painkilling drugs and hot mouthwashes relieve some of the symptoms. A dentist may prescribe an antibiotic drug such as penicillin. The gumboil may burst of its own accord or it may have to be cut open.

Gumma is a soft tumour of the tissues (granulation tissue). The swelling is characteristic of the third stage of SYPHILIS but it is unusual for the disease to reach this stage untreated. A gumma may also occur as a reaction to tuberculosis or yaws. Gummata usually affect the liver. Sometimes the heart, brain, testicles, bone, and skin are affected. On the skin, gummata may ulcerate. Treatment with penicillin is effective.

Guthrie test, or PKU test, is performed on all babies about one week after birth to detect the presence of phenylalanine in the blood. *See* PHENYLKETONURIA.

Gut is a popular term for the INTESTINE.

Gynaecological disorders. The following table lists alphabetically some of the disorders that affect the reproductive organs of women, according to their chief symptoms. Each disorder has a separate entry in the A-Z section of this book. It is important to remember that some of the symptoms are not necessarily abnormal: for example, vaginal discharge is heavier than normal at certain times during the menstrual cycle and before intercourse. Not all of the disorders listed below require medical attention, but if·there is any doubt, a doctor should be consulted. Breast problems are listed under BREAST DISORDERS. Similarly, problems during pregnancy are discussed under the heading PREGNANCY AND CHILDBIRTH. Other relevant sections in the A-Z section of this book are MENSTRUAL PROBLEMS and SEXUAL PROBLEMS.

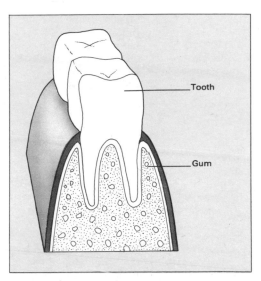

Gum is a fleshy tissue that protects teeth below the level of the hard outer enamel.

Gynaecological disorders

Symptom	Related disorder	Symptom	Related disorder
Absence of, or missed period	Disorders of ADRENAL GLANDS or THYROID GLAND AMENORRHOEA (lack of menstruation) Marked ANAEMIA ANOREXIA NERVOSA (psychological avoidance of eating) CANCER CYST in an ovary ECTOPIC PREGNANCY (development of a foetus outside the womb) Malnutrition (*see* NUTRITIONAL DISORDERS) MENOPAUSE (cessation of periods) Pregnancy (*see* PREGNANCY AND CHILDBIRTH) TUBERCULOSIS	Difficult or painful intercourse	FRIGIDITY (psychological dislike of sexual intercourse) HAEMORRHOIDS (piles) Thick or tough HYMEN (membrane across the vagina) extreme OBESITY PROLAPSE (displacement of the womb) RECTOCELE (HERNIA of the rectum) SALPINGITIS (inflammation of a fallopian tube) VAGINISMUS (spasm in the muscles of the vagina) Atrophic VAGINITIS (inflammation of the vagina after menopause) VULVITIS (inflammation of the vulva) VULVOVAGINITIS (inflammation of the vulva and the vagina)
Aches and pains in abdomen or back	CYST in an ovary ENDOMETRITIS (inflammation of the lining of the womb) FIBROID (benign muscle tumour in the womb) Early GONORRHOEA (a venereal disease) MENSTRUATION (normal) Threatened MISCARRIAGE OVULATION (normal) PREMENSTRUAL TENSION PROLAPSE (displacement of the womb) SALPINGITIS (inflammation of a fallopian tube)	Enlarged womb Genital itching or soreness	CANCER FIBROID (benign muscle tumour in the womb) Pregnancy (*see* PREGNANCY AND CHILDBIRTH) ALLERGY ANXIETY DIABETES MELLITUS LEUKOPLAKIA (itchy white patches on the vulva) LICHEN PLANUS (itchy inflammation) MONILIASIS SCABIES (itchy skin disease caused by mites) STRESS VAGINITIS (inflammation of the vagina)
Bleeding after intercourse	CERVICAL EROSION Chronic CERVICITIS (inflammation of the cervix) POLYP in cervix VAGINITIS (inflammation of the vagina) CANCER of the cervix	Headache, dizziness, moody spells	MENOPAUSE (cessation of menstruation periods in middle age) PREMENSTRUAL TENSION
Difficult or painful intercourse	BARTHOLIN'S CYST (cyst in a gland in the vagina) DYSPAREUNIA (painful intercourse) ENDOMETRIOSIS (displacement of tissue from the lining of the womb) Fissure-in-ano (*see* FISSURE)	Heavy or irregular bleeding	CERVICAL EROSION ECTOPIC PREGNANCY (development of a foetus outside the womb) ENDOMETRIOSIS (displacement of tissue from the lining of the womb)

Symptom	Related disorder	Symptom	Related disorder
Heavy or irregular bleeding	ENDOMETRITIS (inflammation of the lining of the womb) FIBROID (benign muscle tumour in the womb) Onset of MENOPAUSE MENORRHAGIA (heavy periods) METROPATHIA HAEMORRHAGICA (abnormal bleeding from the womb) METRORRHAGIA (irregular periods) POLYP (noncancerous growth in the womb) SALPINGITIS (inflammation of a fallopian tube) TUMOUR in the womb or ovary	Painful period	ENDOMETRIOSIS (displacement of tissue from the lining of the womb)
		Postmenopausal bleeding	CANCER of the womb CYSTITIS (inflammation of the bladder) ENDOMETRITIS (inflammation of the lining of the womb) OESTROGEN drug therapy VAGINITIS (inflammation of the vagina) CYSTITIS (inflammation of the bladder)
		Urinary problems related to genital disorders	"Honeymoon" CYSTITIS NONSPECIFIC URETHRITIS (inflammation of the urethra) STRESS INCONTINENCE (involuntary urination)
Hot flushes	MENOPAUSE (cessation of menstruation periods in middle age)	Vaginal discharge	CANCER of the womb CERVICAL EROSION CERVICITIS (inflammation of the cervix) GONORRHOEA (a venereal disease) LEUCORRHOEA (normal vaginal discharge) POLYP in the cervix SALPINGITIS (inflammation of a fallopian tube) VAGINITIS
Infertility	Extensive ENDOMETRIOSIS (displacement of tissue from the lining of the womb) ENDOMETRITIS (inflammation of the lining of the womb) Failure of ovulation FIBROID (benign muscle tumour in the womb) FRIGIDITY (psychological dislike of intercourse) GONORRHOEA (a venereal disease) Poor or absent sperm count in man SALPINGITIS (inflammation of a fallopian tube)		
Ovarian problems	AMENORRHOEA (absence of periods) CYST in an ovary OOPHORITIS (inflammation of an ovary) TUMOUR in an ovary TURNER'S SYNDROME (sex chromosome abnormality)		
Painful period	DYSMENORRHOEA (medical term for painful periods)		

Pathway of gonorrhoeal infection in the female

① Cervix
② Uterus
③ Fallopian tube
④ Ovary

Gonorrhoea in females may lead to sterility if it is not treated at an early stage.

Gynaecology

Symptom	Related disorder
Vaginal discharge, with inflamed vulva	TUMOUR
	ENDOMETRITIS
	VAGINITIS, including
	TRICHOMONAS VAGINALIS
	infection and vaginal
	MONILIASIS
	VULVITIS

Gynaecology is the branch of medicine that specializes in diseases of women, particularly of the reproductive organs.

Gynaecomastia is the appearance of female breasts in a boy or man.

At puberty, sensitivity to female hormones produces slight gynaecomastia in about thirty per cent of boys. These hormones are produced normally by the adrenal glands before the major development of the testicles. Apart from the embarrassment that the condition may cause, there is no medical need to worry, and no need for treatment. Gynaecomastia at this age disappears naturally after six to twelve months.

In men, gynaecomastia may be the result of some forms of drug treatment, particularly in the treatment of cancer of the prostate.

H

Habit spasm. *See* TIC.

Haemachromatosis. *See* HAEMOCHROMATOSIS.

Haemangioma is a tumour composed of blood vessels. It is usually benign (noncancerous) and generally affects the skin but

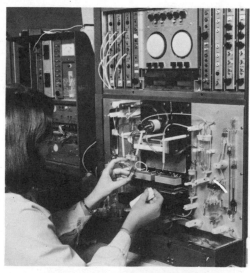

Haematology is the study of blood. Advanced machinery enables accurate blood analysis.

may involve other parts of the body, such as the intestine, or the nervous system. The most common haemangiomas are types of BIRTHMARK.

Haematemesis. *See* BLOOD, VOMITING OF.

Haematocolpos is a rare condition in which menstrual blood is retained because the HYMEN completely closes the entrance to the vagina.

Treatment is to make a small opening in the hymen to allow the blood to escape.

Haematology is the study of BLOOD and blood disorders.

Haematoma is a blood clot in an organ or within body tissues that forms as a result of an accident or surgery. The blood is usually reabsorbed into the body tissues and the clot disappears.

Haematuria is the presence of blood in the urine. It is always a symptom of a disorder, and a person with haematuria must consult a doctor immediately.

Small amounts of blood give urine a smoky or cloudy appearance. Larger amounts make the urine dark red or dark brown. But such discoloration is not always a sign of haematuria: urine that has been standing for a while may naturally become cloudy, and reddish urine may also be caused by the pigments in certain foods, such as beets.

See also HAEMOGLOBINURIA; PORPHYRIA.

Haemochromatosis is a disorder in which there are excessive amounts of iron absorbed by the body. It is more common in men than in women. The skin gradually darkens; diabetes mellitus usually develops because of pancreatic damage; and there may be cirrhosis of the liver.

These symptoms may be accompanied by heart failure, hypopituitarism, and loss of sex drive. Haemochromatosis may be fatal if untreated.

Q: How is haemochromatosis treated?

A: Treatment is directed towards removing the deposited iron. This may be achieved by the weekly removal of a pint of blood, because haemoglobin (the red pigment in blood) contains large amounts of iron. When the patient's iron level returns to normal, removal of blood may be continued to prevent reaccumulation of iron, but at less frequent intervals.

Haemoglobin is the iron-containing protein that occurs in RED BLOOD CELLS. It consists of an iron-containing pigment called haeme, and a simple protein, globin. Haemoglobin carries oxygen in the blood from the lungs to the body tissues, and also carries carbon dioxide from the tissues to the lungs.

Q: Are there different forms of haemoglobin?

A: Yes. More than a hundred types of

abnormal haemoglobin have been identified, produced by rare genetic mutations. SICKLE CELL ANAEMIA and THALASSAEMIA, for example, are caused by different abnormal forms of haemoglobin.

Haemoglobinuria is the presence of the red blood pigment HAEMOGLOBIN in the urine.

See also HAEMATURIA; MALARIA; SICKLE CELL ANAEMIA.

Haemolysis is the breakdown of RED BLOOD CELLS with the release of haemoglobin into the blood plasma. It is caused by poison, abnormal haemoglobins, or infections such as malaria. It results in ANAEMIA. Haemolysis is usually slow enough for the red blood cells to be removed by the liver and spleen. But if haemolysis occurs rapidly, it may produce shivering, fever, and JAUNDICE, and the spleen may increase in size.

Haemolytic disease of the newborn, also known medically as hydrops foetalis, erythroblastosis foetalis (icterus gravis neonatorum), or simply Rh factor incompatibility, is a serious condition affecting a baby before, during, and after birth. It is almost always caused by an incompatibility between the BLOOD GROUPS of mother and child in which the mother is Rhesus negative (Rh−) and the foetus is Rhesus positive (Rh+).

Towards the end of a pregnancy, some of the red blood cells of the foetus escape from the placenta into the mother's bloodstream. With the first child, this need create no immediate problem for either mother or foetus – but an Rh− mother will in fact have formed antibodies to repel and destroy the "invading" Rh+ cells. With the second child, if it is Rhesus positive blood group, the antibodies may cross the placenta and cause breakdown (haemolysis) and destruction of the baby's red blood cells.

Q: Can the disease be prevented?

A: Yes. An injection of anti-Rh gamma globulin is usually given to an Rh− mother within the first 72 hours after delivery of an Rh+ baby, so that any foetal blood entering the mother's circulation is destroyed. This prevents antibodies from developing in most mothers and reduces the chances of haemolytic disease in future pregnancies.

But, if necessary, the severely affected foetus can be given a blood transfusion while still in the womb. All the foetal Rh+ blood is replaced by Rh− blood.

Q: What are the symptoms of the disease?

A: Depending on the severity of the condition, the baby may be anaemic, because of the destruction of the blood's red cells, or have jaundice, because the

yellow pigment bilirubin is released as the red cells break down. If too much bilirubin is released, brain damage (kernicterus) and even death may result, often before birth.

Q: How is a newborn baby with haemolytic disease treated?

A: The baby's blood is exchanged for Rh− blood, an exchange transfusion, two or three times.

Haemophilia is a disease caused by an inherited lack of one of the factors needed for normal blood clotting. This lack is due to a sex-linked recessive genetic defect (*see* GENE). Because the gene is sex-linked, haemophilia occurs in men, whereas women carry the abnormal gene without developing the disease.

Q: What are the symptoms of haemophilia?

A: Haemophilia is characterised by repeated episodes of spontaneous internal bleeding, and prolonged external bleeding following even minor injuries.

Q: How is haemophilia treated?

A: Injections of the missing clotting factor stop any bleeding. But for minor injuries, firm pressure over the affected area may stop the bleeding if it is maintained long enough, often an hour or more.

Q: What precautions should a haemophiliac take?

A: A haemophiliac should avoid contact sports, and any activity in which minor injuries are likely. Any operation, either surgical or dental, requires an injection of the missing clotting factor. Haemophiliacs should wear an identity disc.

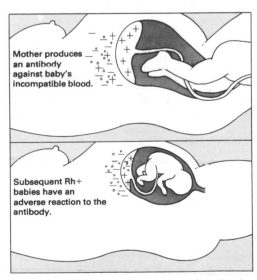

Mother produces an antibody against baby's incompatible blood.

Subsequent Rh+ babies have an adverse reaction to the antibody.

Haemolytic disease of the newborn: first (top), and subsequent pregnancies (foot).

Haemoptysis

Haemoptysis. See BLOOD, SPITTING OF.

Haemorrhage (for EMERGENCY treatment, see First Aid, p.516) is internal or external bleeding. Rapid, heavy bleeding may cause shock; slow continuous bleeding may cause anaemia.

Haemorrhoidal preparations are substances that have a soothing or cleansing action on HAEMORRHOIDS (piles), shrinking them and easing the irritation.

Haemorrhoids (for EMERGENCY treatment, see First Aid, p.586) is the medical name for piles. A haemorrhoid is a mass of distended (varicose) veins just inside the anus. First degree haemorrhoids remain inside the anus; they may bleed from time to time. Second degree haemorrhoids also bleed and may protrude beyond the anus, being felt as a soft swelling during defecation, but spontaneously return inside. Third degree haemorrhoids, once having protruded, remain outside the anus. This type may be accompanied by discharge and itching.

Q: What is the treatment for haemorrhoids?

A: A person suffering from haemorrhoids must eat a high-roughage diet to ensure regular defecation of large, soft stools. This gently stretches the anal sphincter. Ointments, creams, and suppositories may ease the symptoms (see HAEMORRHOIDAL PREPARATIONS). But if the haemorrhoids persist, a doctor should be consulted.

Haemorrhoids can be removed surgically (haemorrhoidectomy).

Haemothorax is blood in the pleural cavity, the space between the lungs and the chest wall. The blood may be removed with a special syringe and needle, or a surgical operation (thoracotomy) may be necessary.

Hair consists of cells of a tough protein called keratin, which grows in the hair follicle. A hair follicle produces and nourishes a hair. The root of the hair (hair bulb) is embedded at the base of the follicle, and it is here that growth takes place. The greasy secretions of a sebaceous gland at the side of the follicle drain into it and lubricate the hair shaft, which can be raised by a muscle attached to the follicle. There are three concentric layers of cells in a hair, and colour is produced in the middle layer.

Q: Why does hair fall out?

A: Hair falls out gradually all over the body to be replaced by new hair. The follicle does not die when hair falls out; it too goes into a static period before then producing a new hair. Baldness results when hair replacement fails to keep up with hair loss (see BALDNESS). Abnormal hair loss (alopecia) may be caused by inflammation of the follicles (see FOLLICULITIS) or some other disorder.

Q: What factors affect the growth and condition of hair?

A: Hair growth is dependent on hormones, particularly the sex hormones. A woman's hair, for example, has a tendency to become greasier just before menstruation, because hormones then stimulate more sebaceous gland secretions, and hormonal changes during pregnancy delay the static phase of hair growth. A decreased thyroid gland or pituitary gland function makes hair become thin, dry, and brittle.

Hair, excess. See HIRSUTISM.

Halitosis. See BAD BREATH.

Hallucinations are false sensory phenomena that have no relation to reality and that may or may not be caused by external stimuli. Hallucinations are different from delusion, which is a positive belief in something unreal. In hallucinations, a person may see, hear, feel, or smell something that does not exist.

Q: What causes hallucinations?

A: Hallucinations may occur as a result of fatigue, particularly if it is accompanied by dehydration, and in an illness that produces a high fever, especially in children. Many drugs produce hallucinations, including sedatives used after a surgical operation, and in drug addiction and alcoholism, the hallucinations may be aggravated by a lack of vitamin B. In some severe forms of mental illness, hallucinations become an integral part of the condition.

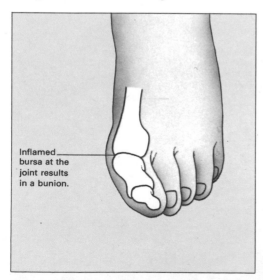

Inflamed bursa at the joint results in a bunion.

Hallux valgus may be caused by badly-fitting shoes that distort the position of the toes.

Hallux rigidus is stiffness and pain in the first joint of the big toe. The condition is usually caused by repeated injury to the joint, but it may be a complication of HALLUX VALGUS.

Hallux valgus is a deformity of the big toe, usually caused by ill-fitting shoes. The toe is angled towards the other toes. The BURSA at the joint becomes inflamed, forming a BUNION. Osteoarthritis may also develop, causing HALLUX RIGIDUS. There are several surgical procedures to correct the condition. Commonly, however, the big toe is straightened, and the arthritic bone and the bunion removed.

Halothane is a gas that is used as a general anaesthetic.

See also ANAESTHETICS.

Hammer toe is a toe deformity in which the first joint is bent downwards at a right angle.

Hamstring is any of the three tendons that connect the muscles at the back of the thigh to the lower leg.

Hand is the end part of the arm. Five long metacarpal bones form the palm of the hand; they are jointed to the bones at the base of each finger. There are three separate bones (phalanges) in each of the four fingers, and two in the thumb. The fingertips are extremely sensitive to pain, temperature, and touch, and are protected by the nails.

Q: How does the hand move?

A: The main muscles that control hand movements are in the forearm, connected to the fingers by long, strong tendons. To prevent friction, the tendons are enclosed in lubricated synovial (membrane lining) sheaths. There are also numerous small muscles in the hand.

Hand-foot-and-mouth disease is a virus infection that occurs in young children, sometimes as a minor epidemic. Small blisters appear on the palms of the hands, the soles of the feet, and in the mouth. It is a mild condition that lasts for about three or four days before recovery occurs naturally.

Hangnail is a partly detached piece of dry skin at the base of a fingernail.

Hangover is the common name for a collection of symptoms caused by drinking an excessive amount of alcohol. These symptoms often include a severe headache, nausea, vomiting, stomachache, dizziness, thirst, and fatigue.

Hansen's disease. *See* LEPROSY.

Hardening of the arteries. *See* ARTERIO-SCLEROSIS.

Hare-lip is a congenital cleft in the front of the upper lip. The cleft may vary in size from a notch to a fissure that extends across the whole lip. Usually it extends from the mouth up into the nostril and can be on one or on sides of the midline. Hare-lip may be associated with CLEFT PALATE.

The treatment for hare-lip is surgery.

Hashimoto's thyroiditis is an inflammation of the THYROID GLAND producing an increase in the fibrous tissue and an infiltration of white blood cells. It is more common in women than in men, and usually develops during middle age. The symptoms, which develop slowly, include lethargy; loss of appetite; dry skin; underactivity of the thyroid gland; and eventually MYXOEDEMA.

Hashish. *See* MARIJUANA.

Hay fever is an allergic condition characterized by irritation of the eyes, nose, and throat, and sometimes a rash. *See* ALLERGY.

Q: What causes hay fever?

A: Dust, grass, flower pollens, and mushroom spores may act as allergens, when they are inhaled, and cause the body to produce an excessive amount of HISTAMINE, a chemical that produces the symptoms of hay fever.

Q: How is hay fever treated?

A: If hay fever is seasonal and not severe, treatment with antihistamine pills and sprays of corticosteroids or sodium cromoglycate may lessen the symptoms. Many cities give a daily pollen count. If the count is high, try to stay indoors, where the air is free from irritants.

If hay fever is severe and long lasting, the cause of the allergy may be found by skin tests, performed by a doctor, to identify the allergen. Following this, a course of desensitising injections may be given before the hay fever season begins.

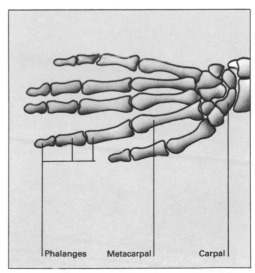

Hand consists of five metacarpal bones and fourteen phalanges.

Headache

A talk about Headache

Headache is a pain or ache across the forehead or within the head itself. It is not a disorder but a symptom. Possible causes of headaches include: (1) conditions associated with emotional disturbances or muscular tension; (2) disorders of the blood vessels of the brain; (3) neuralgia, caused by pressure on nerves; (4) conditions, especially infections, affecting the ears, sinuses, mouth, or the membrane that surrounds the brain; (5) head injuries; (6) conditions that affect the skull; and (7) increased pressure within the brain.

Q: *What are the commonest causes of headache?*

A: One of the commonest causes of a headache is tension in the muscles of the neck and jaw which is associated with fatigue or anxiety.

Another common cause is migraine, in which the headache often occurs in only one half of the head and may be accompanied by nausea and vomiting.

Any generalized infection, such as influenza, may affect the blood vessels and cause a headache. Blood vessels of the brain may also be affected by external factors, such as drinking too much alcohol; smoking excessively; or inhaling or swallowing various chemicals or drugs.

Ear disorders involving inflammation, such as OTITIS and mastoiditis, may cause very severe headaches on the side of the head that is involved. Eye disorders, such as IRITIS, GLAUCOMA, and eye strain, may produce frontal headaches as well as pain around the eye. Sinusitis, particularly of the frontal sinuses above the eyes, may cause a severe ache at the front of the head, usually associated with a respiratory disorder such as a cold or hay fever. Persistent toothache may cause headaches as well as local pain.

A head injury often causes concussion and a generalised headache of variable intensity that seems to get worse during periods of fatigue or emotional stress. It may be accompanied by dizziness, difficulty in sleeping, and loss of concentration. The injured area may also be painful and tender.

Any head injury is potentially serious, especially if there is a history of concussion. A doctor should be consulted so that the skull can be X-rayed and other tests performed.

Q: *How may the common forms of headache be treated?*

A: Aspirin or preparations containing aspirin and paracetamol are usually effective in removing the pain of a normal headache.

A talk about Head injury

Head injury (for EMERGENCY treatment, *see* First Aid, p.552) is damage to the skull or brain. It is one of the most potentially serious types of injury because it threatens the highly complex structure and functioning of the brain.

Q: *What are the various types of skull fractures?*

A: The least serious type is a hairline fracture, in which the skull cracks but the bone does not change position. If a fracture causes the bone to move, the displaced bone may press on to the tissue of the brain. This type of fracture, called a depressed fracture, causes most brain damage.

Q: *What is a brain concussion?*

A: Concussion is a severe jolting of the brain that causes microscopic damage to brain cells. Loss of consciousness may be only momentary, and the patient generally recovers completely. Symptoms of concussion include headache, difficulty in concentrating, blurred vision, feelings of depression and irritability, and, sometimes, nausea. With more serious cases there may also be loss of memory.

Q: *What is a brain contusion?*

A: Contusion of the brain is bruising that damages the nerve centres in the brain. Nerve functioning may become either

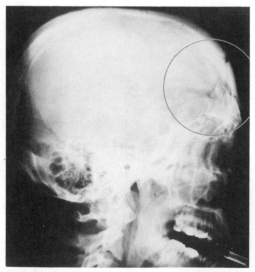

Depressed facture of the front of the skull can be seen on the X-ray photograph

depressed or accelerated.

Q: How are head injuries treated?

A: Although there is little that can be done to repair brain tissue already damaged, there is much that can be done to prevent further harm. Hairline fractures usually heal without complications, and an operation is seldom necessary. A depressed fracture or any type of brain haemorrhage requires an urgent surgical operation. Blood clots are normally removed as soon as possible, bringing about a rapid improvement.

Q: Are there any long-term after effects of head injuries?

A: Yes the brain may become infected as a result of a skull fracture. MENINGITIS is the most serious form of infection, but preventive treatment with antibiotic drugs lessens the risk considerably.

Permanent brain damage can cause a variety of irreversible physical or mental disorders, such as weakness of the limbs (paresis), deafness, blindness, double vision, and speech-related disorders such as APHASIA, are quite common. Possible mental after effects include personality changes and mental impairment. Repeated minor injuries to the head can cause symptoms of disturbed co-ordination, memory, and concentration, and may also affect vision and hearing.

Heaf test is a form of the MANTOUX TEST for TUBERCULOSIS. A drop of tuberculin, prepared from dead tuberculosis, is placed on the skin and is then pricked with special instruments. This will produce a red mark on the skin within a week if the patient has ever had tuberculosis.

Hearing is the perception of sound. For details of how this sense works, *see* EAR.

See also DEAFNESS; EAR DISORDERS.

Hearing aid. *See* DEAFNESS.

Hearing disorders. *See* DEAFNESS; EAR DISORDERS.

Heart is a strong muscular organ the size of a clenched fist, that pumps blood throughout the body. It is situated behind the breastbone (sternum) between the lungs, usually to the left side of the chest.

Q: How does the heart work?

A: There are four chambers in the heart: the right and left atria, and the right and left ventricles. The right and left sides of the heart are totally separate from each other. The atria are thin-walled upper chambers that receive blood from the veins. The ventricles are the lower chambers. The walls of both ventricles are strong, thick, and muscular, but the wall of the left ventricle is thicker and more muscular than the wall of the right ventricle, because it has to pump blood around the entire body, via the AORTA, which is the main blood vessel from the heart.

Deoxygenated blood from the body enters the right ATRIUM from each VENA CAVA, and passes to the right VENTRICLE from which it is pumped through the PULMONARY ARTERY to the lungs. Oxygenated blood from the lungs enters the left atrium from the PULMONARY VEIN, and passes to the left ventricle.

When the atria are full of blood the ventricles relax, allowing blood from the atria to flow into them past the valves that separate the upper and lower chambers. The atria contract and force the rest of the blood into the ventricles. This is called the DIASTOLE. A split second later the ventricles contract, forcing the blood into the arteries past the semilunar valves. This is called the SYSTOLE. Back-flow of blood is prevented by the opening and closing of these valves, which make a characteristic "lub-dub" sound.

A healthy heart can vary in rate from 45 beats a minute to over 180 beats a minute, depending on age.

See also p.8.

Heart attack is the common term for a coronary thrombosis occurring with CORONARY HEART DISEASE. For EMERGENCY treatment, *see* First Aid, p.554.

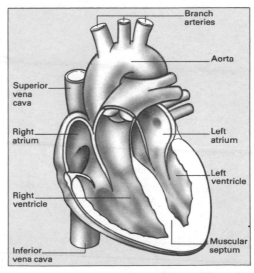

Heart has four chambers: the atria and the ventricles, separated by a muscular septum.

Labels: Branch arteries, Aorta, Superior vena cava, Right atrium, Right ventricle, Inferior vena cava, Left atrium, Left ventricle, Muscular septum

Heartblock

Heartblock is a disorder in the transmission of nerve impulses between the upper chambers (atria) and lower chambers (ventricles) of the heart. A disturbance of this mechanism causes the heart beat to falter or become irregular (arrhythmia).

Q: What are the symptoms of heartblock?

A: A partial heartblock may cause no symptoms, although the irregularity of the heartbeat can be detected with a stethoscope. With a total heartblock, the contractions of the ventricles may not be fast enough to maintain an efficient blood supply. The patient may have bouts of unconsciousness (*see* STOKES-ADAMS ATTACK). At other times, dizziness, faintness, and breathlessness may occur.

Q: What are the causes of heartblock?

A: Heartblock may be associated with congenital heart disease. It can be caused by infection of the heart muscle (myocarditis), damage to heart muscle from rheumatic fever, or a coronary thrombosis.

Q: How is heartblock treated?

A: Patients who have temporary heartblock recover spontaneously when the acute stage of the causative illness has passed. Permanent, complete heartblock may be treated with drugs but the treatment is not curative. The most effective treatment is the addition of an artificial HEART PACEMAKER.

Heartburn, also known as pyrosis, is a burning sensation in the oesophagus (gullet) caused by acid rising from the stomach. It is most frequently associated with INDIGESTION.

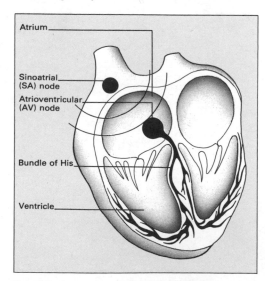

Heartblock occurs when the pacemaker malfunctions, disrupting the heartbeat.

Atrium

Sinoatrial (SA) node

Atrioventricular (AV) node

Bundle of His

Ventricle

Heart disease is the ordinary term used to describe a variety of heart disorders. All the disorders mentioned below are the subjects of individual articles in which symptoms and treatment are discussed.

The sac surrounding the heart, the pericardium, may become inflamed (PERICARDITIS) as a local disease or as part of a general heart inflammation, such as RHEUMATIC FEVER. The heart muscle itself may become inflamed (MYOCARDITIS) or degenerate (CARDIOMYOPATHY) from a variety of causes.

ARTERIOSCLEROSIS can cause CORONARY HEART DISEASE which in turn may lead to coronary thrombosis. The aortic valve is frequently involved, producing narrowing and deformity and, sometimes, backflow of blood because of valvular disease. The distortion of the normal blood flow from valvular disease causes HEART MURMURS.

Hypertension, known commonly as HIGH BLOOD PRESSURE, produces HYPERTROPHY (increase in the size of the heart muscle) and, like other forms of heart disease, may eventually cause heart failure.

Disorders of the normal electrical impulses in the heart may produce atrial FIBRILLATION or HEARTBLOCK, and this can also occur with valvular disease, rheumatic fever, or coronary heart disease.

For further information on other conditions that may affect the heart, *see* ANGINA PECTORIS; BACTERIAL ENDOCARDITIS; BLUE BABY; DEXTROCARDIA; EMBOLISM.

Electrical disorders of the heart include BRADYCARDIA; EXTRASYSTOLE; PAROXYSMAL TACHYCARDIA; STOKES-ADAMS ATTACK; TACHYCARDIA; VASOVAGAL SYNCOPE.

Q: How may a doctor investigate the causes of heart disease?

A: A history of previous illness, such as rheumatic fever or muscle disorder, may help the doctor to interpret any abnormal heart sounds or murmurs. But no specific cause is generally found.

There are many tests that a doctor can use to assess the condition of the heart. Blood tests can detect hormone disorders such as hyperthyroidism (THYROTOXICOSIS) or HYPOTHYROIDISM. An electrocardiogram (ECG) can provide extremely useful information. This information may be supplemented by a BALLISTOCARDIOGRAM, ECHOCARDIOGRAM, and PHONOCARDIOGRAM, all of which detect the effects of the heart's movement and its sounds.

Heart failure occurs when the heart's pumping ability is impaired. The heart continues to beat, but not strongly enough to maintain adequate circulation. This results in a retention of blood in the organs and tissues throughout the body. The reduction of heart function may be due to a variety of conditions including HIGH BLOOD PRESSURE, MITRAL VALVE DISEASE, or CORONARY HEART DISEASE. For symptoms and treatment of chronic heart failure, *see* CONGESTIVE HEART FAILURE.

Acute heart failure may follow a pulmonary embolus (a blood clot blocking an artery in a lung), or coronary thrombosis. The patient experiences shortness of breath, and coughs up bloodstained sputum. (For EMERGENCY treatment, *see* p.554.) Acute congestive heart failure may come on at night because the excess fluid moves from the legs into the circulation when the patient is lying down. This puts further strain on the heart.

Heart massage is a common term for external cardiac compression, a method of maintaining the heart's action by external pressure. For details of the technique, *see* First Aid, p.554.

Heart murmur describes the noise produced by the blood flowing through the chambers and valves of the heart.

With any abnormal murmur, a doctor must be consulted. Many heart murmurs require no treatment although a few may require some form of heart surgery. A person with a serious heart murmur must inform his or her dentist of the condition who will administer drugs before treatment to prevent the possibility of bacterial endocarditis.

Heart pacemaker is a device that gives out electrical impulses to stimulate regular contractions of the heart muscle. The pacemaker's generator and batteries are placed under the skin, either in the armpit or in the abdominal wall, and wires are passed to the heart.

A pacemaker is used during heart surgery, following a cardiac infarction, when an irregular heartbeat is causing episodes of dizziness or faintness, and in some forms of heartblock. *See* STOKES-ADAMS ATTACK.

Heart stoppage, or cardiac arrest, is a temporary or permanent failure of normal heart muscle contraction (for EMERGENCY treatment, *see* First Aid, p.554). When the heart stops, blood ceases to be pumped around the body and various tissues, particularly those of the brain, become adversely affected by the lack of oxygen.

Heart stoppage may be caused by a severe electric shock; coronary thrombosis; or heart disease, particularly when it affects the heart muscle as in CARDIOMYOPATHY and MYOCARDITIS. Heart stoppage may also result from an irregular heart rhythm or Stokes-Adams attack. During heart surgery it is sometimes necessary to stop the heart

deliberately. The heart is restarted by electrical stimulation (cardioversion).

Heart surgery is any operation on the heart. The general procedure during many operations is to cool the patient (hypothermia); connect the patient's blood circulation with a HEART-LUNG MACHINE; and stop the heart beating. This enables the surgeon to operate while the heart is still and empty of blood.

Heart transplant is the replacement of an irreparably diseased heart with a healthy one. *See* TRANSPLANT SURGERY.

Heating pad is an electrical device used to relieve the pain of rheumatic disorders, or to ease stiffness after muscle damage.

Heatstroke, or sunstroke (for EMERGENCY treatment, *see* First Aid, p.566), is an acute and potentially fatal reaction to heat exposure. The onset of heatstroke may be gradual or sudden, with the symptoms of heat exhaustion (headache, weakness, and nausea) occurring in the initial stages. Then the victim ceases to sweat, causing the skin to become hot and dry, and a rapid rise in body temperature to more than 40.5°C (105°F). In the final stage, there is mental confusion, shock, and convulsions, leading to coma and sometimes death.

Hebephrenia *See* SCHIZOPHRENIA.

Heberden's nodes are small, hard lumps that sometimes form next to the joints on the ends of the fingers in people with OSTEOARTHRITIS. There is no cure, but the discomfort of tender nodes may be lessened by heat or corticosteroid injections. Disfiguring nodes can be removed surgically.

Heel is the rear part of the foot, under the

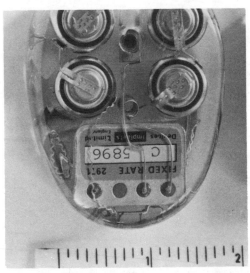

Heart pacemaker produces a series of electrical impulses to stimulate the beats of the heart.

Heliotherapy

ankle and behind the instep. The heel is composed of the heel bone (calcaneus), which bears the full weight of the body when standing, and a thick, firm pad of tissue beneath the calcaneus, which acts as a shock absorber when walking.

Heliotherapy is the use of artificial sunlight in the treatment of disorders such as PSORIASIS and ACNE.

Helminthiasis. *See* WORMS.

Hemianaesthesia is the loss of sensation down one side of the body.

Hemianopia is the loss of half the normal field of vision in one or both eyes. The many types of hemianopia are classified according to which half of the vision is lost and in which eye. The most common are (1) homonymous hemianopia, in which the left (or right) half of each eye is blinded; and (2) bitemporal hemianopia, in which the outer halves of both eyes are blinded.

Hemiparesis is weakness on one side of the body only. It is commonly accompanied by loss of sensation (hemianaesthesia) on the same side. *See* PARALYSIS.

Hemiplegia is total paralysis on one side of the body only. It is commonly accompanied by a loss of sensation (hemianaesthesia) on the same side. Hemiplegia is generally caused by a stroke. *See* PARALYSIS.

Heparin is an ANTICOAGULANT substance found in the liver, lungs, and other tissues. It is prepared from animal tissues for use as a drug, which is injected to prevent thrombosis in an artery or a vein, or to prevent clotting during certain heart and gynaecological operations. Adverse side effects are rare.

Hepatic is the medical term for anything concerning the liver.

A talk about Hepatitis

Hepatitis is inflammation of the liver. There are two types of hepatitis: (1) acute, caused by various viruses (A, B, and non- A non-B); and (2) chronic, caused by excess of alcohol, use of certain drugs, or autoimmune disease. Other infections, such as amoebic dysentery and malaria, may inflame the liver.

Q: What are the symptoms of acute hepatitis?

A: Initially the patient has rapidly fluctuating fever, feels nausea, and may vomit. The patient loses his or her appetite, and a smoker finds that cigarettes taste foul. After about a week these symptoms disappear, and are replaced by JAUNDICE. The skin and the whites of the eyes turn yellow, and the urine is dark coloured. The patient often feels better once the jaundice appears but may still feel tired and weak.

The jaundice lasts for between one and three weeks, after which the patient often becomes depressed. The depression may last for a further one or two months.

The symptoms of all forms of viral hepatitis are similar. However, the symptoms of hepatitis caused by virus B take longer to develop and tend to be more severe. It is this form of hepatitis that is sometimes fatal, with the development of ACUTE YELLOW ATROPHY of the liver.

Some patients experience only mild flu-like symptoms.

Q: How is acute hepatitis treated?

A: In the initial stages, treatment involves bedrest. After the acute stage has passed, the patient can gradually resume normal activities. The patient need not be totally isolated but it is essential that the faeces and urine are carefully disposed of to prevent the spread of infection. Injections of GAMMA GLOBULIN may be given to people who have come into close and prolonged contact with the patient if the doctor advises it.

Q: How is acute hepatitis contracted?

A: The three viruses are transmitted in different ways. Virus A and other viruses are contracted by drinking water or eating food that has been contaminated by the faeces of an infected person. Virus B is usually transmitted either in saliva or in the faeces of an infected person. It is also spread on contaminated hypodermic

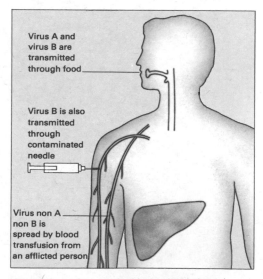

Virus A and virus B are transmitted through food

Virus B is also transmitted through contaminated needle

Virus non A non B is spread by blood transfusion from an afflicted person

Hepatitis may be caused by a viral infection that can enter the body in the ways shown.

needles.

Q: *What are the symptoms of chronic hepatitis?*

A: Chronic hepatitis means liver inflammation lasting for longer than six months. Symptoms include persistent nausea, fatigue, and jaundice. The condition may be mild, or chronic active leading to cirrhosis of the liver.

Q: *How do alcohol and drugs cause hepatitis?*

A: Alcohol leads to the accumulation of fat globules in the liver cells. If large quantities of alcohol are regularly consumed, the cells become distended with fat, burst, and die. The death of the cells produces chemical changes and causes inflammation of the surrounding liver cells. Untreated, alcoholic hepatitis leads to CIRRHOSIS and liver failure.

A talk about Heredity

Heredity is the transmission of mental and physical characteristics from parents to their children. The basic unit of heredity is a gene. Genes, which have the power to pass on hereditary characteristics, appear in strands called chromosomes in the nuclei of every cell in the body, and most importantly in the germ cells (ovum and sperm). The thousands of different genes in the body (perhaps 500 per chromosome) each carry the instructions for one specific characteristic, such as the formation of haemoglobin in the red blood cells. Sometimes the effects of several genes together determine a single characteristic: it is thought, for example, that three or four genes contribute to the determination of eye colour.

Q: *What is a chromosome?*

A: A chromosome is a collection of genes in which each gene occupies a specific position in the strand. Every chromosome consists of a double strand, arranged in a spiral shape, of a protein called deoxyribonucleic acid (DNA). The nucleus of every body cell contains 46 chromosomes arranged in 23 pairs. In a cell that divides to form the sex cells (ovum and sperm), the number of chromosomes is halved, so that each sex cell contains only 23 chromosomes.

At fertilization the sex cells fuse, and the 23 chromosomes from the egg unite with the 23 chromosomes from the sperm to form an embryo with 23 pairs of chromosomes. Hereditary characteristics are those contributed by the mother and by the father. One pair of chromosomes are the sex chromosomes, determining the sex of the new embryo. In males one of these chromosomes is a shorter strand than the other. This short chromosome is called a Y chromosome and contains fewer genes; the longer chromosome is called an X chromosome. Males have XY sex chromosomes, and females XX sex chromosomes.

Q: *What is sex-linked inheritance?*

A: Sex-linked inheritance is the transmission of a characteristic that is controlled by genes on the sex chromosomes. Not all of the genes in the sex chromosomes are paired, because the X chromosome is longer than the Y chromosome. Unpaired genes on the X chromosome exert their influence, even if they are recessive, because there is no corresponding gene to modify their effects. For example, the gene for haemophilia is recessive and is carried on the X chromosome. Haemophilia occurs almost always in males because there is no corresponding gene on the Y chromosome.

Q: *Are genes always inherited in an unaltered form?*

A: No. There may be a fault in the splitting of the sex cells within the parents so that one or more genes in them differ from the genes in the rest of the body. This may result in a child who has characteristics that were possessed by neither parent.

Q: *Can inherited disorders be predicted before birth?*

A: Prediction of some inherited disorders is possible. Through GENETIC COUNSELLING,

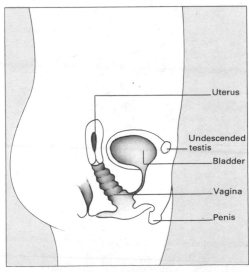

Hermaphrodite (male pseudo-hermaphrodite above) has organs of both sexes.

Hermaphrodite

parents may be advised on the probability of a recurrent, inherited disorder if one has occurred in a previous child or in either of the parent's families. If a pregnancy has started, sampling of the amniotic fluid (amniocentesis) and testing the blood for alpha feto-protein may reveal any of a number of disorders.

Hermaphrodite is a person with both male and female organs. A true hermaphrodite often has sex CHROMOSOMES that are male in the testicular part of the sex glands and female in the ovarian part. This condition is rare in human beings; pseudohermaphroditism is more common. For example, a male may have the appearance of a female, with breasts and a tiny penis, or a female may develop male characteristics. Such a condition is also termed intersex.

Q: *What may make a male appear female?*

A: This rare condition may be caused by a malfunction of the adrenal glands that makes them produce deficient amounts of male sex hormones. Males with this condition may appear females, with breasts, vagina, and vulva, but no womb. A male may also appear female because of an inherited disorder that makes the body fail to respond to the male sex hormone testosterone.

Q: *What condition may make a female appear male?*

A: In some girls, an adrenal gland malfunction may cause the development of male secondary sex characteristics

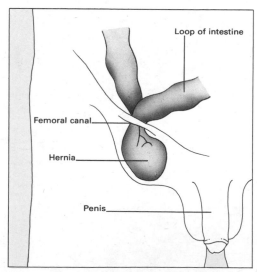

Hernia may occur when part of the intestine protrudes through the femoral canal.

Loop of intestine

Femoral canal

Hernia

Penis

(virilism) with hair growth in unusual places (hirsutism) and voice changes. It is more usual for females to develop male characteristics than for males to develop female ones.

Q: *If there is doubt about a baby's sex, what should be done?*

A: Sex must be determined as early as possible. The sex of a baby can be determined by examination of the cells usually from inside the mouth, or from blood leucocytes, as well as by measurement of hormone levels in the urine, and special tests to examine the vagina.

Hernia, or rupture, is a lump or swelling that is formed when a tissue or organ moves out of its normal position and pushes through adjacent tissues. It may occur internally, as in a HIATUS HERNIA, when the stomach protrudes through the diaphragm muscle into the chest. Or a hernia may be external, when part of the abdominal contents, such as the intestine, protrudes through a weakness in the abdominal muscles causing a local swelling.

Q: *What are the dangers of hernias?*

A: Some hernias can be pushed back into the abdomen by a doctor, and present little danger. If a hernia cannot be pushed back, it is termed irreducible. Abdominal pain, pain over the hernia, and vomiting indicate a condition called strangulation. The blood supply within the hernia is cut off and the herniated tissue dies unless an operation is performed within a few hours. A femoral hernia on the inside of the upper thigh is most likely to become strangulated because the hole is small and the ligament above the femoral artery is strong and tight.

Q: *What is the treatment for a hernia?*

A: Treatment depends on the site of the hernia. In a baby, an umbilical hernia usually disappears by the age of about four; if it does not, an operation can wait until then. In older people, an umbilical, inguinal, or femoral hernia, or one occurring in a surgical scar, is best treated with an operation called a herniorrhaphy, which closes the weakness in the abdominal wall. Hernias in the midline of the abdomen seldom need treatment.

If the patient is too old or not well enough for an operation, a device called a truss can be worn to keep an inguinal or femoral hernia in a reduced position.

Heroin (diamorphine) is an addictive drug that is derived from the opium poppy. Possession of heroin is illegal, but it is used medically to stop pain in the terminal stages of cancer.

Herpes simplex. *See* FEVER SORE.
Herpes zoster. *See* SHINGLES.
Heterograft, or xenograft, is a transplant of tissues from one species to another.
Hiatus hernia is a HERNIA that occurs when a part of the stomach protrudes upward through the sheet of muscle (diaphragm) that separates the chest cavity from the abdomen. If the hiatus hernia is small, there may be no symptoms. Often acid flows into the oesophagus, causing inflammation (oesophagitis). The condition can become serious enough to require a major operation.

Q: *What are the symptoms of a hiatus hernia?*
A: A baby with a hiatus hernia frequently regurgitates food. The baby may appear to have difficulty in swallowing.

In an adult, a typical symptom is heartburn when bending forward or lying down. The pain may spread to the jaw and down the arms, similar to an attack of ANGINA PECTORIS. Food may stick in the oesophagus.

Q: *How is a hiatus hernia treated?*
A: If the hernia is present at birth, the defect usually corrects itself. Until this occurs, the baby should sleep in a cot with the head raised and be given feeds that are thicker than usual.

An overweight adult patient must lose weight, and sleep propped up on a pillow. Drugs can be given to prevent reflux.

If these measures fail to bring adequate relief, or if the symptoms worsen, a surgical operation may be necessary.

Hiccups are repeated involuntary spasms of the diaphragm muscle, accompanied by the closing of the vocal cords. Each spasm causes a sharp inhalation of breath, and a characteristic, abrupt, cough-like noise.

Hiccups are almost always brought on by eating too fast, or swallowing stomach irritants, such as hot or cold food, or carbonated drinks. Occasionally hiccups may be a symptom of a more serious disorder, and a person suffering from a prolonged attack of hiccups should consult a doctor.

A talk about High blood pressure

High blood pressure (hypertension) is a condition in which a person's blood presure is persistently above normal. In a healthy adult, blood pressure is considered to be abnormal if it is above 140/90 when measured while the person is at rest (*see* BLOOD PRESSURE).

Q: *What causes high blood pressure?*
A: In most people, high blood pressure is an inherited variation. The combination of this variation and the tendency of blood pressure to increase with age means that high blood pressure is more common among older people. This is known as essential hypertension.

Sometimes a specific cause for high blood pressure can be found. The known causes of high blood pressure include KIDNEY DISEASE, CUSHING'S SYNDROME, PHAEOCHROMOCYTOMA, and COARCTATION of the aorta.

Q: *What are the symptoms of high blood pressure?*
A: Symptoms are rare. High blood pressure is usually discovered during a routine examination. However, a very high blood pressure may cause headaches, heart failure, and vision disturbances. This is called malignant hypertension, and can rapidly cause the death of the patient from a STROKE, bursting of an ANEURYSM, or URAEMIA.

Less severe forms of high blood pressure produce gradual changes of ARTERIOSCLEROSIS with an increased chance of CORONARY THROMBOSIS or stroke.

Q: *How is high blood pressure treated?*
A: Drug treatment of high blood pressure, which includes the use of DIURETICS and other drugs to lower the blood pressure, has to be continued for the rest of the patient's life. As side effects of drugs are more likely to occur the longer the drugs are taken, drug treatment must be carried out under strict medical supervision. It requires regular assessment and

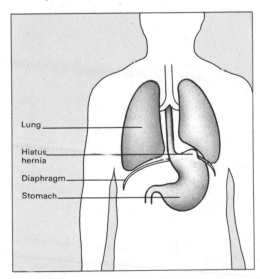

Lung

Hiatus hernia

Diaphragm

Stomach

Hiatus hernia occurs when part of the stomach pushes through an opening in the diaphragm.

occasional adjustment of the drug dosage.

The rare treatable causes of high blood pressure require an operation to remove the coarctation or adrenal gland tumour causing Cushing's syndrome or a phaeo-chromocytoma. Rarely only one kidney is diseased, and when it is removed the blood pressure will stop rising.

Q: What is the danger if blood pressure rises during pregnancy?

A: High blood pressure during pregnancy requires special care and adequate treat-ment to reduce the level to normal. There is an increased chance of de-veloping TOXAEMIA, with the attendant risks of foetal death or of the baby being small.

Hip is the part of the body at the widest part of the pelvis, and the underlying bone. The hip joint at the top of the leg is capable of movement in many directions. It is a ball-and-socket joint in which a ball at the end of the thigh bone (femur) fits into a socket in the pelvis.

Q: What severe disorders can affect the hip?

A: Congenital dislocation of the hip joint occurs spontaneously at, or soon after, birth. It may be caused by an inherited weakness, a breech birth, or slackening of the baby's joints by hormones from the mother. If diagnosed at birth, it can be treated in a plaster-of-Paris cast.

Fractures of the neck of the femur occur commonly in the elderly. Surgical procedures either pin the bones together,

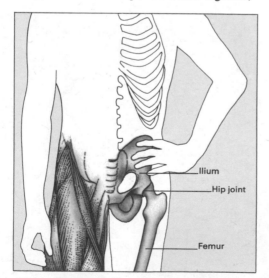

Ilium

Hip joint

Femur

Hip is the strongest joint in the body, supported by large muscles and ligaments.

or replace the head of the femur with a metal head that fits into the hip joint.

The hip may also be involved in rheumatoid ARTHRITIS or OSTEOARTHRITIS, or it may become infected, causing pyogenic arthritis.

Q: How is severe arthritis of the hip treated?

A: If treatment with drugs is not successful, various surgical operations can be performed. The most successful is total replacement of the joint with an artificial one made of metal or plastic and metal.

Hippocratic oath is the vow sworn by stu-dents in some medical schools when they qualify as doctors. The oath is based on the writings of Hippocrates and other Greek physicians and philosophers who lived in the fourth century B.C.

The oath requires a newly-qualified doctor to look after his or her patients to the best of individual ability; not to help a woman to have an abortion; not to take advantage of his or her relationship with a patient to have sexual relations; and to maintain a profes-sional secrecy about anything seen or learned about a patient.

Hirschsprung's disease (megacolon) is a congenital defect of the large intestine in which there is an absence of the nerve fibres within certain segments of the intestinal mus-cles. As a result, the muscles in the affected area do not work and there is no peristalsis (the rhythmic movement by which the intes-tine moves its contents along) in the affected section. This acts as an obstruction.

Q: What are the symptoms of Hirschsprung's disease?

A: There is usually severe, continuous constipation, and the abdomen becomes increasingly distended as the intestine fills with faeces. The affected child may vomit, and growth may be retarded.

Q: How is Hirschsprung's disease treated?

A: Most cases require a surgical operation in which the abnormal section of the intestine is removed, and the two normal ends joined together.

Hirsutism is the excessive growth of hair or the presence of hair in areas that are not usu-ally hairy. Medical conditions that cause excessive hair growth are usually caused by hormonal disturbances and are much more common in females than in males.

Histamine is a chemical that is normally pre-sent in the body. Large amounts are released in response to injury or to antigen-antibody reaction, such as in an allergic reaction. His-tamine is also involved in the secretion of acid by the stomach.

Q: How may the adverse effects of histamine be prevented?

A: The most rapidly effective antidote is adrenaline, which is usually given by injection. ANTIHISTAMINES are better at preventing reactions than treating them, and are useful if an allergic reaction (such as hay fever) is expected.

Histology is the study of the microscopic structure of tissués. Pathological histology is the study of diseased tissues.

Histoplasmosis is a rare infection caused by the fungus *Histoplasma capsulatum.* It originates in the lungs when spores of the fungus are inhaled, and may spread in the bloodstream to other parts of the body. Histoplasmosis may be mild and acute or, rarely, progressive and eventually fatal, if untreated.

The primary acute form of severe histoplasmosis is characterized by a cough, breathlessness, hoarseness, coughing blood, chest pains, and a bluish tinge to the skin. There may also be fever, chills, muscle pains, weight loss, and fatigue. Occasionally, the disease spreads to other parts of the body.

Hives, or urticaria, is a condition characterized by red, slightly swollen eruptions or itchy lumps on the skin. The lumps are called angioneurotic oedema when they occur with excessive swelling of soft tissues.

Q: What causes hives?

A: Hives are caused by an unusual sensitivity to HISTAMINE release, or by an allergic reaction to an insect bite or sting; to a drug; or to certain foods, such as shell fish or eggs. Virus or streptococcus bacterial infection also causes hives in some people.

Q: What are the symptoms of hives and how is the condition treated?

A: Itching is usually the first symptom, followed rapidly by the formation of lumps of various sizes, which may appear anywhere on the skin.

Hives in the mouth or throat may cause respiratory obstructions that require urgent treatment. If the throat is involved, injections of the hormone adrenaline is urgently required, followed by antihistamine drugs. In most cases, hives lasts for only a few days.

Hoarseness is a disorder of voice production that produces a roughness in speech, often accompanying a sore throat. It is the main symptom of LARYNGITIS. If hoarseness continues for more than three weeks, despite adequate treatment for laryngitis, an otorhinolaryngologist should be consulted.

Hodgkin's disease is a malignant (cancerous) condition involving the body's lymph glands. The condition may spread throughout the body to the spleen, liver, and other organs.

As the disease progresses, the patient experiences loss of weight, tiredness, and a general feeling of ill health

Q: How is Hodgkin's disease treated?

A: Radiotherapy may be combined with CYTOTOXIC DRUGS, which may have to be taken for many months. The earlier the diagnosis is made, the more the treatment is likely to be curative.

Homeopathy is a form of medicine in which disorders are treated by giving the patient minute doses of substances that produce the same symptoms as does the disorder. Most of the substances used in homeopathy are derived from herbs that have been repeatedly diluted in a mixture of alcohol and water, sometimes with a little sugar added. The dilution of the mixture is so great that very little of the original substance remains in the final preparation.

A talk about Homosexuality

Homosexuality describes sexual attraction of one person to another of the same sex. A homosexual woman is known as a lesbian.

Q: What causes homosexuality?

A: There are many theories about why homosexuality occurs but there is little real evidence of how sexual object choice is developed.

Normal sexual development includes a transient phase, at about the time of puberty, in which a tendency toward homosexuality is normal. Sometimes, physical homosexual relations take place and sexual tension is relieved, though

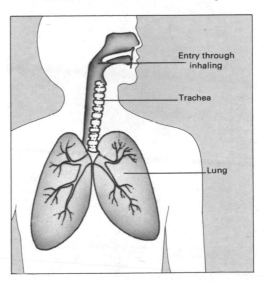

Entry through inhaling

Trachea

Lung

Histoplasmosis is a fungal infection that invades the lung after spores are inhaled.

Hookworm

such relations do not mean that the individuals concerned are permanently homosexual.

In most young people, heterosexual interest develops normally after the homosexual phase.

Q: Is it possible or desirable to treat homosexuality?

A: Many homosexual people are perfectly happy and would not wish to change even if this were possible. Individuals who feel guilty, embarrassed, or abnormal about being homosexual can sometimes benefit from discussions with a sex counsellor or psychiatrist. For homosexuals who really want to become heterosexual, psychoanalysis and psychotherapy may help.

Q: Is everyone who has ever enjoyed physical homosexuality a homosexual?

A: Not necessarily. When men or women are confined together with people of their own sex only, there is no sexual outlet other than masturbation or homosexuality. In such situations, homosexual activity may take place among people who are normally heterosexual. Such individuals usually revert to heterosexuality when they return to the mixed community.

Q: Can homosexuals lead a normal life?

A: Young homosexuals often have a period of promiscuity and then settle down with one partner in a stable relationship. But homosexual partnerships are more subject to turmoil than are heterosexual ones. Older homosexuals, who experience disappointment as they become less physically attractive, may end up feeling rejected and lonely.

Q: How should parents react if they think that their child is homosexual?

A: A parent of a homosexual child should realize that love is more important than condemnation. Trying to persuade a child to change sexual interest often produces problems not solutions. Sympathy and understanding have more effect. Parents who have this concern should seek the help of a psychologist or psychiatrist.

Hookworm. *See* ANCYLOSTOMIASIS.

Hormones are powerful chemical substances produced by cells in one organ that act on other organs to regulate their activity. Several organs produce hormones. The ENDOCRINE GLANDS, such as the thyroid gland, produce hormones that are carried in the bloodstream to effect activities in other parts of the body. Other hormones are produced by the gastrointestinal tract and have a more local effect, stimulating the production of digestive juices from adjacent areas of the small intestines.

See also ADRENAL GLANDS; CORPUS LUTEUM; GONAD; GRAAFIAN FOLLICLE; OVARY; PARATHYROID GLAND; TESTICLE; THYROID GLAND.

Horner's syndrome is a condition that usually affects one side of the face. The pupil of the eye constricts (myosis); the upper eyelid droops (ptosis); and the eyeball is set deeper into its socket than usual. The skin may be red and lose the ability to sweat on the affected side of the face. Horner's syndrome is caused by paralysis of the sympathetic nervous system in the neck. It may result from various rare nervous disorders, occasionally from SHINGLES, or as a result of nerve compression from a tumour in the upper chest.

A talk about Hospitals

Hospitals. The great majority of the nearly 3,000 hospitals in the U.K. are run by the National Health Service. There are a few privately owned and run hospitals which are mainly found in the larger cities. Hospitals vary greatly in size, from a few dozen beds to over 2,000. Most areas will have at least one large hospital with a comprehensive range of specialists and facilities, able to cope with all forms of illness. In addition, there are many small hospitals that specialize in one branch of medicine; these hospitals are commonly concerned with children, childbirth, and mental illness, but most areas also have a

Age	Muscular growth	Height spurt	Pubic hair	Penis	Testes
9					
10					
11					
12					
13					
14					
15					
16					
17					
18					

Androgens such as testosterone are essential hormones for a boy's pubescent growth.

Hormones released in puberty control slow (grey) and fast (coloured) development.

large hospital for the elderly who are unable to be cared for at home. Some large cities have further specialist hospitals, such as those dealing with eyes, ears, and neurological diseases.

Q: How are hospitals organized?

A: The National Health Service organises its hospitals under district administrators, with each hospital having a more junior hospital administrator responsible for the day-to-day running of that hospital.

The nursing staff are organized by the Senior Nursing Officer (Matron), with a Nursing Officer (Sister) in charge of each ward. The staff of most wards also includes qualified nurses (SRN) and nurses who are in training. The State Registered Nurses (SRN) are assisted by a further grade of nurses, the State Enrolled Nurses (SEN).

The senior medical and surgical staff of a hospital are the Consultants, senior doctors who are appointed when they have finished their training until they retire at the age of 65. Each Consultant is responsible for the patients under his or her care, but the patients are jointly cared for by a team of doctors known as the Firm. The team usually includes at least one House Officer, a junior doctor who is appointed for six months or one year and who is supervised by a more senior doctor, the Registrar.

Every hospital also employs a large administrative staff and a variety of other non-medical workers. These include cooks, porters, and the technicians who are required to maintain and service the complicated equipment used in a hospital.

Q: How does a hospital function to benefit a patient?

A: If a patient's GP wants a second opinion before making a definite diagnosis, an appointment will be made for the patient to see a Consultant, a specialist in the problem that has arisen, in the out-patient department of a hospital. The Consultant may be able to make a diagnosis and decide on treatment without admitting the patient to hospital. If hospital admission is necessary, however, the patient's name is registered on the hospital's waiting list. If the illness or condition is a potentially serious one, the patient's name is placed on the urgent waiting list for rapid admission.

A patient who is involved in an accident or who needs immediate hospital attention can go, without referral, to the accident or emergency department of the nearest hospital. Minor treatment may be given in this department, or the patient can be admitted directly into the hospital.

Q: How is a patient admitted to hospital?

A: Only a few patients are admitted directly to hospital as emergency cases. The majority are admitted when their name comes to the top of the waiting list, and they receive a letter or telegram asking them to come to the hospital at a certain time on a particular day.

Many large hospitals now provide information booklets which give new patients the necessary information about visiting hours, meal times, library facilities and other aspects of hospital organization. If patients require information about their illness, and the treatment they are receiving, they should ask the doctor responsible for their care.

Hot flush is a sensation of warmth accompanied by reddening of the skin of the face. It is a common symptom of MENOPAUSE, and may also be symptomatic of various neuroses.

Housemaid's knee. *See* PREPATELLAR BURSITIS.

Humerus is the bone of the upper arm, between the shoulder and the elbow.

Humour is a fluid or semifluid substance in the eyeball. There are two humours, the aqueous humour and the vitreous humour, both of which help to maintain the shape of the eyeball. The aqueous humour fills the region between the cornea at the front of the eye and the lens. The vitreous humour is a transparent, jelly-like substance

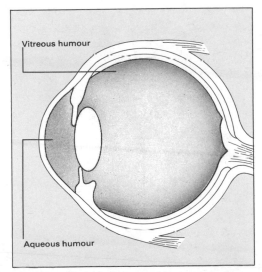

Vitreous humour

Aqueous humour

Humour of two different kinds occurs in the eye – aqueous is fluid, vitreous is jelly-like.

that occupies the region between the lens and the retina at the back of the eye.

Q: *How is the aqueous humour produced?*

A: The aqueous humour is constantly secreted by the tissues of the ciliary body, so there is a continuous flow of the humour from the rear chamber to the front chamber. The aqueous humour is kept at constant pressure by a compensating leakage in the angle between the outer rim of the iris and the back of the cornea.

Q: *What is the function of the aqueous humour?*

A: The aqueous humour carries nutrients and facilitates the exchange of gases (oxygen and carbon dioxide) in the cornea, lens, and other tissues of the eyeball that have no blood supply.

Q: *What disorders may affect the aqueous humour?*

A: Disturbances of the drainage mechanism that maintains a constant fluid pressure in the aqueous humour may cause an increase in the pressure (GLAUCOMA).

Q: *How is the vitreous humour produced?*

A: The vitreous humour is present from birth and remains virtually unchanged throughout an individual's life.

Q: *What disorders may affect the vitreous humour?*

A: Specks or floaters may occur in the vitreous humour caused by the degeneration of its cells with age. This is a normal occurrence and the presence of specks does not noticeably impair vision. Occasionally, a haemorrhage into the vitreous humour may occur, usually caused by an injury. A haemorrhage may also occur in DIABETES MELLITUS, very HIGH BLOOD PRESSURE, and some BLOOD DISORDERS. A doctor should be consulted.

Huntington's chorea is an inherited disorder of the central nervous system that is characterized by involuntary movements and progressive dementia in middle age. *See* CHOREA.

Hutchinson's teeth is a congenital anomaly in which the permanent incisor teeth are narrow and notched. It is usually a sign of congenital syphilis.

Hyaline membrane disease is a respiratory disorder of the newborn. *See* RESPIRATORY DISTRESS SYNDROME.

Hydatid cyst is a kind of CYST that forms in body tissues, especially those of the liver. It encloses the larvae of a type of tapeworm (*Echinococcus granulosus*). This parasite can infest dogs, foxes, wolves, cattle, and sheep. It is passed on to human beings in food that has been contaminated with the eggs of the tapeworm (usually from a dog).

Q: *What are the symptoms of hydatid cysts?*

A: Frequently, there are no symptoms, although there may be a dull ache on the right side of the abdomen and the liver may become enlarged.

Q: *How is hydatid cyst disease treated?*

A: When the condition has been confirmed the only treatment is to remove the cyst, or cysts, by a surgical operation.

Hydatidiform mole is a usually benign (noncancerous) growth of the placenta (afterbirth) that may develop in early pregnancy.

There may be bleeding similar to that from a threatened MISCARRIAGE. The bleeding tends to continue and may result in the spontaneous loss of a mass of small, grape-like tissues from the womb.

Q: *What is the treatment for a hydatidiform mole?*

A: If the growth is not spontaneously expelled, the obstetrician induces labour by infusion of the drug oxytocin, followed by an operation to suck out the uterine contents.

Hydrocele is an accumulation of fluid in any of the body's sac-like cavities. The term is most often used to describe an excess of fluid in the scrotum, the small protective bag that surrounds each TESTIS.

Q: *What causes a hydrocele?*

A: The male embryo has a canal that links the abdominal cavity with the scrotum. This canal usually closes before birth but it occasionally remains open.

A less common cause of hydrocele is inflammation of a testicle or of the epididymis around it. A direct blow to

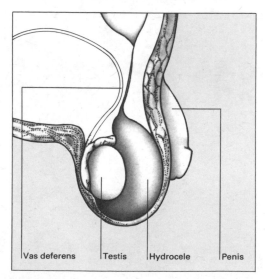

| Vas deferens | Testis | Hydrocele | Penis |

Hydrocele is an accumulation of fluid in a body cavity, especially the scrotum.

the genitals may also cause a hydrocele.

Q: How is a hydrocele treated?

A: Congenital hydrocele in children usually disappears on its own and so does not require treatment. But if it persists for more than a year, a doctor may advise surgery to remove the bag.

Hydrocephalus is the gradual enlargement of a child's skull caused by an increase of cerebrospinal fluid. Brain damage resulting from the excessive accumulation of cerebrospinal fluid produces mental retardation, epilepsy, and finally, in some children, death. Hydrocephalus may be associated with SPINA BIFIDA.

Q: What conditions may cause hydrocephalus?

A: In most cases, the disorder is present at birth (congenital). There is a blockage to the normal circulation and absorption of cerebrospinal fluid in the brain. Or hydrocephalus may be caused by a brain tumour that interferes with the usual circulation of the cerebrospinal fluid. This can also occur because of scarring of the membrane covering the brain following MENINGITIS.

Q: What symptoms appear with hydrocephalus?

A: The chief sign is an abnormally large head. In severe cases, the forehead bulges and the eyes squint and appear to have receded into a face that is disproportionately smaller. The soft spaces between the cranial bones of the skull (fontanelles) may seem unusually tight.

Q: How is hydrocephalus treated?

A: In about one third of babies born with hydrocephalus, the condition does not get worse. There are various forms of brain surgery to bypass the blockage to the flow of cerebrospinal fluid. Usually a tube is run through a tunnel created under the skin to elsewhere in the body where the excess fluid is reabsorbed into the circulatory system.

Hydrocortisone. See CORTISOL.

Hydrogen peroxide (H_2O_2) is a colourless, nontoxic liquid used in a dilute solution in water as a disinfectant to clean wounds, ulcers, abscesses, septic tooth sockets, or inflamed mucous membranes. It may also be used to treat a sore throat, to soften hard wax in the ears, and to bleach hair.

Hydronephrosis is the swelling of a kidney caused by obstruction of urine flow. It causes a gradual destruction of kidney tissues from the increased pressure. Often there are no symptoms, except occasional ache in the lower back, until kidney damage produces chronic kidney failure with an excess of waste materials in the blood.

Q: How is hydronephrosis diagnosed and treated?

A: An X-ray of the kidney, called an INTRAVENOUS PYELOGRAM (IVP), shows the structure of the kidney, and blood tests may reveal uraemia. It is important that any infection be treated immediately to prevent further damage to the kidney. If possible, the obstruction to the urine flow must be removed.

Hydrophobia. See RABIES.

Hydrotherapy is the treatment of a disorder with water: either drinking it or bathing in it.

Hymen, or maidenhead, is a thin fold of mucous membrane and skin surrounding the entrance to the vagina, that may occasionally close it. Despite popular belief, rupture or absence of the hymen is not proof of the loss of virginity. When the hymen takes the form of an unperforated membrane, menstrual blood cannot escape (haematocolpos).

Hyoid bone is a semicircular bone that lies at the base of the tongue, just above the thyroid cartilage (Adam's apple), and partly encircles the epiglottis.

Hyperacusis is an abnormal sensitivity to sound. To a person with hyperacusis, even ordinary levels of sound may cause pain.

Hyperaesthesia is an increased sensitivity of a sensory organ. It occurs most commonly in the skin.

Hyperchlorhydria is an excessive secretion of hydrochloric acid in the gastric juices of the stomach. It may lead to the formation of a PEPTIC ULCER.

Hyperemesis is the medical term for exces-

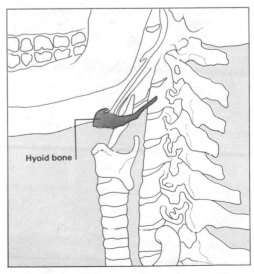

Hyoid bone is a tiny bone that is suspended within the jaw at the base of the tongue.

Hyperglycaemia

sive vomiting. It may be a feature of conditions such as gastric flu and intestinal obstruction. When it occurs in pregnancy it is known as hyperemesis gravidarum, and is a serious form of the early morning sickness that affects fifty per cent of pregnant women.

Hyperemesis gravidarum probably develops because of an oversensitivity of the vomiting centre in the brain to the hormones produced during pregnancy, but may be of psychological origin. The vomiting causes dehydration, and should be treated in hospital with intravenous infusions of glucose, antinauseant drugs, and sedation.

See also VOMITING.

Hyperglycaemia is a condition in which there is an excessive amount of glucose in the bloodstream. It results from diabetes mellitus. *See* DIABETES MELLITUS.

Hyperhidrosis is excessive perspiration. *See* PERSPIRATION.

Hyperkinesis is a disorder in which a child is physically overactive, constantly on the move, touching and feeling things but seldom remaining still enough to play with them. The condition may first be noted in early infancy when a baby cries a great deal, feeds with great difficulty, and seems to sleep less than normal for the age.

Hyperkinesis may be treated with small doses of stimulant drugs. Special teaching methods may help to improve the child's concentration. The condition usually improves spontaneously during early adolescence, before the child leaves school.

Hypermetropia. *See* LONGSIGHTEDNESS.

Hypernephroma, or Grawitz's tumour, is a

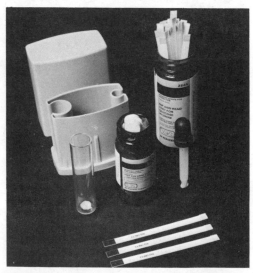

Hyperglycaemia in diabetics may be detected by testing for glucose in the urine.

malignant (cancerous) tumour of the kidney. It is the most common form of kidney cancer, and is twice as common in men as women. It usually occurs after the age of forty.

Hyperopia. *See* LONGSIGHTEDNESS.

Hyperplasia is an overgrowth of cells that results in an increase in the size of an organ.

Hypersensitivity is a state in which the body or part of the body overreacts to outside stimuli. All forms of hypersensitivity are similar to that occurring in an ALLERGY, such as hay fever or asthma.

See also ANAPHYLAXIS; HYPERAESTHESIA.

Hypertension. *See* HIGH BLOOD PRESSURE.

Hyperthyroidism, also known as Graves' disease, or thyrotoxicosis, is overactivity of the thyroid gland, and excessive production of thyroid hormones. *See* THYROTOXICOSIS.

Hypertrophy is an increase in the size of a body tissue or organ. It may occur in the heart muscle of patients with high blood pressure, or in the remaining kidney after one has been removed. Hypertrophy can also occur as the result of changes that take place with age, such as an enlarged prostate gland.

Hyperventilation occurs when a person breathes more rapidly and deeply than normal. This is caused by anxiety or by conditions causing increased acid in the body, such as diabetes or uraemia.

Hypesthesia (hypoesthesia) is a reduction in the normal sensation from the skin or other sense organs. It may result from nerve damage (polyneuritis) or occur with HEMIANAESTHESIA following a stroke.

Hypnosis is an artificially produced trance, similar to light sleep, which makes an individual more susceptible to suggestion. About eighty per cent of all human beings can be hypnotized, but few can be put into a deep hypnotic trance.

Q: What are the medical uses of hypnosis?

A: Hypnosis can be useful in helping patients to give up habits such as smoking, and to overcome phobias such as the fear of flying. If the patient can be induced into a deeper trance, hypnosis can be used to relieve nervous tics and to reduce the awareness of pain experienced during dental operations, childbirth, or even major surgery.

Hypnotics are drugs that induce sleep.

Hypocalcaemia is a condition in which there is a lower than normal level of calcium in the blood. It may occur as a result of underactivity of the PARATHYROID GLANDS, or it may be a consequence of vitamin D deficiency (*see* RICKETS; OSTEOMALACIA).

The condition is extremely serious in newborn babies, particularly those fed on cow's milk. In babies, hypocalcaemia causes vomiting and breathing problems. In adults, there are often no symptoms, and diagnosis is made only after a routine blood test. In severe hypocalcaemia, the patient may suffer a seizure or tetany, with muscular spasms of the hands, feet, and jaw.

Hypochondria is a condition in which a person has an undue concern about his or her physical health and well-being. It is frequently a sign of ANXIETY.

Hypodermic describes anything applied or administered beneath the skin.

Hypoglycaemia is a condition that occurs when the level of glucose (sugar) in the blood is abnormally low. Glucose supplies the body's cells with energy, and a low level of glucose seriously affects the brain cells.

Q: *What are the symptoms and signs of hypoglycaemia?*

A: The patient feels anxious, may behave abnormally, has a rapid, bounding pulse, sweats, feels faint, walks unsteadily, and is is in a generally confused state. He or she may go into a coma.

Hypophysis. *See* PITUITARY GLAND.

Hypopituitarism is decreased function of the pituitary gland that results in an insufficient production of hormones.

Q: *What are the symptoms of hypopituitarism?*

A: Common symptoms of hypopituitarism include loss of weight, tiredness, lack of sex drive (libido), low blood pressure, and a feeling of faintness. Headaches and vision problems (*see* HEMIANOPIA) may also occur, if the cause of the pituitary malfunction is a tumour. Children with hypopituitarism fail to grow normally and remain small but well-proportioned (*see* DWARFISM). In men and women, the normal hair growth becomes sparse. In women, there is a failure to lactate after pregnancy and menstruation ceases.

Q: *What is the treatment for hypopituitarism?*

A: If the cause of the condition is a tumour, treatment is the destruction of the tumour using surgery or radiotherapy. If there is no tumour causing the pituitary insufficiency, or after surgery has been performed, a doctor may prescribe drugs that replace throughout the body the missing hormones normally produced by the various other endocrine glands in response to the pituitary gland's stimulus.

Hypoplasia is the incomplete development of an organ or tissue.

Hypospadias is an opening in the URETHRA on the underside of the PENIS. This condition is a congenital abnormality, and may be corrected by plastic surgery.

Hypostasis is poor circulation in a part of the body, usually the legs.

Hypotension is the medical term for low blood pressure. *See* LOW BLOOD PRESSURE.

Hypothalamus is a part of the brain containing nerve centres that control appetite, thirst, body weight, fluid balance, body temperature, and sex drive (libido). It is located below the THALAMUS and above the PITUITARY GLAND, and acts as a link between the nervous system and endocrine hormone-secreting system.

Hypothermia (for EMERGENCY treatment, *see* First Aid, p.558) is a condition in which the body temperature is lower than normal. The body's normal reaction to cold is to shiver. Hypothermia may take place when the body's ability to produce heat by shivering is reduced, as may happen when the body is excessively chilled, particularly in the young (especially in sick or premature newborn babies) or in the very elderly.

Hypothyroidism is a condition that results from an inadequate supply of hormones from the THYROID GLAND in the neck. When hypothyroidism develops before birth, the infant is retarded both mentally and physically (*see* CRETINISM).

Q: *What are the symptoms of hypothyroidism?*

A: The symptoms of hypothyroidism include tiredness and a sensitivity to cold. The patient's skin becomes dry and puffy, especially on the face, and the hair of the scalp and the eyebrows becomes dry and brittle. The voice may become hoarse and the eyes dry (xerophthalmia). Constipation is common, and in women there are menstrual disorders.

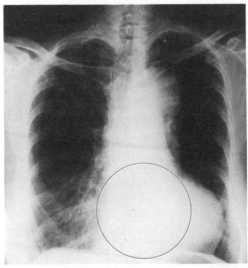

Hypertrophy of the heart: the circle shows the normal size of the heart.

Hypoxia

These symptoms develop gradually. Over a period of time, the individual's personality changes, with a slowing down of the thought processes, sometimes mild confusion and dementia, and occasionally symptoms that suggest paranoia. This severe form of hypothyroidism is called myxoedema.

Q: *What is the treatment for hypothyroidism?*

A: The diagnosis is confirmed with a blood test. A doctor usually begins treatment of hypothyroidism with a small dose of one of the thyroid hormones, and then gradually increases the dose over several weeks, as a sudden change may cause cardiac problems.

Patients who receive appropriate treatment recover completely and can expect to lead a normal life. They will, however, require treatment for the rest of their lives, with occasional blood tests to ensure that the correct amounts of hormones are given.

Hypoxia, or hypoxaemia, is a condition in which there is a lack of, or low content of, oxygen in the body tissues, usually because of a reduction in the oxygen-carrying capacity of the blood.

A talk about Hysterectomy

Hysterectomy is an operation to remove the womb (uterus). In a total hysterectomy, the cervix is also removed.

Q: *Why may a doctor recommend a hysterectomy?*

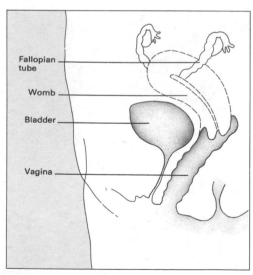

Fallopian tube

Womb

Bladder

Vagina

Hysterectomy patients may keep the fallopian tubes and the ovaries intact.

A: A hysterectomy may be performed for ENDOMETRIOSIS, chronic SALPINGITIS, or continued heavy bleeding (MENORRHAGIA), and sometimes in treating fibroids, a PROLAPSE or ovarian cyst, and cancer of the womb or cervix.

After a hysterectomy, menstruation ceases and conception is no longer possible.

Q: *Are the ovaries removed at the same time as the womb?*

A: In women under the age of about forty-five, the ovaries are usually left if they appear healthy at the time of the operation. In older women, the ovaries are usually removed because they will have no function within a year or two and may cause problems later in life.

Q: *How is a hysterectomy performed?*

A: The operation is usually done through an incision in the abdominal wall. The womb and the fallopian tubes are removed, and the top of the vagina closed to form a blind tube. The patient usually remains in hospital for ten to fourteen days.

The patient is encouraged to get out of bed as soon as possible after the operation to prevent the risk of venous thrombosis in the legs. If the patient has varicose veins or a previous history of venous thrombosis, she may be given small doses of an anticoagulant drug for a day or two after the operation.

Q: *Does a hysterectomy affect a woman's sexual interest?*

A: There should be no effect on the woman's sexual interest. If the ovaries are removed before menopause, the doctor may prescribe a course of hormones, either by implant, by injection, or by mouth. This treatment prevents the sudden onset of the symptoms that are normally associated with MENOPAUSE.

It is advisable not to resume sexual intercourse until the patient has had a post-operative check by a gynaecologist about six weeks after the operation. Initially, there may be some discomfort during intercourse because the top of the vagina is not as elastic as normal.

Hysteria is a form of neurotic disorder that is usually less severe than other mental illnesses. It may present itself at first as an organic disease but later prove to be entirely psychological in origin. Hysteria may be an aspect of the patient's total personality, or it may occur as a sudden (acute) event.

See also MENTAL ILLNESS.

A talk about Hysterical personality

Hysterical personality is a psychological disturbance in which hysteria is a significant aspect of the patient's personality. Hysteria is a form of neurotic mental disorder (*see* NEUROSIS) that may appear as a physical illness, often accompanied by various psychological disturbances, without there being an underlying organic disorder to account for them.

Q: *What are the characteristics of a hysterical personality?*

A: There is no single symptom that characterizes a hysterical personality. Consequently, it is often difficult to identify the condition because the symptoms are so varied and, in some cases, are very subtle.

Hysteria may mimic many types of physical illness, symptoms of which may also be combined with various mental disturbances. The extent to which hysteria affects the patient's personality varies greatly, from continuously involving any physical and mental functioning at one extreme, to relatively infrequent attacks of acute hysterical behaviour at the other extreme.

In general, a person in whom hysteria produces many different symptoms is still able to lead a relatively normal life; in many cases the individual appears superficially as a normal, mature person. However, selfishness is a common trait among hysterical personalities, as is the need to attract attention and admiration from others, which often leads to exaggerated, attention-seeking behaviour in speech, clothing, and mannerisms.

Personality relationships tend to be shallow, and are continually demanding because the hysteric's excessive need for reassurance and praise from friends and relatives can never be completely fulfilled. The hysteric also ignores his or her own mistakes and inconsiderate behaviour, either by appearing to forget them or by blaming other people. (This leads to frequent changes of friends.)

In acute hysteria, the general behaviour patterns and character traits are different. Instead of hysteria affecting large areas of the person's personality, the symptoms occur only in certain circumstances, often relatively specific situations. This is because acute hysteria is an unconscious method of avoiding some unpleasant experience, and the symptoms that appear are those that will help the individual to avoid this situation. In extreme cases, the hysterical symptoms may take the form of blindness, paralysis or weakness of a limb, or loss of speech. Pain may occur in any part of the body and is frequently of a violent or stabbing nature, producing a dramatic sensation that may change considerably from time to time, depending on the patient's need to avoid the frightening situation. Other common symptoms include headache, backache, severe abdominal pain, and the sensation of a lump in the throat (globus hystericus).

Sometimes, the person forgets an unpleasant incident entirely, a form of AMNESIA, and behaves as though it had never happened. Rarely, this form of hysteria may lead to a "double personality" in which the individual switches between two personalities, who may be completely different, to avoid unpleasant situations.

Sometimes the symptoms of an existing physical complaint, such as painful periods (dysmenorrhoea) or migraine, may be aggravated by hysterical symptoms, thereby making it difficult for a doctor to diagnose the main cause of the complaint. Rarely, some people produce symptoms which are so realistic that a succession of doctors are persuaded that there is a serious underlying cause. This condition is known as Münchausen's syndrome. Commonly, the patient complains of abdominal pains and so is repeatedly admitted to hospital for conditions such as appendicitis, cholecystitis, perforated ulcers, and other abdominal disorders that require immediate surgery. Even though the doctor may suspect that the underlying cause is hysteria, it is often very difficult to be certain that a hysterical person is not also suffering from a real life-threatening illness.

Occasionally, a situation that frightens the patient can only be avoided by having "hysterics", a display of extreme behaviour that corresponds to the commonly-held idea of hysteria. If the patient encounters a frightening situation, he or she may fall down screaming and writhing until the situation changes or is removed and the threat no longer exists. The outbursts of extreme behaviour resemble epileptic fits but the patient does not lose consciousness and usually the attacks occur only in the presence of other people.

Isolated attacks of extreme hysterical behaviour that are not related to specific situations do not necessarily signify a hysterical personality.

Q: *What causes a person to develop a hysterical personality?*

A: As with many types of mental disorder, the causative factors of hysteria are not known. In some cases, however, it is thought to be due to a failure of the normal psychological maturation that occurs throughout childhood into adult life and which is responsible for the development of independence. Consequently, a hysteric's personality remains in a rather childish, dependent state. The failure of personality development may result from various factors. For example, a child whose temper tantrums, sleepwalking, or phobias are not handled properly by the parents may become insecure and develop a hysterical personality. Often, unresolved sexual difficulties contribute to the development of a hysterical personality.

In some people, hysteria may develop because of a subconscious conflict resulting from a strong desire to do something that is socially prohibited. For example, an unmarried person's desire for sexual intercourse in a society that condemns such behaviour as immoral may lead to impotence (in a man) or frigidity (in a woman) if the person's sexual feelings are suppresed in a hysterical reaction to the conflict that he or she experiences.

Hysteria may also develop in a normal and mature person, usually as a reaction to prolonged, acute stress. In such cases, the physical symptoms produced by the hysterical response to the stress provide a means of escape from the stressful situation. This may be seen, for example, in soldiers on prolonged, active service who suffer from shell-shock or battle fatigue, and in people who are, or feel themselves to be, trapped in stressful social situtions.

In some circumstances, such as a forthcoming examination, people of low intelligence are particularly likely to develop hysterical symptoms. This is because they may find it impossible to cope with the stresses that people of average intelligence are able to overcome comparatively easily.

Occasionally, individuals develop hysterical symptoms as an unconscious means of escape from normal, everyday stresses with which they are unable to cope when depression occurs.

Q: *How can hysteria be treated?*

A: An outburst of acute hysterical behaviour is often frightening to the onlookers; a calm, reassuring person, preferably somebody who knows the person having the hysterical attack, is needed to take positive action, such as shaking the person or talking to him or her calmly and soothingly until the hysterical attack has passed.

Individuals with the type of hysterical personality in which they try to impress other people are more difficult to treat. The physical symptoms of illness that such hysterics produce are often sufficiently close to the symptoms of genuine disorders to make it difficult for a doctor to arrive at a positive diagnosis without additional investigations. However, too many investigations and hospital admissions may confirm the belief of the individual and his or her relatives that there is a serious underlying disorder which is being missed by the doctors. It is, therefore, important for the person's own doctor to undertake the examination as the doctor knows about his or her medical history and is more likely to arrive at the correct diagnosis than is a doctor who does not know him or her.

Unfortunately, many hysterics are difficult to help because they refuse to believe that they need treatment. In many cases, the best treatment is a form of psychotherapy in which the doctor gives constant reassurance and psychological support, so that the person gradually becomes able to face the situations that he or she finds frightening and which trigger the hysterical symptoms.

Often, however, the hysteric needs prolonged psychotherapy or psychoanalysis to help the individual's personality to develop and mature, so that he or she no longer produces child-like hysterical symptoms as a reaction to stressful situations.

Drugs are rarely of any benefit in the treatment of hysteria, except in cases where anxiety is a major feature. Occasionally, tranquillizers may bring about a dramatic cure when used to treat certain major hysterical symptoms, such as blindness or paralysis. Similarly, sedative drugs may be used to produce a state of half-sleep which, in some cases, may help to cure hysterical amnesia.

Iatrogenic disorder is any disorder brought about as a result of medical treatment.

Ichthyosis is a skin disorder in which the skin becomes dry and scaly, like the skin of a fish. The condition develops either shortly after birth, or between the ages of one and four years. There is no cure for ichthyosis, but a doctor may prescribe ointments to keep the skin soft and supple.

Icterus. *See* JAUNDICE.

Icterus gravis neonatorum. *See* HAEMOLYTIC DISEASE OF THE NEWBORN.

Ictus is a sudden convulsion or seizure, such as may occur at the start of a stroke or an attack of epilepsy. *See* STROKE.

Identical twins are two individuals that have developed from the splitting of a single fertilized egg. *See* TWINS.

Idioglossia is a speech defect characterized by unintelligible pronunciation. The condition may be caused by severe DEAFNESS in infancy, or it may occur after a STROKE.

Idiopathic describes a disorder or condition that occurs for no known reason. Many forms of epilepsy and high blood pressure are described as being idiopathic.

Idiosyncrasy is an unusual and possibly eccentric pattern of behaviour in an individual. Medically, the term is used to describe an unusual reaction to a drug, such as hypersensitivity, or no reaction at all even to a larger than normal dosage.

Ileitis is inflammation of the ileum, the lower part of the small intestine. Symptoms of the disorder include abdominal pain, often with vomiting or diarrhoea, and sometimes blood or mucus in the stool. Malnutrition may result if severe ileitis persists.

Q: What causes ileitis?

A: Infections such as traveller's diarrhoea, cholera, typhoid, salmonella poisoning, viral infections, and tuberculosis may cause ileitis. Acute inflammation of the ileum can also result from food poisoning. Chronic inflammation can occur with COELIAC DISEASE, CROHN'S DISEASE, or tuberculosis.

Q: What is the treatment for ileitis?

A: Drugs are sometimes effective. One form of treatment is to remove the portion of the intestine that is affected. Another is to allow the ileum to heal by surgically by-passing the diseased part.

Ileostomy is an opening into the small intestine that is created surgically by bringing a part of the small intestine (ileum) to the outside surface of the body at the abdomen. An ileostomy may be required as a temporary measure to by-pass the intestine, during the treatment of intestinal obstruction. A permanent ileostomy is necessary following removal of the large intestine.

Q: How are the contents of the ileum collected?

A: The patient must wear a special kind of bag over the ileostomy to collect the liquid that drains from the ileum.

Q: What problems might an ileostomy patient have to deal with?

A: The three main possible problems are skin irritation, odour, and leakage. The skin becomes irritated if it comes into contact with the faeces, or if the patient develops an allergy to the materials of the appliance. Special pastes and ointments can be applied to protect the skin, but the most effective way to prevent irritation is to ensure that the bag fits well over the ileostomy. A secure fit also eliminates any unpleasant odour.

One of the functions of the large intestine is to absorb water from the faeces as they pass along the intestine. An ileostomy patient is unable to reabsorb this fluid, and may become dehydrated. Supplements of salt in the diet and extra fluids are necessary.

Q: Can an ileostomy patient lead a normal life?

A: Yes. Many patients with ileostomies are

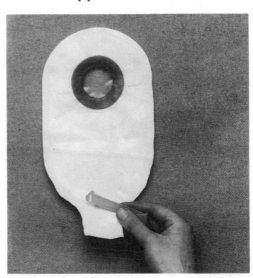

Ileostomy drainage bags fix securely over the stoma and collect the contents of the ileum.

young adults. Once they become adjusted to the minor social inconvenience of an ileostomy, they can lead a normal life.

The various ileostomy associations can give sound, practical advice to new patients.

See also COLOSTOMY.

Ileum is the section of the small intestine that extends from the jejunum to the beginning of the large intestine (colon). It is about 3.9 metres (13 feet) long. (*See* DIGESTIVE SYSTEM.)

Disorders of the ileum, such as chronic ILEITIS, produce malnutrition if they continue for a long time. Tumours of the ileum are rare, but a MECKEL'S DIVERTICULUM may occur as a congenital anomaly.

Ileus is an obstruction of the small intestine. It causes pain and vomiting. Paralytic ileus is an obstruction caused by muscle paralysis that leads to abdominal distension. This commonly occurs after an abdominal operation or peritonitis.

Immersion foot, also known as trench foot, is a serious condition resembling FROSTBITE. If neglected, it can lead to GANGRENE, particularly in a person suffering from arteriosclerosis, diabetes mellitus, or hypothyroidism.

Immersion foot is caused by exposure of the feet to wet, cold conditions, and especially to icy water, for a prolonged period of time.

Immunity is the body's ability to resist invasion by any ANTIGEN (a disease organism, poison, or foreign substance). In defence, the body produces antibodies. These destroy or neutralize antigens. Antitoxins, a type of

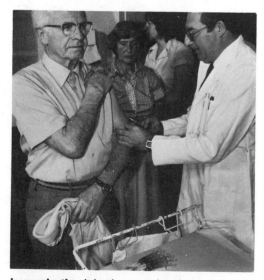

Immunization injections can be given quickly and with relatively little discomfort.

antibody, nullify poisons produced by invading organisms (such as bacteria). The next time that the same organisms invade the body, the defence system recognizes and rapidly destroys them (*see* ANTIBODY). Other foreign substances are dealt with by WHITE BLOOD CELLS (leucocytes). These attack and "swallow up" the invading bacteria, and dispose of it as pus. The role of the leucocytes in the immunity system is not fully understood, but current medical opinion is that one type of white blood cell, the lymphocytes, produce antibodies.

There are two types of immunity: passive immunity and active immunity (*see* IMMUNIZATION).

A talk about Immunization

Immunization is the production of IMMUNITY to various specific diseases and disorders. Such immunization is also known as inoculation or VACCINATION.

Like the body's natural defence system, the immunity gained by immunization may be divided into two types: passive immunity and active immunity.

Q: *What is passive immunity?*

A: Passive immunity following immunization is only temporary and it helps the body to fight a disease possibly contracted. Such immunity to specific diseases is usually provided by injecting gamma globulin containing antibodies from an immunized person or animal. SERUM SICKNESS may occur as a reaction to immunization for passive immunity.

Q: *What is active immunity?*

A: Active immunity provided by immunization is long-lasting in effect and may even be permanent. The immunization stimulates the body's own natural immunity mechanism, and is a precautionary measure to prevent the body contracting a particular disease.

Active immunity is usually provided in one of three ways: (1) by injecting a dead organism of the disease (as against diphtheria, influenza, tetanus, and whooping cough); (2) by injecting a weakened live organism of the disease (as against measles, mumps, tuberculosis, and yellow fever); or (3) by introducing a weakened, live virus through a scratch in the skin (as against smallpox). Some vaccines, such as that against poliomyelitis, can also be taken by mouth.

Q: *Does active immunity give total protection?*

A: Unfortunately not. But if the disease is

IMMUNIZATION

NAME AND DOSE	REACTIONS	NOTES
Diphtheria 3 injections at 5, 6, and 12 months (with Whooping cough and Tetanus). Further injection at age 5.	Rare. Sometimes local soreness.	Usually given with tetanus and pertussis as Triple Antigen. Small dose used for older children and adults preceded by Schick Test for previous immunity or severe reaction.
Tetanus 3 injections at 5, 6, and 12 months (with Whooping cough and Diphtheria). Further injections at age 5 and 10 years.	Rare. Sometimes local soreness.	Usually given with diphtheria and pertussis as Triple Antigen. Further boosters following cuts or animal bites. Antitetanus serum available for injuries in unvaccinated persons.
Whooping cough (Pertussis) 3 injections at 5, 6, and 12 months (with Diphtheria and Tetanus).	Rare. Sometimes local soreness. Very rarely fever; vomiting.	Usually given with tetanus and diphtheria in Triple Antigen. Not advised if there is a history of allergy or convulsions in family, or cerebral palsy.
Poliomyelitis 3 oral vaccine doses at 5, 6, and 12 months (with Diphtheria, Whooping cough, and Tetanus injections). Further doses at age 5 and 10 years.	Rare.	Usually given with Triple Antigen. Not advised during bout of diarrhoea; when taking corticosteroid drugs; in first three months of pregnancy.
Measles 1 injection at 15 months.	Sometimes fever; rash within 8-10 days, for 3-4 days.	May be combined with mumps and/or rubella. Not given to persons taking corticosteroid drugs; suffering from leukaemia or tuberculosis; or during pregnancy.
Mumps Single injection at any age: only if recommended by a doctor.	Rare.	May be combined with measles and/or rubella. Not given to persons with serious illness; allergy to eggs; or during pregnancy. Advised for adult males who have not had the disease, after test to confirm absence of the disease.
German measles (Rubella) Single injection at age 11, for girls only.	Infrequently slight fever; rash; aching joints.	May be combined with mumps and/or measles. Not given to persons taking corticosteroid drugs; suffering from leukaemia or tuberculosis; or during pregnancy.

contracted, the effects are much milder than they would otherwise be.

Q: *Are there any risks in immunization for active immunity?*

A: Statistically, the risks are few. Some people may have allergies to specific vaccines. Rarely, the whooping cough vaccine may lead to brain damage.

Q: *Why are babies immunized?*

A: Diseases such as whooping cough and measles can lead to pneumonia, severe brain damage, permanent disability, or even death. Immunization programmes begin soon after birth, but the older a child is, the more complete is the protection.

Immunosuppressive drugs or treatments suppress the natural immune mechanism of the body. They are used to treat AUTOIMMUNE DISEASE, or after organ TRANSPLANT SURGERY to prevent the body rejecting the foreign tissue of the transplanted organ.

Immunotherapy is a method of treating a patient by conferring passive immunity, usu-

ally by injecting gamma globulin containing antibodies that act on a particular infection or by immunizing a patient with his or her own tumour cells. The term sometimes refers to treatment with IMMUNOSUPPRESSIVE drugs. See IMMUNITY.

Impacted describes body structures that are pressed so closely together that normal movement or growth is impossible.

Imperforate describes any structure in which a natural opening is abnormally closed.

Impetigo is an infectious skin disease that is usually caused by staphylococcus or streptococcus bacteria. It is common among children, and may appear as a complication of an existing skin condition such as eczema or ichthyosis. Chronic impetigo in older persons is known as ecthyma.

Q: *Why is impetigo common among children?*

A: The body's immunity is less well developed in children. Frequent colds with a runny nose move staphylococci from the nose onto the face. Nose-blowing and scratching beneath and around the nose produce minor abrasions on the skin, which allow the bacteria to

Impotence

enter. Other areas, such as the hands and legs, may also become infected.

Q: What are the symptoms of impetigo?

A: Small blisters appear on the skin. These rapidly break down to form pale, crusty, oozing areas that spread. The condition may be complicated by further infection from streptococcus bacteria.

Q: How is impetigo treated?

A: Medical advice should be sought promptly because the infection can spread rapidly to other people. Doctors usually prescribe an antibiotic cream; any crusts should be soaked off with warm water before the cream is applied. If the condition recurs, it may be necessary to use antibiotic cream in the nose, and antiseptic solution in the bath to kill bacteria on the skin.

Q: Are there any complications of impetigo?

A: Yes. If additional streptococcal infection breaks out on the area affected by impetigo, it can cause the kidney disorder acute NEPHRITIS.

Impotence is a man's inability to produce, or maintain, a penile erection. For this reason, an impotent man cannot have sexual intercourse. The condition may be short-lived or may last for a long time. Brief bouts of impotence may follow depression and illnesses, such as influenza, or after taking drugs or alcohol, but in these cases the man can expect a swift return to former potency. Impotence is not the same as INFERTILITY or STERILITY.

Q: What causes impotence?

A: Impotence usually has a psychological origin. There may, however, be a physical cause, such as certain diseases or disorders; for example, Cushing's syndrome, hypopituitarism, polyneuritis, a stroke, diabetes mellitus, or alcoholism. Impotence may also occur as an after-effect of certain surgical procedures, and the patient should be informed of this before such an operation.

Q: How is impotence treated?

A: Where the impotence has a psychological basis, a doctor may arrange for the problem to be discussed with a sex therapist or marriage counsellor. The patient's sexual partner should be involved in such discussion and any consequent treatment.

Where impotence is the result of a physical disease or disorder, the underlying cause must be treated first. Unfortunately impotence caused by some physical disorders may be permanent.

Incision is the cut a surgeon makes at the beginning of an operation. The position of the incision is chosen to cause as little damage to the surrounding structures as possible, and to ensure that the tissues will heal strongly.

Incisor is a chisel-like front tooth used for cutting. There are four incisors at the front of each human jaw. *See* TEETH.

Incontinence is the lack of voluntary control of the bladder or bowels, particularly in an adult. Voluntary control of the bladder during the daytime is not achieved until about the age of two years, and at night may not occur until some years later.

Q: What can cause incontinence of the bladder?

A: Any neurological disorder that interferes with normal sensations from the bladder can prevent control of the sphincter muscle that normally closes it. Such disorders include spina bifida, damage to the spinal cord, multiple sclerosis, and nerve degeneration that occurs with conditions like diabetes mellitus and strokes, or senility. This type of incontinence is also common in attacks of epilepsy.

Incontinence may also result from partial obstruction caused by enlargement of the prostate gland (prostatomegaly) and from disorders of the muscle that controls the outflow of urine; such a muscle disorder may follow an operation or cancer. Some women develop STRESS INCONTINENCE because of prolapse (a displacement) of the womb, which presses on the bladder and changes its anatomy so that urine escapes when the

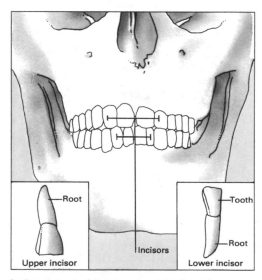

Incisor is one of the four front teeth in the upper and lower jaws of the adult.

Root

Tooth

Root

Incisors

Upper incisor

Lower incisor

woman coughs or laughs. Incontinence may also result from an injury to the spinal cord that prevents impulses between the brain and bladder.

Q: What can cause incontinence of the bowels?

A: In young children, lack of bowel control may simply be resistance to toilet training. But in older children it may be a sign of a serious psychological disorder.

Faecal incontinence is common in the senile, as is constipation. Failure to control the bowels may also be associated with neurological disorders, such as a stroke, multiple sclerosis, or the polyneuritis associated with diabetes mellitus. The condition may follow damage to the sphincter muscle that closes the anus following childbirth or an operation for anal fistula or fissure. Another factor can be cancer of the rectum or simply severe diarrhoea.

Q: How is incontinence treated?

A: The treatment of any form of incontinence must be directed toward the cause. Special bags may be used for urinary incontinence, but faecal incontinence is more difficult to control; absorbent pads have to be worn in waterproof underpants.

A new treatment involves electrical stimulation of the muscles that close the exit from the bladder and rectum.

Incrustation is the formation of crusts or scabs on the skin. *See* SCAB.

Incubation period is the time between exposure to an infectious illness and the appearance of the first symptoms. It is not the same as QUARANTINE. *See* INFECTIOUS DISEASES.

Incubator is a life-support system used in hospitals for rearing premature or seriously ill newborn babies. It is a ventilated, boxlike apparatus in which the atmosphere can be kept sterile and at constant temperature and humidity.

An incubator is also any device used to promote the growth of organisms placed inside it.

Indian hemp is another name for cannabis or marijuana. *See* MARIJUANA.

A talk about Indigestion

Indigestion is incomplete or imperfect digestion. But the condition is poorly defined, and it can vary according to situation and person. Acute indigestion is unpleasant and the chronic form is debilitating. Chronic indigestion is sometimes a symptom of a more serious disorder, such as hiatus hernia, a gall bladder disorder, or a peptic ulcer. It is common during the later stages of pregnancy.

Q: What are the symptoms of indigestion?

A: Usually the person experiences vague abdominal discomfort, and feels generally bloated. Burping may bring temporary relief. The symptoms may be severe enough to produce ill-defined pain that may or may not vary in intensity. Sometimes the feeling of discomfort increases, the patient feels nauseated, and vomits. The symptoms usually last for only about two hours, although a bout of indigestion can last many weeks.

In addition to these symptoms, there may be HEARTBURN. This produces a burning sensation beneath the breastbone that is sometimes accompanied by a bitter taste of fluid rising up into the mouth.

Q: What causes indigestion?

A: Indigestion is usually caused by GASTRITIS (inflammation of the lining of the stomach), often brought on by over-eating or an excess of alcohol. Smoking aggravates the condition. A person who has irregular meals, drinks too much strong coffee, and is anxious or depressed, often develops mild gastritis. The bloated feeling and flatulence may encourage AEROPHAGIA, the habit of swallowing air, which increases the indigestion symptoms. Obesity also aggravates the condition. Chronic indigestion can also be a warning symptom of cancer.

Q: When should an indigestion sufferer consult a doctor?

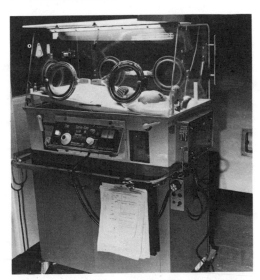

Incubators provide a germ-free environment to help premature newborns survive.

Indigestion

A: If the symptoms are severe enough to interfere with normal life, or to disturb sleep, a doctor should be consulted within twenty-four hours.

Q: Is an upset stomach the same as indigestion?

A: An upset stomach is usually an acute form of indigestion lasting only a few hours and may, in severe forms, be accompanied by diarrhoea and vomiting. This is likely to be a form of GASTROENTERITIS or acute GASTRITIS.

Q: How is indigestion treated?

A: Treatment depends on the cause of the indigestion. Many patients find that the symptoms improve after a light, easily digestible meal, or a glass of milk. Others find that an antacid medicine or tablets bring relief, particularly from heartburn.

In cases of excessive acid production, the doctor may prescribe a new ANTIHISTAMINE that decreases acid production. If anxiety, depression, and tension seem to be the main reasons for the indigestion, the doctor may prescribe tranquillizers or antidepressant drugs. Definite physical causes are treated in the appropriate way.

Induction means causing or producing. The term has several medical applications. In one meaning, induction is the artificial initiation of childbirth. Labour is induced either by surgically rupturing the membrane around the foetus, or by injecting the mother with drugs (*see* PREGNANCY AND CHILDBIRTH).

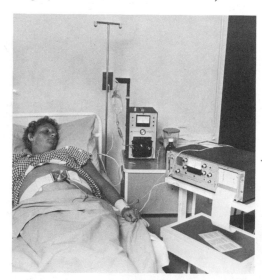

Induction of labour in childbirth can be assisted by complex monitoring equipment.

Induction is also used to describe the beginning of anaesthesia. It may refer to the intravenous injection of a short-acting barbiturate, or the initial inhalation of an anaesthetic gas.

In psychology, induction is a logical process of learning. The term also describes feelings reflected in another person; for example, grief in one person can induce sympathy in another.

Induration is an unusual area of hardness or firmness in a body tissue. The term may refer to bruising, scarring around a wound, or the hardened tissue surrounding an abscess.

Industrial diseases are disorders that are caused by exposure to various toxic substances and microorganisms that are used in industrial processes. *See* OCCUPATIONAL HAZARDS.

Infantile paralysis. *See* POLIOMYELITIS.

Infarction is an area of dead tissue in an organ that has had its blood supply cut off due to blockage in a blood vessel, usually an artery, supplying it. The seriousness of the condition depends on where the infarction occurs.

Q: What causes a blockage in a blood vessel?

A: Thrombosis (blood clotting) in an artery creates a blockage and may be caused by ARTERIOSCLEROSIS or damage to the vessel. A blood clot from another part of the body may become trapped in an artery; this is known as an EMBOLISM.

Q: What are the symptoms of an infarction?

A: These depend on which part of the body is affected. If the infarction is in the heart muscle (myocardial infarction), the patient's symptoms may vary from severe pain radiating from the centre of the chest to the left arm, the neck, shoulders, back, and jaw to a feeling of mild indigestion (*see* CORONARY HEART DISEASE). If the infarction is in the brain the patient suffers a stroke. In both instances, there are no alternative blood supplies, and the tissues die. If the infarction is in the leg, the patient experiences acute cramp-like pain and the leg becomes white and cold. If the patient does not receive immediate surgery, GANGRENE rapidly sets in. An infarction in the kidney produces blood in the urine (haematuria).

Q: Can an infarction be treated?

A: No. Once the tissue has died, it cannot be replaced. It can gradually heal and form scar tissue. Treatment is aimed at preventing an embolism from developing and causing an infarction. Emergency surgery can replace part of the femoral artery with a graft or plastic tubing, but if

INFECTIOUS DISEASES

Disease	Incubation (days)	Quarantine (days)	Infectivity (days)	Duration (days)
Chickenpox	14-21	21	−1 - +6	6-8
Diphtheria	2-5	7	14-28 (until clear)	Until clear
Dysentery (bacillary)	2-7	7	7-21 (until clear)	3-5
German measles (rubella)	14-21	21	7 before rash appears until 5 after	5
Glandular fever	4-14	5+	Not known	7-21
Influenza	1-3	Not necessary	When symptoms appear until 7 after	3-5
Measles	8-14	14	4 before rash appears until 7 after	6-8
Meningitis	3-5	5+	2	Varies
Mumps	14-28	28	7 before symptoms appear until 9 after	10-14
Poliomyelitis	4-13	21	Last part of incubation period and first week of acute illness	10-15
Roseola	2-5	5	Varies	5-7
Scarlet fever	2-5	Until clear	Beginning of incubation period until 14-21 after symptoms appear	7-10
Typhoid fever and Paratyphoid	7-21	Until clear	Until clear	14-21
Whooping cough (pertussis)	7-21	21	21	42

the tissues have already died (gangrene), amputation is the only treatment.

Infection is the invasion of the body by disease-producing organisms. There are five main types of infective organisms: (1) viruses (*see* VIRUS); (2) BACTERIA; (3) fungi (*see* FUNGAL DISORDERS); (4) PROTOZOA; and (5) WORMS. Infection may enter the body in the air that is breathed; in food or water that is eaten or drunk; directly through the skin; or from another part of the body in which the organism produces no ill effects (*see* CONTAGIOUS DISEASES).

Infectious diseases are those diseases that are transmitted from one person to another, possibly causing an epidemic. For this reason, such diseases are also called COMMUNICABLE DISEASES. CONTAGIOUS DISEASES are caught by direct physical contact with the diseased.

The table on this page lists common infectious diseases, each of which has a separate article in the A-Z section of this book.

There are many other less common infectious diseases, and the following also have articles in the A-Z section of this book: AMOEBIC DYSENTERY; BORNHOLM DISEASE; BRUCELLOSIS; CHOLERA; ENCEPHALITIS; HAND-FOOT-AND-MOUTH DISEASE; HEPATITIS; RABIES; SMALLPOX; TOXOPLASMOSIS; TUBERCULOSIS; TYPHUS; VENEREAL DISEASES; YAWS; YELLOW FEVER.

Infectious mononucleosis (glandular fever) is an acute infectious disease. *See* GLANDULAR FEVER.

Inferiority complex is a state of mind in which a person believes himself or herself to be inferior to others. *See* COMPLEX.

A talk about Infertility

Infertility is the inability to produce offspring. It is not the same as STERILITY, because an infertile person may have no physical disorder of the reproductive system.

Many couples are temporarily infertile. The likelihood of becoming pregnant on any one occasion is only about one per cent. However, over a period of two years, ten per cent of couples are infertile.

Fifty per cent of women under the age of thirty who have regular intercourse can become pregnant within six months. Nearly eighty per cent may be pregnant within a year, the remainder within two years. Older women usually take longer.

Q: *What should a couple do if they believe they are infertile?*

A: Taking into consideration the above statistics, it is advisable for a couple to delay any kind of investigations for at least a year. During this time they can work out the exact OVULATION day of the woman. To do this, the woman takes her temperature first thing in the morning before having anything to eat or drink. Fourteen days before the onset of menstruation, the temperature rises by about 0.5°C (1°F). The rise in temperature occurs twenty-four hours after ovulation. If a temperature chart is kept for three to four months, a woman can estimate the day of ovulation.

The ovum is ready for FERTILIZATION for twenty-four hours. It is not known for

Infertility

certain how long a sperm can survive in the womb, but it is thought to be up to three days.

Q: *Why are some couples infertile?*

A: A SEXUAL PROBLEM, such as complete ignorance about the mechanics of intercourse, is a more common factor than is realized. Other sexual difficulties that disrupt fertility include FRIGIDITY and IMPOTENCE.

Sometimes a woman who ovulates only occasionally has a partner with a low sperm count. This means the chance of fertilization is greatly reduced.

In fifty per cent of infertile couples, both partners are affected because of some physical reason. In the remaining fifty per cent, half the men and half the women are physically incapacitated.

Q: *What conditions can make a man infertile?*

A: Apart from sexual problems, infertility results if a condition or disorder affects (1) the total number of sperm produced during ejaculation; or (2) the number of viable, or normal, sperm produced. Such disorders include any infection of the sexual organs, for example, epididymitis; venereal disease; prostatitis; mumps; or a blockage of the vas deferens (sperm duct).

The temperature of the testicles affects the production of sperm. Undescended testicles are too warm to function. In the same way, some obese men become temporarily infertile in hot environments, or from wearing tight underpants

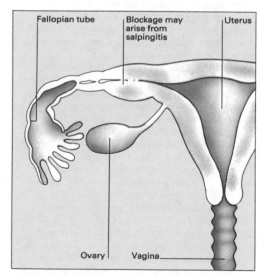

Infertility in women may be caused by a blockage in the fallopian tube.

that hold the testicles too close to the body. More rarely, varicose veins of the spermatic cord, known as varicoceles, increase the blood flow of the testicles, and keep them too warm. Other causes of infertility include certain chromosome abnormalities, Klinefelter's syndrome, cystic fibrosis, certain drugs, and irradiation of the testicles.

Q: *How is a man's fertility assessed?*

A: A doctor examines the man's testicles and then the prostate gland during a rectal examination. A sample of semen is collected and examined within two hours using a microscope to determine the sperm count. If any abnormality is noticed, the test is repeated two or three times to ensure an accurate diagnosis.

Q: *How is infertility in a man treated?*

A: General attention to health is essential. If the man is overweight, he must diet to lose weight. He should not smoke and should moderate his drinking, if necessary. Loose underpants often help to increase the number of sperm produced, and sometimes the doctor recommends bathing the testicles in cold water twice a day. If the sperm count is low, abstinence from sexual intercourse three to four days before the expected day of ovulation should increase the number of sperm ejaculated.

Infections of the reproductive organs must be treated; a varicocele can be removed by a minor operation. If no sperm are being produced, or if there is a blockage in the vas deferens, it is seldom possible to cure the condition, although sometimes an operation can unblock the sperm duct. Undescended or retractile testicles have to be treated during childhood.

Sexual problems, such as impotence or premature ejaculation, need sympathetic discussion with a sex therapist or the family doctor.

Q: *What conditions make a woman infertile?*

A: Infertility in women results if a condition or disorder affects (1) ovulation; (2) the movement of the ovum along the fallopian tube; (3) the ability of the fertilized ovum to implant in the wall of the womb; or (4) normal sexual intercourse.

Ovulation may be disrupted by anxiety, or one of various hormone disorders. A hormone imbalance may occur for a few months following a course of contraceptive pills. Illnesses such as tuberculosis or diabetes mellitus affect ovulation, and it is also thought that obesity, smoking, and alcohol affects it. An ovarian cyst also disrupts ovulation.

The movement of the ovum is restricted by any infection of the fallopian tube, including salpingitis, venereal diseases, or an abscess. The lining of the tube becomes scarred, and even if an egg is successfully fertilized, an ECTOPIC PREGNANCY is likely.

Disorders that affect the womb include endometriosis, endometritis, polyps, and fibroids. In some women, a congenital anomaly results in a deformed womb.

The presence of an intact hymen or VAGINISMUS may indicate problems with techniques of sexual intercourse. Dyspareunia (painful intercourse) may indicate a gynaecological infection.

Sometimes cervical secretions kill the sperm even when intercourse is successful.

Q: *How is infertility in a woman assessed?*

A: Some tests can be carried out at home, for example, the temperature test for the day of ovulation described above. A gynaecological examination is necessary to see if there is any local infection in the vagina, cervix, or fallopian tubes. It is usual for a doctor to check general health with a chest X-ray, blood test, and urine sample. A cervical smear is taken to eliminate the possibility of local infection due to cervicitis as well as cancer.

A postcoital test may have to be done. Vaginal secretions are examined two to three hours after intercourse to make sure that the sperm are still moving vigorously, and are not being killed by the secretions.

If the results of these tests are normal, a D AND C operation is usually performed to examine the lining of the womb. This may be followed by a salpingogram to show the shape of the womb and the condition of the fallopian tubes.

Q: *How is infertility in a woman treated?*

A: Anxiety is a cause of infertility among many couples who have not been able to have children for a few years. Medical investigations often act as a form of psychotherapy, which has led some infertile couples to conceive even before treatment begins.

If an infection is discovered during the investigations, it is promptly treated. However, repair operations on already scarred fallopian tubes are rarely successful. Adjustment of a womb abnormality is also difficult, but is sometimes successful.

Hormone disorders are easier to treat. Ovulation can be stimulated with a drug called clomiphene, combined with a small dose of oestrogen. Care is taken to prevent multiple pregnancy.

In a technique introduced in Britain during the late 1970s, infertile women have become pregnant after having a fertilized ovum implanted in the womb. The ovum is taken from the woman at ovulation, fertilized in a laboratory by sperm taken from the husband, and then replaced in the woman's womb. But this method is still in its experimental stages.

Q: *How successful are treatments for infertility?*

A: Of those couples who seek treatment, twenty per cent of the women conceive before treatment is started. A further twenty per cent become pregnant within two years of treatment. It is important, however, that each partner follows the doctor's advice. Conception may occur after years of infertility. This may happen after the adoption of a child, but there is no scientific explanation for it.

Infestation is the harbouring of animal parasites, such as ticks, mites, and fleas, on the skin or in the hair, or worms in the body tissues or organs.

Inflammation is a localized reaction of body tissue to injury or disease. Inflammation may result from physical damage, infection or surgery, or exposure to electricity, chemicals, heat, cold, or radiation. It may also occur in

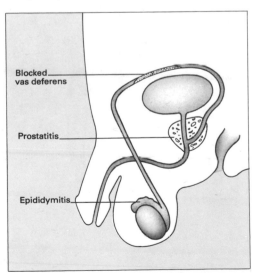

Infertility in men may arise from prostatitis, epididymitis, or a blocked vas deferens.

Blocked vas deferens

Prostatitis

Epididymitis

Influenza

AUTOIMMUNE DISEASE and with cancer.

Q: *What are the symptoms of inflammation?*

A: The affected area becomes swollen and painful, and the skin becomes red and warm. If the inflamed area is large, there may also be a slight rise in body temperature, headache, and a loss of appetite. As the body repair processes start to heal and replace injured tissue, the inflammation gradually disappears. However, a collection of pus may remain. This usually discharges through the skin, with the final disappearance of all the symptoms. If the pus is not discharged, it acts as a barrier to healing. In this case, a tough capsule may form around the pus, causing an ABSCESS.

Occasionally, chronic inflammation may occur. Some infections, such as tuberculosis, act slowly, and the process of healing keeps pace with the damage. If this happens, fibrous tissue may form around the centre of infection. The fibrous tissue may cut off the blood supply, so that the central area of affected tissue dies. If this occurs internally, a chronic abscess is formed; if it involves the body surface, an ulcer or festering sore results.

Q: *How does the body respond to inflammation?*

A: After the initial injury or infection, damaged tissue releases a chemical, probably a HISTAMINE, that causes the blood vessels in the area to expand and leak. This increased blood flow causes redness and warmth. The escape of fluid from the blood vessels causes the swelling. Pain is partly caused by compression of the nerve endings that accompanies the swelling, and partly by irritation of the nerve endings by substances causing or resulting from the inflammation.

The inflow of blood carries additional WHITE BLOOD CELLS and ANTIBODIES. These remove damaged tissue and attempt to destroy any invading micro-organisms by engulfing them. However, in engulfing the micro-organisms, the white blood cells themselves may be destroyed. Pus is composed of dead white blood cells.

Q: *How is inflammation treated?*

A: Because inflammation is a natural healing process, it is advisable to interfere as little as possible. The injured area should be washed and a mild antiseptic applied. Any foreign bodies or chemicals should be carefully removed or washed away. The inflamed part should be rested. A doctor should be consulted if the area of inflammation is extensive; if it becomes extremely painful; if it persists for a long time; or if an abscess or a festering sore forms.

A talk about Influenza

Influenza is an acute viral infection caused by any of several closely related viruses. There are three major groups of these viruses, designated A, B, and C. Infections with the influenza A virus tend to be more severe and to last longer than those caused by the milder B and C viruses. Major influenza epidemics are usually caused by a strain of the influenza A virus.

Q: *What are the symptoms of influenza?*

A: After an incubation period of about two days there is a sudden onset of shivering, sometimes with a chill; headache; weakness and fatigue; aching in the muscles and joints; a sore throat; and a dry, painful cough. At the beginning of the illness there may also be vomiting and an aversion to light and noise. Initially, the body temperature may rise to about 40°C (104°F), dropping to between 38°C (102°F) and 39°C (103°F) for two or three days, then settling at between 37.5°C (100°F) and 38°C (102°F).

As the illness progresses, the cough may become less dry and painful because of the production of sputum. If no complications develop, the fever generally lasts for about five days. Recovery is usually rapid and without

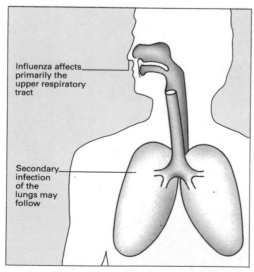

Influenza affects primarily the upper respiratory tract

Secondary infection of the lungs may follow

Influenza is a viral infection that may lead to secondary infection of the lungs.

relapse, although it may be accompanied by some weakness and depression.

Q: Can influenza have any complications?

A: Yes. Influenza lowers the body's resistance to infection. This makes the patient vulnerable to invasion by other organisms that may cause secondary infections, especially of the throat, sinuses, and ears, such as laryngitis, sinusitis, and otitis media. With such relatively minor complications, the original symptoms of influenza are intensified, and may be accompanied by bronchitis and a persistent cough. Pneumonia may also occur.

Q: How is influenza treated?

A: Influenza should be treated as any other fever. The patient should go to bed as soon as symptoms appear, and should remain there until a complete recovery has been made. The patient should drink plenty of fluids, especially while there is a fever. Aspirin may help to relieve muscle and joint pains, and to reduce fever. The patient should be isolated, both to prevent the spread of infection and to reduce the risk of secondary infections. If any complications develop, a doctor should be consulted. Antibiotics are often prescribed, but these are of no value against influenza itself, although they may be useful for treating secondary infections.

Q: Can influenza be prevented?

A: Injections of dead influenza virus may confer immunity to that particular strain of influenza. The vaccination is neither immediately nor totally effective: it confers immunity about seven days after injection and protects about 70 per cent of those immunized. But the influenza virus tends to change and produce new strains, so vaccination with one strain does not give immunity to all of them. For this reason, vaccinations must be given each year as new strains develop. Experiments have been performed using a modified live virus, but these have not proved as effective as vaccinations with the dead virus.

The drug amantadine hydrochloride, has proved useful in preventing respiratory infections due to A_2 strain of influenza virus. Amantadine hydrochloride should not, however, be used by pregnant women.

Q: How does influenza spread?

A: Influenza is an infectious disease, that may cause an epidemic. It is spread by inhaling infected droplets in the air, which are produced by coughing and sneezing. Influenza may occur at any time of the year, but is most common during winter.

Infra-red treatment is the use of infra-red radiation to treat various disorders. Infra-red is invisible heat radiation beyond the red end of the visible spectrum. Infra-red treatment may be used by physiotherapists for muscle disorders and rheumatic diseases, or to help in relieving the pain caused by minor muscle damage, such as sprains and strains. A device called an infra-red thermograph, which detects and photographs infra-red rays, may be used in the diagnosis of some disorders, particularly breast cancer. *See* THERMOGRAM.

Infusion is the introduction of a sterile fluid into a vein. Drugs may be administered by this method, and it may also be used to maintain the balance of salts within the body.

Infusion is also a method of extracting chemicals by soaking a substance, usually a plant, in water.

Ingrown toenail is a tendency for the edge of a toenail to grow into the adjacent soft tissue, producing infection and inflammation. This condition most commonly develops on the big toe from a combination of factors, including tight shoes; the tendency to cut the nail in a semicircular shape; and, in many people, having nails with an inverted U-shape rather than a flat surface, so that the edges point down into the toe.

Q: What is the treatment for an ingrown toenail?

A: The first essential remedy is to wear

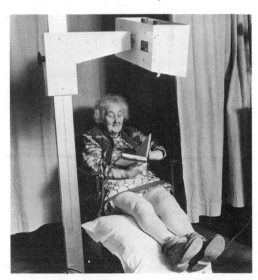

Infra-red treatment may be used to relieve pain from osteoarthritis of the knees.

259

loose-fitting, round-toed shoes to remove pressure from the nail. The toenail should be cut straight across and not in a curve. The toe should be thoroughly cleaned at least twice a day, when the edges of the nail can be gently lifted. Regular cleaning helps to reduce minor infection, and a small plug of cotton, soaked in surgical spirit, can be used as an antiseptic.

If these simple measures fail to control the infection, and PARONYCHIA (chronic infection) develops, then antibiotic creams and lotions may be tried. If infection still persists, a surgical operation may be performed to remove the side of the nail and part of the skin of the toe.

Inguinal describes anything pertaining to the groin. For example, the inguinal glands are lymph nodes situated in the groin.

Inhalation therapy is the drawing in of breath, vapour, gas, smoke, drugs, or powder into the lungs to treat various respiratory disorders.

Inherited disorders are abnormalities that may be passed on from parents to children. *See* CONGENITAL ANOMALIES; HEREDITY.

Inhibition is the prevention or restraint of some bodily activity by another bodily process. For example, fear may inhibit gastric secretions.

In psychiatry, inhibition refers to the restraints against performing antisocial acts. For example, in adults, anger at another person seldom leads to violence as it usually does in children; most adults are inhibited against violence. In this sense, inhibition is different from repression: inhibition may be a conscious or an unconscious process; repression is always unconscious and automatic.

See also AUTONOMIC NERVOUS SYSTEM; PERISTALSIS.

Injection is a method of forcing a fluid into the body. It is usually performed using a needle and a syringe, but may also be done using compressed air. An injection may be intradermal, in which fluid is injected into the superficial skin layers; subcutaneous, injected between the skin and underlying muscle; intramuscular, into a muscle; intravenous, into a vein; intra-arterial, into an artery; epidural, around the nerves of the spinal cord; intrathecal, under the meninges of the brain; or intra-articular, into a joint.

Inner ear is the part of the ear that consists of the cochlea, semicircular canals, and auditory nerve. *See* EAR.

Innocent. *See* BENIGN.

Inoculation is a method of IMMUNIZATION in which a micro-organism or toxin is injected into the body to produce immunity.

Insanity is a legal term for any mental disorder that results in a person being unaware of the consequences of his or her actions, and in not being held responsible for them. Various legal procedures may be necessary before a person can be certified as legally insane and before medical treatment for a specific mental disorder can be started. *See* MENTAL ILLNESS.

Insect bites. *See* First Aid, pp.514-515.

Insecticide is any substance that kills insects. Many insecticides are also poisonous to animals and human beings. The newer insecticides lose their potency and are destroyed more quickly, so that long-term hazards are less likely.

Insidious describes any condition that comes on so gradually that the affected person is unaware of its onset. Cancer is often insidious, whereas the onset of influenza is sudden or acute.

Insomnia is the inability to sleep, or difficulty in sleeping, resulting in long periods of wakefulness. Some people require less sleep than others, and the inability to sleep continuously through the night is not an illness in itself. Because of great individual differences in sleep patterns, what one person considers to be insomnia another may regard as normal.

Q: What causes insomnia?

A: Insomnia may be a symptom of almost any disease or disorder. Physical causes of insomnia include overeating, hunger, cold, heat, noise, excessive tea or coffee before going to bed, or an uncomfortable bed. Pain is a common cause of insomnia, and a cough, particularly when combined

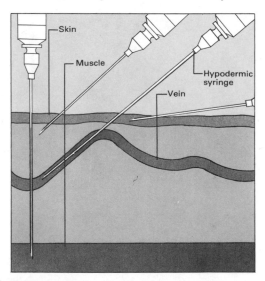

Skin

Muscle

Hypodermic syringe

Vein

Injections can be given in many ways, including intramuscularly and intravenously.

with a fever, often causes difficulty in sleeping. Persistent insomnia is often caused by anxiety or depression.

Q: *How is insomnia treated?*

A: It is important to ensure that there is a warm, comfortable bed in a quiet room. Pain should be treated with painkillers, such as paracetamol or aspirin. A hot bath, a warm, milky drink, or a light snack may also help. Some people find that plenty of physical exercise during the day and a short walk before going to bed make sleeping easier.

If sleeplessness is caused by anxiety or depression, it may help to discuss the problems with a doctor who may then prescribe sleeping drugs for a short period during the initial treatment of depression. Sleeping drugs should not be taken without consulting a doctor.

See also SLEEP.

Insufflation is the blowing of a fluid, gas, or powder into a body cavity. Insufflation may be used in the treatment of inflammations of the external tube of the ear, and as a method of unblocking the Eustachian tube in the treatment of middle ear diseases.

Insulin is a hormone produced by the ISLETS OF LANGERHANS, clusters of cells within the pancreas, a gland situated behind the stomach. Insulin controls the use of glucose, fats, and lipids by the body. An excess of insulin, sometimes caused by a pancreatic tumour, causes HYPOGLYCAEMIA (a low level of sugar in the blood), and a lack of insulin produces hyperglycaemia, which is a symptom of DIABETES MELLITUS.

Insulin, obtained from the pancreases of cattle or pigs, is used in the treatment of diabetes mellitus and is given by injection. The animal insulin is prepared in various ways to make it act quickly (soluble insulin) or slowly, in combination with zinc or other substances, so that only one or two injections a day are necessary. The strength of insulin is expressed in units of activity in each ml (cc), and is given in syringes calibrated in units.

Integument. *See* SKIN.

Intelligence quotient (IQ) is an index of intelligence based on the results of a variety of tests of verbal, writing, and mathematical ability, together with physical performance at set tasks. Standard intelligence tests include the Babcock-Levy, Binet, and Stanford-Binet tests, although most of these have been superseded by the Wechsler test.

The IQ of a child taking a test is compared with others of the same age in percentage terms. For example, a child may score between 90 and 110 per cent of what would be expected of someone of his or her age group,

and so is said to be of normal average intelligence. Any score above 110 ranges from superior intelligence to near genius or genius, whereas a score below 90 ranges from dull normal to profoundly mentally retarded. Tests for adults are different from those for children, and are not otherwise age-related.

Q: *Are IQ tests always accurate?*

A: No. There are many reasons why such tests may be inaccurate. Much depends on the way a child has been educated and on his or her social and cultural background.

Intercostal means situated between the ribs.

Intercourse. *See* SEXUAL INTERCOURSE.

Interferon is a protein substance that is produced by body cells to help to combat virus infection by preventing the growth of viruses. Research is now under way into methods of stimulating interferon production by the body. Efforts are also being made to isolate and synthesize interferon, so that it can be administered at the onset of a virus infection.

Intermittent claudication is pain or cramp in the calf muscle during exercise. Relieved by rest, the pain recurs when the muscle is again exercised.

Q: *What causes this form of pain?*

A: The cramp-like pain is the result of an inadequate blood (and therefore oxygen) supply to the calf muscles, caused by a disorder of the blood vessels. The disorder is usually ARTERIOSCLEROSIS, or may follow blockage of an artery by an embolus (clot of blood or other material from elsewhere in the body), or by BUERGER'S DISEASE (chronic inflammation

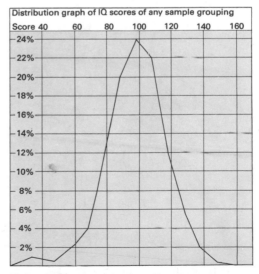

IQ (intelligence quotient) levels in any given group can be represented by this graph form.

of the blood vessels). Occasionally, intermittent claudication occurs following an injury to the leg and subsequent blood vessel damage.

The condition commonly develops in smokers, and in those with diabetes mellitus. The symptoms become worse if the patient becomes anaemic or develops HYPOTHYROIDISM.

Unless the onset is sudden because of an embolus or thrombosis, there is a gradual deterioration in blood supply to the muscles. The symptoms tend to become worse, and, finally, any form of activity causes pain.

Q: *Are there any dangers in intermittent claudication?*

A: Yes. The condition is a sign of poor blood supply to the leg, and other tissues also suffer, possibly resulting in gangrene of the toes and feet. Sudden blockage of the blood vessel may lead to an INFARCTION (area of dead tissue) and gangrene in the muscles and the gradual deterioration may result in peripheral NEURITIS (inflammation of nerves).

Q: *How is intermittent claudication treated?*

A: It is essential that a patient who smokes should stop smoking, because this may prevent any further progress of the condition and allow him or her to lead a relatively normal life without further discomfort. A doctor may prescribe a drug that makes the blood vessels widen (vasodilator), but such drugs are seldom successful because the disease of the arteries prevents their expansion.

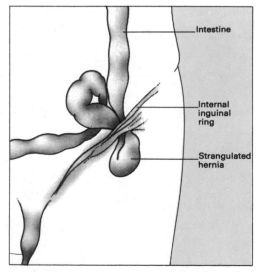

Intestinal obstruction may be caused by a strangulated hernia and requires surgery.

If the symptoms are severe and the patient is suffering from considerable incapacity, surgery is indicated. An arteriogram locates the diseased section, and arterial surgery is performed to graft in a new segment of artery or plastic tubing. This treatment often gives complete relief from symptoms.

Intersex is an individual with both male and female characteristics. *See* HERMAPHRODITE.

Intertrigo is the soreness and inflammation that occur between layers of skin which rub together; it is a form of DERMATITIS. The skin becomes soft and peels off to expose reddened, sore areas that are vulnerable to infection. Intertrigo usually occurs in the creases of the neck, beneath large breasts, and in the groin. In obese people, intertrigo may also occur in the abdominal creases.

Treatment involves dieting and exercise to lose weight, and keeping the skin clean and dry, with frequent washing and powdering.

Intestinal flu, also called gastric flu, is a popular name for viral GASTROENTERITIS.

Intestinal obstruction is a complete or partial blockage of the intestine. It may occur at any time and for a variety of reasons. An intestinal obstruction interferes with the normal passage of the products of digestion through the digestive system.

Q: *What are the symptoms of an intestinal obstruction?*

A: The first symptom is usually abdominal pain, followed by swelling (distention) of the abdomen. The swelling is more marked if the obstruction occurs in the lower parts of the intestine. There may also be constipation and failure to pass internal gas. Vomiting may occur, although not for some hours after the initial symptoms, unless the obstruction is in the small intestine.

Q: *What causes an intestinal obstruction?*

A: There are various conditions that may cause an intestinal obstruction. Some are comparatively simple to treat, such as an accumulation of hard faeces or infestation with parasitic worms. Others are more serious, such as tumours, a strangulated hernia, or intestinal adhesions.

Q: *How is an intestinal obstruction treated?*

A: The treatment depends on the cause of the obstruction. If the large intestine is obstructed and the symptoms are not severe, there may be time for various tests, such as SIGMOIDOSCOPY and X-ray examination following a barium enema. If the symptoms are acute, an urgent surgical operation is required.

Surgery is not always necessary, but other treatments are given only if the cause is comparatively simple to treat or if the intestine can overcome the obstruction without the need for surgery. For example, if the obstruction is caused by the twisting of the intestine around an adhesion or a scar, it may untwist on its own without treatment. In all such cases the stomach is kept empty by sucking fluid up a gastric tube, and intravenous fluids are continued until it is certain that either the obstruction has disappeared or that surgery is necessary.

See also ADHESION; CROHN'S DISEASE; DIVERTICULITIS AND DIVERTICULOSIS; HERNIA; HIRSCHSPRUNG'S DISEASE; INTUSSUSCEPTION; MECKEL'S DIVERTICULUM; MECONIUM; VOLVULUS.

Intestine is the part of the digestive tract that extends from the outlet of the stomach to the anus. It is commonly called the gut, or bowel.

The intestine has two parts: the small intestine and the large intestine (the terms refer to their diameters, not to their lengths). The small intestine is the longer of the two, made up of the short DUODENUM and the JEJUNUM, which make up about two-fifths of the small intestine; and the ILEUM, which makes up three-fifths.

The large intestine is made up of the CAECUM (with the appendix), and the COLON, which ends at the RECTUM.

The contents of the intestine are moved by a series of muscular contractions and relaxations known as peristalsis. In the small intestine, food is digested and absorbed and the excess waste products and water pass into the large intestine. In the large intestine, excess fluid is reabsorbed, and bacterial action on the faeces produces some of the essential vitamins B and K for the body. *See* DIGESTIVE SYSTEM.

The intestine is covered by the peritoneum which, in many places, combines to form a membrane (the mesentery). The mesentery allows the ileum and parts of the colon freedom of movement and position while, at the same time, holding the intestine in the correct position. Blood vessels and nerves as well as many lymphatic vessels and lymph nodes occur in the mesentery. The veins in the mesentery join the hepatic portal vein that carries blood to the liver.

Intoxication is a state of being poisoned. The term is commonly applied to the condition produced by an excess of alcohol, but it can also refer to poisoning by drugs, and the confusion and delirium caused by fever.

Intradermal means within the skin layer. For example, rashes that occur within the substance of the skin are termed intradermal rashes.

Intramuscular means within a muscle. For example, an intramuscular injection is one in which a solution of a drug is injected directly into a muscle.

Intrauterine device (IUCD, IUD) is a plastic or metal and plastic device that can be inserted into the womb (uterus) as a form of contraceptive. The intrauterine contraceptive device is more correctly called an IUCD rather than an IUD. (In medical terminology, IUD can also mean intrauterine death.)

There are at least four main kinds of intrauterine contraceptive device, most of which are in the shape of a double S, the figure 7, the letter T, or are like a ram's horn.

Q: *How does an IUCD work?*

A: The way an IUCD works is not exactly known. It is now thought that the principal effect takes place within the womb, either by creating an environment hostile to sperm or to the blastocyst, or by interrupting the process during attachment of the blastocyst.

One type of IUCD is activated by the hormone progestagen and is usually effective for a year, after which it should be changed. Other types should be changed every two years or are effective indefinitely.

Q: *Does an IUCD cause pain or discomfort?*

A: In general, no. But unfortunately, pain and heavy periods may occur for several months after an IUCD is inserted. Some IUCD's have been known to puncture the lining of the womb and cause heavy bleeding or haemorrhage. This form of contraception does not suit every woman,

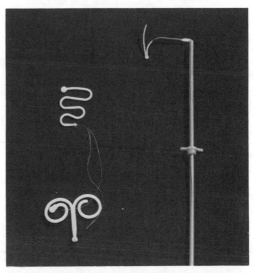

IUDs of various shapes; the one on the right is attached to the introducing instrument.

and should be considered only on a doctor's advice.

See also CONTRACEPTION.

Intravenous means within a vein. For example, an intravenous injection is made directly into a vein.

Intravenous cholangiogram is a special X-ray of the gall bladder and bile ducts taken after an intravenous injection of an iodine salt that contains a radiopaque solution. *See* CHOLANGIOGRAM.

Intravenous pyelogram (IVP) is a special X-ray of the kidneys taken after an intravenous injection of an iodine salt that contains a radiopaque solution.

Introvert is a personality type characterized by an introspective attitude, as opposed to an extrovert, who has an outgoing and sociable personality.

See also EXTROVERT.

Intussusception is a form of intestinal obstruction in which one section of the INTESTINE telescopes into the next section, like the finger of a glove being turned inside-out, and is drawn increasingly farther in by the action of the intestinal muscles. Most intussusceptions occur in children.

Q: What causes intussusception?

A: In most cases, the cause is not known. It has been suggested that intussusception occurs most often in children who have had a recent infection that causes a swelling of lymphoid tissue in the intestinal wall. The body treats the swelling as part of the intestinal contents and pulls it along by the action of the intestinal muscles. Occasionally a polyp,

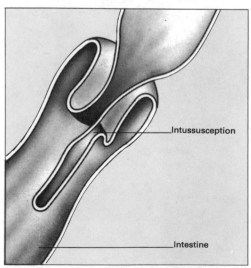

Intussusception

Intestine

Intussusception is an obstruction caused when a part of the intestine folds in upon itself.

tumour, or MECKEL'S DIVERTICULUM may cause intussusception in adults.

Q: What are the symptoms of intussusception?

A: In children, intussusception usually occurs suddenly, with severe pain, vomiting, and pallor. The affected child may draw up the knees and scream with the pain. As the attacks become more severe, the straining to expel faeces may cause blood and mucus to be passed from the rectum. But between attacks, the child may be calm and relaxed and may appear to have recovered.

Q: What is the treatment for intussusception?

A: Immediate hospitalization is vital. The patient is first given a barium enema, to prove the diagnosis. The pressure of the enema sometimes restores the affected parts of the intestine to their normal positions. But if this does not happen, a surgical operation is necessary.

In vitro is a term applied to reactions that occur outside a living body. For example, drugs are often tested in vitro ("in glass") before being tested on a living body.

In vivo is a term applied to reactions that occur within a living body.

Iodine is a non-metallic element. It is essential in the human diet for the correct functioning of the THYROID GLAND. Lack of iodine in the diet leads to the formation of a GOITRE and HYPOTHYROIDISM.

Q: Is iodine used in medical treatment?

A: Yes. Iodine salts may sometimes be given in the early treatment of hyperthyroidism (THYROTOXICOSIS), excessive activity of the thyroid gland. Iodine dissolved in an alcoholic solution or combined with povidone (povidone-iodine) is used as an antiseptic skin preparation before surgical operations or to clean wounds. Iodine preparations are also used as a diagnostic aid in special X-rays, such as a cholecystogram (of the gall bladder), intravenous pyelogram (of the kidney), and arteriogram (of an artery).

Radioactive iodine is used in the diagnosis of thyroid gland disease as well as in investigations of liver, lung, and kidney disorders. The preparation loses half its radioactivity within eight days. In larger doses, it may also be used in the treatment of hyperthyroidism and cancer of the thyroid gland.

Ionizing radiation is any radiation that causes substances to break up into ions (charged atoms or molecules). Gamma rays and X-rays are two examples of ionizing radiation. *See* RADIATION.

IQ is an abbreviation of intelligence quotient. *See* INTELLIGENCE QUOTIENT.

Iridectomy is an operation to remove part of the iris in the eye. It is most commonly performed as a treatment for acute GLAUCOMA to reduce the build-up of fluid pressure in the eyeball. An iridectomy may also be done to create an artificial pupil.

Iris is the coloured ring that surrounds the pupil of the eye. The iris is positioned in front of the lens and behind the cornea. Within the iris are muscle groups that by contracting or relaxing regulate how much light passes through the pupil. In bright light, some muscles of the iris relax and the pupil becomes smaller; in dim light, these muscles contract and the pupil becomes larger to admit as much light as possible.

Q: What determines the colour of the iris?

A: Eye colour, produced by pigment cells in the iris, is an inherited characteristic. (*See* HEREDITY.)

Q: What disorders can affect the iris?

A: The iris can become inflamed (iritis, choroiditis, or uveitis). A cleft iris is a congenital anomaly known as a COLOBOMA. An albino has very little pigmentation in the iris, and so the eyes look pink because the small blood vessels are visible.

Iritis is inflammation of the iris of the eye. The iris appears muddy in colour and smaller than usual. The pupil is also small and it changes size slowly in reaction to light variations, and so vision tends to be blurred. The eye waters continually. Pain in and above the eye, sensitivity to light (photophobia), redness, and soreness are other symptoms.

Iron is a metallic chemical element. It occurs in HAEMOGLOBIN, the constituent in red blood cells that carries oxygen, and so iron is an essential element in the human body. Iron is also present in enzymes (substances that produce chemical change) associated with respiration and in myoglobin, an important protein in muscle. The body gets its iron from foods. Those rich in iron include liver, eggs and lean meat. Pregnant women need more iron than do other adults. Growing children also need more iron to help to build new body tissue.

Q: What happens if there is insufficient iron in the body?

A: Iron deficiency ANAEMIA occurs. The condition may be caused by a gradual loss of iron from the body because of a bleeding peptic ulcer, menstrual problems, or bleeding from a cancer. Iron deficiency may be caused by a sudden and severe haemorrhage.

Q: How is iron deficiency treated?

A: The body is able to absorb iron, in almost any form, when taken orally. If iron deficiency does not improve after iron has been taken orally, as may happen in conditions in which there is absence of acid in the stomach, then iron may be given by intravenous or intramuscular injection. Adverse side effects from taking a normal dose of iron are rare but, occasionally, a patient has constipation or diarrhoea with mild symptoms of indigestion.

Irradiation is the application of any form of radiation to a tissue or substance. In medical treatment, irradiation may be in the form of X-rays, radioactive particles, heat, or ultra-violet light. *See* RADIATION.

Irrigation is the washing out of a body cavity or a wound with water or an antiseptic fluid. *See* ENEMA.

Ischaemia is a decreased blood supply to a particular part of the body. It is caused by spasm or disease in the blood vessels.

The condition most commonly develops in ARTERIOSCLEROSIS. This may result in cramp (*see* INTERMITTENT CLAUDICATION) in the legs, or ANGINA PECTORIS if it affects the heart, or a mild STROKE (transient ischaemia), if it affects the brain. Such strokes may be followed by complete recovery, because there is sometimes no brain damage.

Ischaemia may also result from acute blockage of an artery either following injury or because of a blood clot (*see* EMBOLISM). Some tissues die much more quickly than others when they become ischaemic. The brain survives for only about five minutes whereas the kidneys can continue to function for one to two hours.

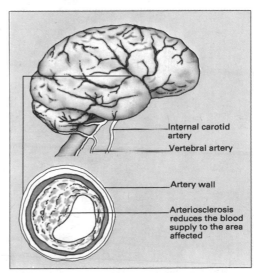

Internal carotid artery

Vertebral artery

Artery wall

Arteriosclerosis reduces the blood supply to the area affected

Ischaemia is a reduced blood supply. When it occurs in the brain, it causes a mild stroke.

Ischiorectal abscess

Ischiorectal abscess is an infection between the ischium bone of the pelvis (part of the hip-bone) and the adjacent area of the intestine, more usually the anus than the rectum. The abscess is painful, with local swelling and extreme tenderness. An ischiorectal abscess requires surgical treatment.

Ischium is one of the three bones that form the pelvis. It joins the ILIUM near the hip joint and the PUBIS at the front. The ischium is a strong bone with a protuberant lower part, which is covered by a fluid-filled cavity (bursa) that counters pressure. This is the area that supports the body when sitting.

Ishihara's test is a method of detecting colour blindness. *See* COLOUR BLINDNESS.

Islets of Langerhans are clusters of cells within the pancreas, a gland located behind the stomach.

Q: What is the function of the islets of Langerhans?

A: They secrete insulin and glucagon. The most important is INSULIN, which reduces the level of glucose in the bloodstream by helping to convert glucose to glycogen. GLUCAGON increases the level of glucose in the blood.

Q: What happens if the islets of Langerhans fail to function normally?

A: The production of the pancreatic hormones is upset, resulting in various disorders. Lack of insulin causes DIABETES MELLITUS.

　　Rarely, a tumour of the pancreas may cause overproduction of insulin, causing HYPOGLYCAEMIA; or excess glucagon, producing HYPERGLYCAEMIA.

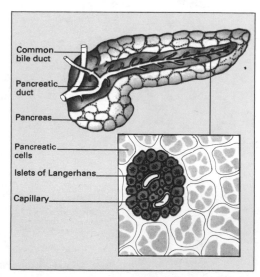

Common bile duct

Pancreatic duct

Pancreas

Pancreatic cells

Islets of Langerhans

Capillary

Islets of Langerhans are pancreatic cells that secrete insulin and glucagon.

Recurrent attacks of PANCREATITIS damage the islets of Langerhans and may cause diabetes mellitus.

Isolation has various medical meanings. The most common use of the term describes the situation of a patient who is kept apart from other people to prevent the spread of an infectious disease, such as smallpox. A patient may also be kept in isolation during the treatment of various diseases, such as leukaemia, in which the treatment itself reduces the patient's resistance to infection.

Isolation also describes the extraction and identification of bacteria or viruses that cause a particular disease.

In psychiatry, isolation describes a patient's state of loneliness or solitude.

Isotonic describes anything, particularly muscles, that have equal tone or tension. An isotonic solution is a solution of salts in water that closely matches the body's normal fluids in strength.

Isotope is an individual form of a chemical element that differs from others like it only in the composition of the nucleus of its atoms. All isotopes of a single element have similar chemical properties. But all their physical properties may vary; for example, some isotopes are radioactive. Radioactive isotopes are used in the investigation and diagnosis of many disorders. They are also used in treatment, for example, to destroy cancerous tumours.

See also RADIOLOGY.

Itching, known medically as pruritus, is a symptom that is produced by a disturbance to the nerve endings just under the skin. The reasons for itching are not fully understood. Some people feel itching sensations much more easily than others, and an itching skin condition such as measles can cause much more distress in one patient than another.

Q: What conditions may cause itching?

A: Itching may be a symptom of dry skin following sunburn or ICHTHYOSIS. There are many other skin disorders that may be accompanied by itching, including ECZEMA, URTICARIA, SCABIES, and LICHEN PLANUS. Generalized itching, which is often worse when the person is tired or warm in bed, may occur for no obvious reason. Various investigations may be carried out to discover if the cause is URAEMIA, or a liver disorder such as JAUNDICE or CIRRHOSIS. Sometimes continued itching or itching that stops and starts again is a symptom of underlying anxiety or depression. Occasionally, a malignant disease, such as HODGKIN'S DISEASE, produces itching for some months before the disease itself appears. Rarely itching occurs during pregnancy, when it may be accompanied by urticaria.

Q: *Why do areas of itching occur?*

A: Itching in one spot may be caused by sensitivity to chemicals or materials. Examples include perfume behind the ears, nickel on jewellery, or clothing made of wool or an artificial fibre.

Local itching around the anus (pruritus ani) may be associated with the slight moist discharge from a HAEMORRHOID (piles), following diarrhoea or, quite commonly, as a form of allergy to anaesthetic ointments used in the treatment of haemorrhoids. In children, anal itching, particularly at night, may be caused by THREADWORM.

Itching of the vulva (pruritus vulvae) may occur with any form of local infection, such as VULVITIS or VAGINITIS; or it may be associated with skin infections, such as MONILIASIS (thrush). Genital itching is a common symptom of DIABETES MELLITUS and may occur with LEUKOPLAKIA, a condition that develops before cancerous changes in the vulva.

Q: *How is itching treated?*

A: Areas of irritation that occur after sunburn or dry skin from any cause may be helped with soothing creams and lotions, such as calamine. If the itching persists a doctor may carry out investigations to discover the cause and prescribe the appropriate treatment.

Antihistamine and antipruritic drugs and creams may aid in controlling the symptoms and sometimes the doctor may prescribe corticosteroid creams or ointments to be used for a short time.

IUCD. *See* INTRAUTERINE DEVICE.

IUD. *See* INTRAUTERINE DEVICE.

IVP. *See* INTRAVENOUS PYELOGRAM.

J

Jacksonian epilepsy is a form of epilepsy in which only one half of the brain is involved, generally because a scar or a tumour there acts as a focal point for irritation. As a result, when a grand mal attack (a major seizure) occurs, only limited areas of the body are affected at first: for example, one side of the face or one hand. The seizure may then progress and affect the whole of one side of the body before finally causing loss of consciousness and the typical convulsions. Sometimes, however, the attack remains localized and the patient does not lose consciousness. *See* EPILEPSY.

Jaundice, known medically also as icterus, is a condition characterized by a yellowing of the skin and the whites of the eyes. It is a symptom, not a disease in itself. The yellow colour is caused by an excess in the body of the BILE pigment bilirubin. Normally, bilirubin is formed by the breakdown of haemoglobin during the destruction of worn-out red blood cells. It is then excreted by the liver into the bile via the bile ducts.

Q: *What causes an excess of bilirubin in the body?*

A: An excess can be caused by (1) overproduction of bilirubin; (2) the failure of the liver to metabolize bilirubin or to excrete it; or (3) a blockage of the bile ducts.

Overproduction of bilirubin may be caused by the destruction of an excessive number of red blood cells (haemolytic anaemia). The liver cannot then excrete bilirubin fast enough. This occurs in malaria, thalassaemia, and haemolytic disease of the newborn.

Mild jaundice occurs as a common and normal condition in newborn babies, because at birth there is a deficiency in the enzyme that helps to excrete bilirubin. Rarely, this enzyme deficiency can also cause jaundice in adults. But in babies, the condition disappears within a few days as the enzyme is formed.

Jaundice may also result from diseases of the liver such as hepatitis or cirrhosis.

If the bile ducts become blocked, bile

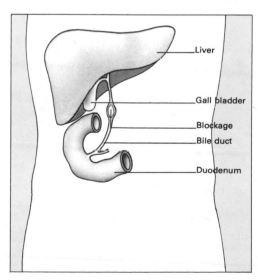

Jaundice is a symptom of many disorders, one of which is blockage of a bile duct.

Jaw

cannot be excreted, and jaundice occurs. The ducts may be blocked by (1) inflammation and infection (cholangitis); (2) a gallstone (cholelithiasis); or (3) cancer of the pancreas or the common bile duct. Occasionally, drugs such as chlorpromazine may inhibit bilirubin excretion by the liver.

Q: *What other symptoms can occur with jaundice?*

A: Other symptoms depend on the specific cause of the jaundice. In many forms of the condition, bilirubin is excreted in the urine, which becomes dark brown in colour. If the excretion of bile is obstructed, stools are almost white and the digestion of fat is impaired. If the condition has been present for some time, intense itching may occur due to excess bile in the skin.

Q: *How are the causes of jaundice diagnosed?*

A: Diagnosis requires special blood tests, in which a doctor determines whether the liver is diseased, whether the bilirubin is being correctly metabolized by the liver cells, and whether there is any abnormal weakness in the red blood cells. The urine is examined for bilirubin, and the faeces for pale coloration (which would indicate an obstruction to bile excretion). It is sometimes necessary to perform a liver BIOPSY to examine cells under a microscope.

Jaw is the name of each of the two large bones in which the teeth are embedded. Each jaw represents two bones that fuse before

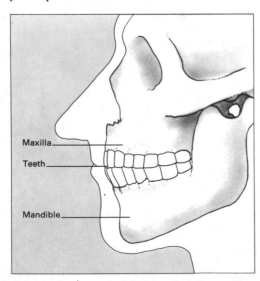

Jaw, the framework of the mouth, is formed by the maxilla and mandibular bones.

Maxilla

Teeth

Mandible

birth: the mandibles join in the front to form the chin, and the maxillae form most of the roof of the mouth and contain the two sinuses that open into the nose.

The upper jaw is stationary and the lower jaw is hinged from it at small hinge joints situated in front of the ears. Powerful cheek muscles pull the lower jaw up to the upper jaw for biting. For chewing, the muscles move the lower jaw backward and forward or from side to side.

Q: *What medical problems can occur with the jaw?*

A: Because the hinge joints are small, the most common jaw problem is dislocation, resulting in the inability to close the mouth. A sudden blow is the usual cause, but dislocation may occur from yawning while leaning with the chin on one hand. Careful manipulation by a doctor replaces a dislocated jaw.

Fractures of the jaw may require dental and facio-maxillary surgery to reposition either jaw in the correct biting position. Because the upper jaw extends upward as far as the floors of the eye sockets, fractures of the maxilla may also cause a change in the position of the eye, resulting in visual problems.

Minor arthritis in a jaw joint causes a clicking sensation, and sometimes pain when the jaw is moved up and down.

Infection of the jaw may follow dental disorders, and may cause inflammation of the nasal sinuses (sinusitis) or, rarely, inflammation of the bone (osteomyelitis).

Q: *How can a person eat with a fractured jaw?*

A: A person with a fractured jaw cannot eat solid food: it is impossible to bite. The broken jaw is usually wired to the other jaw to re-establish the correct biting position. For this reason, all food has to be sucked through a straw. Great care must be taken to ensure that choking and vomiting do not occur, because a person whose jaws are wired together cannot expel the vomit and may choke to death. A doctor may advise the patient to carry wire cutters to use in such an emergency.

Jejunum is part of the small intestine. It is about 1.2 metres (four feet) long and connects the duodenum and the ileum. Enzymes in the small intestine continue the breakdown of food (from the stomach), which can then be absorbed through its wall into the lymphatic vessels and the hepatic portal vein.

COELIAC DISEASE is a disorder of the mucous lining of the jejunum.

See also INTESTINE.

Jet lag is the disorientation in the normal biological CIRCADIAN RHYTHM that is experienced by a person who travels quickly from one time zone to another of more than four hours' difference. The greater the time difference, the more serious is the disorientation. Because of jet lag, a person may feel sleepy during the day, alert during the night, and hungry at inconvenient hours. The body temperature may no longer be synchronized with day and night requirements.

Q: What is the best way to deal with jet lag?

A: The body may take a long time to adjust to a new circadian rhythm, possibly as many as ten days. If the stay in the new time zone is to be short, it is often advisable not to adapt, but to retain the familiar rhythm, even at the expense of unusual hours. On a business trip this generally means that at least some working hours fall within commercial times. A longer visit requires adaptation, which may mean taking sedatives for a few nights to ensure enough sleep.

Jigger (or chigger, or chigoe) is the common name of the burrowing flea, *Tunga penetrans*, which occurs in tropical India, Africa, and America. The female flea burrows under the skin, generally of the legs and feet and especially between the toes, where it causes intense local itching. A swelling forms where the insect lays its eggs, and the swelling often becomes ulcerated and infected. Treatment is to open the swelling with a sterilized needle to remove the jigger and the eggs and then to apply antiseptic cream.

Dirt that enters the skin as the jigger burrows its way in may cause tetanus.

Joint is medically defined as an area in the body at which two bones are in contact. At a joint, the bones may be freely mobile under the control of muscles, ligaments, and tendons; they may be only slightly mobile; or they may be fixed so as to be immobile.

Q: What are mobile joints?

A: At a typical mobile joint, the ends of the bones are covered with tough cartilage and lined with a membrane (the synovial membrane) containing a small amount of lubricating fluid. The joint has stabilizing ligaments limiting the directions and the extent to which the bones can be moved.

Q: Are there different kinds of mobile joints?

A: Yes, there are several different kinds. A hinge joint acts like a hinge: examples include the elbow and the fingers. A ball-and-socket joint, in which the rounded end of one bone fits inside a concave socket of the other, allows good rotation: examples are the shoulder and the hip. A saddle joint allows sliding movement in two directions: the ankle and thumb are saddle joints. A plane joint permits only slight sliding movement, as in the wrist bones. An ellipsoid joint allows circular and bending movements but no rotation: the fingers have ellipsoid hinge joints. A pivot joint, allowing rotation and no other movement, is found solely between the two top vertebrae of the neck.

Mobile joints are more complex than the slightly mobile or immobile joints.

Q: What are slightly mobile joints?

A: At a typical slightly mobile joint, the bones have a layer of cartilage between them and are held firmly together by strong ligaments. Such joints are found between the pubic bones (symphysis pubis) and the discs between the vertebrae of the spine.

Q: What are immobile joints?

A: Immobile joints occur where two bones are fused or fixed together before or shortly after birth. Examples are the ilium, pubis, and ischium, which together form the pelvis, and the many flat bones that combine to make up the skull.

Joint disorders. There are many conditions that may involve joints: degenerative conditions, such as osteoarthritis; inflammatory conditions, such as rheumatoid arthritis; conditions involving the membranes surrounding the joints, such as synovitis; generalized disorders involving the joints, such as gout; damage to the joint involving dislocation or complicated fracture; congenital disorders, including congenital dislocation of the hip and clubfoot; and, sometimes,

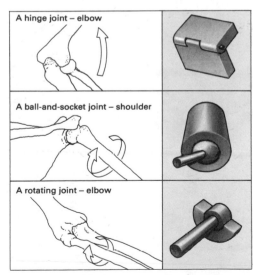

A hinge joint – elbow

A ball-and-socket joint – shoulder

A rotating joint – elbow

Joints of several different types allow the human skeleton freedom of movement.

disorders of the cartilage, such as a slipped disc and a torn cartilage in knee disorders.

Each of the following joint disorders has a separate article in the A-Z section of this book:

ANKYLOSING	GOUT
SPONDYLITIS	HAMMERTOE
ANKYLOSIS	OSTEOARTHROPATHY
ARTHRITIS (including	OSTEOARTHROSIS
rheumatoid	OSTEOCHONDRITIS
arthritis and	PERTHES' DISEASE
osteoarthritis)	POLYARTHRITIS
ARTHRODESIS	RHEUMATIC FEVER
BURSITIS	SLIPPED DISC
CAPSULITIS	SPONDYLITIS
CERVICAL SPONDYLOSIS	SPONDYLOLISTHESIS
CLUBFOOT	SPONDYLOSIS
DISLOCATION	SUBLUXATION
FROZEN SHOULDER	SYNOVITIS

Jugular vein is any one of four veins in the neck. They are: the internal jugular veins, one on each side of the neck; and the external jugular veins, one at the front of the neck and the other at the side of the neck.

K

Kahn test is a blood test for detecting the presence of the venereal disease syphilis. *See* SYPHILIS; WASSERMANN TEST.

Kaolin, or china clay, is a naturally occurring form of aluminum silicate used medically in many antidiarrhoeal mixtures. It has absorbent properties.

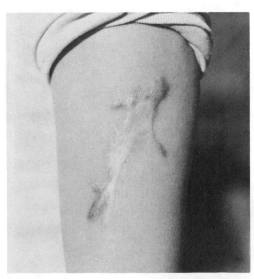

Keloid scar occurs when the body's healing process overresponds following an injury.

Keloid is a mass of excessive fibrous tissue that develops at the site of a scar. Black people are more likely to form keloids than are people of other races.

Keratitis is an inflammation of the cornea, the transparent membrane that forms the front of the eye. If the condition occurs suddenly, it causes pain, sensitivity to light (photophobia), and watering of the eye. If keratitis develops gradually, only minor discomfort may result. Opaque patches in the cornea can cause the patient's vision to blur.

Q: What causes keratitis?

A: Keratitis is often a symptom of a more general disorder. Virus infections, such as TRACHOMA (chronic conjunctivitis) or herpes simplex, may infect the cornea. Bacterial infection may follow any eye wound. Keratitis is also a consequence of congenital syphilis or, rarely, tuberculosis. Occasionally a form of keratitis occurs in middle-aged women with ROSACEA. A deficiency of vitamin A causes dryness of the cornea which makes it more susceptible to infection.

Q: How is keratitis treated?

A: Further damage to the cornea can be prevented with eye drops containing the drug atropine to dilate the pupil. Corticosteroid drugs reduce the inflammation. It is essential for the eyes to be examined by an ophthalmologist.

Kernicterus is a serious form of haemolytic disease of the newborn, a condition in which brain damage occurs. *See* HAEMOLYTIC DISEASE OF THE NEWBORN.

Kernig's sign may be seen as a result of a neurological test in which the patient lies flat on the back after bending the knee. The doctor then tries to straighten the leg. If the patient unconsciously resists, it may indicate irritation of a nerve where it passes out of the spine, as may occur with a slipped disc or meningitis.

Ketones are substances formed by the body during the breakdown of fats and fatty acids into carbon dioxide and water. Acetone is an example of a ketone.

Excessive amounts of ketones are formed when fat is used, instead of sugar, for providing energy. This condition, called ketosis, occurs during starvation and, sometimes, during high fevers when large amounts of heat energy are needed. It may also happen in diabetes mellitus, when the body has difficulty in using sugar normally.

Ketosis. *See* KETONES.

Kidney is one of a pair of organs located at the back of the abdomen, against the strong muscles next to the spine, and behind the intestines and other organs. The adrenal glands lie on the top of the kidneys.

Each kidney weighs about five ounces (150 grams) and is about 10 cm (four inches) long in the average adult. Its inner side forms the renal pelvis, which collects urine as it is formed and passes it out of the kidney to the bladder via the ureter. The inner side is also joined to the artery and vein that carry blood to and from the kidney.

Q: *What is the function of the kidneys?*
A: The kidneys filter out water and also unwanted substances in the blood. These substances are produced by the normal working of the body. They are excreted by the kidneys in the form of urine. The kidneys also keep the salts and water of the body in the correct balance.

Q: *How do the kidneys work?*
A: Blood passes through each kidney under high pressure. The blood is filtered by the glomeruli, special structures in the kidney containing clusters of capillaries that collect water, salts, and unwanted substances. The filtrate passes along a fine tube, the nephron (of which there are approximately one million in each kidney), which reabsorbs any of the water, glucose, and salts that the body still requires and allows the rest to pass into the pelvis of the kidney as urine.

See also p.14.

Kidney dialysis (medically known as haemodialysis) is a method of filtering unwanted substances from the blood using a machine that acts as an artificial kidney. It is used for patients whose own kidneys are damaged or malfunctioning.

Q: *How does a kidney dialysis machine work?*
A: Blood from an artery passes into the dialysis machine and over a thin sheet of membrane that acts as a filter for unwanted substances. The purified blood is then fed back into one of the patient's veins.

A variety of machines are available, some of which are small and safe enough to be used by the patient at home. The most modern machine is portable.

Q: *Are there any problems in using such a machine?*
A: Yes. Many of the problems are associated with maintaining sterility, but most of these have been overcome by the use of machines with disposable parts. It can be difficult to find suitable veins and arteries in the patient, but it is now possible to implant a small plastic tube (called a shunt) in the blood vessels that can be connected to the machine.

Q: *How often should dialysis be performed?*
A: It is usually necessary to perform dialysis for periods of four to six hours, three times a week, in hospital, at a special dialysis centre set up for the purpose, or at the patient's home.

Q: *When may kidney dialysis be used?*
A: Dialysis is used to treat acute or chronic kidney failure. In acute renal failure, dialysis continues until the kidneys recover their normal function. In chronic renal failure, dialysis continues either for the rest of the patient's life or until a kidney transplant is performed.

See also KIDNEY; KIDNEY DISEASE; TRANSPLANT SURGERY.

Q: *Can dialysis be carried out without the use of a machine?*
A: Yes. Peritoneal dialysis does not require a machine. It is performed by inserting a sterile plastic catheter into the abdominal cavity and irrigating the peritoneum with an isotonic solution that extracts the unwanted substances from the blood.

A talk about Kidney disease

Kidney disease. The body depends on the kidneys to excrete many waste products and to maintain the correct balance of water and salts, and any kidney disorder interferes with these important functions.

Q: *What are the symptoms of kidney disease?*
A: The symptoms of kidney disease depend on the underlying cause. They are often

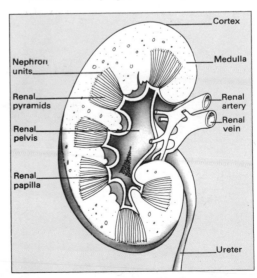

Kidney filters body fluids within the nephron units and expels wastes via the ureter.

Kidney disease

mild and vague until a late stage in the disease. Kidney disease may cause an increased amount of urine to be formed, leading to abnormally frequent urination (polyuria). Or the formation of urine may be diminished, leading to abnormally infrequent urination (oliguria).

Some kidney diseases, such as acute nephritis, may cause blood in the urine (haematuria). Other symptoms of kidney disease include acute abdominal pain (colic); and generalized oedema, which is swelling due to the accumulation of water in the body tissues.

If both kidneys stop working completely, waste products accumulate in the body and poison the patient. This can be fatal and requires urgent medical attention.

Q: *What causes kidney disease?*

A: Kidney disease may be caused by many factors, such as injury; infection; cancer; or disorders in other parts of the body. In some cases, kidney disease may occur without apparent cause.

The kidney may be damaged in a serious accident, causing a rupture of its surrounding capsule and leading to severe haemorrhage. The damaged kidney may have to be surgically removed (nephrectomy). Rarely, the kidney may be damaged by radiotherapy treatment carried out for cancer. This may eventually result in high blood pressure and kidney failure.

Stones may form in the kidneys (nephrolithiasis) and cause kidney damage. This may occur without apparent cause, or it may be due to an underlying

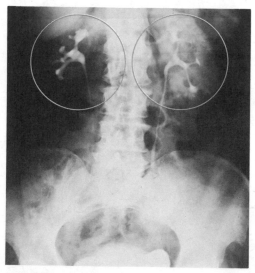

Kidney disease may be detected with an intravenous pyelogram, a form of X-ray.

metabolic disorder. Occasionally, microscopic crystals form in the kidney substance itself (nephrocalcinosis). These may occur for the same reasons as do stones, or, rarely, in babies who are given excessive amounts of vitamin D.

The kidney may become infected and inflamed. This may result in various kidney diseases, such as nephritis; glomerulonephritis; or pyelonephritis. Infection of the kidneys often results from the spread of infection from the bladder.

Cancer of the kidney may occur in the renal pelvis, the collecting area for urine, or in the kidney itself (hypernephroma). The latter is most common in adults, but a nephroblastoma (Wilms' tumour) may occur in young children.

Many disorders in other parts of the body have an effect on the kidney. High blood pressure gradually damages the kidneys. Because of such damage, high blood pressure often continues to be a problem after the original cause has been found and treated. Various hormone disorders, such as parathyroid gland hyperactivity, Cushing's syndrome, and diabetes insipidus, affect kidney function. Diabetes mellitus not only causes sugar in the urine (glycosuria) but may eventually cause damage to the glomeruli or to the blood supply to the kidney. A stone in the ureter may cause urinary obstruction. This may result in reverse pressure of the urine into the kidney, producing distention and progressive loss of function (hydronephrosis).

Q: *What tests are carried out to diagnose kidney disease?*

A: Suspected kidney disease can be investigated in various ways. Chemical testing of the urine detects the presence of any abnormal substances, such as protein (albuminuria), sugar (glycosuria), or haemoglobin (haemoglobinuria). The concentration of salts and urea also can be determined. Examination of urine through a microscope may detect blood (haematuria) or white blood cells resulting from infection. Tests that measure the amount of urea and creatinine (two waste products that should be excreted by the kidney) in the blood help detect kidney disease.

The kidneys also may be given either an INTRAVENOUS PYELOGRAM (IVP), a form of X-ray, or, a retrograde pyelogram. Both procedures outline the urine collecting system and help to detect abnormalities of kidney size and shape.

An ARTERIOGRAM shows the blood supply to the kidney; and occasionally a renogram, using radioactive iodine, is carried out.

Finally, if the diagnosis still is in doubt, a renal biopsy may be performed, using a long needle to obtain a small sample of kidney tissue for examination with a microscope.

Q: *How are kidney diseases treated?*
A: The treatment of kidney diseases depends on their cause, and may involve the skilled care of a nephrologist, a specialist in kidney diseases.

For details of individual kidney disorders, *see* ALBUMINURIA; CALCULUS; DIABETES MELLITUS; GLOMERULONEPHRITIS; GLYCOSURIA; HAEMATURIA; HAEMOGLOBIN-URIA; HYDRONEPHROSIS; NEPHRITIS; NEPHROTIC SYNDROME; NOCTURIA; OLIGURIA; POLYURIA; PYELONEPHRITIS; URAEMIA.

Kidney stone. *See* CALCULUS.

Kleptomania is a compulsive and uncontrollable desire to steal. The stolen objects often have little intrinsic value. It is a form of mental illness and may be a symptom of depression in which the stealing continues, in an obvious manner, until the patient is caught. In such cases there is probably an unconscious desire to be caught and to receive appropriate treatment.

Klinefelter's syndrome is a genetic disease seen in males, caused by the presence of one or more extra (female sex) X chromosomes. It is not true hermaphroditism. It is not usually diagnosed until after puberty, at which time the male breasts may become enlarged and the testicles remain small. Varying degrees of mental retardation may also be present. There is no specific treatment.

See also HERMAPHRODITE.

Knee is the hinge joint between the lower end of the thigh-bone (femur) and the upper end of the shin-bone (tibia). The front of the knee is covered by the lower tendon of the quadriceps femoris, a massive group of muscles that extend to the top of the thigh. The broad tendon that attaches this muscle to the front of the tibia contains the patella (kneecap). The patella forms a protective shield in front of the knee joint, behind which pass the main artery, vein, and nerve of the leg.

There are strong ligaments on each side of the knee which prevent its dislocation outward or inward. Inside the joint are two ligaments (cruciate ligaments) that protect the joint from dislocation forward or backward. There are also two semilunar cartilages attached to the outer edges of the internal surface of the joint on top of the tibia.

When the leg is extended to straighten it at the knee, the bones work together so that they lock into a rigid structure.

See also KNEE PROBLEMS.

Kneecap. *See* PATELLA.

Knee jerk may be seen as the result of a neurological test in which the tendon of the large muscle in front of the thigh (quadriceps femoris) is tapped with a small hammer just below the kneecap (patella). This produces an involuntary kicking movement of the leg. The manner and speed with which the reaction takes place help a doctor to diagnose certain neurological disorders. *See* REFLEX.

Knee problems. The knee is a complex joint capable of a large range of movements and it has to support the full weight of the body. For this reason, it is particularly vulnerable to injury, degenerative changes, and joint disorders. With increasing age, degeneration of the knee joint through osteoarthritis becomes more likely. It occurs particularly in those who are overweight or who have a previous history of knee injury. A form of bursitis (housemaid's knee) occurs particularly in persons who have to kneel frequently or continually while working.

Damage to the semilunar cartilages within the knee joint is a common occurrence that often results from excessive rotation when "locking" the leg straight (*see* KNEE). Sometimes the surface lining the knee can degenerate (osteochondritis), and a fragment can break off inside the joint. This causes pain, further damage, and a tendency for the knee

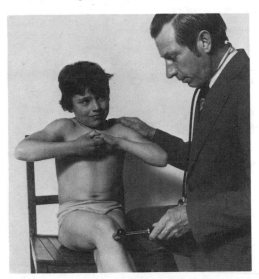

Knee jerk is a reflex reaction that is obtained by tapping the knee just below the patella.

Knock-knee

to lock, thereby preventing the leg from being fully extended.

Occasionally, the quadriceps muscle (which passes over the knee) ruptures and causes an unstable knee joint. This condition is usually associated with a sudden strain, but sometimes there is little obvious reason. This is particularly likely to happen in the elderly.

See also BOW-LEGS; BURSITIS; JOINT DISORDERS; KNOCK-KNEE; MENISCUS; PATELLA.

Knock-knee (medically known as genu valgum) is a disorder in which the lower legs are curved outward so that the knees touch each other and the ankles are apart. This condition commonly occurs in childhood as a normal stage of development between the ages of about two and a half and four years. As the child continues to grow, the legs gradually straighten.

Koilonychia is a deformity of the nails. The nail becomes thin and the normal curve of the outer surface is reversed, giving the nail a spoon-shaped appearance. This uncommon condition may occur in patients with iron-deficiency anaemia.

Koplik's spots are a sign of measles. They are tiny red spots with white centres that appear on the palate, inside the cheeks, and on the tongue; they may also occur on the internal surface of the eyelids.

See also MEASLES.

Korsakoff's syndrome is a form of mental illness. It is commonly found in brain-damaged patients suffering from ALCOHOLISM, but it may also accompany other forms of brain damage, for example, cerebral tumours, head injuries, and minor strokes.

Q: What are the symptoms of Korsakoff's syndrome?

A: The patient is unable to remember recent events and tends to invent plausible accounts of what he or she has been doing during the past few days or weeks. Memory for distant events is normal and any skills learned in the past can be performed with ease. This is in contrast to the patient's ability to learn a new skill which, being difficult to remember, is consequently difficult to perform.

Q: What is the treatment for Korsakoff's syndrome?

A: The treatment depends on the cause. Alcoholism should be treated appropriately, and large amounts of B vitamins often produce a slow improvement.

See also ALCOHOLISM.

Küntscher nail is a tubular metal nail that is inserted into the centre of a bone in the treatment of a fracture.

Kwashiorkor is a form of severe malnutrition in children. There is a characteristic loss of pigmentation of the hair giving it a reddish-brown appearance. The children have dry, scaling, pale skin, as well as a protuberant abdomen, and they fail to grow normally. There is also often swelling (oedema) of the feet and legs. Severe cases may lead to extreme emaciation.

Kymograph is an instrument that records movements such as blood pressure changes, muscle contractions, respiratory movements, or changes in pressure in the intestine. The recording is called a kymogram.

Kyphosis is either an excessive curvature of the spine, such as that of a "hunchback," or a more gradual, but still abnormal, curvature. It commonly affects the spine behind the chest, but may affect the lower or upper spine if there is an excessive amount of bending forward.

It is frequently associated with scoliosis (sideways curvature of the spine), and with bone disorders that affect the vertebrae, osteoporosis in the elderly, ankylosing spondylitis, and a form of osteochondritis that affects the bones of the spine.

See also LORDOSIS; SCOLIOSIS.

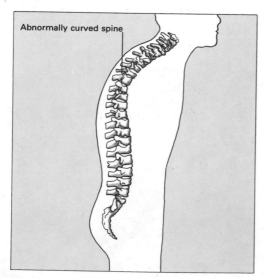

Abnormally curved spine

Kyphosis produces a stooping posture by exaggerating the spine's posterior curve.

L

Labial describes anything pertaining to the lips, either of the mouth or vulva.

Labium is a lip or edge of a body structure. The term is used to describe the thick edge of a bone, the cervix (neck) of the womb, or one of the lips of the mouth. *See* VULVA.

Labour is the process of childbirth by which the baby and placenta (afterbirth) are delivered. *See* PREGNANCY AND CHILDBIRTH.

Labyrinth is the inner ear, consisting of the three semicircular canals and the cochlea. *See* EAR.

Labyrinthitis is inflammation of the inner ear. Labyrinthitis is accompanied by extreme dizziness and vomiting, and sometimes causes deafness.

Bacterial or viral infection may spread to the inner ear from a middle ear infection (OTITIS media); occur with MENINGITIS; or follow an operation on the ear, such as FENESTRATION or STAPEDECTOMY. The disorder requires urgent treatment from a specialist in ear diseases.

Laceration is a tear in any tissue in the body. It may be external or internal. External lacerations are often caused by a cut from a sharp object (for EMERGENCY treatment, *see* First Aid, p.582). Internal lacerations may occur when an organ is damaged by a violent blow, and an emergency operation is often necessary.

Lacrimal apparatus is the anatomical name for the structures in each eye that produce and distribute tears. The lacrimal gland lies in a notch in the upper, outer corner of the bony eye socket. The tears it secretes are carried in twelve small ducts to the surface of the eyeball. They are washed across the eye by the action of blinking. Two ducts at the inner corner of the eye drain the tears into the lacrimal sac and then into the nose.

Lacrimation is the medical term for the production of tears by the lacrimal gland of the eye. *See* LACRIMAL APPARATUS.

Lactation is the secretion of milk from the female breasts, and the period of lactation is the length of time for which breast-feeding continues.

Q: What makes the breasts start producing milk at the end of pregnancy?

A: Throughout pregnancy, the breasts develop and increase in size in response to increased amounts of the hormones oestrogen, progesterone, and chorionic gonadotrophin (the chorion is the membrane that encloses the foetus). These hormones are produced by the placenta, the organ of chemical interchange between mother and foetus. The increase in breast size is caused partly by the larger number of ducts that form in the breast and partly by an increase in the amount of fatty tissue.

Milk is not formed until after the baby is born. Milk production is stimulated by the hormone PROLACTIN produced by the

pituitary gland at the base of the brain, which in turn is stimulated by changes that take place at the onset of labour.

But "first milk" or COLOSTRUM, a fluid rich in fat and proteins, is secreted near the end of pregnancy. It contains antibodies from the mother that help to protect the baby against disease. As soon as the baby is born, the mother's hormone levels drop rapidly, prolactin secretion starts, and milk is produced. *See* PREGNANCY AND CHILDBIRTH.

Q: Why does milk secretion sometimes occur before the baby starts sucking?

A: The contraction of the breast tissue to expel milk is partly a reflex to the baby sucking and partly a response to the presence of the hormone OXYTOCIN (also secreted by the pituitary gland). This hormone may be produced in response to the mother's emotional reaction when she hears the baby crying. Oxytocin also causes contraction of the womb, and this accounts for an increase in vaginal flow when breast-feeding takes place.

Q: How may lactation be stopped?

A: If the woman does not want to breast feed, firm binding of the breasts is usually sufficient to stop lactation after the birth of the baby. If milk appears later, further oestrogens should be given.

The problem is more difficult if lactation needs to be stopped once it has started. A combination of oestrogens, restricted fluid intake, and a firm brassiere may stop lactation.

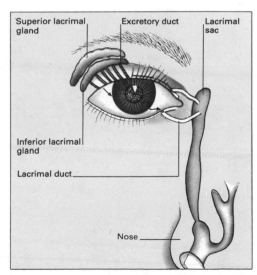

Superior lacrimal gland

Excretory duct

Lacrimal sac

Inferior lacrimal gland

Lacrimal duct

Nose

Lacrimal apparatus is the structure from which tears flow to wash over the eyes.

Lactic acid

Q: *Are there any dangers in using oestrogens to stop lactation?*

A: Yes, although risks are small and probably affect only women who are over the age of thirty-five, those who smoke, or those who have had an operation, such as a Caesarean section. There is also a slightly increased risk of venous thrombosis because of the effect of the oestrogens.

Q: *Can anything be done if lactation does not begin?*

A: Little can be done because the reasons for failure to start lactation are not fully understood.

Q: *Are there any problems that may occur during lactation?*

A: Yes. Gradual failure of lactation, once it has started, is usually caused by a combination of the mother's fatigue and anxiety as well as lack of sufficient fluid. This may occur when the mother returns home from hospital, and it is relatively easy to treat.

Other problems include engorgement of the breasts, failure to produce sufficient milk, or MASTITIS (inflammation of the breasts). Infection of the breast ducts usually results from a cracked nipple, but it may occasionally be a complication of PUERPERAL FEVER, a condition that can develop after a woman has given birth. Part of a breast becomes tender, swollen, and inflamed, and a sudden fever occurs, often starting with a shivering attack. A doctor may prescribe antibiotics and painkilling drugs. If possible, breast-feeding should continue because this empties the affected area. If an abscess forms, it will have to be incised.

Lactic acid is a colourless substance produced by the fermenting action of bacteria on milk or milk sugar (lactose). It occurs in sour milk and certain other foods. It is also produced during glucose and fat metabolism in the human body.

Lactose is a sugar found in milk. In the human digestive system, it is broken down into simpler substances by an enzyme (lactase) in the small intestine.

Lameness. *See* CLAUDICATION.

Laminectomy is a surgical operation in which a plate of bone (lamina) is removed from the back of one or more vertebrae to expose the spinal cord. It is performed during any operation on the spinal cord.

Lance is a double-edged surgical knife. The term is also used for a minor surgical operation in which a lance is used to open an abscess or boil.

Langerhans' islands. *See* ISLETS OF LANGERHANS.

Lanolin is a pale yellow fatty substance obtained from the grease of sheep's wool. It is used in various skin preparations because it mixes with oils and with water to produce ointments that penetrate the skin and so help in the absorption of drugs.

Lanugo is the fine, downy hair that covers a foetus.

Laparoscopy is an examination of the interior of the abdomen with a lighted tube called a laparoscope. Laparoscopy is also known as peritoneoscopy.

Q: *How and why is laparoscopy performed?*

A: The examination can be carried out under local or general anaesthesia. A small incision is made, usually next to the navel; the instrument is then passed through the peritoneum, the membranous sac that lines the abdominal cavity. Carbon dioxide or nitrous oxide gas is passed into the peritoneal cavity through a needle to swell the abdomen and make it possible to examine the organs.

Disorders such as cancer, CROHN'S DISEASE, and cysts of the ovary can be diagnosed using this technique.

Q: *Can any operations be performed with a laparoscope?*

A: Yes. A surgeon can take a small piece of tissue for microscopic examination (biopsy), or perform a STERILIZATION operation in a woman.

Q: *Is laparoscopy a safe procedure?*

A: Yes, the examination is relatively safe and simple to perform.

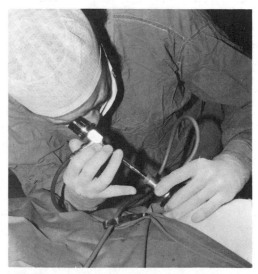

Laparoscope is used under general anaesthetic to illuminate and explore the inner abdomen

Laparotomy is a surgical operation to open the abdomen. It may be performed to inspect the internal organs (exploratory laparotomy), or as a preliminary to further surgery.

Laryngectomy is an operation to remove the voice box (larynx), usually performed in the treatment of cancer. An opening is made in the windpipe (TRACHEOTOMY) so that the patient can breathe, and many of the nearby lymph glands are removed at the same time if they are malignant.

Q: *Can a patient with a laryngectomy talk?*

A: Not immediately, and never normally as before. But a patient with no larynx can learn OESOPHAGEAL SPEECH, in which sounds are produced in the oesophagus.

Laryngitis is inflammation of the vocal cords. It may be acute or chronic.

Q: *What causes acute laryngitis?*

A: Any sudden respiratory infection, such as the COMMON COLD or INFLUENZA, or infection of the back of the throat, such as TONSILLITIS or PHARYNGITIS, can cause acute laryngitis. Diphtheria used to be a common cause of laryngitis, but is now extremely rare in Western countries.

   Overuse of the voice, heavy smoking, and habitual alcohol consumption all tend to produce a hoarse voice made rapidly worse by any minor infection.

Q: *What are the symptoms of acute laryngitis?*

A: The voice is husky and sometimes disappears completely (aphonia). Talking may cause pain in the throat.

Q: *What is the treatment for acute laryngitis?*

A: It is essential to attempt to stop talking for at least forty-eight hours. Steam inhalations may help, and treatment of the causative condition, such as tonsillitis, may be necessary.

Q: *Are there any complications of acute laryngitis?*

A: Yes. In babies and young children, the infection may occasionally spread to the windpipe (tracheitis) and bronchi (bronchitis) causing a syndrome called laryngotracheobronchitis, or croup. This is a potentially serious complaint and often needs treatment in hospital. The child usually has a high fever and a barking cough.

   In adults the condition is seldom serious. It usually interferes with normal speech for about one week.

Q: *What are the symptoms and causes of chronic laryngitis?*

A: The chief symptom is continued hoarseness, accompanied by a slight cough and a tendency for the voice to become weaker with use. Drinking alcohol, smoking, and overuse of the voice are all factors that can produce these symptoms.

Q: *How is chronic laryngitis diagnosed and treated?*

A: The diagnosis is made by a throat specialist, who examines the vocal cords to make sure that there is no other cause for the hoarseness.

   See also HOARSENESS.

Laryngoscopy is the examination of the interior of the voice box (larynx) using an instrument called a laryngoscope.

In the technique known as indirect laryngoscopy, the laryngoscope consists of a rod with a small mirror at one end. It is passed down the throat and gives a reflected view of the larynx.

In direct laryngoscopy, performed under a general anaesthetic, the laryngoscope is a rigid, illuminated tube which is passed down the throat to give a direct view of the larynx.

Larynx is the structure in the front of the neck that is commonly known as the voice box. It extends from the root of the tongue to the entrance of the windpipe (trachea). Until puberty, the larynx of a male person differs little in size from that of a female. At puberty, it enlarges considerably in males but only slightly in females.

The "box" that makes up the larynx consists of nine cartilages that are connected by ligaments and membranes, and are moved by several muscles. The largest of the cartilages, the thyroid cartilage, protrudes at the front of the neck to form the Adam's apple.

Q: *What are the functions of the larynx?*

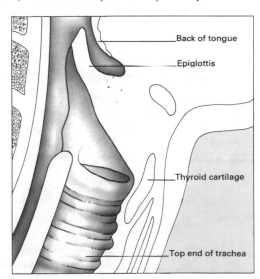

Larynx, or voice box, is made up of nine cartilages joined by ligaments and a membrane.

Laser

A: The larynx forms part of the airway to the lungs. One of the nine cartilages, the epiglottis, closes the larynx during swallowing to prevent food from entering the windpipe.

The other main function of the larynx is the production of speech. Inside the larynx are two vocal cords; the space between them is called the glottis. At rest, the vocal cords are open and allow breathing to occur. During speech, the vocal cords come together, leaving only a narrow space between them. When air breathed out from the lungs passes through the cords, they vibrate and produce the sounds of speech.

Q: What disorders can affect the larynx?

A: An infection may cause LARYNGITIS (inflammation of the larynx). Diphtheria is particularly dangerous if it involves the larynx, because the airway can become blocked by a membrane produced by the infection. Other infections elsewhere in the airway, such as a common cold or bronchitis, may spread and also affect the larynx.

The vocal cords may be damaged by overuse. This may cause small swellings on the vocal cords, often resulting in hoarseness or even a temporary loss of voice (*see* LARYNGITIS). Cancer and other tumours of the vocal cords and larynx may also occur. In such cases, surgical removal of the larynx (laryngectomy) may be necessary if radiotherapy is ineffective.

Laser is a device that amplifies light to produce an extremely intense beam. It is used in

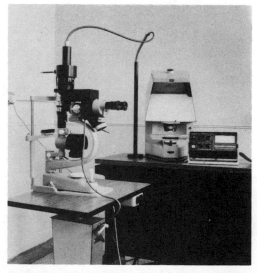

Laser apparatus can be used to perform highly accurate and specialized surgical procedures.

the treatment of various disorders, such as a DETACHED RETINA, certain conditions resulting from diabetes mellitus, and small tumours in the eye.

Lassa fever is an acute viral illness that is often fatal. It is most common in West Africa, but cases have occurred elsewhere. The onset of the symptoms is usually gradual, with high fever, headache, severe muscle pains, loss of appetite, an abnormal decrease in the number of white blood cells, and a slow pulse rate. These symptoms may last for one or two weeks, after which there is a slow recovery, or there may be a deterioration. In about half of all cases, these initial symptoms are followed by confusion, coma, and death.

Q: How is Lassa fever treated?

A: There is no cure for Lassa fever. The treatment involves complete bed rest and careful monitoring of all the bodily functions. The patient must be isolated to ensure that the infection does not spread to other people. Injections of GAMMA GLOBULIN from a person who has recently recovered from Lassa fever may be given, both to the patient and to anyone who may have come into contact with the illness.

Laughing gas is the common name for the anaesthetic gas nitrous oxide. *See* NITROUS OXIDE.

Lavage is the washing out of a body cavity. Gastric lavage is the washing out of the stomach with water, sodium bicarbonate, or some other fluid.

Laxatives are any substances that cause emptying of the bowel. They are often used in the treatment or prevention of CONSTIPATION.

Q: What substances are used as laxatives?

A: There are three main groups of laxatives. Those most commonly used act by irritating the bowel wall, causing a contraction and forcible expulsion of the faeces. But continued use of this kind of irritant laxative leads to a gradual loss of effectiveness. Senna, cascara sagrada, and phenolphthalein are examples of this group and are found in many commercial preparations.

The second group of laxatives acts by attracting water from the body into the intestine, increasing the volume of faeces. Milk of magnesia, Epsom salts (magnesium sulphate), and Glauber's salts (sodium sulphate) are common examples. More recently, vegetable substances that swell when they are swallowed have been used.

The third group is called bulk laxatives, and they include bran, vegetable fibre, and general roughage. Bulk swells the contents of the large intestine and acts as a stimulant to defecation as well as resulting in a bulkier stool. The diet of many people in Western countries is deficient in these substances. This may lead to constipation as well as other disorders.

Q: *What are the dangers in using laxatives?*

A: Laxatives should be used only in cases of severe and prolonged constipation and under a doctor's orders. Laxatives that act by irritating the bowel may become habit-forming so that the bowel may not function well without the irritant stimulus. In order to produce a laxative effect, gradually increasing doses have to be used. If they are taken over a pro-longed period of time, the bowel wall may become damaged.

Other kinds of laxatives are safer to use, but may need to be taken in larger amounts than is first realized.

Q: *Should laxatives be used to treat any form of constipation?*

A: No. Laxatives should never be used if constipation suddenly occurs or is accompanied by abdominal pain or fever. In such a case, there may be an INTESTINAL OBSTRUCTION or APPENDICITIS and laxatives are likely to make the condition worse. A doctor should be consulted.

L-dopa is another name for the drug levodopa. *See* LEVODOPA.

Lead poisoning occurs most commonly in children, usually from eating lead-containing paint. It is also found among workers in the lead industry. Lead is excreted very slowly and so tends to accumulate in the body tissues, especially in the nervous system, bones, liver, pancreas, teeth, and gums. A small amount of lead can circulate in the body without causing any ill effects. But when the safe limit is exceeded, normal bodily functions are disturbed. This occurs slowly and cumulatively if the lead poisoning is chronic, or rapidly and sometimes fatally if it is acute.

Q: *What are the symptoms of lead poisoning?*

A: The symptoms of chronic lead poisoning appear gradually and include fatigue; headache; irritability; dizziness; and breathlessness, caused by anaemia. If the intestine becomes involved, there may also be constipation, nausea, and severe abdominal pain. Nerve damage and permanent brain damage may also result.

Acute lead poisoning causes severe cramp, vomiting, black or bloody diarrhoea, acute abdominal pain, convulsions, delirium, and coma. The first sign is a metallic taste in the mouth, then signs of burns in the throat and oesophagus.

The diagnosis of lead poisoning is confirmed by the presence of anaemia with excessive amounts of lead in the blood and urine.

Q: *How is lead poisoning treated?*

A: Acute lead poisoning requires emergency medical treatment. Initially, the stomach is often washed out. Special drugs, called CHELATING AGENTS, help to remove lead from the tissues. This lead is then excreted by the kidneys in the urine. If lead poisoning has caused anaemia, a special diet with supplementary iron may be prescribed. Any brain damage requires expert psychological assessment and help.

Q: *Can lead poisoning be prevented?*

A: Yes, if precautions are followed strictly in industries that use lead. Also only lead-free paint should be used indoors or on surfaces accessible to children.

A talk about Learning disabilities

Learning disabilities are a group of disorders that interfere with a child's ability to learn. They may, therefore, cause a child to do poorly in school, or not to do as well as the child otherwise might.

There are many types of learning disabilities. A learning-disabled child may, for example, have difficulty concentrating, memorizing, or co-ordinating certain kinds of physical movements. A learning disability may also interfere with a child's ability to speak, spell, understand spoken language,

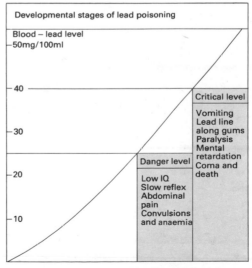

Developmental stages of lead poisoning	
Blood – lead level —50mg/100ml	
—40	Critical level
	Vomiting Lead line along gums Paralysis Mental retardation Coma and death
—30	
—20	Danger level
	Low IQ Slow reflex Abdominal pain Convulsions and anaemia
—10	

Lead poisoning is at a critical level when there is 40mg lead content per 100ml of blood.

Learning disabilities

or solve mathematical problems.

Q: *What are the causes of learning disabilities?*

A: Finding the exact cause of a child's learning disability is not always easy. Researchers believe, however, that most learning disabilities result from damage to major nerves leading to the brain or from minor damage to the brain itself. The nervous-system damage interferes with the ability to receive and use information transmitted from the disabled child's senses to his or her brain. Many children suffering from a learning disability nevertheless tend to be of average or above-average intelligence, and they do not seem to have an unusual incidence of abnormal hearing or vision.

Q: *What might cause nerve or brain damage?*

A: Such damage can occur before birth, during the birth process, or after birth. Damage before birth can result from poor nutrition and illness in the mother, which may affect the foetal nervous system. Certain injuries during pregnancy, particularly those involving the abdomen or pelvis, can also result in nervous-system damage to the unborn child. In addition, some hereditary defects in the mother or the father, or both, can cause nerve or brain damage before birth.

During the birth process, nerve or brain damage can occur if labour is prolonged or particularly difficult, causing temporary lack of oxygen supply to the brain.

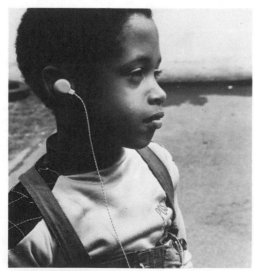

Learning disabilities can sometimes be overcome by specialized equipment.

Nerve or brain damage after birth can result from many causes, including injuries to the skull or spinal cord, malnutrition, inherited chemical imbalances, or disease. Research suggests that certain chemicals, especially lead, may also contribute to learning disabilities after birth.

Q: *Can a learning disability be present when there is no damage to nerves or to the brain?*

A: Yes. Although research into this phenomenon continues, scientists are generally of the opinion that a learning disability can come about without nervous-system damage. Scientists have found, for example, that continued absence of various early learning experiences, such as hearing language or handling objects, can result in certain learning disabilities in children.

Q: *What are the symptoms of a learning disability?*

A: The symptoms of a learning disability depend on the type of disorder involved. The symptom of one type of learning disability, DYSPHASIA, is a child's difficulty in speaking or in understanding oral language. DYSLEXIA, on the other hand, shows itself as a difficulty in reading and writing. DYSGRAPHIA, a third type of learning disability, is likely when a child is unable to control the finger muscles used in writing.

Still other types of learning disability interfere with a child's power to concentrate or to behave in a socially acceptable manner. Such a child is considered to suffer from hyper-activity, or HYPERKINESIS. Hyperactive children—who are more often boys than girls—tend to speak and to act impulsively and boisterously. These children are also usually impatient. Their conduct, whether at home or at school, is generally looked upon by peers and adults as disruptive and uncontrolled.

Other learning disabilities display themselves as a lack of distinguishing left from right or of distinguishing between letters of the alphabet that have some similarities in form, such as *b* and *d*.

Q: *How are learning disabilities diagnosed?*

A: The parent is usually the first person to suspect that a child has a learning disability. The parent usually alerts the family doctor.

Upon examination, the doctor may refer the child to other specialists for further testing and evaluation. The specialists may include a neurologist, a psychologist, a child psychiatrist, an eye specialist, an ear specialist, and a speech therapist. In addition, one or more of these may recommend that a social worker become involved in the evaluation of the child to try to determine if some factor in the home environment is contributing to, or even causing, the child's learning disability. Some schools provide for the diagnosis and treatment of children with learning disabilities.

Q: *How are learning disabilities treated?*

A: The kind and extent of treatment of a child with a learning disability depends on the individual diagnosis. In sum, there is no one form of treatment that seems to work well with all of the various types of learning disabilities. Doctors and educationalists therefore continue to study the effectiveness and safety of many of the treatment methods presently used.

Leech is a bloodsucking parasite that was formerly used in medicine, until the early twentieth century when it was abandoned, as a means of bloodletting.

Infestation with leeches is called hirudiniasis, and it can result in a considerable blood loss. It is rare.

Q: *What is the treatment for hirudiniasis?*

A: If a leech is still on the skin surface, a lighted cigarette, match, or salt applied to the leech causes it to release its hold. The wound should be washed with an antiseptic, and a sterile dressing applied. If a leech is attached internally, expert medical attention is required.

Various repellent substances are available to protect against leeches.

Left-handedness, a tendency to use the left hand in preference to the right, is found in about eight per cent of people. In most people, the left side of the brain is "dominant," and controls the right side of the body; in left-handed people, the right side of the brain is dominant. Left-handed people are usually left-footed also, and they may stutter or suffer from dyslexia if they are forced to write with the right hand.

Legionnaire's disease is a potentially fatal bacterial disorder, named for an outbreak at the 1976 American Legion conference in Philadelphia where 182 people succumbed, 29 of whom died. The disease was previously unknown, and it is not known how it is transmitted. It seems probable that the bacteria cause a mild illness with fever, cough, and signs of pneumonia in some people, who then transmit it more seriously to others.

Leiomyoma is a benign (noncancerous) tumour of smooth muscle, commonly called a fibroid when it occurs in the womb. Leiomyomas may also occur in the gastrointestinal tract where they generally produce no symptoms, although occasionally they cause an INTESTINAL OBSTRUCTION.

Leishmaniasis is a group of infectious diseases of the skin and internal organs caused by various protozoan parasites of the genus *Leishmania*. Leishmaniasis is usually transmitted by sandflies.

There are two main types of leishmaniasis: visceral leishmaniasis, also called kala-azar; and cutaneous leishmaniasis, also called Delhi boil or oriental sore. Various forms of leishmaniasis are endemic to tropical and subtropical regions throughout the world.

In American leishmaniasis, one of the two varieties of leishmaniasis of the skin, the ulcers form in a similar way to those of oriental sore. But the ulcers usually form in the nose and throat and tend to be more destructive; also they commonly become infected. This can cause serious complications and may even be fatal. American leishmaniasis may last for several years.

Q: *How is cutaneous leishmaniasis treated?*

A: Many cases of oriental sore and some of American leishmaniasis heal spontaneously and do not require treatment. When spontaneous recovery does not occur, the treatment is similar to that for visceral leishmaniasis: with antimony drugs, or amphotericin B for resistant infections only, and antibiotic drugs to treat secondary infection.

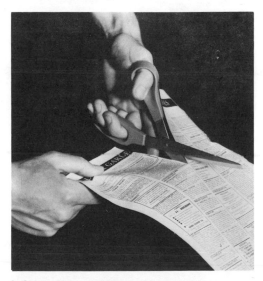

Left-handed people sometimes need to use specially adapted utensils and equipment.

Lens

Lens is a curved piece of transparent material that causes light rays passing through it to converge or diverge. The lens in the eye is a transparent, colourless, biconvex disc that helps to focus light onto the retina (for details, *see* EYE). Glass lenses are used in CONTACT LENSES, SPECTACLES, and various medical instruments.

Leontiasis is a thickening of the tissue or bones of the face. It causes considerable swelling and an alteration in appearance, giving a lionlike expression. Leontiasis may be a symptom of LEPROSY or it may be caused by an underlying bone disease (leontiasis ossea), which is probably a form of PAGET'S DISEASE OF BONE.

Leprosy is a slowly progressive infection caused by the bacterium *Mycobacterium leprae*. The disorder is common in Central and South America, in the Far East, in tropical countries of Asia and Africa, and in some of the Pacific Islands.

Leprosy is not infectious in adults unless they have been in close contact for long periods. But it is infectious in children, and they should be kept out of contact.

There are two main forms of leprosy, tuberculoid leprosy and lepromatous leprosy. Often, both occur in the same patient.

Q: *What are the symptoms of tuberculoid leprosy?*

A: Tuberculoid leprosy appears as an infection around nerve endings, causing gradual loss of feeling and also the appearance of pale areas on the skin where sensation is disordered. The nerves may be felt as thickened, tender rope-like

structures. This may lead to paralysis producing WRIST DROP or FOOT DROP, and sometimes local areas of ulceration because of the lack of normal sensation.

Q: *What are the symptoms of lepromatous leprosy?*

A: The normal pigmentation in some areas on the skin is lost and becomes slightly reddened, because of inflammation. There are usually many such areas scattered symmetrically across the body, and the edges merge into the normal skin so that they may not be obvious in a pale-skinned person. Occasionally there is thickening of the skin of the face, often involving the ears, to produce the "lion face" (LEONTIASIS).

As the disease progresses, the membranes of the nose, mouth, and throat may ulcerate producing distorted lips and loss of cartilage in the nose.

Q: *How does leprosy progress?*

A: The progress is extremely variable. Patients with tuberculoid leprosy often overcome the infection without much damage. Lepromatous leprosy progresses slowly, with increasing episodes of fever, enlargement in the size of affected skin areas, eye infection (IRITIS), lymph gland enlargement and, sometimes, involvement of the testes (ORCHITIS). Reactions like this ultimately lead to death.

Q: *How is the condition diagnosed and treated?*

A: For a doctor, diagnosis is simple, and can be confirmed by examining a biopsy of the edge of an affected skin area or nerve.

Drugs such as DAPSONE are successful in the treatment of leprosy, but must be used initially in small doses. The drug may otherwise cause the symptoms to become worse, with pain in the nerves. Treatment must be given for at least two years, generally longer.

Leptospirosis is an infectious disease caused by spirochaete bacteria of the group called leptospira. It is passed on to humans from dogs, pigs, or rats that are carriers of the disease. There are about 130 kinds of leptospira bacteria.

Q: *How is leptospirosis transmitted?*

A: A human becomes infected with bacteria through direct contact with the animal's urine or with water or soil contaminated by it. The infection penetrates scratches on the skin or may enter through the mucous membranes of the mouth or vagina. Infections occur most commonly in sewer workers, veterinary

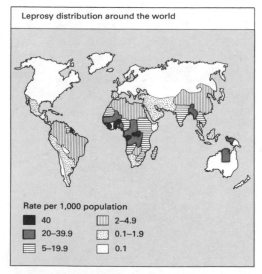

Leprosy distribution around the world

Rate per 1,000 population

- ■ 40
- ▨ 2–4.9
- ■ 20–39.9
- ▦ 0.1–1.9
- ▤ 5–19.9
- □ 0.1

Leprosy, now an easily treatable disease, is still endemic in some parts of the world.

surgeons, and farmers, but anyone can catch leptospirosis by swimming in contaminated water.

Q: *What are the symptoms of leptospirosis?*

A: After an incubation period of up to three weeks, there is sudden onset of severe headache, muscular aching (myalgia) with shivering attacks (rigor), and fever that may last about a week. The whites of the eyes often become red and inflamed.

The fever then settles slowly, and about ten days later the symptoms return with neck stiffness and mental confusion. The patient has a dislike of bright lights (photophobia), caused by a mild or severe form of MENINGITIS.

In severe forms of the illness, JAUNDICE and bleeding occur, mental confusion is common, and urinary output is greatly reduced resulting in uraemia (a toxic condition caused by failure of the kidneys). Death may result.

Q: *How is leptospirosis diagnosed and what is the treatment?*

A: The leptospira bacteria may be cultured from a sample of the patient's blood, urine, or spinal fluid. The blood may also contain antibodies that indicate the presence of leptospira.

Leptospirosis is a serious illness and the patient must be admitted to a hospital for antibiotic treatment.

Lesbian is a woman who has a sexual preference for women, and practises lesbianism, the female form of homosexuality.

Lesion is any damaged or abnormal area of tissue, such as a wound, injury, or an area altered by infection.

Lethargy is a feeling of fatigue and listlessness, both physical and mental. It may occur for no particular reason, or following any illness or operation. Continued lethargy, for no obvious reason, is abnormal and a doctor should be consulted.

Leucocyte. *See* WHITE BLOOD CELL.

Leucocytosis is an increase in the number of white blood cells (leucocytes) in the blood. It is a normal response to infection and also to bodily damage, such as that caused by surgery or by an accident. An increase in abnormal leucocytes may occur in conditions such as GLANDULAR FEVER, LEUKAEMIA, and some forms of ANAEMIA.

Leucopenia is a reduction in the normal number of white blood cells (leucocytes) in the blood. It may occur in any acute virus infection or in forms of chemical poisoning, with agranulocytosis.

See also AGRANULOCYTOSIS.

Leucotomy is the cutting of the nerve fibres that lead from the middle to the front part of the brain. It is usually known as lobotomy.

A talk about Leukaemia

Leukaemia is a malignant disease of the white blood cells (leucocytes), which play a key part in the body's defence mechanism against infection. It is a type of cancer that affects the bone marrow and other blood-forming tissues throughout the body. The cause of leukaemia is not known, but seems to be associated with a failure of the developing leucocytes to mature.

Normal mature leucocytes cannot reproduce and are replaced at the ends of their lives. Leukaemic cells, however, have the ability to reproduce but do not develop sufficiently to act as a defence against infection. As leukaemia progresses, the leukaemic cells displace normal leucocytes, leaving the patient extremely vulnerable to infection.

There are several forms of leukaemia, both acute and chronic, which are classified according to the type of leucocyte affected. The major types of leucocytes involved in leukaemia include lymphocytes, polymorphonuclear leucocytes, and granulocytes.

Q: *What forms of acute leukaemia are there?*

A: There are two main forms of acute leukaemia: acute lymphoblastic leukaemia (ALL), and acute myeloblastic leukaemia (AML). ALL affects lymphocytes and occurs usually in children. AML affects the cells that form polymorphonuclear leucocytes and is more common in adults.

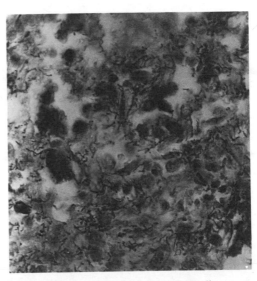

Leptospira bacteria can be seen as small irregular lines in this picture of blood.

Leukaemia

Q: *What are the symptoms of the acute leukaemias?*

A: The symptoms of both forms of acute leukaemia are similar. The patient usually has a sudden high fever and a severe throat infection. There may also be nosebleeds, bruising under the skin, and pain in the joints. In some patients, the onset of symptoms is slower, with lethargy, anaemia, and increasing weakness.

Q: *What forms of chronic leukaemia are there?*

A: There are two main forms of chronic leukaemia: chronic myeloid leukaemia (CML), and chronic lymphocytic leukaemia (CLL). CML affects immature polymorphonuclear leucocytes, and usually occurs after the age of thirty five years. CLL affects lymphoid tissue and lymphatic cells, and usually occurs in men over the age of fifty years.

Q: *What are the symptoms of the chronic leukaemias?*

A: The symptoms of both forms of chronic leukaemia are similar. The onset is usually slow, with increasing fatigue, lethargy, and weakness. The patient may also lose weight and suffer from loss of appetite. The course of the illness is also slow and may last for several years without causing major problems. However, there may be various complications, such as anaemia; bleeding under the skin; recurrent fever; and the formation of nodules and ulcers under the skin.

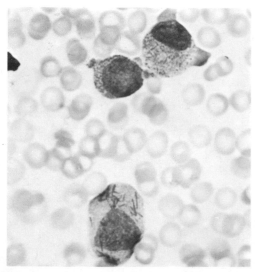

Leukaemia affects the white blood cells, which are displaced by leukaemic cells.

Q: *How is leukaemia diagnosed?*

A: The specific diagnosis of leukaemia requires a blood test and a bone marrow BIOPSY. Leukaemia is confirmed by the presence of large numbers of abnormal leucocytes in the blood, and the typical leukaemic cells in the bone marrow. With the chronic leukaemias, the patient may be unaware of the disease, and a diagnosis is often made only when the patient is examined for another reason, such as a routine check-up.

Q: *How is leukaemia treated?*

A: The treatment of acute and chronic leukaemia is often similar, but it is dependent on varying factors involved in each case. The aim of treatment is to suppress the reproduction of leukaemic cells. CYTOTOXIC DRUGS, which prevent cell multiplication, are used for this purpose. The rapidly-dividing leukaemic cells are more susceptible to these drugs than are normal leucocytes.

The treatment of the acute leukaemias usually involves the use of several cytotoxic drugs together. Once the number of leukaemic cells has been reduced, CORTICOSTEROIDS and only one or two cytotoxic drugs need be used to maintain the improvement. With the chronic leukaemias, cytotoxic drugs and corticosteroids may also be used. In some cases, blood transfusion may be necessary.

Research into leukaemia is very active. Several new drugs are being tested and many of the latest techniques are available only in leukaemia research centres. For this reason, a patient with any form of leukaemia should obtain advice and treatment from an expert in this field.

Q: *Can leukaemia be cured?*

A: No cure has yet been found for most forms of leukaemia. A large number of children treated for ALL have survived for over five years without any further symptoms, and may be cured. Most patients (about eighty per cent) can resume normal life for some time before a relapse occurs. The problem is to ensure that every leukaemic cell has been destroyed.

AML is invariably fatal, but the symptoms can be controlled and the patient's life extended, especially the period of useful life. The prognosis for those with the chronic leukaemias is largely dependent upon the age at which the disease occurs; as with AML, the symptoms can be controlled and life extended. Patients with CML are more likely to die as a result of leukaemia than are those with CLL, because CML usually starts at an earlier age.

Leukoderma is the loss of the normal skin pigmentation, resulting in the appearance of pale patches. This may occur temporarily following the treatment of any skin infection, such as DERMATITIS. Leukoderma may also be caused by handling chemicals that remove the pigment from the skin. Less commonly it may be caused by LEPROSY. VITILIGO is a form of leukoderma for which the cause is unknown.

Leukoplakia is a condition in which thickened white patches develop on the tongue and inside the cheeks or other mucous membranes, such as those of the vulva or penis. It is a disorder of the cells of the mucous membrane that may be a prelude to cancer.

Q: *What causes leukoplakia of the mouth and how is it treated?*

A: Smoking, drinking alcohol, and chronic irritation from damaged teeth or badly fitting dentures are thought to be some of the causes. The causes should be eliminated or treated and small lesions removed by surgery.

Q: *How is leukoplakia of the vulva treated?*

A: Itching irritation of the vulva may be the symptom that makes a woman consult a doctor. An examination may reveal the white patches of leukoplakia. The area should be examined regularly to see if there are any malignant changes. In the rare cases in which cancer is thought to be developing, parts of the vulva may be surgically removed.

Levodopa (L-dopa) is a drug used in the treatment of PARKINSON'S DISEASE. It is thought to increase the amount of dopamine, a chemical necessary for the normal working of brain tissue which is lacking in this disorder. Initial small doses of levodopa are usually increased to larger doses, which may produce toxic symptoms. These include loss of appetite and nausea with, occasionally, abdominal pain, constipation, and diarrhoea. Lowered blood pressure may cause a feeling of faintness and dizziness, often accompanied by excessive sweating and palpitations. The patient may also show neurological symptoms such as involuntary chewing and twisting movements of the limbs.

Psychiatric problems such as drowsiness, depression, and (sometimes) paranoia and hallucinations, may also arise. Even less commonly, there are problems with passing urine and, in men, sexual problems.

Q: *How are the toxic effects of levodopa treated?*

A: The toxic effects of levodopa are seldom a major problem if the dosage of the drug is increased slowly. A small temporary reduction in dosage causes the symptoms to disappear.

Q: *Are there any conditions in which levodopa should not be used?*

A: Yes. Care must be taken with patients who have a psychiatric history or the eye disorder glaucoma, or who are taking certain other drugs, such as MAO inhibitors for depression. Persons with disease of the heart, liver, or kidneys are more likely to develop toxic effects. Levodopa should not be taken by pregnant women.

LGV is an abbreviation of lymphogranuloma venereum, a venereal disease. *See* LYMPHO-GRANULOMA VENEREUM.

Libido is a psychological term for the conscious or unconscious sexual drive, the desire of an individual for another person. The form and force of psychosexual libido depends, in part, on cultural conditioning and psychological education. It also depends on biological effects produced by the sex hormones.

Libido may be increased by visual and sensory impulses, and reduced by fear, anxiety, or depression. Sexual drive and desire can be altered by hormonal changes that occur during the menstrual cycle and by hormone disorders, such as HYPOPITUITARISM.

Lice are a group of parasitic insects that live on various animals, including humans. There are three main types of lice that infest human

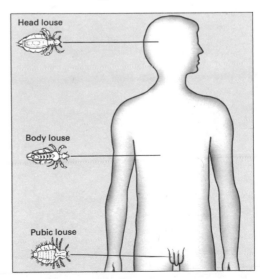

Head louse

Body louse

Pubic louse

Lice of three main kinds infest the head hair, the body hair, and the pubic hair.

Lichen planus

beings: the two varieties of *Pediculus humanus*, which live in the hair or on the body, and the crab louse, *Phthirus pubis*, which lives in the pubic hair. The head louse belongs to the same species as the body louse, but it confines itself to the scalp.

Q: What symptoms do head lice cause?

A: Often there are no symptoms, although in severe cases there is itching of the scalp, which can cause secondary infection through scratching with dirty fingernails. Crusting and oozing then occur, similar to that of impetigo.

Head lice are most common among schoolchildren because of the frequency with which they put their heads together during work projects and games. If one child is infected, then all the other children are likely to be infected.

Q: How is the condition diagnosed and treated?

A: In severe cases, the lice can be seen. But in most children, the diagnosis is made after finding small, shiny, pearl-coloured eggs (nits) attached to the hairs.

Treatment involves careful washing of the hair with a medicated shampoo, prescribed by a doctor. After washing, the hair should be combed to remove any nits. The procedure should be repeated a week later and, on each occasion, the shampoo should be left to dry on the hair before it is washed off the next morning.

Q: What symptoms indicate the presence of crab lice?

A: There is intense itching in the pubic area and possible secondary infection in scratch marks. In severe infestations, the hair in the armpits, eyebrows, and eyelashes may also be involved.

Q: What is the treatment for crab lice?

A: The diagnosis is made in the same way as for head lice by finding nits on the hairs or lice on the body. Treatment involves washing the body from the neck downward with a special solution each day for three days, and leaving it to dry. Prolonged treatment may cause dermatitis. The patient's sexual partner should also be treated.

See also RELAPSING FEVER; TYPHUS.

Lichen planus is a skin inflammation of sudden onset that usually starts at the wrists and spreads to the trunk. The condition may last many weeks or months.

Q: What are the symptoms of lichen planus?

A: The skin lesions are small, slightly raised purple or red areas that glisten. They occur on the front surfaces of the forearms, trunk, and shins. In severe cases, the lesions may occur anywhere on the body. The lesions itch and are often surrounded by scratch marks. They may even occur in the mouth, or on the vulva or penis. Occasionally, the nails may be involved, resulting in ridging and splitting.

Sometimes the symptoms subside within three months; the patches lose their shiny colour and become brown and scaly, before disappearing. In some patients, the condition lasts for many years.

Q: What is the treatment for lichen planus?

A: As the cause is not known, there is no specific treatment, although usually the lesions can be kept under control with creams or lotions containing corticosteroid drugs.

Life expectancy is the length of time for which, according to statistics, an individual may expect to live. In Britain, the life expectancy of a child born between 1975 and 1980 is estimated to be 73.1 years.

Ligament is a supporting band of fibrous tissue that holds a joint or body organ in place. Ligaments give support and at the same time allow movement.

Ligation is the application of a ligature. *See* LIGATURE.

Ligature is a thread made of catgut, silk, nylon, or steel that is used to tie round and close a blood vessel or any body tube.

See also SUTURE.

Lightening is the sensation of reduced abdominal swelling or distension that usually occurs during pregnancy about two to four weeks before the onset of labour. *See* PREGNANCY AND CHILDBIRTH.

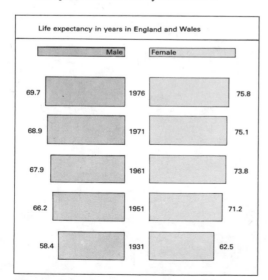

Life expectancy in years in England and Wales

	Male		Female	
69.7		1976		75.8
68.9		1971		75.1
67.9		1961		73.8
66.2		1951		71.2
58.4		1931		62.5

Life expectancy has steadily increased as general health standards have improved.

Limping, or lameness. *See* CLAUDICATION.

Lipaemia is the presence in the bloodstream of large amounts of the fatty substances called LIPIDS (which include cholesterol). There is strong evidence that extremely high levels of such substances, the condition called hyperlipaemia or hyperlipidaemia, is a factor in the cause of ARTERIOSCLEROSIS and therefore of coronary heart disease, strokes, and disorders of peripheral arteries.

Q: What causes an increase of the fatty substances in the blood?

A: There is a normal increase in the lipids (particularly triglycerides) after any meal. For this reason, in a medical test the level of lipids is measured after a patient has been fasting for at least eight hours.

Hyperlipaemia detected in this way may be caused by such disorders as HYPOTHYROIDISM, DIABETES MELLITUS, and a rare condition present at birth called XANTHELASMA, in which the body is unable to metabolize cholesterol normally.

More commonly, hyperlipaemia is associated with a combination of factors, such as a mild inherited tendency towards the condition, cigarette smoking, a diet containing excessive amounts of animal fats, lack of physical exercise, and obesity.

Q: What is the treatment for high lipid levels?

A: Treatment of any specific cause found may reduce the level of lipids. But, more usually, treatment is directed at the individual's life-style. A doctor may recommend special drugs and a diet low in animal fats and carbohydrates. The person should stop smoking, reduce weight if obese, and exercise regularly.

Lipid is any one of a group of fats or fatlike substances that occur in the body. Lipids include TRIGLYCERIDES and cholesterol as well as fatty substances that are combined with sugars and phosphates.

Lipids are easily stored in the body, where they are an important part of cell structure and a source of reserve energy.

Lipoma is a benign (noncancerous) tumour that is made up of fat cells. Lipomas commonly occur under the skin and may be felt as diffuse, soft swellings, particularly over the shoulders and trunk. They seldom cause problems, but can be removed surgically.

Lips, the fleshy structures round the mouth, are where the normal skin of the face joins the mucous membrane that lines the mouth.

See also CHEILOSIS; HARE-LIP.

Lisp. *See* SPEECH DEFECTS.

Listlessness is a vague feeling of lack of energy, fatigue, and other symptoms suggestive of mild depression. Listlessness is similar to LETHARGY.

Lithiasis. *See* CALCULUS.

Lithium is a metallic chemical element used medically as lithium carbonate or lithium citrate in treating MANIC-DEPRESSIVE ILLNESS.

Litholapaxy is an operation to remove a stone (calculus) from the bladder without making an incision. First a surgeon makes a cystoscopic examination of the bladder, and then crushes the stone by LITHOTRITY. The fragments are flushed out immediately.

See also CALCULUS; LITHOTOMY.

Lithotomy is an operation to remove a stone (calculus), usually from the bladder or salivary glands, through a surgical incision.

See also CALCULUS; LITHOLAPAXY.

Lithotrity is the use of a special instrument, called a lithotrite, to crush a stone (calculus) in the bladder or urethra.

See also LITHOLAPAXY.

Little's disease is a form of CEREBRAL PALSY in which the legs are particularly affected. It is often accompanied by epilepsy, writhing movements of the limbs (athetosis), and mental retardation.

A talk about the Liver

Liver is the largest and most complex organ in the body. Most of it lies in the right upper side of the abdomen under the diaphragm and ribs, and it extends across to the left side of the body, overlying the upper part of the stomach.

The liver in the average adult weighs about

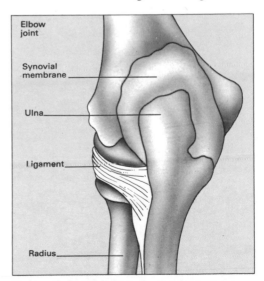

Elbow joint

Synovial membrane

Ulna

Ligament

Radius

Ligaments bind together the bones at a joint, such as at the elbow.

Liver

three pounds (1.5 kilos). It is covered by a tough, fibrous capsule. The gall bladder and its ducts lie beneath the right side of the liver.

The products of digestion are absorbed by capillaries in the intestinal wall and carried in the hepatic portal vein to capillaries within the liver. The liver is composed of up to 100,000 branched and interconnected cells (lobules). Each lobule is surrounded by capillaries from the hepatic portal vein and the hepatic artery. More than a litre (two to three pints) of blood passes through the liver each minute. The blood leaves along the hepatic vein to join the inferior vena cava and pass to the heart.

See also DIGESTIVE SYSTEM; GALL BLADDER.

Q: What is the function of the liver?

A: The cells of the liver process digested food, storing as much of it as is required and converting the remainder into substances the body needs. For example, the sugar glucose is converted into glycogen and stored in the liver until the body needs extra energy.

The liver stores vitamins (except vitamin C) until they are required, and its reserves can last for many months. Iron and several other minerals are also stored in the liver. Liver cells also manufacture PROTEINS and LIPIDS.

Liver cells also recycle various substances, such as haemoglobin, that are needed by the body. In addition, the liver destroys many poisonous substances that may be absorbed into the body and acts as an organ of excretion. BILE salts and bilirubin are formed in the liver and

pass into the bile ducts, to be excreted into the duodenum or stored in the gall bladder. Unwanted proteins are destroyed and changed into urea, which is carried in the bloodstream to the kidneys and excreted in the urine.

All these metabolic processes produce a considerable amount of heat that helps to maintain the body's normal temperature.

Q: What disorders may affect the liver?

A: The liver is a complex organ that can be disrupted by a number of disorders, of which the major causes include infection; poisoning; excessive alcohol; metabolic abnormalities; obstruction; and deficiency diseases. Many disorders do not produce any symptoms until they have reached an advanced stage because the liver has large reserves that can be used if it is damaged.

Infection of the liver may cause it to become swollen, and may produce a dull ache in the upper right part of the abdomen. Usually, however, pain does not occur with liver disorders. Instead, the first symptom of many disorders is JAUNDICE, which occurs when the bile pigment bilirubin accumulates in the blood. This may be caused by an inability of the liver to metabolize bilirubin, or by an obstruction to the flow of bile from the liver to the intestines.

Abdominal swelling, resulting from fluid in the peritoneum (ascites), may be caused by obstruction of the hepatic portal vein. Such obstruction may also cause varicose veins to form at the lower end of the oesophagus and burst, causing blood to be vomited (haematemesis) and blood in the faeces (MELAENA). The sudden blood loss and influx of protein into the intestines may cause hepatic encephalopathy.

Other causes of this disorder include CIRRHOSIS and acute viral HEPATITIS, which are themselves caused by infection or poisoning. The symptoms include confusion; flapping movements of the hands; and lack of co-ordination (ataxia). The patient may lapse into a coma, which may be fatal.

Cancer of the liver may also occur. Liver tumours are usually malignant and result from the spread of cancer from other parts of the body (metastasis). Occasionally a primary tumour may occur in the liver, called a hepatoma. Hepatomas are usually associated with cirrhosis, caused either by alcoholism or by nutritional deficiency.

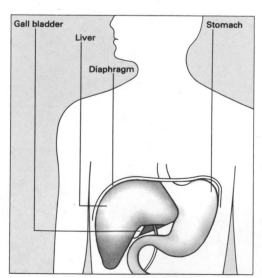

Liver is the largest organ in the body and lies below the diaphragm protected by the rib cage.

See also BUDD-CHIARI SYNDROME;
CHOLANGITIS; HAEMOCHROMATOSIS;
HYDATID CYST; LEPTOSPIROSIS; MALARIA.

Liver fluke. *See* FLUKES.

Loa loa, or loiasis, is a form of filariasis transmitted by the flies of the genus *Chrysops*, which occur in Central and Western Africa.

Lobectomy is an operation to remove a lobe from any organ, usually of the lung.

Lobotomy is a surgical incision into the rounded, projecting part (lobe) of an organ. The term usually refers to a psycho-surgical operation known in full as a prefrontal lobotomy, in which nerve fibres leading to the frontal lobes of the brain are severed. The operation may be performed in the treatment of severe forms of mental illness, such as schizophrenia and obsessive or compulsive neuroses. But it is done only for the most disabling disorders, and only after all other forms of treatment have failed.

Prefrontal lobotomy may cause adverse and irreversible side effects, such as disturbed reasoning and a blunting of the emotions. The operation is now rare.

Lochia is the vaginal discharge that occurs for three to four weeks after childbirth. During the first few days the discharge is mainly bright red blood that gradually becomes reddish-brown in colour, to brownish-yellow and then to white over the next three weeks. The amount of lochia varies.

Lockjaw. *See* TETANUS.

Locomotor ataxia is a loss of muscular co-ordination caused by advanced syphilis. *See* TABES DORSALIS.

Logorrhoea, also known as logomania, is extremely rapid speech that may be incomprehensible and over which the speaker seems to have little or no control. In a mild form, logorrhoea may occur with anxiety. But, in a more serious form, obsessive talkativeness is a symptom of MANIA and, occasionally, SCHIZOPHRENIA.

Longsightedness (hyperopia, or hypermetropia) is a disorder of vision in which distant objects are seen clearly, but closer objects appear blurred. The blurring occurs because light rays from nearby objects are not focused normally on the retina, either because the refractive power of the eye lens is too strong, or (more commonly) because the eyeball is not long enough from front to back. Longsightedness may be inherited or it may develop after the age of 40 as the lens of the eye becomes less elastic (presbyopia). Corrective SPECTACLES or CONTACT LENSES may be prescribed to restore normal vision.

Lordosis, also known as hollow back or saddle back, is an excessive curvature of the spine with the bend towards the front. The condition affects the lumbar region (between the ribs and the pelvis), and is the opposite in deformity of KYPHOSIS or hunchback.

Q: What causes lordosis?

A: Lordosis commonly occurs in obese people with weak back muscles and heavy abdomens. It may also develop in pregnant women. And any hip deformity, such as that caused by osteoarthritis, tends to make the body lean forward, which may produce lordosis.

Q: How is lordosis treated?

A: Treatment must be directed toward the cause; this is the only way of encouraging the spine to return to normal shape.

Loss of appetite is known medically as anorexia. It is a common symptom in most illnesses and usually precedes the onset of nausea. The patient's appetite returns when he or she recovers from the illness.

Q: Are there any more serious causes?

A: Yes. Loss of appetite in the elderly must always be taken seriously if it continues for more than a week or two.

It is more commonly a symptom that occurs with depression, and may be accompanied by a slight loss of weight. In younger patients, loss of appetite may also be related to psychological factors, and may occur with alcoholism, because of chronic gastritis (inflammation of the stomach).

Females more commonly than males suffer from ANOREXIA NERVOSA, a serious

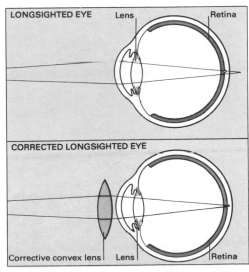

Longsightedness occurs when the lens fails to focus light at one point on the retina.

Loss of hearing

disorder that may not be detected until weight loss has been considerable.

Q: *How is loss of appetite treated?*

A: In most cases, the cause is obvious and the treatment is directed toward the main problem; the appetite then improves in due course. But any patient who has lost his or her appetite for more than two weeks should consult a doctor in case there is a more serious underlying cause.

Loss of hearing. *See* DEAFNESS; HEARING DISORDERS.

Loss of memory. *See* AMNESIA.

Loss of sensation. *See* NUMBNESS.

Loss of sight. *See* BLINDNESS.

Loss of weight. Like loss of appetite, loss of weight occurs with many acute or prolonged illnesses and may be one of the obvious signs of the disorder. Continued loss of weight for no obvious reason must always be considered a serious symptom.

Q: *What may cause unexplained loss of weight?*

A: ANOREXIA NERVOSA may be a cause particularly in young girls and women, but in older people an underlying chronic disorder, such as tuberculosis or cancer, must always be considered. Hyperthyroidism (overactivity of the thyroid gland) increases the body's rate of metabolism and this may cause unexplained loss of weight. Depression and anxiety are also commonly accompanied by weight loss.

Q: *How should weight loss be treated?*

A: If the cause of weight loss is not obvious and is rapid or continues for more than a month, the individual must consult a doctor. A thorough physical examination, with various tests and X-rays, may have to be carried out to discover if there is any serious cause.

See also WEIGHT PROBLEMS.

Louse. *See* LICE.

Low back pain. *See* LUMBAGO.

Low blood pressure (hypotension) is a condition in which the blood pressure is below normal or reduced. Most doctors in the English-speaking world consider low blood pressure to be a symptom of some other disorder. But, in many parts of the world, low blood pressure is itself considered to be a disorder that can cause various symptoms, including depression, lethargy, and fatigue.

This strikingly different attitude is probably the result of different methods of medical training. In a patient recovering from influenza, for example, low blood pressure may accompany the depression and the lower than normal temperature that usually occurs with this disorder. In other words, the symptoms may not be caused by the low blood pressure itself.

Q: *What conditions may be accompanied by low blood pressure?*

A: Like high blood pressure, slightly low blood pressure may be a particular person's normal pressure. Provided there are no other symptoms and the individual feels well, the low blood pressure can be considered a chance variation from average, probably associated with a prolonged life expectancy. But if low blood pressure occurs in an individual whose blood pressure is normally higher, it may be caused by some recent illness. In this case, it should be only temporary and should improve spontaneously. Some kinds of drugs, particularly antidepressants, may cause low blood pressure.

A more serious possible cause of low blood pressure is peripheral neuritis, in which the autonomic nervous system is affected so that blood accumulates in the veins of the legs because of the absence of the normal nervous response that causes the veins to contract. Disorders such as diabetes mellitus, tabes dorsalis, and Parkinson's disease may result in low blood pressure. Patients who have had a coronary THROMBOSIS or who are in a state of shock also have low blood pressure.

Q: *What are the symptoms of low blood pressure?*

A: Frequently there are no symptoms and the condition is found at a routine physical examination. The person may

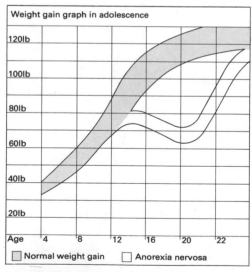

Loss of weight caused by anorexia nervosa and normal weight gain is contrasted.

feel dizzy and a sudden change in position, such as standing up quickly, may cause fainting. Serious low blood pressure may bring on the symptoms of shock, pallor, and a feeling of coldness.

Q: *How is low blood pressure treated?*

A: There is a spontaneous improvement in most individuals, although treatment of the cause helps the return to normal. Drug treatment that may cause the low blood pressure should, if possible, be discontinued. Patients with peripheral neuritis are more difficult to treat. An improvement may be made by an increase in blood volume, achieved by additional salt in the diet and, sometimes, with corticosteroid drugs.

Low blood sugar. *See* HYPOGLYCAEMIA.

LSD is an abbreviation of lysergic acid diethylamide. It is a drug that, even in minute doses, produces disturbances of the autonomic nervous system and the brain. It may produce apprehension, hallucinations, and various states of anxiety and depression. Persons who take LSD claim that it may also produce elation and heightened perception.

One possible result of taking LSD is a flashback. This is an episode in which an unpleasantness experienced while on LSD is reproduced when the person has not taken the drug, with all the upsetting symptoms of the original experience. For example, a person on LSD may become frightened in a crowd, and he or she may later feel exactly the same when in a crowd again, even though the drug has not been taken.

LSD is not a truly addictive drug. But experimenting with it can be dangerous, especially for those who are not mentally or emotionally stable, and long term damage may be done. Some LSD takers have developed a persistent psychosis.

LSD has been used medically in psychological research into various forms of mental illness, such as psychotic disorders, as well as in the treatment of chronic alcoholism.

See also DRUG ADDICTION.

Lues is a medical term for SYPHILIS.

A talk about Lumbago

Lumbago is low backache, in the lumbar region of the spine. It is an extremely common symptom and can be caused by various conditions. These may be related directly to the spine, or they may originate elsewhere in the body with pain being referred to the lumbar region.

Q: *What spinal conditions may cause lumbago?*

A: The ligaments holding the lumbar vertebrae may become strained when the muscles are weakened or the spine has an abnormal curvature. This produces deep pain that is made worse by movement. It may occur with LORDOSIS or SCOLIOSIS caused by poliomyelitis, or be caused by differences in the lengths of the legs. Occasionally, particularly in women, the vertebrae are not formed correctly so that there is partial dislocation of the spine (spondylolisthesis).

Lumbago can result from bone problems that affect the spine, such as ankylosing spondylitis in young men, or osteoporosis, osteoarthritis, or cancer of the vertebrae in the older age groups.

A SLIPPED DISC can cause low back pain. If the disc puts pressure on the sciatic nerve, the condition is made worse by the addition of sciatica, in which there is pain down one or both the legs.

Q: *What other conditions may cause lumbago?*

A: Lumbago may result from muscular disorders such as fibrositis, or slightly strained or torn muscles. Generalized muscle disorders, such as polymyalgia rheumatica in the elderly, may also cause lumbago.

Kidney disorders can frequently produce backache. Gynaecological disorders such as painful periods (dysmenorrhoea) are often accompanied by dull, persistent lumbago.

Occasionally, shingles is preceded by considerable pain in the lower back

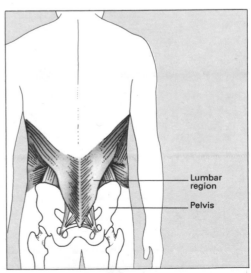

Lumbar region

Pelvis

Lumbago is a term used to describe pain in the muscles of the small of the back.

Lump

before the typical rash appears.

Lumbago is a common symptom with depression, but all other causes must be eliminated before the backache can be considered to be of psychological origin.

Q: How is lumbago treated?

A: A doctor decides on the appropriate treatment after diagnosing the cause. Diagnosis may require a full physical examination accompanied by appropriate blood tests, spinal X-rays, and, if necessary, a kidney X-ray (IVP).

A firm mattress, heat, and exercises to strengthen the back muscles and, if obesity is producing chronic strain of the spinal ligaments, a weight-reducing diet, all help. Painkilling drugs and those that produce muscle relaxation help to relieve many forms of lumbago; antirheumatic drugs, such as indomethacin, may be prescribed if bones and ligaments are involved. Manipulation may help if lumbago is of sudden onset and caused by spinal problems, and a surgical corset is also sometimes required to give the spine support and limit movement.

If all treatments fail and pain continues, it may be necessary to consider some form of surgical operation to stabilize the spine. This may be the only way to deal with a slipped disc or spondylolisthesis, for example.

If lumbago persists, its psychological aspects must be considered and anti-depressive treatment may be needed. It is understandable if patients wish to try some form of unorthodox treatment, such as acupuncture, although it is essential to make sure first that the condition does not require surgery.

See also BACKACHE.

Lumbar puncture is the insertion of a long needle to extract cerebrospinal fluid from around the nerves below the spinal cord in the lumbar region.

Lump is any abnormal swelling. Most lumps are benign (noncancerous), but some are malignant (cancerous) and for this reason anyone with a persistent unexplained lump should consult a doctor without delay. *See* CYST; FIBROMA; GANGLION; HERNIA; LIPOMA; NEUROMA; OSTEOMA; TUMOUR; VON RECKLING-HAUSEN'S DISEASE.

Lumpy jaw is a form of actinomycosis, a chronic fungus infection of the mouth, jaw, face, and neck. *See* ACTINOMYCOSIS.

Lung is the organ concerned with respiration (breathing). There are two lungs, sited within the thorax (chest cavity), a protective cage formed by the ribs and breastbone in front and the spine at the back. Between the lungs lies the heart, major blood vessels, and the oesophagus.

Air enters the body through the nose and mouth and passes into the throat. From there it enters the larynx and then into the trachea (windpipe) which divides into two bronchi, each of which leads to a lung.

Inside the lungs, oxygen in the air breathed in enters the bloodstream. At the same time, carbon dioxide leaves the blood and enters the lungs to be breathed out.

Q: What is the internal structure of the lungs?

A: The right lung, consisting of three lobes, is slightly larger than the left lung which has only two lobes. Each lobe is further divided into segments.

As the two main bronchi enter the lungs they divide into five narrower bronchi, one for each lobe. These bronchi then divide and subdivide into narrower and narrower tubes, called bronchioles. The bronchioles terminate in tiny and extremely thin-walled air sacs called alveoli. The oxygen-carbon dioxide exchange takes place through the moist walls of the alveoli.

The lungs and the inner surface of the thorax are covered by a thin membrane called the pleura. A small amount of lubricating fluid on the pleura allows the lungs and rib-cage to move against each other without friction.

The bronchi and bronchioles are lined with cells that keep them moist. These cells have small hairlike projections that

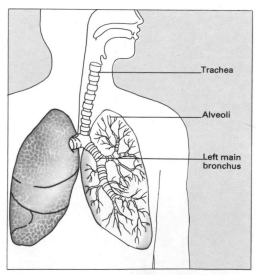

Trachea

Alveoli

Left main bronchus

Lungs are the ogans in which oxygen from the air is transferred to the bloodstream.

sweep mucus and debris to the trachea, and eventually to the oesophagus.

See also LUNG DISORDERS.

Lung cancer is the presence of a malignant (cancerous) tumour in the lung. The tumour usually forms in a bronchus (one of the tubes that carries air to and from the lungs), although it may grow in the alveoli that form the lung tissue itself. It is a serious disorder, usually not detected until the disease has already spread and it is too late for effective treatment. Most people who contract lung cancer are heavy cigarette smokers. Compared with a nonsmoker, a heavy smoker (more than twenty cigarettes a day) a 20 times greater chance of developing lung cancer. Regular chest X-rays may increase the chance of early detection.

Q: *What are the symptoms of lung cancer?*

A: Cancer of the bronchus does not always produce symptoms until it has been present for some time. The first symptom is usually a cough, with only a little sputum which may be blood-stained (haemoptysis). This may be followed by pneumonia or collapse of a segment of the lung (atelectasis) caused by partial blockage of the bronchus. The later symptoms include weight loss and increasing weakness and lethargy. Breathlessness is a feature and is usually caused more by general weakness than by damage to the lung tissue.

Q: *How is lung cancer diagnosed and treated?*

A: The diagnosis may be made by chest X-ray as well as by the detection of cancer cells in the sputum. It can be confirmed by means of bronchoscopy, which enables a surgeon to determine the exact position of the tumour. Unfortunately, treatments for lung cancer are not likely to be successful. The average survival time for an untreated patient is less than a year, and even with treatment only ten per cent survive for five years.

Fewer than a quarter of patients have a tumour that can be treated with surgery (either lobectomy or pneumonectomy). The usual alternative treatments are radiotherapy and the use of cytotoxic drugs, although such drugs are seldom effective.

Q: *How can lung cancer be avoided?*

A: Because of the association between cigarette smoking and lung cancer, the best way to avoid the disease is not to smoke. If smoking is stopped, the chance of developing lung cancer drops at a steady rate.

See also CANCER.

Lung disorders. The lungs have great reserves of capacity for air. Disorders of slow onset may therefore not cause symptoms until they have progressed for some time and caused considerable damage.

Disorders of the lung include those affecting: (1) the trachea and bronchi (the tubes that carry air in and out of the lungs); (2) the bronchioles (the narrower tubes within the lungs); (3) the lung fabric itself, where the exchange of oxygen and carbon dioxide takes place between the air and blood; and (4) the surrounding pleura and ribcage (thorax). Each of the disorders listed has a separate article in the A-Z section of this book.

Area affected	Possible disorder
Trachea and bronchi	ABSCESS of the lung
	BRONCHIECTASIS (scarring of bronchi preventing proper drainage of mucus)
	BRONCHITIS (inflammation of the bronchi)
	CANCER of the bronchus
	TRACHEITIS (inflammation of the windpipe)
Bronchioles	ASTHMA
	CYSTIC FIBROSIS (formation of abnormally sticky mucus)
Lung fabric	ACTINOMYCOSIS (fungal infection of the lung)
	ATELACTASIS (complete or partial collapse of the lung)
	EMBOLISM (blockage of an artery)

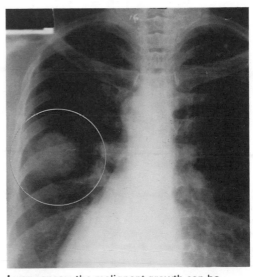

Lung cancer: the malignant growth can be seen on the left of the X-ray photograph.

Lung function tests

Area affected	Possible disorder
Lung fabric	EMPHYSEMA (destruction and enlargement of lung's air sacs)
	LUNG CANCER
	PNEUMOCONIOSIS (inflammation of the lung caused by inhaling dust)
	PNEUMONIA
	TUBERCULOSIS
Pleura and thorax	EMPYEMA (pus in the pleural cavity)
	HAEMOTHORAX (blood in the pleural cavity)
	LUNG CANCER
	PLEURISY (infection of the pleura)
	Epidemic PLEURODYNIA (Bornholm disease, a virus disorder)
	PNEUMOTHORAX (air in the pleural cavity)
	TIETZE'S SYNDROME (inflammation of the cartilage)
	TUBERCULOSIS

Lung function tests (pulmonary function tests) assess the condition and functioning of the lungs. They may be used as part of an investigation into a respiratory disorder. The various tests help a doctor to diagnose a condition and determine its severity; they may also establish whether a particular treatment is effective. Some lung function tests can be performed using simple equipment, such as a spirometer and a peak flow meter. Other tests, such as the analysis of gases in

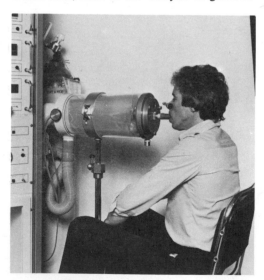

Lung function test is carried out on a piece of apparatus called a respirometer.

exhaled air and the measurement of oxygen and carbon dioxide levels in the blood, require sophisticated equipment and a detailed analysis of the results.

Lung machine. *See* HEART-LUNG MACHINE.

Lupus erythematosus (LE), one of a group of disorders known as the collagen diseases, takes two distinct but unrelated forms: discoid or cutaneous lupus erythematosus (DLE) and systemic lupus erythematosus (SLE). Both conditions affect the skin; SLE is probably an autoimmune disease.

Collagen is a fibrous insoluble protein in connective tissue. Both DLE and SLE affect the connective tissue, but are of unknown cause or causes. It is often difficult to distinguish between the two conditions; much confusion has arisen because the skin lesions are the same in both diseases. But other features are completely distinctive.

Q: What are the symptoms of DLE?

A: DLE is a chronic skin disorder that occurs most commonly in middle-aged women. It produces thickened, slightly scaly, reddened patches on the face, cheeks, and forehead. The characteristic is known as "butterfly rash." The patches sometimes spread to the scalp and cause hair loss. Sunlight makes the condition worse, so in some patients it virtually disappears during the winter months. Nearly all patients with DLE remain in good health apart from the skin disorder. It is exceptionally rare for patients with DLE to develop SLE.

Q: How is chronic DLE treated?

A: Patients with DLE should wear hats and sunlight barrier creams to protect their skins. Also, the use of corticosteroid skin creams may be helpful. Ultimately, some of the lesions heal on their own.

In severe cases, chloroquine (a drug used to treat malaria) may be beneficial. But, because chloroquine sometimes has an effect on the eyes, it should be used with great caution.

Q: What are the symptoms of SLE?

A: The patient may have a similar kind of butterfly rash as in DLE. There may also be fever, arthritis and signs of problems with lung and heart function.

Unlike DLE, SLE, also known as disseminated lupus erythematosus, is a generalized condition that may affect not only the face, but many tissues of the body, especially the kidney.

Q: How is SLE diagnosed and treated?

A: A knowledge of the patient's history combined with discovery of abnormalities in blood tests will help diagnosis. Treatment with corticosteroids may help.

Luxation. *See* DISLOCATION.

Lymph is the clear fluid that is drained from around the body's cells into the lymphatic system. It carries away bacteria and waste products.

See LYMPHATIC SYSTEM.

Lymphadenitis is inflammation of a lymph node, which causes it to swell. It is a normal reaction to any nearby infection. For example, any infection of the upper respiratory tract is accompanied by swelling of the tonsillar glands and other glands in the neck.

Lymphadenoma is a malignant (cancerous) tumour that affects the lymph nodes. *See* HODGKIN'S DISEASE.

Lymphangitis is inflammation of the lymphatic vessels. It occurs, to a certain extent, with LYMPHADENITIS. It may also develop in serious infections of the skin, for example in a septic wound, when red lines can be seen in the skin running from the wound to the nearest lymph nodes. This is a serious sign and requires urgent medical treatment.

Lymphatic leukaemia. *See* LEUKAEMIA.

Lymphatic system is a network of thin-walled vessels found throughout the body which drains fluid (lymph) from between the body cells into the bloodstream. The lymph vessels contain small valves, similar to those in veins, which prevent the backflow of lymph.

Rounded bean-shaped structures called lymph glands are situated at frequent intervals along the lymph vessels.

Most of the lymph vessels eventually converge to form the thoracic duct, a major lymph vessel that runs alongside the descending aorta. It connects to one of the main branches of the superior vena cava, a main vein carrying blood to the heart.

Lymphatic vessels are important to the mechanism by which fats are processed by the body. Vessels draining the small intestine collect the digested fat and pass it directly into the main blood circulation so that it bypasses the liver.

See also LYMPH GLAND.

Lymph gland, or node, is a small bean-shaped structure that forms part of the LYMPHATIC SYSTEM. Lymph glands are found throughout the body, particularly in places where lymph vessels unite.

The lymph glands have three main functions: (1) to filter out and destroy foreign substances such as bacteria and dust; (2) to produce some of the white blood cells called lymphocytes; and (3) to produce antibodies to help in the body's IMMUNITY system.

Specialized lymphoid tissue, similar to lymph glands, includes the tonsils, adenoids, and areas of the body such as the Peyer's patches in the wall of the small intestine.

Lymphocyte is one of the two main types of WHITE BLOOD CELLS. Lymphocytes are made in the lymph nodes, bone marrow, and thymus gland. They are concerned with the formation of antibodies and IMMUNITY.

See also LEUKAEMIA.

Lymphogranuloma venereum (LGV) is a venereal disease caused by bacteria related to those that cause psittacosis and trachoma. Symptoms include enlargement of the lymph nodes in the groin and the appearance of small ulcers on the surrounding skin.

Lymphoma is any form of growth connected with lymphoid tissue. A growth of this kind occurs, for example, with HODGKIN'S DISEASE.

See also LYMPHOSARCOMA.

Lymphosarcoma is a kind of malignant (cancerous) LYMPHOMA. Its symptoms are very similar to those of lymphatic LEUKAEMIA.

Lysol is an antiseptic solution of cresols and soap used as a general disinfectant. Lysol cannot be used to disinfect wounds because it is damaging to the skin.

M

Macula is the medical term for either a flat blemish or spot on the skin, or the part of the retina of the eye containing the FOVEA, on which light is focused.

Madura foot is a chronic fungus infection that occurs most commonly when fungi spores enter a wound in the foot.

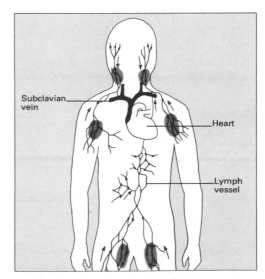

Lymphatic system drains fluid from around body cells back into the circulation.

Magnesia, Milk of

Magnesia, Milk of, is a suspension of magnesium hydroxide in water. It is used as a mild LAXATIVE or to treat indigestion.

Magnesium sulphate, commonly known as Epsom salts, is generally used as a LAXATIVE.

Magnesium trisilicate is a chemical compound of magnesium oxide, silicon dioxide, and water. It is used as an antacid in various preparations for treating indigestion.

Maidenhead. *See* HYMEN.

Malaria is a serious disease caused by a PROTOZOA called plasmodium. The disease is transmitted by the anopheles mosquito. The female mosquito bites an infected human and sucks the blood into its stomach, where the protozoa develop; when the mosquito next bites a human, these protozoa are injected into the bloodstream and reach the liver. Finally, they are released back into the blood to infect the red blood corpuscles; when these burst, further red blood corpuscles are infected and a recurring cycle of symptoms is started. The most severe form of malaria is called malignant tertian malaria (because the symptoms recur every three days) and is frequently fatal. It is caused by the parasite *Plasmodium falciparum.* The other three, milder forms are caused by *P. vivax, P. ovale,* and *P. malariae.*

Q: *What are the symptoms of malaria?*

A: After an incubation period of two to five weeks, there is a sudden attack of shivering followed by a high fever of at least 40°C (104°F). This is often accompanied by confusion, headache, and vomiting that lasts for several hours. These symptoms may occur at intervals of two to three days, depending on the type of malaria, and, if the disease is not treated, they will recur at irregular intervals throughout the person's life.

Q: *How is malaria diagnosed and treated?*

A: The diagnosis is made by examination of a blood sample, which reveals the presence of malarial parasites.

Initial treatment with the drug CHLOROQUINE may have to be supplemented by using QUININE or other drugs.

Q: *What measures can be taken to prevent malaria?*

A: Any person travelling to a malaria-infected area must take antimalarial drugs, usually chloroquine or primoquine, every week, throughout the stay and for one month after returning to a nonmalarious area.

Malignant describes any condition or disorder that has a tendency to become worse. *See also* BENIGN.

Malnutrition describes the physical deterioration of the body caused by following a diet that is deficient in nutrients, or by disorders in which the body fails to absorb nutrients. *See also* ANOREXIA NERVOSA; KWASHIORKOR; NUTRITIONAL DISORDERS; SPRUE.

Malocclusion is the failure of the teeth of the upper and lower jaws to meet correctly. It may cause problems with biting and chewing, but can usually be corrected with a brace on the teeth and proper orthodontic care. *See also* DENTAL DISORDERS; ORTHODONTICS.

Malpresentation describes an abnormal position of a foetus in the womb, possibly making natural delivery difficult. *See* PRESENTATION; PREGNANCY AND CHILDBIRTH.

Malta fever. *See* BRUCELLOSIS.

Mammogram is a specialized X-ray examination of breast tissue that is performed to investigate unidentified lumps in the breast. *See also* THERMOGRAM.

Mammoplasty is an operation to change the size and shape of the breasts. In reduction mammoplasty, the breasts are made smaller by removing some tissue. To increase the size of the breasts, an inert fluid-filled bag is implanted behind each breast.

Mandible is the lower jawbone. *See* JAW.

Mania is a form of mental disorder characterized by emotional excitement and lack of self-control, often resulting in rapid, irregular speech, overactivity, and violent behaviour.

Mania is also an uncontrollable desire to do something: for example, dipsomania is an abnormal and excessive desire to drink alcohol. *See also* DEPRESSION; MANIC-DEPRESSIVE ILLNESS.

Manic-depressive illness is a form of mental

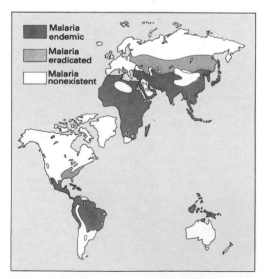

Malaria
endemic

Malaria
eradicated

Malaria
nonexistent

Malaria still persists in areas of uncleared swampland where the carrier mosquitos breed.

disorder that affects at least one per cent of the population. The first attack most commonly occurs in early middle-age, and it is more likely to occur in women than in men.

There are apparently two forms of this disorder: (1) the type in which depression is the only form of illness – periods of normal mood and behaviour are followed by a prolonged downswing of depression; and (2) the less common form in which mania alternates with depression.

Q: How is manic-depressive illness treated?

A: Hospitalization, with drug treatment and, sometimes, electroconvulsive therapy (ECT), is needed for severe cases.

The controlled use of lithium often prevents recurrences of mania. If it is combined with an antidepressant drug, given on maintenance therapy, it helps to lessen the mood swings of manic-depressive illness.

See also DEPRESSION; MANIA.

Mantoux test is a method of determining whether a person has at some time been infected by tuberculosis. A positive reaction generally indicates that the person has acquired partial immunity to the disease. A negative reaction indicates lack of immunity.

See also HEAF TEST; TINE TEST.

MAO inhibitors (monoamine oxidase inhibitors) are a group of drugs that are used in the treatment of DEPRESSION, particularly if other antidepressant drugs have not been effective.

Q: What adverse reactions can occur with the use of MAO inhibitors?

A: These drugs make the body destroy adrenaline, noradrenaline, and similar substances at a slower rate than usual. In a patient taking an MAO inhibitor, any drug or food that contains adrenaline-like substances or that stimulates the body to form adrenaline may cause a sudden and dramatic rise in blood pressure. This results in a severe headache and the danger of rupturing a blood vessel which, in turn, could lead to a stroke. For this reason, a psychiatrist may be wary of prescribing such drugs to a patient with a history of stroke, high blood pressure, or heart or liver disease.

Apart from these serious side effects, MAO inhibitors cause few of the other side effects that are associated with other antidepressant drugs.

Q: What precautions should be taken by patients taking MAO inhibitors?

A: Patients must obtain from the prescribing doctor a list of foods that must be avoided while taking MAO inhibitor

drugs and for at least two weeks afterwards. These foods contain substances that may form adrenaline-like factors; they include cheese, broad beans or their pods, protein and yeast extracts, and alcohol.

Patients taking MAO inhibitor drugs are advised not to take any additional drugs without consulting their doctor.

Marburg disease is a rapidly fatal form of virus ENCEPHALITIS that was first imported from Africa to research laboratories at Marburg, West Germany. The disease cannot be cured. Treatment involves complete isolation to prevent the spread of infection, and injections of GAMMA GLOBULIN prepared from a patient who has recently recovered from the disease.

Marijuana is a drug made from the dried leaves or flowers of the cannabis plant. It is usually smoked in cigarettes and is regarded as only mildly addictive. Other names for marijuana include cannabis, Indian hemp, kif, bhang, and dagga. The possession or use of marijuana is illegal in most Western countries.

Q: What are the effects of taking marijuana?

A: Mild drowsiness is often accompanied by an increased awareness of colour, sounds, and taste, which fluctuates in accordance with complex mood changes.

Many people who smoke marijuana tend to become listless and may have difficulty in concentrating. Physical inertia is commonly accompanied by loss of appetite, loss of weight, and a general lack of care about physical appearance.

Q: Is there any harm in smoking marijuana?

A: When marijuana is smoked occasionally by an otherwise well-adjusted individual there appears to be little harm.

Continued frequent use of marijuana, however, produces physical changes, and, sometimes, a true state of addiction. Physical changes include loss of weight, loss of sex drive, and a reduced sperm count in men.

Q: Can the use of marijuana lead to other, more serious forms of drug abuse?

A: It is unlikely that marijuana leads to dependence on any other drug. But the social situation in which illegal drugs are used means that marijuana smokers can be in association with persons who use "hard" drugs such as heroin and cocaine. This creates the opportunity to experiment with the other drugs.

See also DRUG ADDICTION.

Marrow is the soft, central part of bone. There are two types of marrow: (1) red marrow and (2) yellow marrow. *See* BONES.

Masochism

Masochism is a psychiatric term for a feeling of sexual satisfaction derived from being hurt. It is named for the Austrian novelist von Sacher-Masoch. It is manifested in many minor ways, for example, lovers' bites. But in its severer forms, such as whipping, it can cause physical harm and suffering. A doctor may recommend psychiatric counselling.

See also SADISM.

Massage is a therapeutic treatment in which the muscles are rubbed and manipulated for the relief of local pain and for relaxation. It is often used to remove excess fluid and to break up small adhesions under the skin.

Mastectomy is an operation to remove a breast. A partial mastectomy is the removal of one section of the breast, simple mastectomy is the removal of the whole breast, and radical mastectomy is the removal of the breast as well as some of the underlying muscle and the lymph glands in the armpit.

Q: Why is a mastectomy performed?

A: The operation is performed to remove breast tumours. Simple and radical mastectomies are performed as treatments for breast cancer, where the tumour is malignant and there is a danger of cancerous cells invading other parts of the body.

Q: Is any further treatment given for breast cancer?

A: Yes, sometimes, but this depends on the type and stage of the cancer. If the cancer is localized in the breast tissue, further treatment may not be required. Radiotherapy and chemotherapy are often used in conjunction with the operation.

Q: What problems may occur after a mastectomy?

A: As fluid may gather under the wound, drainage tubes are normally left in place for a few days. Apart from the physical discomfort associated with the operation, a woman who has had a breast removed also has to face major psychological problems. Discussion with a doctor may help to relieve anxiety but, frequently, a talk with another woman who has had the same operation is most helpful. She knows and understands the underlying fears and anxieties that are likely to arise. The woman's husband is often also given counselling. His understanding and reassurance will help to restore her confidence.

Mastitis is inflammation of the breast. It may be acute (occurring suddenly) or chronic (long-lasting).

Q: What causes acute mastitis?

A: Acute mastitis is caused by an infection, which occurs most commonly during lactation after childbirth when the breast is swollen with milk. Infection usually enters through a cracked nipple.

Q: How is acute mastitis treated?

A: If possible, breast-feeding should be continued, because this keeps the breast ducts clear. Firm bandaging of the breast and a reduction in the amount of fluid consumed help to reduce any excessive swelling (engorgement). A doctor may prescribe antibiotic drugs and painkillers until the infection is under control.

Occasionally, these treatments fail and an abscess starts to form. In such cases, breast-feeding must be stopped and the abscess incised and drained.

Q: What is chronic mastitis?

A: It is not an infection. It is caused by hormones in the body that affect the breast tissues so that they become swollen and tender. It is quite common just before a menstrual period and, in women who generally suffer from premenstrual tension, it can last from several days to two weeks. Chronic mastitis frequently occurs in women who are approaching menopause. This form of the disorder ceases after menopause is complete.

Q: How is chronic mastitis treated?

A: A firm, well-fitting brassiere may be all that is necessary. If the discomfort persists, fluid-removing (diuretic) pills are frequently helpful. The regular use of hormones is sometimes necessary.

Mastoid is a part of the temporal bone that is located behind the ear. The mastoid is filled

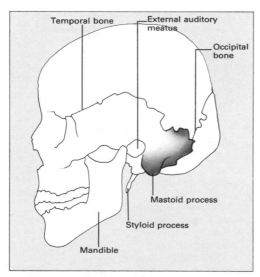

Labels: Temporal bone; External auditory meatus; Occipital bone; Mastoid process; Styloid process; Mandible

Mastoid is a projecting bone on the skull that is located behind the ear lobe.

with air cells arranged like a honeycomb that communicate with the middle ear. *See* MASTOIDITIS.

Mastoiditis is an infection of the mastoid bone behind the ear. It is usually caused by the spread of an infection from the middle ear, which occurs if a middle ear infection is inadequately treated. The symptoms include fever, a throbbing earache, a discharging ear, and deafness. In some patients the bone behind the ear may be painful.

Early treatment with antibiotic drugs cures most patients, and is essential to prevent damage to the mastoid bone. If bone damage has occurred, or if the infection does not respond to antibiotics, part of the mastoid bone may be surgically removed to prevent deafness.

Masturbation is the stimulation of one's own genitals to produce an ORGASM.

Q: Why do people masturbate?

A: Masturbation is a normal activity when it reduces sexual tension if, for cultural or social reasons, sexual intercourse is not possible. It is usually practised for the first time in early puberty, boys tending to start at an earlier age than girls. Full sexual maturity and regular sexual intercourse reduces the need for, and the frequency of, masturbation. Masturbation continues, however, as a common outlet for sexual relief, particularly during times of marital stress or illness, following the break-up of a marriage, and in people who have never had sexual intercourse.

Q: Is masturbation harmful?

A: Blindness, mental illness, and impotence are still sometimes believed to be the consequences of masturbation: there is absolutely no evidence to support these theories. The anxiety and feeling of guilt, aroused because the person feels that he or she is doing something wrong, are much greater problems.

Maxilla is the upper jawbone. *See* JAW.

Measles, also known as rubeola morbilli, is a highly contagious virus disease that causes fever and a characteristic rash. It occurs most commonly before adolescence and one attack usually confers immunity for life. The incubation period varies between eight and fourteen days. Measles is contagious during a period that lasts from four days before until five days after the rash appears. The quarantine period is fourteen days from the date of last contact with measles.

Q: What are the symptoms of measles?

A: The initial symptoms include fever, which may reach 40°C (104°F); a sore throat; coughing; and a running nose. These symptoms usually last for about four

days. About two days before the rash breaks out, small white spots (Koplik's spots) may appear inside the mouth and eyelids. These usually fade when the rash appears. The characteristic rash of measles is blotchy and orange-red in colour. It usually appears first behind the ears, then spreads to the face and neck. About twenty-four hours after its first appearance, the rash has usually covered the whole body. During the next three or four days, the rash and fever gradually disappear, although the cough may persist for an additional ten to fourteen days.

Q: How is measles treated?

A: There is no cure for measles. Treatment is directed at reducing the fever, and preventing the development of complications such as otitis media, sinusitis, bronchitis, and, rarely, encephalitis.

Q: Can measles be prevented?

A: Yes. A vaccine of a mild form of the measles virus will protect 97 per cent of children against the disease. They should be vaccinated no earlier than twelve months but no later than fifteen months.

Meckel's diverticulum is a small pouch near the end of the ileum. It is the remains of a branch of the gut that extended into the umbilical cord in the foetus. It is present in about two per cent of the population.

See also DIVERTICULUM.

Meconium is the greenish brown, thick faeces that a baby passes in the first few days after birth. It consists mainly of the cell debris and bile that a baby swallows in the womb.

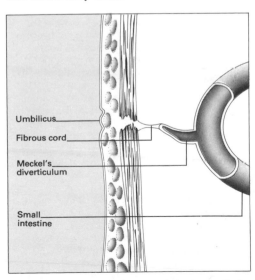

Umbilicus

Fibrous cord

Meckel's diverticulum

Small intestine

Meckel's diverticulum is a pouch in the wall of the intestine that may become inflamed.

Medical insurance

Medical insurance. The two main benefits provided by medical insurance are (1) the payment of an income when the insurer's normal income is lost because of illness, and (2) the payment of medical fees and other expenses incurred by the insurer.

Q: *What forms of state medical insurance benefits may be obtained?*

A: In the U.K., the weekly National Insurance contributions that are paid partly by employers and partly by employees entitle all employed people to sickness benefit. This benefit does not cover the cost of prescription charges, unless the individual concerned has a certificate of exemption or is included in one of the categories of people who are automatically exempt from prescription charges. These categories include children, the elderly, and those with low incomes.

Benefit cannot be obtained until the individual has been ill for at least three days. The doctor will sign a certificate giving the diagnosis of the illness and the length of time that the patient is expected to be away from work. The back of this form (MED 3) must then be completed by the patient before it is handed to the employer or sent to the local Social Security office. Many employers will continue to pay the individual's full basic salary while he or she is ill, and will then obtain the sickness benefit from the Social Security office.

Q: *Can this sickness benefit be obtained indefinitely?*

A: In exceptional cases, yes. However, anyone who claims sickness benefit for more than a few weeks will have his or her case reviewed by a medical board (appointed by the Ministry for Social Security), and it may be necessary for the patient to appear before this board. The hospital or GP will be asked to supply a detailed report on the patient's condition.

Those in financial difficulty may apply for Supplementary Benefit on a form supplied by the Social Security office. In certain cases, a Disablement Allowance will be paid for those who are permanently incapacitated.

Q: *What forms of medical insurance exist in industry?*

A: All companies have some form of accident insurance in case an employee is injured while at work or at the place of work. In addition to this compulsory accident insurance, certain trade unions provide their members with private sickness benefit and can arrange for their members to be treated at a trade union hospital.

Many companies offer their executives private medical insurance as one of the benefits of employment. Certain trade unions now offer similar benefits to their members.

Q: *How do private medical insurance schemes work?*

A: The largest private medical insurance companies are the British United Provident Association (BUPA) and the Private Patients' Plan (PPP). The Western Provident Association (WPA) and Lloyd's of London also operate medical insurance schemes. There are slight differences between all of these schemes.

Generally, the benefit obtained depends on the premium, the amount of money that is paid into the scheme each year. At the highest premium rate all medical expenses in the most expensive hospitals are covered, but the benefit for consultations and medical tests outside hospitals is usually less than the fees that are charged.

Individual premiums are usually lower if insurance is obtained through a company scheme.

Q: *What points should be considered when choosing private medical insurance?*

A: Most medical insurance schemes are complicated, and it is often wise to discuss the matter with a friend who has experience of one or other of the schemes. It is important to read the details of each scheme carefully, and to understand exactly which medical expenses the insurance covers.

Many of the available insurance schemes provide comprehensive cover for in-patient hospital treatment, but will only pay a proportion of the fees for any out-patient consultations and treatment. Also, not all the schemes provide cover for medical tests and investigations that are carried out outside a hospital.

Very few insurance schemes provide cover for fees charged for private treatment by GPs, although specialists' fees are usually covered.

All private medical insurance schemes stipulate a maximum amount of benefit that a patient can claim in any one year. For expenses above this amount, which may be incurred by a long-lasting serious illness, the patient is not insured.

Even under the most comprehensive and expensive schemes there are always certain expenses, such as drugs obtained outside a hospital, that are not covered.

Q: *Is it advisable to obtain medical insurance when travelling abroad?*

A: Yes. Although there are reciprocal arrangements for health care between most European countries, the procedure for obtaining treatment is often difficult. It is sometimes necessary to pay the full cost of treatment, and claim a reimbursement later.

Private medical insurance schemes generally provide cover for medical expenses incurred abroad up to certain limits, but people travelling to North America, or to non-European countries that do not have special health agreements with the U.K., should obtain additional insurance.

Medical social worker, formerly an almoner, is a trained member of a hospital staff who is concerned with the social welfare of patients. The duties of a medical social worker include helping with the claiming of any relevant Social Security benefits, and ensuring that adequate arrangements are made for the patient's convalescence at home, when the services of a health visitor, district nurse, or home help may be required.

Medical tests are physical examinations that ascertain the state of a person's general physical health or confirm a provisional diagnosis. The following is a list of medical tests, each of which has a separate entry in the A-Z section of this book.

AMNIOCENTESIS	GENETIC COUNSELLING
ANGIOGRAM	GLUCOSE TOLERANCE
AORTOGRAM	TEST
ARTERIOGRAM	HEAF TEST
AUDIOGRAM	INTELLIGENCE
BARIUM	QUOTIENT (IQ)
BASAL METABOLIC	INTRAVENOUS PYELO-
RATE	GRAM (IVP)
BIOPSY	ISHIHARA'S TEST
BLOOD PRESSURE	KAHN TEST
BODY TEMPERATURE	LARYNGOSCOPY
BRONCHOGRAM	LUNG FUNCTION
CAT SCANNER	TESTS
CERVICAL SMEAR	MAMMOGRAM
CHOLANGIOGRAM	MANTOUX TEST
CYSTOGRAM	MYELOGRAM
CYSTOSCOPY	ORAL CHOLE-
ECHOCARDIOGRAM	CYSTOGRAM
ECHOGRAM	PALPATION (breast
ELECTROCARDIOGRAM	examination)
(ECG)	PHONOCARDIOGRAM
ELECTROENCEPHALO-	QUICK'S TEST
GRAM (EEG)	RINNE'S TEST
ELECTROMYOGRAM	SCHICK TEST
(EMG)	SEDIMENTATION RATE
ENDOSCOPY	(ESR)
GASTROSCOPY	SPINAL TAP

TINE TEST	URINALYSIS
TSH TEST	VENOGRAM
TUBERCULIN TEST	WASSERMANN
ULTRASOUND	TEST
TECHNIQUES	WIDAL'S TEST

Mediterranean anaemia. *See* THALASSAEMIA.

Mediterranean fever is a type of intermittent fever that is usually caused by brucellosis. *See* BRUCELLOSIS.

Medulla is the inner part of a structure in the body, in contrast to the outer part (which is called the cortex).

Megacolon is an extremely enlarged colon that usually results from HIRSCHSPRUNG'S DISEASE, which is a congenital abnormality of the large intestine. Rarely, a megacolon may be caused by chronic constipation or by damage to the intestinal wall, as may occur with ULCERATIVE COLITIS and DIVERTICULITIS.

Megaloblast is a large, immature type of cell that is found in the bone marrow. It forms abnormal red blood cells, particularly those associated with PERNICIOUS ANAEMIA.

Megalomania is an unrealistic and unshakable belief that one is of great importance, usually associated with the conviction that others do not recognize this importance. It is also known as delusion of grandeur. *See* MANIA.

Meibomian cyst. *See* CHALAZION.

Melaena are faeces that are black and tarlike. The condition is caused by the action of the intestinal enzymes on blood, which may come from bleeding anywhere in the body.

Melancholia. *See* DEPRESSION.

Melanin is the dark pigment that is found in the skin, hair, and the CHOROID of the eye.

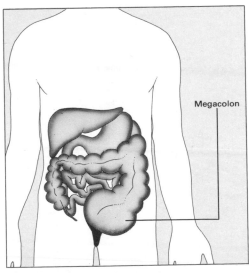

Megacolon usually affects the whole of the large intestine above the part without nerves.

Melanoma

See also CHLOASMA; MELANOMA; MELANURIA; MELASMA.

Melanoma is a brown pigmented lesion. A cancerous pigmented tumour is called a malignant melanoma. Most malignant melanomas arise from pigment cells in normal skin; a few may develop from pigmented moles. They are extremely rare in children. People who have been exposed to strong sunlight throughout their lives are more likely to develop malignant melanomas than those who have not. Pigmented growths on the legs, particularly in women; under the nails; on the palms of the hands and soles of the feet; or on the mucous membranes inside the mouth are particularly likely to become malignant. Malignant melanomas may also occur in the pigmented choroid layer of the eyeball.

Q: What are the symptoms of a malignant melanoma?

A: Most melanomas do not produce any definite symptoms, especially when they are in the early stages of development. For this reason a doctor should be consulted when any naevus, whether pigmented or not, forms a scab; bleeds; becomes surrounded by an inflamed area; becomes larger; or changes colour.

Q: How is a malignant melanoma treated?

A: It is usually necessary for the malignant melanoma to be removed surgically. If it has spread, it may also be necessary to remove any lymph glands affected.

Chemotherapy may be used if a malignant melanoma is situated on a limb. CYTOTOXIC DRUGS are usually injected into an artery to give a high concentration of the drug in the affected area. By the time the drug has reached the rest of the body, it has been greatly diluted; this method keeps any adverse effects to a minimum.

Melanuria is abnormally dark urine. It is found in cases of jaundice; haemoglobin in the urine (haemoglobinuria); certain malignant melanomas; and some rare congenital metabolic disorders, such as porphyria.

Melasma is pigmentation of the skin in which brown patches occur on the forehead and cheeks. It affects some women who take contraceptive pills or who are pregnant. In such women the condition is called chloasma. Melasma is increased by sunlight. The skin patches fade naturally when the woman stops taking the pills or after childbirth.

Membrane is a thin tissue layer that covers the surface of an organ, lines the inside of a tube or cavity, or separates one organ from another.

Memory, loss of. *See* AMNESIA.

Menarche is the onset of menstruation at puberty. *See* MENSTRUATION.

Menière's disease is a disorder of the inner ear arising from changes in the pressure of fluid within the ear's semicircular canals. It is commonest in those over the age of forty, and in 25 per cent of patients it will eventually affect both ears.

Q: What are the symptoms of Menière's disease?

A: Symptoms include attacks of dizziness, vertigo, nausea, vomiting, and sudden increases of deafness in the affected ear. The attacks occur in bouts, with periods of months or even years between them. They last several hours, and often leave a continued buzzing (TINNITUS) in the ear.

Q: How is Menière's disease treated?

A: There is no single effective method of treatment. Acute attacks are treated with antinausea drugs, and others drugs may reduce the frequency of the attacks. If treatment with drugs is ineffective, surgery may be necessary.

Meninges are the three membranes that cover the surface of the brain and spinal cord and follow the nerves for a short distance outside the central nervous system.

See also MENINGIOMA; MENINGITIS; SUBARACHNOID HAEMORRHAGE; SUBDURA.

Meningioma is a tumour that arises from the MENINGES, usually those around the brain and most commonly those above the CEREBELLUM. Multiple meningiomas may occur in VON RECKLINGHAUSEN'S DISEASE. They are usually benign (noncancerous) but may occasionally form a SARCOMA.

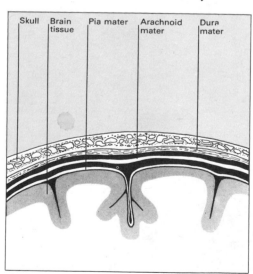

| Skull | Brain tissue | Pia mater | Arachnoid mater | Dura mater |

Meninges surround the brain in three layers: pia mater; arachnoid mater; and dura mater.

Meningitis is inflammation of the membranes (meninges) that cover the brain and the spinal cord. The symptoms of meningitis usually appear suddenly (acute meningitis) but, in some forms of the disorder, the onset of symptoms may be gradual. If untreated, acute meningitis is rapidly fatal.

Q: What are the symptoms of meningitis?

A: Acute meningitis is often preceded by a minor, influenza-like infection or by a sore throat. After one or two days, there is a sudden onset of a severe headache, vomiting, fever, and mental confusion. In severe cases, the patient goes into a coma. The patient may also have a stiff neck; be unable to straighten the leg after bending it at the hip joint (Kernig's sign); and be abnormally sensitive to light (photophobia). Some infections that cause meningitis, such as meningococcal meningitis, may produce skin rashes.

　　If the onset of meningitis is gradual, the symptoms are similar to those of the acute form, but develop over a period of one or two weeks.

Q: What causes meningitis?

A: Meningitis may be caused by a wide variety of viral, fungal, protozoan, or bacterial infections.

Q: How is meningitis treated?

A: The treatment of meningitis depends upon the cause. But meningitis may be fatal if treatment is not started in the early stages; immediate hospitalization is necessary. A lumbar (spinal) puncture is then performed and the cerebrospinal fluid examined to determine the cause of the meningitis.

　　Most patients with acute bacterial meningitis respond well to treatment with powerful antibiotics. Intravenous infusions may also be necessary if the patient is dehydrated.

　　The treatment of protozoan and viral meningitis depends upon the symptoms. Patients with viral meningitis usually recover, but they may be extremely ill during the early stages of the disorder.

Meniscus is a thin, crescent-shaped cartilage that is attached to the upper end of the shin-bone (tibia) within the knee joint. There are two menisci: the lateral meniscus and the medial meniscus. Collectively, they are called the semilunar cartilages. They form an important part of the mechanism by which the knee is locked to produce a strong and stable straight lower limb (*see* KNEE).

　　The most common disorder that affects the meniscus is tearing of the cartilage. It is a common sporting injury and usually occurs when the knee is twisted violently while in a half-bent position. There is usually pain as soon as the cartilage is torn. The victim often falls down and is unable to straighten the leg. The following day the knee is usually swollen and painful. The swelling may disappear after resting the knee for one or two weeks. But when normal activity is resumed, the knee may give way or may suddenly lock so that the leg cannot be straightened normally. The usual treatment is to remove the cartilage surgically (meniscectomy).

A talk about Menopause

Menopause is the end of menstruation. By popular usage, the term has come to be synonymous with climacteric. Menopause is a combination of physical and psychological changes.

Q: At what age does menopause usually occur?

A: Menopause occurs most commonly between the ages of 45 and 55 years, but it may occur earlier or later without there being any abnormality. As a general rule, the younger a woman was when she began to menstruate, the older she will be at the start of menopause.

　　Menstruation ceases at any age after the surgical removal of the womb (hysterectomy). But the symptoms of menopause occur only if both ovaries as well as the womb are removed and menopause has not already taken place naturally.

Q: How does menstruation cease?

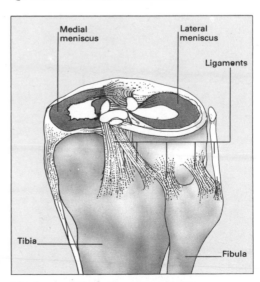

Meniscus cartilage is composed of strong fibres; it helps to lock the leg straight.

Menopause

A: This varies greatly from woman to woman. Some women menstruate normally and regularly, then stop suddenly. But in most women, menstruation becomes irregular during menopause. The periods themselves may be shorter than usual, and the interval between them may vary from about two weeks to ten weeks. The periods may be heavy or light.

Any bleeding that occurs more than six months after the last period, even if it seems like a normal period, should be regarded as abnormal and reported to a doctor.

Q: *What are the symptoms associated with menopause?*

A: The most common symptoms are hot flushes, sweating, palpitations, depression, irregular menstruation, fatigue, headache, and sleeping difficulties.

Q: *Do all women suffer from menopausal symptoms?*

A: No. In many women the symptoms are absent or extremely mild. But most women do have some symptoms, although many do not consider the problems serious enough to consult a doctor. It is often difficult to be sure that the symptoms are associated with menopause and not with other problems. For example, headaches are common at any age and depression may have various other causes.

Q: *Why do menopausal symptoms occur?*

A: The symptoms are caused by hormonal changes that occur gradually over several years. In a woman of childbearing age, the ovaries secrete the oestrogen hormones in response to FOLLICLE-STIMULATING HORMONE (FSH) from the pituitary gland. At the approach of menopause, the ovaries become less responsive to FSH and secrete less oestrogen. As a result, the pituitary gland produces more FSH to try to maintain oestrogen levels.

As a direct result of these hormonal changes, ovulation becomes infrequent, periods become irregular and menopause finally occurs. However, the pituitary gland still secretes large amounts of FSH, which affect the blood vessels in the skin, causing them to dilate. This in turn produces the hot flushes, sweating, palpitations, and headaches, all common menopausal symptoms.

The hormonal changes also cause the breasts and womb to become smaller after menopause. The lining of the vagina becomes thinner and drier, and the muscles that support the womb become weaker, so that a PROLAPSE may occur.

Q: *How can the symptoms of menopause be treated?*

A: Medical treatment is not usually necessary. A doctor may be able to help by explaining what happens during menopause and by dispelling the anxieties that a woman may have about loss of femininity and the expectation of years of depression and unhappiness.

If treatment is after all necessary, the doctor may prescribe a mild tranquillizer or an antidepressant. If the hot flushes are severe, drugs may be prescribed to reduce the sensitivity of the blood vessels.

Sometimes these treatments are ineffective, in which case hormone replacement therapy (HRT) may be recommended. This involves giving small doses of oestrogen, with or without progesterone, by mouth, injection, or implantation of an oestrogen-containing pellet. HRT increases the amount of oestrogen, thus adjusting the hormonal balance by decreasing the FSH.

Q: *What other changes may occur after menopause?*

A: Apart from gradual reduction in size of the breasts and womb, the vagina and the vulva also change. These changes may cause discomfort and pain during sexual intercourse. If this occurs, oestrogen-containing suppositories or creams, used regularly, restore the thickness and moistness of the vaginal lining.

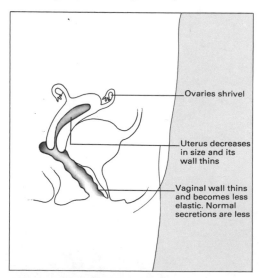

Ovaries shrivel

Uterus decreases in size and its wall thins

Vaginal wall thins and becomes less elastic. Normal secretions are less

Menopause is accompanied by changes in the female reproductive system.

Q: *Should a woman still have regular gynaecological examinations after menopause?*

A: Yes. Regular gynaecological examinations, including a CERVICAL SMEAR test, are as important after menopause as before it.

Q: *Is there any change in attitudes to sex after menopause?*

A: This varies among individual women. Most women do not notice any change in their sex drive. Some find that their sex drive is increased after menopause, when the risk of an unwanted pregnancy has definitely disappeared. However, women who become depressed find that often their sex drive is reduced.

Q: *What form of contraception should be used during menopause?*

A: A doctor should be consulted about contraception during menopause. Contraceptive pills are inadvisable for women over the age of forty years. An intrauterine contraceptive device (IUD) or a diaphragm with a spermicidal cream or jelly probably give the best protection (*see* CONTRACEPTION). Contraceptive measures should be used for at least six months and, sometimes, up to one year after menopause to make sure that periods have finally stopped, and that the woman is no longer fertile.

Menorrhagia is the medical term for heavy periods; that is, regular menstruation that involves greater than normal blood flow and that usually lasts longer than normal. *See* MENSTRUAL PROBLEMS.

A talk about Menstrual problems

Menstrual problems may occur at any time between menarche (when periods first begin) and MENOPAUSE (when they end).

During puberty, many girls have irregular periods. But as a rhythm becomes established, problems become less common, and the absence of periods (AMENORRHOEA) is usually a sign of pregnancy or of a psychological problem.

The most common problem during the early years of menstruation is pain (*see* DYSMENORRHOEA), and in later years there may be feelings of irritation and depression, breast tenderness, and ankle swelling because of PREMENSTRUAL TENSION. Also, fluid retention may occur for a few days before menstruation.

Bleeding between periods may occur at any time, but is most common during the few years before menopause. If it persists, you should consult a doctor. Heavy periods (*see* MENORRHAGIA) or irregular periods (*see* METRORRHAGIA) also commonly occur.

A threatened MISCARRIAGE may simulate a menstrual problem when in fact it is caused by a pregnancy.

Q: *What conditions cause abnormal menstrual bleeding?*

A: Heavy periods may be caused by various conditions that affect the womb, such as ENDOMETRIOSIS, ENDOMETRITIS, FIBROIDS, or SALPINGITIS. Occasionally, general disorders, such as hypothyroidism or thyrotoxicosis, CIRRHOSIS of the liver, and blood disorders involving a reduction in clotting ability, may cause abnormal menstrual bleeding. More frequently, heavy periods are associated with the hormone imbalance related to menopause or, less frequently, to an OVARIAN CYST.

At any age, one of the most common causes of abnormal bleeding is psychological disturbance because of ANXIETY, DEPRESSION, or SEXUAL PROBLEMS.

Q: *How is abnormal menstruation treated?*

A: Treatment depends on the cause. A woman experiencing this problem should consult a doctor. A diagnosis will be made after physical and gynaecological examinations. If necessary, it will include a CERVICAL SMEAR test and a vaginal swab to discover if any infection is present. A pregnancy test reveals if pregnancy is the cause of lack of menstruation.

Menstrual problems	Associated symptoms
Amenorrhoea	Absence of menstruation. Commonly due to pregnancy, menopause, and emotional disturbance.
Dysmenorrhoea	Pain starting just before or with menstruation.
Ectopic pregnancy	A missed period followed by severe pain. Fallopian tube may rupture. Internal haemorrhage may result.
Menorrhagia	Prolonged and heavy periods.
Metrorrhagia	Bleeding between periods. Possibility of uterine fibroids or cancer of the uterus.
Premenstrual tension	Irritability, depression, fatigue, headaches, breast tenderness, abdominal swelling.

Menstrual problems can usually be easily identified and treated by a doctor.

Menstruation

If no physical cause can be found for the absence of menstruation, a hormonal disturbance may be the cause. This is frequently of a temporary nature and no treatment is needed. However, if there is no return of natural menstruation, a doctor may prescribe hormones that usually produce a type of menstruation.

Q: *What are other treatments if diagnosis is uncertain or hormone therapy is unsuccessful?*

A: A diagnostic D AND C (dilation and curettage) is a simple and minor operation that allows a general gynaecological examination as well as a microscopic examination of the lining of the womb. Often this simple operation is in itself sufficient to return menstruation to normal. The woman does not need to remain hospitalized for more than a day.

If abnormal bleeding continues, either because of hormonal disturbance, fibroids, or cancer, a HYSTERECTOMY (surgical removal of the womb) may have to be performed. But this operation is becoming less common. Hysterectomy induces menopause. Troublesome symptoms occur only if the ovaries are removed as well as the womb.

Menstruation is the shedding of the lining of the womb (endometrium) that occurs regularly in women between menarche (the beginning of menstrual periods) and menopause (the end of periods). It produces a vaginal bleeding that lasts for three to seven days and occurs every twenty-four to thirty-four days – the length of the menstrual cycle. About half-way through the cycle, an egg is released from an ovary to travel along a fallopian tube to the womb. This process is called OVULATION.

Q: *How is the length of a menstrual cycle calculated?*

A: The menstrual cycle is the time between the first day of one period and the first day of the next, including the days when bleeding occurs.

Q: *Are all menstrual cycles the same?*

A: No. Most women have a slight variation, within a day or so, in the length of their menstrual cycles, and each woman's cycle can also vary from month to month. The cycle tends to be the same length, usually about twenty-eight days, but some women have a cycle that is consistently longer or shorter than this.

Q: *Is menstruation always the same?*

A: Like the menstrual cycle, the period may have slight variations in individual women. Bleeding is usually heavier in the first day or two and then becomes lighter for the next two or three days.

Q: *How does the body control menstruation?*

A: Regularity of menstruation is a complex balance between the levels of hormones produced by the ovaries (oestrogens and progesterone) and those produced by the pituitary gland at the base of the brain, the follicle-stimulating hormone (FSH) and the luteinizing hormone (LH). FSH stimulates the ovary to produce oestrogen in the first half of the menstrual cycle. Oestrogen causes a thickening of the lining of the womb. In mid-cycle, a sudden increase in LH causes ovulation and production of progesterone, which alters the womb lining in preparation for a fertilized egg.

Fertilization produces an embryo that stimulates another hormone to maintain the womb lining. If fertilization does not take place, the womb lining is shed as the menstrual flow, and the cycle of events begins all over again.

Q: *How are the hormones from the pituitary gland involved in menstruation?*

A: As the production of oestrogen increases from the ovaries, its rising concentration diminishes the level of FSH from the pituitary by a mechanism known as a "feedback." The pituitary gland then releases LH.

The feedback of the various hormones is detected by the hypothalamus in the brain. The hypothalamus can also be affected by other factors, such as

Menstrual cycle			

Days				
1	7	14	21	28

Graafian follicle matures	Ovulation occurs	Corpus luteum develops and later degenerates

Menstruation

Uterine wall

1	7	14	21	28
Days				

Menstruation normally occurs during the first five days of the menstrual cycle.

emotions, anxiety, or depression, and the effects of other hormones in the bloodstream.

Q: *Why do menarche and menopause occur?*

A: The onset of menstruation is associated with the hormonal changes of puberty, and the final end of menstruation is caused by aging of the ovaries. But in neither case is the exact mechanism fully understood.

Q: *What care should a woman take during menstruation?*

A: There is no need to restrict any activities during menstruation unless the blood flow is extremely heavy. Absorbent pads (sanitary napkins) or internal tampons may be worn. Sanitary napkins are more obtrusive and may cause vulval soreness, but they are more absorbent than tampons. Tampons left in the vagina for a long time may produce offensive discharge because of vaginitis. Menstrual blood has no harmful effects on the woman or anything that it may touch.

Q: *At what age may a girl use internal tampons?*

A: This depends on her size. It is often advisable to attempt to insert the first tampon when she is not menstruating, because the technique is sometimes difficult to learn.

    See also AMENORRHOEA; MENOPAUSE; MENSTRUAL PROBLEMS.

Mental defect is a deficiency of one or several areas of brain function. It may be a general lack of intelligence (mental retardation), or it may affect only one type of mental ability without affecting the overall level of intelligence.

A talk about Mental illness

Mental illness is an abnormality of thinking or behaviour without any obvious physical cause. Mental illness is a relative term. It refers to the behaviour of those who deviate from what is normally expected of them by others. Because of this and also because the normal range of behaviour is so wide, it is often extremely difficult to establish that a person is mentally ill. If the abnormality is so great or if the history of the disorder is obviously one of profound mental disturbance, then a doctor may be able to make a diagnosis. Diagnosis and treatment are made easier if a patient consults a doctor voluntarily.

Q: *What types of mental illness may occur?*

A: There are several different ways of classifying mental illness, none of which is completely satisfactory. One of the most widely used systems of classification divides mental illness into three main categories: (1) psychoses, (2) neuroses, and (3) personality disorders.

    In addition to these main categories are sexual disorders, mental retardation, and the dementias.

Q: *What are psychoses?*

A: Psychoses are gross disturbances of mental functioning and behaviour accompanied by a distintegration of the personality and loss of contact with reality. Psychoses are characterized by persistent delusions and hallucinations. The patient usually has no insight into the disorder. Psychoses are thought to be caused by a chemical or hormonal disorder that affects the brain in genetically vulnerable individuals. The main psychoses are schizophrenia; manic-depressive illness; and paranoia.

Q: *How are psychoses treated?*

A: Psychoses may be treated with tranquillizers, such as chlorpromazine and haloperidol, which may be combined with electroconvulsive therapy (ECT). Because many patients with psychotic disorders do not realize that they are mentally ill, such treatment often has to be given after compulsory admission to hospital. Treatment of psychoses is not always effective, although the symptoms can usually be alleviated. Some patients respond well and become normal for long periods. However, the condition may return at any time after treatment ceases.

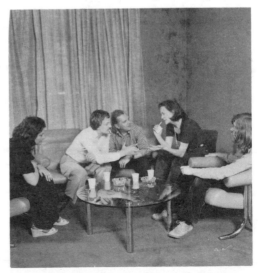

Group therapy can help many patients bring their difficulties out into the open.

Mental retardation

Q: *What are neuroses?*

A: Neuroses are an exaggeration of the normal responses to the stresses of life. In a patient with a neurosis, the reaction interferes with normal activities. Unlike a psychotic patient, however, a person with a neurosis is aware of the disorder and usually seeks medical help. Anxiety, depression, hypochondria, hysteria, obsession, and phobias are all neuroses.

Q: *How are neuroses treated?*

A: The treatment of neuroses is often difficult. Symptoms, such as hysteria, may be controlled with tranquillizing drugs. If such treatment is given early in the disorder, the symptoms may disappear spontaneously. However, it is usually necessary to combine drug treatment with PSYCHOTHERAPY or behaviour therapy.

Q: *What are personality disorders?*

A: There are several different types of personality disorders:(1) personality pattern disturbances, including schizoid (shy and seclusive), cyclothymic (alternations of depression and elation), and paranoid behaviour (delusions of persecution); (2) personality trait disturbances, which have a single dominant characteristic, such as compulsiveness; and (3) psychopathic personality disturbances, which are marked by antisocial behaviour without feelings of guilt. ALCOHOLISM and DRUG ADDICTION are also considered to be personality disorders.

Q: *How are personality disorders treated?*

A: Most personality disorders need expert psychiatric treatment, which may involve behaviour therapy using de-sensitization methods that expose the patient to the conditions inducing the disorder.

Q: *Can mental illness occur in children?*

A: Yes. Apart from mental retardation and certain types of MENTAL DEFECT, children may also become depressed. AUTISM is a rare condition that some psychiatrists believe to be a form of juvenile schizophrenia.

Q: *How can the community and the family help a patient who is mentally ill?*

A: It is important that the family, friends, and the family doctor are aware that some forms of mental illness, such as schizophrenia and manic-depressive psychosis, are more common in certain families. An awareness of this possibility means that treatment can be started early, even if it requires compulsory admission to hospital.

Provisions should be made for those who are so mentally ill that they are a danger to themselves or to others. Most patients with depression are aware of their condition and realize the need for treatment. However, those with a psychotic illness may not be aware of their disorder, and compulsory admission to hospital is needed. A doctor will be able to give advice about the necessary procedures.

Most people with hysterical or mildly paranoid personalities are able to adapt to normal life, although their behaviour may seem strange.

Co-operation between hospitals, the family, and the community means that fewer patients are compulsorily detained for psychiatric treatment than previously. Many patients are encouraged to lead as normal a life as possible while under overall supervision of a psychiatrist or a social worker, which may include some form of psychotherapy.

See also ANOREXIA NERVOSA; DEMENTIA; HOMOSEXUALITY; MASTURBATION; MENTAL RETARDATION; PERSONALITY DISORDERS; SEXUAL PROBLEMS.

Degrees of mental retardation as measured by IQ score	
110 score	Average and above intelligence
100	
90	
80	Below average but not retarded
70	
60	Mildly retarded
50	Moderately retarded
40	
30	Severely retarded
20	Profoundly retarded
10	

Mental retardation (shaded) is graded by IQ. A person below 90 is educationally subnormal.

Mental retardation is subnormal intelligence. It may be caused by lack of brain development, or brain damage from injury or illness.

Q: *What causes mental retardation?*

A: In most cases the cause is unknown but the normal variation in intelligence that occurs in the population can produce persons with below average as well as above average intelligence. Several rare inherited disorders, such as phenylketonuria, Tay-Sachs syndrome, and von Recklinghausen's disease may cause mental retardation.

Chromosomal abnormalities (of which Down's syndrome, or mongolism, is the most common) and antenatal infection (such as German measles and toxoplasmosis) may also result in brain damage. Smoking during pregnancy and various disorders, such as pre-eclampsia and placenta praevia, may reduce the blood flow to the developing foetus. This may produce a mild form of foetal malnutrition that may affect development of the brain.

Brain damage may occur at birth. It may, for example, be caused by asphyxia or haemolytic disease of the newborn. Premature babies, especially if their birth weight is less than 3lb (1.5kg), are more likely to be mentally retarded during infancy and childhood. Such damage may be caused by a serious head injury; a serious infection, such as meningitis; or poisoning, especially with heavy metals such as lead. Chronic malnutrition, such as kwashiorkor, can also prevent normal brain development, thereby reducing intelligence.

In many cases of mild mental retardation, social and economic factors are more significant than medical causes. These factors include poverty, social isolation, and cultural deprivation during early childhood. It has also been shown that if an infant is separated from its mother for a continuous period during its first year of life, mental retardation may result. If the separation lasts for longer than six months, the mental retardation may be irreparable.

Q: *How is mental retardation assessed?*

A: In some cases, mental retardation may be detected at birth or soon afterward. For example, Down's syndrome is usually apparent at birth. However, mental retardation, particularly if it is mild, is often detected first by the parents, who may notice that their child has problems with feeding; lacks normal responses, such as smiling; or is slow in learning to crawl or walk. In such cases, the parents should consult a doctor, who will examine the baby to try to find a cause. The examination usually includes a full neurological investigation, sometimes with an electroencephalogram (EEG), skull X-rays, hearing tests, and vision tests. From these, a doctor may be able to give the parents an indication of the degree of the child's retardation and the problems that they may encounter. Many parents find it difficult to accept that their child may be mentally retarded, and, even if they suspect that this may be the case, refrain from seeking expert confirmation. Professional advice, however, is essential if the child's learning potential is to be developed as fully as possible, and will help the parents to cope with the strain and responsibility of bringing up a mentally retarded child.

An accurate assessment of an infant's intelligence is impossible. When the child is about three years old, an intelligence test may be given. This can give a reasonable indication of the severity of mental retardation, which may help the parents to plan for the child's future.

Mental retardation is generally classified as mild, moderate, or severe. Individuals are assessed according to their degree of subnormality and their potential for learning social, occupational, and academic skills.

Children with mild retardation (with an INTELLIGENCE QUOTIENT in the range of 50-70) can usually be taught to do simple mathematics, to read and write, and to perform uncomplicated tasks. Those with severe retardation may have difficulties with speech, co-ordination, bladder control, and bowel control. The most severely retarded seldom learn to walk and usually remain incontinent, needing lifelong supervision.

Q: *Can mental retardation be prevented?*

A: In some cases it is possible to prevent mental retardation. At present, however, it is not possible to prevent most cases of mental retardation. If any inherited disorder has occurred in the family of either of the potential parents, a genetic counsellor may be able to give advice about the likelihood of retardation in their children. Some chromosomal abnormalities can be detected by testing fluid from the womb during pregnancy (amniocentesis). If this indicates that the baby will be retarded, an abortion can be performed if the parents wish it.

The possibility of brain damage caused by malnutrition of the foetus can be reduced by stopping smoking before pregnancy, and by skilled antenatal care during pregnancy.

Tests for phenylketonuria are performed routinely within ten days of birth. If these are positive, a special diet will prevent brain damage. Early

Menthol

diagnosis and treatment of hypothyroidism prevents cretinism.

Q: *Are there other problems that are
associated with mental retardation?*

A: Yes. Cerebral palsy and epilepsy, which
are also caused by brain damage, often
occur in the mentally retarded. The drugs
that are used to control epilepsy may
further impair mental functioning.

It is difficult to teach mentally retarded
persons about safety precautions, and so
they are more likely to be hurt in
accidents.

Q: *How can the mentally retarded be helped?*

A: Skill, patience, and understanding from
the parents, doctors, and educators who
specialize in teaching the mentally
retarded can enable retarded children to
be educated to their fullest capabilities.

The severely retarded often have other
disorders, such as spina bifida and
hydrocephalus, cerebral palsy, or
congenital heart disease. Such disorders
may prevent them from being educated
to the fullest extent, and they may need
lifelong hospital care.

Home care of the mentally retarded is
extremely demanding on other members
of the family, even with the support and
encouragement of relatives and friends.
Societies that have a special interest in a
particular disorder can often give expert
advice, and may be able to put parents in
contact with others who have similarly
retarded children.

Menthol is an alcohol that is obtained from
the oils of several kinds of mint. It may be

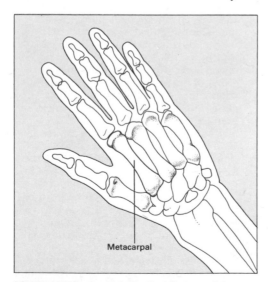

Metacarpal

Metacarpal bones link the five fingers of the
hand with the small bones of the wrist.

used alone or in steam inhalations to treat
sinusitis and bronchitis. Menthol is often
combined with camphor or eucalyptus to produce creams, lotions, and ointments.

Meprobamate is a tranquillizing drug that is
used mainly to treat mild anxiety.

Meprobamate may produce loss of appetite, nausea, vomiting, diarrhoea, and headaches. Large dosages may cause dizziness,
drowsiness, lack of co-ordination, and a decrease in blood pressure.

Mercury is a liquid metallic substance that is
commonly used in thermometers and other
instruments. Some mercury compounds are
still used in antiseptics and eye ointments,
but teething powders containing mercury are
no longer used as they were found to be a
cause of PINK DISEASE.

Mercury poisoning may occur from pollu-
tion of food (*see* MINAMATA DISEASE), from the
use of mercury in industrial processes that
may be inhaled, or from skin contact over a
period of time. If mercury has been swallowed, treatment must include washing out
the stomach and swallowing an egg white to
absorb the mercury.

Mescaline is an alkaloid that is the active hal-
lucinogenic substance of the peyote or peyotl
cactus (*Lophophora williamsii*). The effects of
mescaline are similar to those of LSD and
include visual and auditory hallucinations,
distortions of time sense, feelings of anxiety
or even persecution, and feelings of elation.
Not all of these effects necessarily occur,
because the reaction to mescaline varies
considerably among individuals, as well as in
the same person at different times.

See also DRUG ADDICTION.

Mesentery is a membrane-like fold of tissue
attached to the back of the abdominal wall. It
supports the intestines and contains the blood
vessels, nerves, and parts of the lymphatic
system that connect with the intestines.

Metabolism is the sum of all the chemical and
physical processes that occur within the body.
It includes the repair and replacement of
dead or damaged tissues, and the production
of energy.

Metabolism involves two basic processes:
anabolism and catabolism. Anabolism is the
synthesis of complex substances from simpler
ones, which occurs during the growth of body
tissues. Catabolism is the reverse process: the
breakdown of complex substances into simpler substances. The BASAL METABOLIC RATE is
a measure of the body's energy expenditure
when at complete rest.

Metacarpal is any one of the five bones that
form the structure of the palm of the hand.

See also HAND.

Metastasis is the spread of a disease from one

part of the body to another. The term usually refers to the spread of cancer, although metastasis may also occur in some infections, such as endocarditis and tuberculosis.

In cancer patients, cells that have separated from a primary tumour may spread through the lymphatic system, into the veins, or, more rarely, into an artery. These cells (metastases) may also spread across the surface of a structure, such as the peritoneum lining of the abdomen or the pleura surrounding the lungs. Occasionally, metastases result from surgery, and may be found in the scar of the wound through which a tumour has been removed. *See* CANCER.

Metatarsal is any one of the five bones that form the main part of the arch of the FOOT. *See* BUNION; HALLUX VALGUS; METATARSALGIA.

Metatarsalgia is pain in the front of the foot. The most common cause is a form of flatfoot in which the arch between the bases of the big and little toes is deformed, and the heads of the metatarsal bones rest on the ground. This pressure on the bones produces pain, causes the skin to thicken, and may eventually cause the toes to curl. Metatarsalgia may also be caused by pressure on a nerve (neuralgia), or by a stress fracture, which can occur after prolonged walking or running.

Resting the injured foot and wearing a soft-soled shoe is usually the only treatment required while the fracture heals. Prolonged physiotherapy to strengthen the underlying muscles may be effective in patients under the age of forty years. But if the pain is severe, it may be necessary to wear a plaster cast for about one month.

Methadone is a synthetic painkiller similar to morphine. It may be used as a cough suppressant and in the treatment of heroin addiction. Methadone blocks the effects of heroin withdrawal and, although methadone itself is addictive, it is thought to be easier to withdraw from than is heroin. Use of methadone in heroin withdrawal should be under expert medical supervision in a centre that specializes in control of drug addiction.

Methamphetamine is a stimulant drug that has effects similar to those of amphetamine. *See* AMPHETAMINE.

Methaemoglobin is a compound form of HAEMOGLOBIN that prevents the haemoglobin in red blood cells from carrying adequate amounts of oxygen to the body tissues. The presence of methaemoglobin is usually caused by poisoning with aniline dyes, potassium chlorate, or various other chemicals, including nitrites in drinking water. But it may also be caused by a hereditary deficiency of the substance that helps convert methaemoglobin to haemoglobin.

Methyl alcohol. *See* ALCOHOL.

Metropathia haemorrhagica is bleeding from the womb for which a cause cannot be found. *See* MENSTRUAL PROBLEMS.

Metrorrhagia is the medical term for bleeding from the womb, either during menstruation or at other times. *See* MENORRHAGIA; MENSTRUAL PROBLEMS.

Microbes are microscopic living organisms. The term is often applied to any organism that causes disease. *See* GERMS.

Microcephalic describes an individual whose head is disproportionately small in comparison with the rest of the body. The abnormally small head, present at birth, is usually associated with mental retardation.

Microsurgery is any surgical technique that requires the use of a microscope and specially adapted instruments. It is used for operations that require extreme delicacy, as in surgery of the ears, the eyes, or the brain.

Micturition is the medical term for the act of passing urine. *See* BLADDER DISORDERS; URINE.

Middle ear is the part of the ear that transmits sounds from the outer ear to the inner ear (*see* EAR).

Midwife, or nurse-midwife, is a person skilled in caring for women in normal pregnancy, during labour, and following childbirth.

A talk about Migraine

Migraine is a recurring severe headache, often affecting only one side of the head and accompanied by a variety of other symptoms. It occurs more commonly in women than in

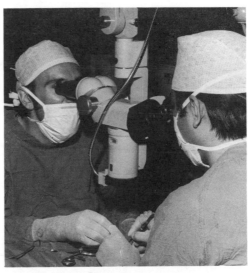

Microsurgery permits surgeons to perform operations of extreme delicacy.

Migraine

men and usually first appears between the ages of ten and twenty years.

Q: What are the symptoms of migraine?

A: The initial symptoms are usually mild fatigue and depression. These may be accompanied by visual disturbances with irregular, flashing patterns of light; temporary blindness in one half of the visual field (hemianopia); or double vision (diplopia) because of eye muscle weakness. Sometimes there is also weakness or loss of sensation in a limb (hemiparesis or hemi-anaesthesia).

The symptoms may last a few minutes and disappear before the beginning of the typical throbbing headache. The pain is frequently accompanied by nausea and vomiting, aversion to light (photophobia), and sensitivity to noise.

The headache may last several hours, or even a day or two, before disappearing and allowing the individual to fall asleep and then to awake refreshed. Migraine attacks may occur daily or as infrequently as once every few months.

Q: What causes migraine?

A: The cause is not known, although about half of all migraine sufferers have another member of the family who has similar headaches. Sometimes there is an association with certain foods, such as chocolate, cheese, or cured meats, suggesting an allergy. The initial symptoms result from a narrowing of the blood vessels that supply the brain, followed by an expansion that produces the headache.

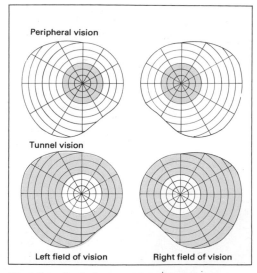

Peripheral vision

Tunnel vision

Left field of vision   Right field of vision

Migraine: shaded area of this diagram shows areas of defective vision.

Q: Does migraine last for life?

A: Usually migraine becomes less frequent with increasing age, and is relatively uncommon after the age of fifty. Some people, however, continue to suffer from migraine into old age.

Q: Can migraine occur in young children?

A: Yes. A child may not complain of a headache, but suffer from recurrent attacks of malaise accompanied by nausea and vomiting. The child may be able to describe the first symptoms of distorted vision and flashing lights, which can be extremely frightening if neither the child nor the parents understand what is happening.

Q: Can anything increase the likelihood of migraine?

A: Yes. Apart from certain foods that may cause migraine in some individuals, there are other factors that may bring on the symptoms. Many women experience a migraine a day or two before menstruation and the headache is associated with premenstrual tension. Some people develop a migraine when they are under emotional stress or after a period of stress, typically during the weekend. Some people find that particular wines can produce a migraine, probably because of a combination of alcohol and other wine ingredients.

Q: Why does alcohol cause migraine?

A: It is not known why alcohol causes migraine. But there is a particular kind of migraine, sometimes called a cluster headache, in which a one-sided headache is accompanied by a running nose and a sore, reddened eye on the affected side. Several attacks occur within a few days and then there is a prolonged period without headaches. This type of migraine is more common in middle-aged men and may be triggered by alcohol.

Q: How is migraine treated?

A: The usefulness of drugs is limited and many people learn to cope without them. Some migraine sufferers merely go to bed in a darkened room until the headache passes. Painkilling drugs, such as aspirin, are useful in relieving the headaches.

The drug ergotamine may be prescribed for acute attacks. It must be taken at once in the dosage prescribed. It works effectively if sucked, but it can also be given by injection, especially if nausea or vomiting is occurring.

Q: Can migraine be prevented?

A: If attacks occur frequently, treatment of premenstrual tension or anxiety and depression may produce an improvement.

If this does not work, a doctor may prescribe one of the drugs that can be effective in preventing migraine.

Migraine sufferers should learn to keep track of things and conditions that normally precede their attack. Steps can then be taken in the future to prevent similar attacks.

Miliaria is an intensely irritating, fine red rash on the body, especially round the waist, and in the bends of the knees and elbows. *See* PRICKLY HEAT.

Milk is the secretion from the female breast that feeds a newborn baby. Human breast milk contains the right balance of ingredients, such as water, organic substances, antibodies, enzymes, and mineral salts, for the infant's well-being, although human milk varies in quantities of nutritive ingredients week by week during lactation. An alternative is cow's milk, modified by processing. Untreated cow's milk should not be fed to babies.

See also LACTATION.

Milk of magnesia. *See* MAGNESIA, MILK OF.

Milk teeth are the first, temporary set of teeth to appear. They are also called deciduous teeth. The teeth are present, hidden in the jaws, in a newborn baby and they begin to grow through the gums by the end of the first year. A child has twenty milk teeth. *See* TEETH.

Milroy's disease is an inherited disorder in which there is an absence of lymph vessels in one part of the body, such as an arm or a leg. There is generalized swelling of the area that becomes worse in hot weather; when the limb is allowed to hang down unsupported; or, in women, before menstruation.

Treatment is to wear a tight stocking or bandage and to take precautions against skin infections, because any resultant scarring may be increased by the swelling. Operations to remove the swollen tissues are seldom successful.

See also LYMPHATIC SYSTEM.

Minamata disease is a form of MERCURY poisoning that first occurred in the late 1950s among the population of Minamata Bay, Japan, after eating fish contaminated by mercury compounds discharged into the bay by local industry. Symptoms included trembling, weakness, and anaemia, as well as mental disturbances. Death occurred in the severest cases.

Mineral oil (liquid paraffin) is a preparation of light petroleum oils sometimes used in medicine. The oil is used on the skin and as a lubricant for catheters (tubes passed into the body to inject or remove fluid) and surgical instruments. Taken internally, mineral oil acts as a laxative and is used in the treatment of chronic constipation.

Minerals are inorganic elements or compounds. Minerals in the diet are important to good health. Various elements are essential parts of body cells, including calcium, chlorine, copper, fluorine, iodine, iron, magnesium, manganese, phosphorus, potassium, and sodium. The chief mineral salts in the body are chlorides and phosphates. Some minerals are incorporated into body tissues, but others are excreted.

See also DIET.

Miotic is any substance that makes the pupil of the eye constrict. Pilocarpine and eserine are miotics.

Mirror writing is writing formed from right to left (instead of left to right) so that it appears normal when seen reflected in a mirror. Mirror writing commonly occurs in left-handed children who are attempting to write with their right hand. Learning problems can be avoided if the trait is recognized and help is obtained for the child.

See also LEARNING DISABILITIES.

Miscarriage is the spontaneous termination of pregnancy before the embryo or foetus can live independently. In medical terminology, miscarriage and ABORTION have the same meanings. The usual reason for a miscarriage is a defect in the embryo or foetus that prevents its natural development. This defect may be inherited, caused by injury to the mother, or the result of infectious illness. The first symptom of a threatened miscarriage in a pregnant woman is vaginal bleeding, and

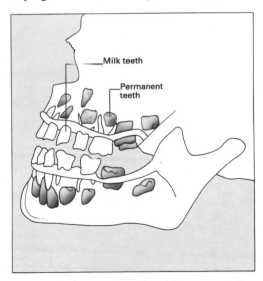

Milk teeth begin to be replaced by permanent teeth when a child is about five years old.

Mites

this requires immediate medical attention. A miscarriage is most likely to occur in the third or fourth month of pregnancy. Expulsion of a foetus from the womb after approximately the twenty-eighth week of pregnancy is known as a stillbirth if the foetus is dead, and as a premature birth if the foetus is alive.

See also ABORTION.

Mites are minute arachnids related to spiders. They belong to the animal order Acarina, which includes a great number of different species, and includes the ticks. Mites may exist on the skin or in the hair as parasites and can transmit disease.

See also RICKETTSIA; SCABIES; TICKS.

Mitral valve disease is a disorder of the heart caused by damage to the valve between the upper chamber (atrium) and the lower chamber (ventricle) on the left side of the heart. The opening in the valve may be narrower than normal (mitral stenosis) or wider than normal (mitral incompetence). Commonly these conditions result from scarring caused by RHEUMATIC FEVER, or, rarely, they may be present at birth.

Q: *What are the symptoms of mitral stenosis?*

A: The first symptoms are usually shortness of breath during exercise and, sometimes, episodes of breathlessness at night because the lungs become congested with blood. The symptoms begin gradually, because it takes many years for the scarring to take place. As scarring worsens, the symptoms become more severe so that acute breathlessness may occur on the slightest exertion, and there may be signs of heart failure because of

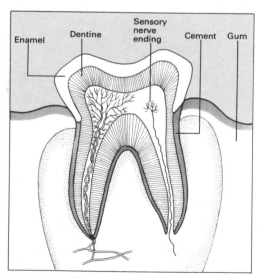

Molar is a large, deep-rooted tooth at the back of the jaw used for chewing and grinding.

back pressure of blood into the right side of the heart. Signs may include a bluish tinge to the lips (cyanosis) and swollen ankles.

Many patients develop a rapid irregular heartbeat called atrial FIBRILLATION. Sometimes the shortness of breath is accompanied by coughing attacks that may produce bloodstained sputum (haemoptysis).

Q: *What is the treatment for mitral stenosis?*

A: Initially, a doctor may prescribe diuretic drugs and digoxin to help to control the heart failure. If atrial fibrillation has recently occurred, beta-blocking drugs or a controlled electric shock (cardioversion) may restore normal heart rhythm.

Moderately severe or severe mitral stenosis may be treated by surgery. The valve can be enlarged by cutting the scarred tissue (valvotomy), or replaced with an artificial valve or one obtained from a pig's heart.

Q: *What are the symptoms of mitral incompetence and how is it treated?*

A: The symptoms are less severe than those of mitral stenosis, but increasing fatigue and shortness of breath commonly occur. Usually drug treatment with diuretics and digoxin is sufficient to control the symptoms. However, if this fails, the damaged valve can be replaced by surgery, as in mitral stenosis.

Molar is a broad tooth at the back of the mouth used for chewing and grinding. An adult has twelve molar teeth, with three upper and three lower molars on each side of the mouth. The back four molars are also known as wisdom teeth. *See* TEETH.

Mole is a coloured area or spot on the skin. Moles vary in size, may be flat or raised, and may have various shades of colour or pigmentation. Some are covered with hair.

Moles are formed from cells containing the dark pigment melanin. Some may be present at birth, although many develop during childhood or early adult life. A mole that is present at birth is usually called a birthmark.

Q: *Do moles require treatment?*

A: Treatment is not necessary unless the mole is disfiguring, for example, a large hairy mole on the face. Treatment may also be necessary if the mole is situated where clothing irritates it, such as around the waist, possibly resulting in infection and inflammation. Moles can usually be removed, under a local anaesthetic, by plastic surgery.

Q: *Can moles become cancerous?*

A: Yes, but this is extremely rare. A mole that changes in size, colour, or shape should be examined by a doctor. Bleeding moles may be malignant (cancerous), and they should be reported to a doctor at once.

See also MELANOMA.

Molluscum contagiosum is a virus skin infection that is often caught in swimming pools, or through sexual intercourse. Small, firm, pearly warts commonly occur in one region of the trunk, near the armpit or groin, and may spread elsewhere on the body. They usually disappear spontaneously after a few months, but a doctor may treat them by freezing, cautery, or applying a caustic.

Molluscum fibrosum. *See* VON RECKLINGHAUSEN'S DISEASE.

Mongolism. *See* DOWN'S SYNDROME.

Moniliasis, also called candidiasis and thrush, is an infection caused by the microorganism *Candida albicans,* a yeast fungus that is normally found in the intestine and on the skin. A change in environment, for any reason, can allow the microorganism to increase in number and cause the infection.

Q: What environments encourage moniliasis?

A: Antibiotic treatment for some other condition, such as bronchitis, kills many of the bacteria normally present on the skin and in the intestine. This allows the fungus to grow and cause moniliasis. Altered hormone levels in the body, such as those that occur during pregnancy and in women who take contraceptive pills, also make it easier for monilial fungi to grow. The infection may accompany other disorders, such as diabetes mellitus, leukaemia, or conditions that require treatment with corticosteroid drugs, all of which alter the body's immunity to monilia.

Q: Which parts of the body are affected by moniliasis?

A: Moniliasis mostly affects areas of the body that are moist and warm. In babies, the mouth is a common area for thrush, where moniliasis results in small white patches on a red, inflamed background. Similar conditions occur in the vagina, and this is a common area for the infection in women.

There are various areas on the skin that can commonly become infected. These are the groin, around the anus, beneath the breasts (particularly in heavily built women), and in folds of skin in people who are obese.

Moniliasis may occur as a form of nappy rash in babies when the buttocks are allowed to remain moist with urine.

Q: Can moniliasis occur elsewhere?

A: Yes. It may infect the nail folds, particularly in those whose hands are often in hot water, and this can form a kind of PARONYCHIA. Occasionally, moniliasis can invade the body to infect the lungs, the intestine, or the urinary tract; this occurs particularly in those who are seriously ill or who have undergone prolonged courses of powerful antibiotics.

Q: Can moniliasis be sexually transmitted?

A: Yes. Inflammation of the end of the penis (balanitis) may occur in uncircumcised men after intercourse with a woman with moniliasis. Both partners must be treated (*see* BALANITIS).

Q: How is moniliasis treated?

A: Skin infections are treated with fungicidal creams or lotions, and vaginal infections may be treated with pessaries. The rare internal forms of moniliasis have to be treated with potent fungicidal drugs, under the care of a doctor.

Q: Are there any serious complications with moniliasis?

A: Serious complications only arise when moniliasis invades the body, and these are rare. Commonly, however, moniliasis recurs after treatment. In this situation, it may be necessary to give fungicidal drugs by mouth to kill any excess of monilia in the intestine.

Monoamine oxidase inhibitors. *See* MAO INHIBITORS.

Monocyte is a type of white blood cell that has a single nucleus and a relatively large amount of surrounding cytoplasm. *See* WHITE BLOOD CELL.

Mononucleosis. *See* GLANDULAR FEVER.

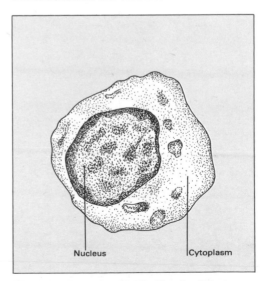

Monocyte is a type of white blood cell that contains a large nucleus and cytoplasm.

Monoplegia

Monoplegia is paralysis of one limb. *See* PARALYSIS.

Morbidity is the state of being ill. The term is also used to describe the proportion of sick people in a particular community.

Morbilli is a medical word for MEASLES.

Morning sickness affects about fifty per cent of women in early pregnancy. They experience nausea and vomiting, usually beginning about the sixth week of pregnancy and finishing by the twelfth week. A headache often occurs with morning sickness, and a feeling of dizziness and exhaustion. The symptoms usually occur in the morning, but may be present at any time during the day.

Q: What causes morning sickness?

A: Morning sickness probably results from an increased sensitivity of the vomiting centre in the brain, caused by the hormonal activity of early pregnancy. These hormones also have an effect on the gastrointestinal tract, so that the movement of faeces along the colon is slowed down. As a result, some food and gastric secretions remain in the stomach in the morning.

Q: How is morning sickness treated?

A: Many women find that nausea can be prevented by eating a few biscuits and drinking a glass of milk first thing in the morning. This is because the gastric secretions are absorbed by the food.

If this simple measure fails, a doctor may prescribe an antinausea drug to be taken before going to bed at night. B complex vitamins may also be prescribed.

Q: Can morning sickness ever be serious?

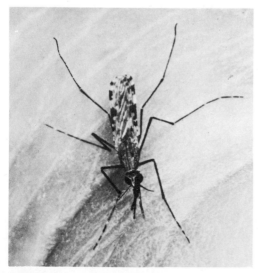

Mosquito can carry the infective organisms that cause malaria and yellow fever.

A: Yes. In a few women, vomiting and nausea occur so frequently that loss of weight occurs.

Rarely, a condition of excessive vomiting known as HYPEREMESIS gravidarum occurs. Continued vomiting produces dehydration, and the condition requires hospital treatment with intravenous infusions of glucose, antinauseant drugs, and sedation.

Morphine is an ALKALOID drug derived from the opium poppy. It is a powerful painkiller and cough suppressant. Morphine relieves anxiety as well as inducing contentment and even happiness in patients suffering from severe pain. It is also used in the treatment of acute heart failure and shock. Prolonged use of morphine can result in psychological and physical dependence.

Morphine is seldom prescribed in tablet form because, although it may be absorbed through the intestine, its action is slow and uncertain. Morphine is injected to produce a predictable result, and rapid action follows an intravenous injection. The drug is often prescribed for patients with terminal cancer.

Morphine should not be prescribed for the elderly or the very young, because they are particularly sensitive to the drug's effects. Nor should it be used in those who have lung disease, such as asthma, because of its depressant effect on breathing.

See also METHADONE; OPIATE.

Mosquito is a bloodsucking insect. It can carry parasites that cause diseases in human beings. There are many species of mosquitoes. Those of the Anopheles group carry MALARIA; the Aedes mosquito carries YELLOW FEVER and dengue fever, as well as viruses that cause encephalitis in some tropical countries; and the Culex mosquito carries a form of filaria that causes ELEPHANTIASIS.

Infections transmitted by mosquitoes can be prevented by spreading the breeding grounds of the mosquito with a thin film of oil; this prevents the larvae, which grow in water, from breathing. Insecticides sprayed at night and the use of mosquito nets over beds provide personal protection, and insect repellant creams may be effective during the day.

Motion sickness is nausea and vomiting caused by violent or repeated movement of the body. Motion sickness may be preceded by sweating, yawning, and fatigue. It is more common in children and often disappears with age as the organ of balance (the semicircular canals within the ear) becomes less sensitive to movement. Airsickness, carsickness, and seasickness are all examples of motion sickness. It may be caused by any form of transport, as well as by amusement rides at fairs or playgrounds.

Q: How can motion sickness be prevented?

A: A person who suffers from motion sickness should take antinausea drugs before starting any journey, but not if they are driving. During the journey, the person should lie with the head slightly raised, preferably in the part of the vehicle that experiences the least movement.

Small amounts of food and drink should be taken at regular intervals, but alcohol should be avoided.

Motor describes any body structure that is concerned with movement. For example, a motor nerve carries the "instructions" that make a muscle move.

Motor neuron disease is a group of similar disorders of unknown origin that cause degeneration of the nerve cells in the spinal cord or brain and affect muscle activity. There is increasing muscle weakness and wasting, usually beginning in the hands and feet and spreading to involve the shoulders and buttocks. It usually affects adults in late middle age.

The type of motor neuron disease called amyotrophic lateral sclerosis is usually fatal within three years, whereas progressive muscular atrophy may last for as long as twenty years. The condition known as progressive bulbar palsy affects the throat muscles and causes difficulty with talking, chewing, and swallowing. Death often occurs within a year or two from pneumonia.

There is no effective treatment for motor neuron disease, although physiotherapy may help to maintain mobility.

See also MUSCULAR DISORDERS.

Mountain sickness. *See* ALTITUDE SICKNESS.

Mouth is formed by the bone structure of the jaws. The upper part is formed by the upper jawbone (maxilla) and the lower part by the lower jawbone (mandible). The entrance to the mouth is surrounded by the skin and muscles that form the LIPS, and the interior contains the GUMS, PALATE, TEETH, and TONGUE. The MUCOUS MEMBRANE, the soft skin lining the mouth, is kept moist by the secretions of the SALIVARY GLANDS and heals rapidly if damaged.

See also CHEILITIS; CLEFT PALATE; DENTAL DISORDERS; GINGIVITIS; HARE LIP; LARYNGITIS; MOUTH ULCER; SORE THROAT; STOMATITIS; TONSILLITIS.

Mouth breathing is breathing through the mouth when the nose is blocked, perhaps as a result of an infection, such as a cold or an injury to the nose, such as a fracture. In children, mouth breathing is often caused by swollen ADENOIDS.

Mouth breathing may cause snoring and disturbed sleep. The mouth may also become dry, which increases the probability of gum infection. Treatment is not necessary to stop a person breathing through the mouth, if the cause is obvious. Normal breathing is resumed when the cause disappears.

Mouth-to-mouth resuscitation is a form of artificial respiration in which the victim's lungs are inflated with air breathed out by the rescuer. For details, *see* First aid, p.518.

Mouth ulcer is an open sore that affects the mucous membrane that lines the inside of the mouth. It is known medically as aphthous ulcer. It is possibly caused by a virus that normally lives in the body cells without causing symptoms. But in the presence of a disorder, such as a common cold, ulcers form. Throat drops and ointments may help mouth ulcers to heal. A doctor may prescribe tablets that can be sucked for rapid healing.

MS. *See* MULTIPLE SCLEROSIS.

Mucopurulent describes a discharge from the body that contains both mucus and pus. Such a discharge may occur as mucus from the nose, sputum from the lungs, or fluid from the anus in disorders that involve inflammation of the colon or rectum, such as ulcerative colitis and diverticular disease.

Mucous colitis, also called SPASTIC COLON and irritable bowel syndrome, is a recurrent intestinal disorder in which there are bouts of abdominal pain with diarrhoea or constipation in an apparently healthy person. There is an abnormality of the muscular action that passes food along the colon, and this causes the constipation or diarrhoea.

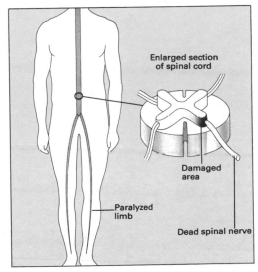

Enlarged section of spinal cord

Damaged area

Paralyzed limb

Dead spinal nerve

Motor neuron disease affecting the spinal nerves results in leg paralysis.

Mucous membrane

Q: *What causes mucous colitis?*

A: Mucous colitis may develop during emotional stress, such as studying for examinations, or anxieties associated with work or domestic problems. There is a tendency for it to occur in individuals who are obsessional, but it may also appear for no apparent reason. Sometimes a food allergy may be involved.

Q: *What are the symptoms of mucous colitis?*

A: The disorder first appears in young adults and it is variable, with long periods in which there are no symptoms. Abdominal pain may occur as a dull ache over one area of the colon or, occasionally, there may be intermittent colic that is relieved by a bowel movement. Sometimes there is constipation or a form of diarrhoea in which frequent small amounts of faeces with a thin tape-like or pellet-like appearance are passed. The faeces may be covered with mucus. Diarrhoea is often the principal symptom, usually occurring first thing in the morning or immediately after a meal. The rest of the day may be free from pain or diarrhoea. The person may feel tired and mildly depressed. Weight loss is unusual.

Q: *How is mucous colitis diagnosed and treated?*

A: A doctor makes a diagnosis after excluding other possibilities, such as gastroenteritis, ulcerative colitis, amoebic dysentery, or other intestinal disorders that cause abdominal pain and diarrhoea. If necessary, the doctor may arrange for faecal analysis, sigmoidoscopy, and a barium enema to make sure there is no underlying disease of the intestine.

Once the doctor has made the diagnosis, the patient can be reassured that there is no serious disorder. This reassurance combined with a diet containing additional bulk (such as bran or methyl cellulose) and the use of antispasmodic drugs usually produce an immediate improvement.

Mucous membrane is a thin layer of cells containing glands that secrete a sticky fluid called MUCUS. Mucous membranes line the internal passages and cavities of the body, such as the bladder, bronchial tubes, intestine, mouth, and vagina.

Mucus is a clear, slime-like fluid that is continually secreted by glands within any of the body's mucous membranes. Mucus acts as a protective lubricant barrier.

Multipara is the medical term for a woman who has had two or more pregnancies that lasted for more than twenty weeks. A grand multipara is a woman who has had six or more children.

Multiple sclerosis, or disseminated sclerosis, is a disorder of the brain and spinal cord in which scattered areas of damage to nerve cells occur. The nerve damage results in a great variety of symptoms, sometimes followed by recovery or marked improvement. Further damage may occur at irregular intervals over many years, causing increasing disability in some, but not all, patients.

The cause of multiple sclerosis is not known, but it may be associated with some kind of altered immunity to a virus infection.

Q: *What are the symptoms of multiple sclerosis?*

A: The first symptoms usually occur between the ages of twenty and forty and are slightly more frequent in women. The onset is usually gradual and may include slight, temporary weakness in one arm or leg; tingling or numbness in a limb or on one side of the face; double vision (diplopia) because of a weakness of an eye muscle; blurred vision (amblyopia); or frequently pain in one eye because of neuritis affecting the optic nerve (retrobulbar neuritis). Other symptoms that may occur at the same time or in later attacks include incontinence of urine; unsteady gait (ataxia); giddiness (vertigo); and sometimes emotional disturbance with sudden tears or laughter, depression, or cheerfulness.

As the disorder progresses, these symptoms recur along with various others that involve the nervous system. They tend to last longer and may not disappear

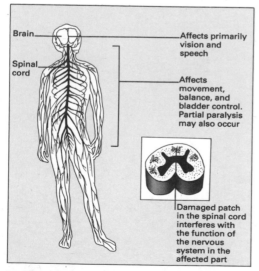

Brain — Affects primarily vision and speech

Spinal cord — Affects movement, balance, and bladder control. Partial paralysis may also occur

Damaged patch in the spinal cord interferes with the function of the nervous system in the affected part

Multiple sclerosis is slow damage of areas of nervous tissue causing progressive paralysis.

completely, so that the patient may be left with a limp, a hesitation in speech or a flickering movement of the eye.

Some patients are never disabled by their symptoms, but in others the symptoms may be severe enough to confine them to bed, and make them unable to walk or maintain bladder control. As the disorder progresses, recovery from each attack is less complete. The patient may be left with stiff limbs, often accompanied by intermittent, painful spasms of the muscles. Eventually, urinary or lung infections may occur, and one of these complications usually causes death.

Q: *What is the treatment for multiple sclerosis?*

A: There is no treatment for this·disorder. A few patients have a rapid, progressive disease with frequent relapses that lead to death within one or two years. Others may have only one or two minor problems followed by complete, spontaneous recovery without further trouble. Most patients, however, have recurring symptoms for fifteen to twenty-five years, and may then stabilize.

The diagnosis is made on the basis of a history of the recurrent attacks and a doctor's examination of the patient. Prompt administration of corticosteroid drugs may produce a rapid improvement in symptoms, but does not affect the progress of the disorder.

Physiotherapy, massage, and treatment of any infection all help to maintain reasonable health. It is important to keep up the morale of the patient.

Mumps, also called epidemic parotitis or infective parotitis, is a virus infection that causes painful inflammation and swelling of the salivary glands. Mumps is most common among children, but it may also affect adults.

Q: *How long is the incubation period and quarantine for mumps?*

A: The incubation period is between fourteen and twenty-five days; usually twenty-one days. Quarantine should last for twenty-eight days after the last contact. The disorder is infectious for about two days before the swelling appears and for three days after the swelling goes down or for a total of ten days, whichever is longer.

See also INFECTIOUS DISEASES.

Q: *What are the symptoms of mumps?*

A: There is usually an initial period of one to two days of headache, malaise, and fever. This stage is followed by a sudden rise in temperature to about 40°C (104°F),

which accompanies the onset of painful swelling of the salivary glands. The parotid glands in front of the ears are the glands most commonly involved in the early stage, but swelling may spread to the glands under the jaw. The swollen glands are tender to touch and may cause difficulty in opening the mouth. The extent of the swelling may vary from day to day. Only one side may be affected. The acute stage of the illness usually lasts five to six days, with a gradual reduction in the swelling as the patient improves.

Mumps in adults may cause inflammation of the pancreas; of the testicles in men, which may lead to sterility; or of the ovaries in women.

Q: *What is the treatment for mumps?*

A: There is no cure for mumps. Therapy is directed toward making the patient comfortable, reducing fever, and ensuring adequate fluid intake. Painkilling and sedative drugs may be prescribed.

Q: *Can mumps be prevented?*

A: Yes. A vaccine containing a mild, living virus is available and it may be used to immunize children at the age of twelve to fifteen months. It is not often recommended in the U.K. except for adults who have not had the disease. Occasionally, mumps vaccine produces a mild illness. It is thought that immunity lasts for life and the vaccine certainly protects about 95 per cent of children.

Münchausen's syndrome is a mental disorder in which the patient persuades doctors that he or she has a real physical disease when no

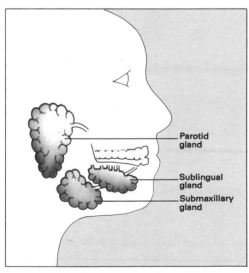

Mumps usually affects the parotid salivary glands but can cause other inflammation.

Murmur

disease is present. It can be regarded as an extreme form of malingering. The disorder is named after Baron Karl F. H. von Münchausen, who was known for his tall tales of courage and skill on the battlefield, none of which were true.

Patients with Münchausen's syndrome are skilled at mimicking the physical signs and symptoms of a disorder, such as myocardial infarction, appendicitis, and cerebral tumour. Such pretended complaints may lead to hospital admission, multiple tests, and even surgical operations to try to determine the cause of the "disorder." Despite having a definite desire for medical treatment, the patient may be unaware of his or her underlying need for sympathy and care.

Murmur. *See* HEART MURMUR.

Muscle is a tissue composed of fibres that can contract and relax to produce movement in a part of the body. There are three kinds of muscles: striated, smooth, and cardiac.

Disorders that can affect muscles or are associated with muscular disorders include: CUSHING'S SYNDROME; FRIEDREICH'S ATAXIA; HYPERTHYROIDISM (THYROTOXICOSIS); HYPOTHYROIDISM; LUPUS ERYTHEMATOSUS; MUSCULAR DYSTROPHY; MYALGIA; MYASTHENIA GRAVIS; MYOCARDITIS; MYOSITIS; MYOTONIA CONGENITA; and TETANY.

Muscle relaxants are drugs of two main types, those that relax muscles and those that relieve painful muscle spasms.

Drugs of the first type are used in general anaesthesia to produce complete relaxation of the muscles before surgery, and may be short-acting or long-acting. Drugs of the

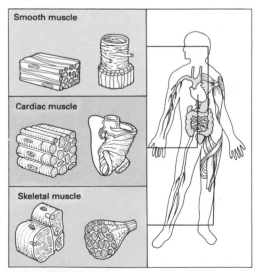

Muscle may be smooth (involuntary); specialized (cardiac); or striped (skeletal).

second type are used to relieve the muscle spasms that sometimes occur in spastic conditions, such as those following a stroke, or in some muscle and rheumatic disorders.

Muscular dystrophy is the name of a group of progressive disorders the symptoms of which include weakness and gradual wasting away of muscles. There are various classifications of these disorders, but the terms most usually applied to the three main types are: pseudohypertrophic muscular dystrophy, facioscapulohumeral muscular dystrophy, and limb-girdle muscular dystrophy.

There is no specific treatment but physiotherapy can help in the slowly progressive forms of muscular dystrophy. Corrective surgery can also be considered as treatment for the slowly progressive forms.

Mutation is a sudden change in some characteristic. In genetics, mutation describes a permanent change in one of the genes of a chromosome (*see* HEREDITY).

Mute describes someone who is unable to speak. A person may lose the power of speech following a stroke (the condition called aphasia) or disease or injury to the vocal cords.

See also DEAFNESS.

Myalgia is pain in a muscle. Such pain may occur after excessive physical exercise. Myalgia may also develop during any acute virus illness and is an indication of mild inflammation of the muscles (myositis). It is frequently associated with inflammation of fibrous tissue (fibrositis).

The pain is usually made worse by movement and the muscles are frequently tender. Treatment with mild painkilling drugs and the application of heat is usually effective.

See also RHEUMATIC DISEASES.

Myasthenia gravis is a disorder that affects the nerve impulses that control the movement of muscles. It is a form of AUTOIMMUNE DISEASE. The muscles become weak, although temporary recovery slowly takes place if affected muscles are rested.

Q: What are the symptoms of myasthenia gravis?

A: The onset is often sudden, producing a drooping eyelid (ptosis) and double vision (diplopia) because of weakened eye muscles. These symptoms may be accompanied by difficulty in swallowing or speaking. Weakness of a limb may occur, particularly after the limb has been exercised. On some days the symptoms may not be noticeable, whereas on others they may become severe. Occasionally, the muscles involved in breathing become affected, producing the risk of asphyxiation.

Q: How is myasthenia gravis diagnosed and treated?

A: A doctor may suspect the presence of myasthenia gravis and the diagnosis can be confirmed by the improvement that takes place after use of a drug that helps to improve nerve transmission to the muscles. In many patients the surgical removal of the thymus gland is curative (*see* THYMUS).

Some patients improve naturally, and in these no treatment is required.

Mycetoma is a chronic fungal infection that produces festering swellings, often on the feet. *See* ACTINOMYCOSIS; MADURA FOOT.

Mycobacteria are a group of microorganisms, two of which cause leprosy and tuberculosis. *See also* BCG.

Mycosis is any infection caused by a fungus, such as actinomycosis and blastomycosis.

Mydriatic is any substance that makes the pupil of the eye dilate.

Myelin is a fatty substance that forms a sheath around many of the body's nerves.

Myelocele is an opening in the lowest part of the spine that exposes the underlying spinal cord. Myelocele is the most serious form of spina bifida. *See* SPINA BIFIDA.

Myelogram is an X-ray of the spinal cord. It is used in the diagnosis of spinal tumours, slipped discs, and other spinal problems.

Myeloid leukaemia. *See* LEUKAEMIA.

Myeloma is a malignant (cancerous) tumour of the bone marrow. The tumour usually occurs first in one bone, but soon spreads to many other bones (multiple myelomatosis). The bones of the skull, ribs, spine, and pelvis are usually involved, although myelomas may occur in any bone. Myelomatosis is most common in the elderly.

Q: What are the symptoms of myelomatosis?

A: Backache or pain in the affected bone is a common symptom, although fatigue and shortness of breath caused by anaemia may be noticed first. The patient's resistance to infection is lowered, allowing chest and urinary infections to develop. The tumours weaken the bones, and fractures commonly occur.

Q: How is myelomatosis diagnosed and treated?

A: Many patients with myelomatosis produce an abnormal type of gamma globulin (Bence Jones protein) that can be detected in the urine. The presence of this protein, anaemia, and a high ESR (red blood cell sedimentation rate) all suggest multiple myeloma. The diagnosis can be confirmed by a bone marrow biopsy, in which a sample of bone marrow is examined using a microscope.

Treatment with chemotherapy, corticosteroids, and radiotherapy may greatly prolong the patient's life, but the disease is eventually fatal. Treatment of secondary infection with antibiotics and blood transfusion for severe anaemia improve the patient's general health and vitality.

Myocarditis is inflammation of the heart muscle. The symptoms are often vague and mild at first. Fatigue, shortness of breath, and sometimes palpitations (rapid, irregular heart beat) occur. Heart failure may develop and sometimes blood clots in the heart. The clots (emboli) may travel in the blood circulation to other parts of the body and cause strokes or sudden obstruction of an artery to a limb, resulting in gangrene.

Q: What causes myocarditis?

A: Various infections can affect the heart muscle, either because of the infection or the toxins that it produces, such as those from diphtheria. Many other conditions, such as disseminated lupus erythematosus, and rheumatic fever, can also involve the heart.

Various chemicals and some drugs, particularly those used in the treatment of cancer, can damage the heart muscle. Care must also be taken during radiotherapy of lung cancer to insure that the heart does not become inflamed.

Q: How is myocarditis diagnosed and treated?

A: A doctor makes an initial diagnosis from the symptoms and confirms it with an electrocardiogram (ECG) and other

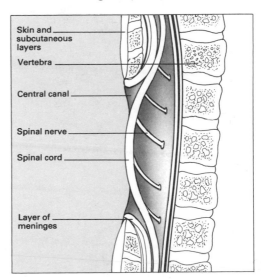

Skin and subcutaneous layers

Vertebra

Central canal

Spinal nerve

Spinal cord

Layer of meninges

Myelocele is a condition in which the spinal cord protudes through the vertebrae.

321

heart investigations. Treatment is directed at the cause, once it has been discovered. The patient must have complete rest, oxygen if necessary, and corticosteroid drugs.

Myoclonus is a brief spasm of muscular contraction that may involve a group of muscles, a single muscle, or even only a number of muscle fibres. Often the contractions occur rhythmically, producing a regular twitching of the affected muscle. If myoclonus involves several muscles, it may be sufficiently violent to cause the person to fall over. The treatment depends on the cause, but there is a variety of antispasmodic drugs that may help to reduce the likelihood of myoclonus.

Myoma is a muscle tumour. Most myomas are benign (noncancerous), although a few may become malignant (cancerous).

Myopathy is any muscular disorder that results in weakness and degeneration of the muscle tissue that is not caused by a defect in the nervous system. The muscular dystrophies are classified as myopathic disorders. *See* MUSCULAR DYSTROPHY.

Myopia is the medical term for shortsightedness. *See* SHORTSIGHTEDNESS.

Myositis is inflammation of the muscles. It may be caused by injury, infection, exposure to cold, or parasitic infestation.

Myotonia congenita is a rare, inherited muscular disorder in which muscles relax slowly after contraction. This causes stiff movements; for example, difficulty in relaxing the grip after shaking hands. The throat muscles may be affected, causing difficulty in speaking or swallowing. There is no cure, but drug treatment can control the disorder.

Myringotomy is surgical perforation of the eardrum, usually performed under a general anaesthetic. This is done for acute otitis media or when the middle ear is filled with thick mucus (glue ear). This may occur following antibiotic treatment for otitis media, and may cause deafness.
See also MASTOIDITIS.

Myxoedema. *See* HYPOTHYROIDISM.

Myxovirus is a family of viruses that includes those that cause mumps and influenza.

N

Naevus. *See* BIRTHMARK.

Nail is the hard semitransparent tissue that covers the upper surfaces of the fingers and toes. It is also the medical term for a metal rod used in orthopaedic surgery to stabilize a fracture.

Fingernails and toenails are dead tissue, without nerves or blood supply. They are a modification of skin, and they grow from a groove that is overlapped by a fold of the skin, the nailfold. The semicircular paler area near the base of the nail is called the lunula. The thin outer layer of skin adjacent to the nail is known as the cuticle.

Fingernails grow at an average rate of about one fiftieth of an inch (0.5mm) per week; toenails grow at about a fourth of this rate. The rate of growth may be altered by the season of the year, any acute illness, or damage to the nail bed.

Q: What conditions affect the nails?

A: Bitten fingernails are commonly a sign of anxiety. Ridging or grooving on the nails is evidence of altered growth because of illness or damage to the nail bed. The nail bed may become infected with tinea or monilia (both fungal diseases), causing deformity of the nail with discoloration and splitting. The nails of psoriasis patients are frequently pitted and often split easily. A similar condition may be seen in patients with rheumatoid arthritis. Nails can also be affected by certain hormone deficiencies.
See also CLUBBING; INGROWING NAIL; KOILONYCHIA; PARONYCHIA.

Nappy rash is inflammation of a baby's skin in the area covered by the nappy. The red inflamed area round the buttocks and genitalia may ooze and crust. Nappy rash is usually caused by faecal bacteria reacting with the urine to produce ammonia. The longer a baby lies in a wet, dirty nappy the stronger the ammonia becomes. The rash may be aggravated by the nappy's moisture, monilial infection and also the chemical effect of any detergents or soaps left in a nappy that has not been properly rinsed after washing. Nappies may be kept free from bacteria by soaking them in a sterilizing solution or boiling them.

Q: What is the treatment for nappy rash?

A: Frequent changing of the nappy is essential. Exposure to the air without any covering is the surest way to heal the skin. The urine in the nappy must be able to evaporate, so plastic pants should not be worn until the rash has disappeared. Various soothing applications, such as calamine lotion, zinc compound cream, or petroleum jelly, are effective, and should be applied frequently after careful washing of the inflamed area. If the area becomes infected, a doctor may prescribe antibiotic or antifungal creams.
See also BABY CARE.

Narcoanalysis is a form of psychotherapy in which a patient is questioned while under the influence of sedative or hypnotic drugs that help to reduce the patient's conscious and unconscious resistance to questioning.

Narcolepsy is a syndrome characterized by recurrent and overpowering attacks of sleep at unexpected or inappropriate moments. It usually happens after a sudden burst of emotion, but may also occur without warning, or after the psychic or sensory awareness of an impending attack (the aura). The sleep pattern is shallow, and the normal need for sleep is not disturbed. Narcoleptic people sometimes also suffer from cataplexy, an emotional seizure that causes the victim to fall to the floor without losing consciousness.

Narcotics, or more correctly narcotic analgesics, is a term that refers to the naturally occurring opiates morphine and codeine; derivatives of these substances; and totally synthetic compounds that produce effects similar to morphine and codeine. The term narcotics, when properly used, does not include sedatives or hypnotics such as the barbiturates.

See also DRUG ADDICTION; DRUGS.

Nares is the medical name for the nostrils, the external openings of the nose.

Nasal describes anything pertaining to the nose.

Nasopharynx is the small space, above the soft palate at the back of the roof of the mouth, that connects the nasal cavities with the throat. Also known as the postnasal space, it contains the ADENOIDS and the openings of the two Eustachian or auditory tubes that lead to the ears. The nasopharynx is closed during swallowing by the muscles of the soft palate.

Natural childbirth is a term that describes several methods of childbirth in which the mother actively co-operates and consciously enjoys the birth and delivery of her baby. Natural childbirth reduces, and occasionally makes it possible to avoid altogether, the need for painkilling drugs or anaesthesia and makes the delivery a more natural event.

There are many myths about childbirth that can produce anxiety in a woman when she discovers that she is pregnant. Her whole attitude to pregnancy may be modified by increasing fears based on these myths.

Q: *How can these anxieties about labour be changed?*

A: Antenatal classes explain what is happening at the various stages of pregnancy and exactly what happens during labour. It is explained that the hard effort that is necessary during labour is similar to that needed for any athletic

sport, a mixture of physical and psychological stress. The basis of the instruction in the classes is to teach the woman how to help herself and her attendants during labour.

Q: *In what ways can a woman help during labour?*

A: Muscular tension can be lessened by special exercises, such as breathing in a manner that relaxes. In the first stage of labour, before the neck of the womb is open, breathing during contractions should be a series of deep breaths that become rapid and more shallow as the pains increase, and return to slower, deeper breathing as the pains lessen. This difficult stage, which is often lengthy and tiring for the mother, can be made easier by applying gentle pressure to the area over the sacrum bone. Such pressure shifts the weight of the body from the spinal column to the pelvis.

In the second stage of labour, when the foetus is being expelled from the womb and down through the pelvis, the breathing pattern is different. Rapid, short puffing breaths are taken and then the breath is held for a few moments while the mother pushes down with her abdominal muscles during contraction.

The obstetrician indicates when to "push," and this pattern of puffing and pushing alternates until the baby is expelled from the birth canal. During this second stage, if the father is present, he can help by supporting the mother's back with his arm and holding her legs bent.

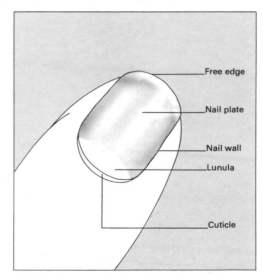

Free edge

Nail plate

Nail wall

Lunula

Cuticle

Nail injuries, especially to the nail wall or to the cuticle, can be extremely painful.

Naturopathy

The third stage of labour is the expulsion of the placenta. This is not a lengthy process and the woman should be asked to give a further push or cough as the placenta is expelled.

Q: What are some methods of natural childbirth?

A: There are many different methods of natural childbirth, often called after the doctor who first advocated the particular regimen. Examples are the Leboseyer, Lemaze, and Dick-Read methods.

Whatever method is taught, it is essential for the woman to realize that everything is being done to help her and that some labours are much more difficult than others, even when perfectly normal. Many women do need painkilling drugs, but this is not a sign of failure on the part of the mother or of the method. Other problems may arise so that the obstetrician may use forceps, vacuum extraction, or perform a Caesarean section.

Q: Can all women be helped by learning one of the methods of natural childbirth?

A: Unfortunately not. Some women find it impossible to overcome their fears about labour and are not helped by antenatal classes that teach natural childbirth methods.

See also PREGNANCY AND CHILDBIRTH.

Naturopathy is an alternative method of treatment using diet, herbal medicines, and physical treatments such as hydrotherapy and exercise. Conventional drugs are not used.

Naturopathy has a long history and has recently been enjoying a revival. But nature cures are considered to be outside the sphere of normal medical practice. Naturopathists believe that nature treatments are the only way to deal with disease.

Q: What sort of remedies do naturopathic practitioners use?

A: Herbal remedies are common, and many can be effective. Most aperients (senna, cascara, and other vegetable laxatives) are of herbal origin. Digitalis and quinidine, which are derived from plants, are used in orthodox medicine to treat heart conditions; peppermint may be prescribed for digestive disorders; and extracts of the poppy (opium and morphine) are commonly prescribed by doctors as painkillers. Other herbal remedies are still being discovered or reintroduced into medical practice as the basis for their action becomes understood. Naturopathic practitioners have used many of them for centuries.

Q: What other forms of treatment are used in naturopathy?

A: Faith healing is used by some naturopathic practitioners, and, it would seem, healing can take place whether the patient believes in it or not. Many patients have reported remarkable improvements, but the benefits of natural healing have not yet been scientifically proven.

Nausea is the sensation of feeling sick in the stomach. Many conditions can cause nausea, which is a preliminary symptom before vomiting. Nausea may also accompany any sudden shock, either from a physical cause, such as an accident, or emotional shock, such as revulsion on seeing something unpleasant.

Q: What physical conditions cause nausea?

A: Any digestive disorder, particularly acute or chronic gastritis, may be accompanied by nausea. Probably the most common cause is eating too much rich, fatty food, or drinking too much alcohol, particularly on an empty stomach. Nausea may precede vomiting in MOTION SICKNESS and is a frequent symptom of early pregnancy (*see* MORNING SICKNESS).

Q: How is nausea treated?

A: The treatment of nausea depends on the cause. A severely nauseated person may be more comfortable lying down in a quiet place, possibly with head and shoulders raised. Anyone with persistent nausea should consult a doctor.

Navel. *See* UMBILICUS.

Nearsightedness. *See* SHORTSIGHTEDNESS.

Neck is any narrow region between two parts of an organ or body, although the term usu-

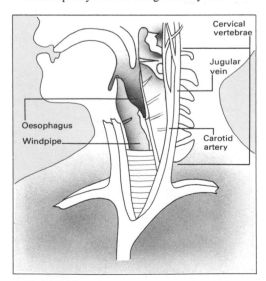

Neck contains many arteries, veins, nerves, and muscles supported by cervical vertebrae.

Cervical vertebrae

Jugular vein

Oesophagus

Windpipe

Carotid artery

ally applies to the part of the body between the shoulders and the head.

The neck is a flexible structure that supports the head and contains major blood vessels and separate tubes for air and food. The seven bones in the neck, called cervical vertebrae, form the upper part of the spine. The two top cervical vertebrae, the atlas and axis, are pivoted to allow rotation of the head.

Strong muscles on each side of the spine partly protect the structures in the front part of the neck. These structures include the oesophagus, the trachea (windpipe), and the larynx (voice box). The carotid arteries and jugular veins in the neck carry blood to and from the head and brain. There is also a series of lymph glands that guard against the entry of infection from the throat. The salivary parotid glands, below the ears and adjacent to the jaw, produce saliva. The thyroid gland, just below the larynx in front of the trachea, produces hormones that control the body's metabolism.

See also SLIPPED DISC; STIFF NECK.

Necrosis is the death of a small area of tissue within an organ. It may occur as a result of an accident, such as a burn, or of a disease, such as tuberculosis. Necrosis often follows obstruction of an artery that supplies a particular area of tissue, as in GANGRENE.

Neisseria is a group of bacteria that includes the organisms that cause GONORRHOEA and one of the common forms of bacterial MENINGITIS.

Nematode is a type of parasitic roundworm. *See* WORMS.

Neonatal describes any event occurring in the first four weeks after birth. *See* ANTENATAL.

Neoplasm is the medical name for any new growth, but in common usage it frequently refers to a tumour. Doctors distinguish between malignant (cancerous) neoplasms and benign (noncancerous) neoplasms.

See also CANCER.

Nephrectomy is an operation to remove a diseased kidney. A partial nephrectomy is performed when only part of the kidney is diseased.

A nephrectomy may be necessary if there is a kidney tumour such as HYPERNEPHROMA; if the kidney is severely damaged by disease, for example, HYDRONEPHROSIS, or a CALCULUS (stone); or following an accident in which the kidney is badly damaged. Recovery from the operation is quick, and the remaining kidney increases in size to cope with the increased demands on it.

Nephritis is a general term for any inflammation or infection of the kidney. The condition may involve the kidney's filtration unit (glomerulus) producing GLOMERULONEPHRITIS.

Or nephritis may involve the tubules within the kidney, causing problems in reabsorption of water and salts (interstitial nephritis). Inflammation affecting the drainage area of the kidney, with damage to the kidney pelvis and surrounding tissue, leads to PYELO-NEPHRITIS.

Disease of the kidney tissue may be an allergic reaction, or may be caused by blood vessel disorders, or the result of high blood pressure (hypertension). Certain drugs may also damage the kidneys. Kidney damage may follow a rise in the level of calcium in the blood associated with parathyroid gland disorders or other disorders, including gout. Damage can also be caused by poisoning with lead or by radiation.

See also NEPHROTIC SYNDROME; PYELITIS; URAEMIA.

Nephrolithiasis is the formation of stones (calculi) in the kidney.

Q: Why do kidney stones form?

A: Stones may form if there is obstruction of the normal urine flow, as in HYDRONEPH-ROSIS. They may result from an excess of certain chemicals in the bloodstream, such as uric acid in gout and calcium in parathyroid gland disorders.

Q: What are kidney stones made of?

A: There are three common forms of stones: those formed from uric acid; those that are calcium oxalate; and mixed stones composed of calcium, magnesium, and ammonium phosphates. *See* CALCULUS.

Q: What are the symptoms of nephrolithiasis?

A: Often there are no symptoms until the stone moves from its usual position.

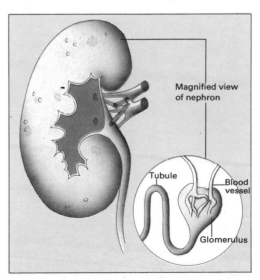

Magnified view of nephron

Tubule

Blood vessel

Glomerulus

Nephritis may affect the nephrons or other parts of the kidney, such as the pelvis.

Nephrosis

Rarely, large stones can form in the kidney (staghorn calculi), causing kidney damage without any obvious symptoms.

When a stone moves from the pelvis of the kidney into the ureter (the tube that carries urine to the bladder), there are severe spasms (renal colic) of pain from the lower back to the groin, with vomiting and sweating. There may also be blood in the urine (haematuria).

Q: *How is nephrolithiasis diagnosed and treated?*

A: A history of pain and haematuria suggests a stone, and its presence can usually be detected by an X-ray. An INTRAVENOUS PYELOGRAM (IVP) reveals where the stone is causing an obstruction.

A small stone may eventually pass down the ureter and out through the bladder. But large stones either remain in the kidney (and may have to be removed surgically) or become stuck in the ureter. A special instrument can be used to extract the stones stuck in the ureter during CYSTOSCOPY (an examination of the bladder). If this measure fails, surgery has to be done to remove the stone.

An acute attack of pain requires urgent treatment with strong painkilling and antispasm drugs prescribed by a doctor. Large quantities of fluid should be drunk, because this helps to make the stone pass down the ureter. All the urine that is passed must be filtered through a fine cloth so that the stone can be seen. It is usual to have an X-ray a few weeks later to make certain that a second stone has not stuck in the ureter.

Q: *Apart from pain, what are the dangers of kidney stones?*

A: The stone may obstruct urine flow and cause hydronephrosis or frequent attacks of PYELONEPHRITIS (inflammation of kidney substance).

Q: *Why do some people develop stones more easily than others?*

A: Apart from the reasons already mentioned, stones may develop from drinking water with a high concentration of salts. Stones more commonly occur in hot climates as the urine is more concentrated. It is necessary for people to drink plenty of fluid in tropical countries.

Nephrosis is any disorder of the kidney that is caused by degeneration and not by inflammation, for example, HYDRONEPHROSIS (obstructed outflow) and the NEPHROTIC SYNDROME (degenerative kidney change). It may also occur with AMYLOIDOSIS and some forms of poisoning.

Nephrostomy is an operation to drain urine from the pelvis of the kidney, usually performed because the ureter is blocked by a stone or a tumour.

Nephrotic syndrome is a kidney disorder in which too much protein is excreted in the urine. This results in decreased protein in the blood, OEDEMA (swelling of the body tissues), and disturbances of body fats. In rare cases the disorder may be present at birth or occur spontaneously in early childhood.

Q: *What are the symptoms of nephrotic syndrome?*

A: Symptoms include fatigue, weakness, and loss of appetite. A physical examination by a doctor may reveal a sudden or slow accumulation of fluid in the body tissues.

Q: *What causes nephrotic syndrome?*

A: Acute or chronic GLOMERULONEPHRITIS may result in the disorder. Also, any abnormality that causes an increase in the back pressure of blood in the veins leaving the kidney produces congestion in the kidney tissue. This can happen in heart failure or following a thrombosis in the renal vein.

Nephrotic syndrome may be a result of some systemic disease such as POLYARTERITIS NODOSA, AMYLOIDOSIS, DIABETES MELLITUS, MALARIA, or MYELOMA (bone marrow tumour). It may also be caused by an allergic reaction to drug treatment (*see* SERUM SICKNESS). The cause of the most common form of nephrotic syndrome in children is not known.

Q: *What is the treatment for nephrotic syndrome?*

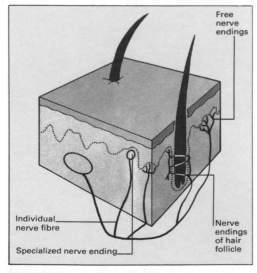

Free nerve endings

Individual nerve fibre

Specialized nerve ending

Nerve endings of hair follicle

Nerve is a number of fibres bundled together that carries electrical impulses.

A: Nephrotic syndrome requires careful and skilled attention from a specialist in kidney disease, with repeated tests to assess the effect of treatment. The more serious causes make treatment difficult, and the outcome is more likely to be fatal. Corticosteroid drugs are particularly useful for treating children and chemotherapy is sometimes effective. DIURETIC drugs to increase urine flow reduce the swelling of oedema.

Nephrotomy is a surgical operation to cut into kidney tissue. It is sometimes performed as part of the treatment for a kidney stone (NEPHROLITHIASIS).

Nerve is a part of the body's "communications system," which carries messages between the brain and spinal cord and various other parts of the body. It consists of bundles of nerve fibres covered with a sheath of connective tissue and sometimes by a layer of fatty cells (myelin). Nervous impulses are transmitted by a weak electrical current that results from chemical changes taking place through the nerve wall. The final transmission, from one nerve to another or from a nerve to another structure, is carried out by a chemical reaction.

Sensory nerves collect information from the body and transmit it in the form of electrical impulses to the central nervous system for action. Other nerves pick up the impulses at nerve junctions (synapses) and trigger appropriate responses. For example, specialized nerve endings in the skin may detect a sensation such as cold, and pass the information to the brain. The brain may cause other nerves to stimulate shivering.

Motor nerves cause movement through the action of muscles. A reaction to intense heat, for example, causes the brain to stimulate motor nerves that cause the part of the body to be jerked away from the source of heat.

The main nerves are named according to the region from which they branch off. There are twelve pairs of cranial nerves, and thirty-one pairs of spinal nerves. The spinal nerves consist of eight pairs of cervical nerves, twelve pairs of thoracic nerves, five pairs of lumbar nerves, five pairs of sacral nerves, and one pair of coccygeal nerves.

See also AUTONOMIC NERVOUS SYSTEM; NERVOUS SYSTEM.

Nervous breakdown is a nonmedical term for any form of incapacitating mental illness. *See* MENTAL ILLNESS.

Nervous diseases. *See* MENTAL ILLNESS; NEUROLOGICAL DISORDERS.

Nervous system is a network of millions of interconnected nerve cells (neurons) that receive stimuli, co-ordinate this sensory information, and cause the body to respond appropriately. The individual nerve cells transmit messages by means of a complicated electrochemical process.

The nervous system is comprised of two main divisions: the central nervous system (CNS), which consists of the BRAIN and the SPINAL CORD; and the peripheral nervous system (PNS), which consists of spinal nerves and cranial nerves. These nerves link the CNS with the body's receptors and effectors.

Q: What are receptors and effectors?

A: The receptors include the various sensory cells and sense organs, whose function is to respond to various types of stimulation. For example, eyes respond to light, and ears respond to sound.

The effectors are all of the parts of the body, such as muscles and glands, that respond to instructions from the CNS.

Q: What are the functions of the CNS?

A: The CNS integrates the information from the PNS and sends instructions to various parts of the body so that appropriate responses are made to continually changing conditions. The brain is also involved in the processes of thinking, learning, memory, and intelligence.

Q: What are the functions of the PNS?

A: The PNS signals changes in the environment, as registered by the receptors, to the CNS. The instructions from the CNS to different parts of the body are also carried by the PNS.

Anatomically, the autonomic nervous system (ANS) is part of the PNS. However, in terms of function, the ANS

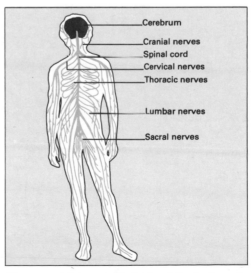

Nervous system runs throughout the body and relays information to the brain.

Nettle rash

can be considered as a separate system. The ANS is concerned with controlling the body's involuntary activities, such as the beating of the heart, intestinal movements, and sweating. The actions of the ANS can be modified by the CNS, but it also has a degree of independence.

Nettle rash. *See* HIVES.

Neuralgia is any form of pain along a nerve. Pressure on a nerve, such as from a slipped disc in the neck, may produce continuous pain in the shoulders and arms. Neuralgia may also occur as a result of inflammation, as may occur in shingles (herpes zoster). The pain may persist in the trunk area after the attack because of scarring around the nerve endings. This condition is known as postherpetic neuralgia.

Another type of neuralgia is known as metatarsalgia, in which the bones in the foot press on a nerve. Trigeminal neuralgia is a rare and acute form involving severe spasms of pain in the nerve endings of the face (*see* TRIGEMINAL NEURALGIA).

Q: How is neuralgia treated?

A: Treatment is directed at finding the cause, which may be difficult because some causes are not well understood. Painkilling and muscle relaxant drugs frequently give relief until the cause can be identified and treated. If drugs are not effective, some types of neuralgia may be treated surgically.

Neurasthenia is a term, no longer in use, that describes a condition in which a person complains of lack of energy, loss of appetite, and, frequently, loss of weight; it is often

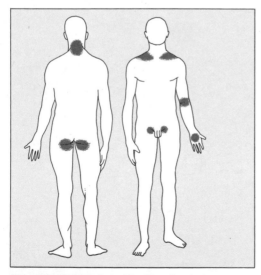

Neurodermatitis is a skin disorder that most commonly affects the sites shown.

accompanied by insomnia, fatigue, and a feeling of inadequacy. These are usually symptoms of DEPRESSION, but they may signal the onset of any chronic illness. The symptoms may have an underlying physical cause, and a doctor should be consulted. The doctor may suggest psychotherapeutic help.

Neuritis is inflammation of a nerve. If neuritis affects many nerves, the condition is called polyneuritis. *See* POLYNEURITIS.

Neurofibroma is the swelling of a peripheral nerve, caused by a thickening of the nerve sheath or connective tissue. If a neurofibroma occurs in soft tissue, such as that of the mouth or stomach, there may be only slight symptoms. But neurofibromas that develop on nerves leaving the skull or spine, or on nerves adjacent to bones, may cause loss of sensation or paralysis as a result of pressure on the nerve. *See* VON RECKLINGHAUSEN'S DISEASE.

Neurofibromatosis is a disorder in which pigmented areas form on the skin. It is associated with multiple neurofibromas. *See* NEUROFIBROMA; VON RECKLINGHAUSEN'S DISEASE.

Neurodermatitis is a skin disorder in which recurrent irritation occurs for no obvious reason. It causes an intense desire to scratch, resulting in inflammation and possibly infection. Continued scratching may lead to local thickening of the skin, which may develop a brownish pigmentation.

Q: What causes neurodermatitis?

A: An allergy, eczema, and congenital dry and scaly skin may be contributory factors. But anxiety, mental tension, and emotional disturbances are probably the main causes. The condition is more common in women than in men and in families with a history of allergy. Before diagnosing neurodermatitis, a doctor makes sure that there are no other skin conditions such as scabies, lichen planus, or local vaginal or anal infections that may produce irritation in those areas.

Q: How is neurodermatitis treated?

A: Corticosteroid creams usually give relief and an antipruritic drug may be prescribed to combat itching.

Neuroglia is the connective or supporting tissue between nerve cells within the central nervous system of the brain and spinal cord.

Neurological disorders. There are many disorders that affect the nervous system. The brain is concerned with both physical control of the body and with mental activities, such as reasoning. For disorders of mental activity, *see* MENTAL ILLNESS.

The following table lists some disorders of

the nervous system according to the structures involved. Each disorder has a separate article in the A-Z section of this book.

Structure	Disorder
Meninges (membranes surrounding the brain and spinal cord)	MENINGIOMA (a tumour of the meninges) MENINGITIS (inflammation of the meninges) SPINA BIFIDA (a congenital defect of the spinal canal)
Central nervous system (brain and spinal cord)	ALZHEIMER'S DISEASE (presenile dementia) BRAIN DISORDERS CEREBRAL HAEMATOMA ENCEPHALITIS (inflammation of the brain) ENCEPHALITIS LETHARGICA (epidemic encephalitis) EPILEPSY EXTRADURAL HAEMORRHAGE (external bleeding around the brain) GLIOMA (tumour of supporting cells of the brain) HYDROCEPHALUS (build-up of fluid within the brain) KORSAKOFF'S SYNDROME (generalized brain dysfunction) MICROCEPHALY (incomplete brain development) MIGRAINE MOTOR NEURON DISEASE (degeneration of brain cells) POLIOMYELITIS STROKE SUBARACHNOID HAEMORRHAGE (bleeding around the meninges) SYRINGOMYELIA (cavity formation in spinal cord) TABES DORSALIS (brain dysfunction due to syphilis)
Peripheral nervous system	BELL'S PALSY (facial paralysis) NEUROFIBROMA (a tumour of the connective tissue of a nerve) POLYNEURITIS (inflammation of several nerves) RETROBULBAR NEURITIS (inflammation of the optic nerve) TRIGEMINAL NEURALGIA (facial pain) VON RECKLINGHAUSEN'S DISEASE (multiple tumours of the nerve sheaths)

Neurology is the study of the nervous system and its disorders.

Neuroma is a tumour that is made up of nerve cells. A mature nerve cell cannot reproduce, and so cannot form a tumour. But the connective tissue (neuroglia) that supports the nerve cells can form tumours.

Some neuromas occur singly, others may be found throughout the body with pigmented patches on the skin. This condition is called VON RECKLINGHAUSEN'S DISEASE.

Neuropathy is a general term for any disorder of the peripheral nerves, including the autonomic nervous system. For example, pressure on one of the peripheral nerves in the hand (the median nerve) may cause CARPAL TUNNEL SYNDROME.

See also POLYNEURITIS.

Neurosis is a term used to describe a mental disorder that has no physical cause and that does not produce gross disturbances of the mental processes. *See* MENTAL ILLNESS.

Neurosurgery is the specialized branch of surgery that deals with the nervous system.

Neurotic is a person who is suffering from a NEUROSIS or in whom emotions overcome the normal steadying effect of reason.

Neutropenia is a decrease in the number of neutrophils, the most common white blood cell. It may be caused by any of several factors, but most commonly results from a viral infection.

See also AGRANULOCYTOSIS

Niacin is the chemical name for one of the vitamin B complex. It is also called nicotinic acid. *See* VITAMINS.

Nicotinamide is a derivative of niacin or

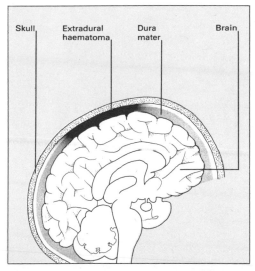

| Skull | Extradural haematoma | Dura mater | Brain |

Extradural haematoma is bleeding between the dura mater and the skull.

Nicotinic acid

nicotinic acid, and is a member of the vitamin B complex. *See* VITAMINS.

Nicotinic acid is an alternative name for niacin, one of the vitamin B complex. *See* VITAMINS.

Night blindness is an eye disorder in which vision is abnormally impaired in dim light or at night. It is caused by a deficiency of visual purple (rhodopsin) in the light-sensitive rods of the retina at the back of the eye. Visual purple is decreased if there is a dietary deficiency of vitamin A – its principal component. Another cause may be the slow regeneration of visual purple after exposure to bright lights, which causes the supply to be used up. Night blindness may also occur in other eye disorders, such as retinitis pigmentosa, choroidoretinitis, glaucoma, and xerophthalmia.

Q: How is night blindness treated?

A: Night blindness caused by vitamin A deficiency can be treated with therapeutic dosages of the vitamin, sometimes in the form of halibut liver oil. Treatment of the cause of the disorder may improve the condition, but there is no treatment for retinitis pigmentosa. Some types of damage to the retina, such as retinitis pigmentosa, are usually irreversible.

Nightmare is any frightening dream. Nightmares are most common in young children, who may find difficulty in distinguishing between fantasy and reality.

Frightening mental stimulation may also cause night terrors, in which a child wakes screaming but cannot remember the cause. Gentle reassurance is all that is usually needed to help the child return to sleep. Night terrors follow a specific pattern.

Q: Why do adults have nightmares?

A: Nightmares sometimes occur in adults who are depressed or anxious about something with which they feel incapable of dealing. Such nightmares are often accompanied by the physical signs of fear, such as palpitations and sweating, and may wake the individual. Antidepressant drugs may help those whose nightmares result from depression.

Nightmares may also result from a traumatic experience, such as a serious accident, or a death in the family.

Night sweat is profuse sweating during sleep. It is common in children and normal when caused by vigorous activity before going to bed. Night sweats, in both adults and children, may also be caused by a chronic disease in which the body temperature rises during the night and falls during the following morning. Some diseases that may cause night sweats include tuberculosis, brucellosis, malaria, and, occasionally, cancer. The treatment of night sweats depends upon the cause. Most cases are harmless and require only fewer bedclothes and a change of night clothes. However, if night sweats persist, it is advisable to consult a doctor.

Night terror is a severe form of nightmare in which a child wakes up screaming and extremely frightened. It may be accompanied by SLEEPWALKING. *See* NIGHTMARE.

Nipple is the raised area in the centre of the breast. It is surrounded by a disc-shaped pigmented area called the areola. In a woman, about twenty milk ducts join in the nipple, and it is from these that milk is secreted by a mother who is breast-feeding a baby. *See* LACTATION.

Any bleeding from the nipple should be discussed immediately with a doctor, because it may indicate breast cancer. Skin diseases can also affect the nipple; the most serious of these is a moist, red eczema called PAGET'S DISEASE OF THE NIPPLE.

Nit is the egg of a louse. Nits may be seen as small white spots on the hair of an infested person. *See* LICE.

Nitrate is a salt of nitric acid. Some nitrates, such as glyceryl trinitrate, cause the blood vessels to dilate, and are used to treat angina pectoris. Others, such as potassium nitrate (saltpetre), are used as food preservatives.

Nitrous oxide is a colourless gas with a faint, characteristic odour that is used as a general anaesthetic in minor operations. However, in combination with another anaesthetic, it can be used for major surgery. Recovery from nitrous oxide anaesthesia is often accom-

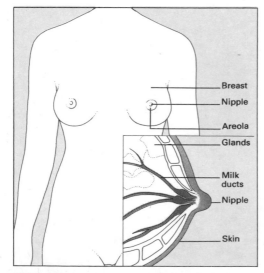

	Breast
	Nipple
	Areola
	Glands
	Milk ducts
	Nipple
	Skin

Nipple is surrounded by a pigmented areola and contains ducts from the mammary glands.

panied by a period of confusion, during which the patient alternates between tears and laughter. For this reason, nitrous oxide is commonly called laughing gas.

Nocturia is the need to pass urine at night. It is differentiated medically from involuntary urination at night (nocturnal enuresis).

Nocturia commonly occurs in the elderly because the kidneys are less able to concentrate urine, and it becomes necessary to empty the bladder once or twice a night. In pregnant women, nocturia results when the enlarged womb presses on the bladder.

Nocturia may be a symptom of DIABETES MELLITUS, prostate problems, or a kidney disorder, such as chronic NEPHRITIS, NEPHROTIC SYNDROME, or PYELONEPHRITIS. Nocturia often occurs in HEART FAILURE or liver disease when there is OEDEMA (fluid retention).

Treatment depends on the cause. Assessment may involve kidney function measurements and other tests.

Nocturnal enuresis. *See* BED-WETTING.

Nonspecific urethritis (NSU) is inflammation of the urethra (the tube through which urine passes from the bladder) that is not known to be caused by a specific organism. It may be caused by various infections, including a viral infection similar to trachoma and the protozoan infection trichomoniasis. Nonspecific urethritis is a form of venereal disease and can be transmitted only by sexual contact.

Q: *What are the symptoms of nonspecific urethritis?*

A: The main symptoms in men are pain on urination and a discharge from the penis that is usually worse in the morning. In severe cases, urination is extremely painful, and there may be a thick white discharge similar to that in gonorrhoea.

Most women show no symptoms. Rarely, there may be mild pain during urination, a slight vaginal discharge, and pain during sexual intercourse. In most women, the only sign of nonspecific urethritis is infection of the neck of the womb (cervicitis).

Q: *How is nonspecific urethritis treated?*

A: Nonspecific urethritis is usually treated with an antibiotic drug; tetracycline is the most effective. Treatment lasts for two or three weeks. Alcohol should not be drunk for at least two weeks after the start of treatment, and sexual intercourse should be avoided until a doctor considers that the patient is cured.

Q: *Can nonspecific urethritis cause any complications?*

A: Yes. A relapse may occur before the patient is cured. This is especially likely if the patient has had sexual intercourse or has drunk alcohol during treatment. Nonspecific urethritis may also cause EPIDIDYMITIS, PROSTATITIS, or SALPINGITIS. The most serious possible complication is REITER'S DISEASE, which may cause inflammation of the iris of the eye (iritis) and swelling of the joints (arthritis).

Noradrenaline is a hormone that is secreted by the sympathetic nervous system. Produced at nerve endings, it is the main chemical transmitter from sympathetic nerves to smooth muscle, heart muscle, and glands. It is also produced by the central part (medulla) of the adrenal glands, from which it passes into the bloodstream. Noradrenaline is a hormone that prepares the body for "fight or flight" in situations of stress. Circulating in the blood, it constricts the blood vessels and so reduces the blood flow to the brain, intestine, liver, and kidneys; relaxes the pupils of the eyes; and soothes movement of the smooth muscle of the gut. Another of its actions, when a large dose is given, is to stimulate the release of glucose from the liver, causing a rise in blood sugar level.

Noradrenaline can be released by stimulating the nerves or by the action of drugs such as amphetamines. It is given by intravenous infusion to treat shock.

See also ADRENAL GLAND; ADRENALINE; PHAEOCHROMOCYTOMA; SHOCK.

Nose, an external protrusion in the centre of the face, is the major organ of smell, and has an internal part that extends backward, as two channels, through the front of the skull. It extends as far as the nasopharynx at the

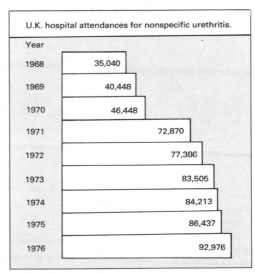

U.K. hospital attendances for nonspecific urethritis.	
Year	
1968	35,040
1969	40,448
1970	46,448
1971	72,870
1972	77,306
1973	83,505
1974	84,213
1975	86,437
1976	92,976

Nonspecific urethritis is spreading more quickly than other venereal diseases.

Nosebleed

upper, back part of the throat. The two channels from the nostrils are separated from each other by a thin partition bone called the nasal septum. On each side are openings into air spaces within the cheekbones, the maxillary sinuses, and there are connections with the two sinuses in the frontal bone of the skull located at the top of the nose. There are other, smaller sinuses in the centre of the skull (see SINUS).

The external nose is formed by two small nasal bones, which can be felt at the bridge of the nose, and pliable cartilage covered with more mobile areas of skin that form the flare of the nostrils.

Q: *What are the functions of the nose?*

A: The nose has several functions. The hairs at the entrance filter out large dust particles, and the adenoids at the back of the nose combat disease organisms. The mucous membrane lining the nose warms and humidifies the air before it passes into the throat. And at the top of the nose, adjacent to the frontal sinuses, sensitive endings of the olfactory nerve detect smells. In addition, the cavities of the nose and sinuses help to give the voice its characteristic resonance.

Q: *What disorders may affect the nose?*

A: The COMMON COLD is the most usual infection that affects the nose, although an allergy such as HAY FEVER or VASO-MOTOR RHINITIS may be another cause of a running nose. A nosebleed may occur spontaneously, or following infection or an accident. Chronic nasal infections produce CATARRH and a postnasal

drip. The skin on the surface of the nose may become swollen and reddened, a condition known as RHINOPHYMA.

A blow to the front of the face may break the nose bones and damage the cartilage. Often the structures return to their natural positions after healing and, provided the nasal septum is straight, no permanent damage results. If, however, the nose is deformed, it should be set in the correct position by surgery. Sometimes the nasal septum is deformed, either as a result of a congenital anomaly or following an accident (see DEVIATED NASAL SEPTUM).

Occasionally small, soft swellings called polyps occur in the nose, causing obstruction to one or both nostrils. These may result from an allergy or a chronic infection. They can usually be removed under local anaesthetic.

It is usual for the sense of smell to deteriorate with age and to be lost whenever the nose is blocked, either because of infection, injury, or on the rare occasions when a foreign body is pushed into a nostril. Smoking may also reduce the sense of smell.

Nosebleed. For EMERGENCY treatment, *see* First Aid, p.590. Bleeding from one or both nostrils may occur for various reasons. Causes include an accident; an infection, such as the common cold; the result of a blood disorder, such as HAEMOPHILIA or LEUKAEMIA, or a side effect of taking anticoagulant drugs; because of repeated picking of the nose with the fingernails; or high blood pressure. Some nosebleeds happen spontaneously for no apparent reason.

Q: *Why do nosebleeds occur spontaneously?*

A: Spontaneous nosebleeds that occur in the elderly may be associated with deterioration of the blood vessels in ARTERIOSCLE-ROSIS, and are not really linked with high blood pressure (hypertension), as is commonly believed. Spontaneous nosebleeds are also common at puberty, particularly in boys, when they are thought to be caused by an expansion of the blood vessels in the nose from the stimulus of the sex hormones.

Q: *How should a nosebleed be treated?*

A: There are two procedures to be followed, depending on the age of the victim. The individual can sit in a chair with the head bent over a bowl and with a finger pressed to the bleeding nostril for at least ten minutes. Following an accident, and particularly with elderly people, lay the victim down with the head and shoulders supported on pillows or cushions, and

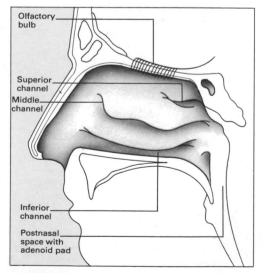

Olfactory bulb

Superior channel

Middle channel

Inferior channel

Postnasal space with adenoid pad

Nose is a large cavity in the skull lined with mucosa, communicating with the throat.

see that the nostril is compressed. An ice pack on the bridge of the nose helps to reduce the blood flow.

If these simple measures fail to work, consult a doctor.

Q: *How is a persistent or recurring nosebleed treated?*

A: If the nosebleed is caused by a ruptured blood vessel, an E.N.T. specialist may be able to cauterize it with chemicals or by electricity, thus stopping the bleeding. If this is not possible, the nose can be packed with adrenaline-soaked gauze for at least twenty-four hours. It is rarely necessary to do more than this, although occasionally the victim needs a transfusion and a further operation to stop the bleeding.

Nostril is one of the two external openings of the nose. *See* NOSE.

Nucleus is a central point of a body around which matter is concentrated. For example, every body cell has a nucleus, which contains CHROMOSOMES and various other minute structures (*see* CELL) that control its activity.

The term nucleus is also used to describe a collection of nerve cells in an area within the brain.

Nucleus pulposus is the central part of an intervertebral disc; it is surrounded by a ring of tough, fibrous cartilage. At birth, the nucleus pulposus is a soft, jelly-like material, but with increasing age it is gradually replaced with fibrocartilage of the surrounding ring and thus loses much of its elastic quality. *See* DISC; SLIPPED DISC.

Nullipara is the medical term for a woman who has never given birth. The term covers those whose pregnancy has been terminated naturally or under medical supervision.

Numbness is complete or partial loss of sensation in an area of skin.

There are many conditions that may cause numbness and most of them involve the nervous system. Intense cold also produces numbness of the hands and feet and other skin areas, particularly in persons with poor peripheral circulation. Numbness may also be a symptom of an acute emotional upset, such as hysteria.

Q: *What are the neurological causes of numbness?*

A: Neurological causes of numbness include those caused by pressure on a nerve, such as sciatica, spondylosis (a degenerative condition of the spine), carpal tunnel syndrome (a disorder in the wrist), as well as polyneuritis. Other causes of numbness may involve the central nervous system as a result of a stroke or multiple sclerosis, syringomyelia (a

disorder of the spinal cord), tabes dorsalis, or locomotor ataxia (a disorder of the nervous system). Numbness may also be caused by a deficiency of vitamin B_{12}, resulting in polyneuritis and degeneration of the spinal cord.

Q: *How is numbness treated?*

A: The treatment depends on a correct diagnosis of the cause. This can be made only by a doctor, who should be consulted when any numbness persists.

Nutrition is the sum total of the processes of eating, digesting, and assimilating food to obtain the carbohydrates, proteins, vitamins, and minerals necessary to maintain growth and health. *See* DIET; MALNUTRITION.

A talk about Nutritional problems

Nutritional problems may develop if food does not contain the essential nutrients or if a disorder interferes with the normal digestion or absorption of food.

Q: *What are the likely causes of nutritional deficiency?*

A: Nutritional disorders occur because of either a deficiency of the correct nutrients in food needed to maintain normal working and repair of the body, or a failure of the body to assimilate the correct nutrients. Everyone needs a certain balance of trace elements, vitamins, and other nutrients in his or her diet to maintain normal body activities.

There can also be too much of a nutrient in the diet, such as excessive

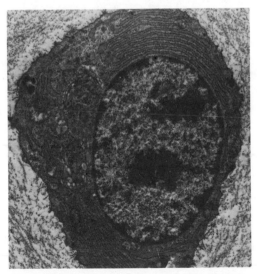

Nucleus of a cell controls and co-ordinates its chemical activity.

Nymphomania

carbohydrate, resulting in such problems as obesity. Much of the excess is stored in the body as fat.

Q: *Why do nutritional disorders occur?*

A: Nutritional disorders will result from excessive fasting, from failure to eat the correct food during times of increased need, such as pregnancy and lactation, and during childhood, when growth is most rapid. Nutritional disorders also result from a voluntary or psychological refusal to eat some or all foods, as with total vegetarians and in anorexia nervosa; or from an increased intake of food, as occurs in any chronic disorder. This is particularly noticeable when it is accompanied by a fever or loss of protein from the body because of burns or wounds.

Q: *Are there any other medical causes of nutritional disorders?*

A: Yes. Medical causes of nutritional disorders include liver disease (cirrhosis), malabsorption from the intestine because of conditions such as Crohn's disease (inflammation of the ileum) and sprue (malabsorption). Other medical causes include genetic anomalies (such as phenylketonuria), and disorders that sometimes develop following gastro-intestinal surgery during which part of the intestine is removed or by-passed (such as gastroenterostomy).

Q: *What are some symptoms of nutritional disorders?*

A: The symptoms depend on which nutrient the body lacks. For example, lack of iron produces anaemia and nail deformity (koilonychia); lack of calcium causes osteomalacia (bone softening); and deficiencies of protein, carbohydrate, and fat result in weight loss. *See* DEFICIENCY DISEASE; VITAMINS.

Q: *How are nutritional disorders prevented and treated?*

A: Where there is no underlying medical problem, nutritional disorders can be prevented by eating a varied, well-balanced diet. This is especially important for pregnant women, who need a good, balanced diet because it also provides for the nutritional demands of the foetus.

A person suffering from a nutritional disorder usually recovers quickly when the diet improves, unless there is an underlying disease. A doctor can help in planning an appropriate diet.

When a nutritional disorder is well advanced and serious, it may be necessary to hospitalize the patient and to supply a diet of protein concentrates given by gastric tube or intravenously.

Q: *What disorders other than obesity are caused by an incorrect diet?*

A: It is probable that conditions such as appendicitis, constipation, diverticular disease, and mucous colitis are aggravated by a diet rich in refined carbohydrates and containing little vegetable fibre. It cannot be emphasized enough that roughage is an important ingredient of any balanced diet. A diet rich in saturated fats causes an increase in the levels of cholesterol and fats in the blood, exposing the person to the risks of arteriosclerosis.

Many people drink too much alcohol and eat too little food. Alcohol is a common substitute for energy foods and is the cause of many health problems. In some parts of the world, people drink large quantities of herbal teas that can cause cirrhosis and liver cancer.

Some food fads cause nutritional disorders if they are indulged in. Vegans may develop vitamin B_{12} deficiency with pernicious anaemia.

See also KWASHIORKOR; MARASMUS.

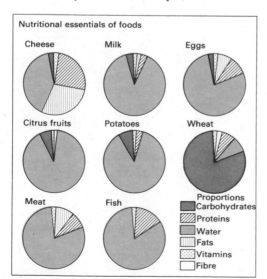

Nutritional essentials of foods

Cheese   Milk   Eggs

Citrus fruits   Potatoes   Wheat

Meat   Fish

Proportions
■ Carbohydrates
▨ Proteins
□ Water
▥ Fats
▦ Vitamins
□ Fibre

Nutrition is the process by which the body extracts and uses food constituents.

Nymphomania is an abnormally excessive desire in females for sexual intercourse. It may sometimes be associated with an inadequate personality development. Such a personality is unable to sustain a deep, lasting commitment and is able only to support superficial and transient relationships.

Nystagmus is a disorder that involves

involuntary eye movements. The eyes move rapidly and constantly from side to side or, less commonly, up and down or rotationally.

Q: *What causes nystagmus?*

A: Congenital nystagmus may be caused by an eye defect such as a cataract, coloboma, or severe nearsightedness (myopia). It often affects albinos, and also miners who have worked for long periods in badly-illuminated conditions. It can be an indication of a disorder of the organ of balance (such as labyrinthitis or Ménière's disease) or of the centre in the brain associated with balance (for example, caused by a brain tumour or a stroke). Other causes include motion sickness, drugs such as alcohol or barbiturates, chorea, and multiple sclerosis.

Q: *How is nystagmus treated?*

A: The treatment of nystagmus is directed at the cause.

O

Obesity is the condition of being overweight because of excess body fat. Strictly, the term obesity is used to denote a body weight that is twenty per cent or more over the average for a person's age, build, sex, and height. The degree of obesity can be determined by measuring the thickness of the fat over the muscles of the fold in front of the armpit. *See* WEIGHT PROBLEMS.

Obsession is a state of anxiety in which an individual is preoccupied with an idea or an action to the exclusion of all else. The action or idea may bring no benefit to the individual, but he or she is nevertheless abnormally concerned by it.

Q: *Is obsession a form of mental illness?*

A: Everyone has or has had mild obsessions about something or somebody, and it could be argued that obsession is an essential factor in creativity. But obsession in a pathological form that interferes with normal life is a form of mental illness and should be treated. When the obsession totally controls the behaviour of a person, he or she is said to be suffering from an obsessional neurosis. Psychoanalysts identify some people as obsessional types because they are controlled by anxiety. In such cases obsession is considered to be a personality disorder, or a feature of one.

Q: *What forms does obsession take?*

A: An obsession may be impulsive,

inhibitory, or compulsive. Impulsive obsession is characterized by some form of action and can become a MANIA. Inhibitory obsession usually takes the form of a phobia, in which the individual cannot do something because of a fear that is often irrational.

In compulsive obsession, the individual may become extremely anxious if he or she is unable to carry out the obsessional desire. For example, a person may feel compelled to wash his or her hands constantly in the belief that they will never be clean. Other people may develop an obsession for locking doors. They may return again and again to make sure the door is locked before leaving, or find themselves unable to leave home for fear that the door can never be locked properly. This may be because the person feels vulnerable to hurt or harm.

Q: *Can obsessions be treated?*

A: Treatment is difficult. In mild cases, the use of tranquillizers can sometimes be helpful. Psychotherapy or psychoanalysis is seldom successful; behaviour therapy may help some people. The symptoms frequently lead to depression, which makes the obsession worse. Treatment of the depression with antidepressant drugs or electric shock therapy, or, occasionally, pre-frontal lobotomy, sometimes improves the condition.

Obstetrics is the branch of medicine that is concerned with pregnancy, labour, and the period just after childbirth (*see* PUERPERIUM). Obstetricians also specialize in GYNAECOLOGY.

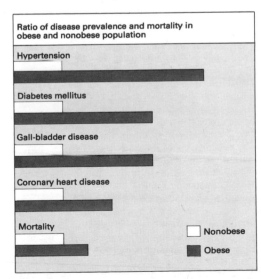

Ratio of disease prevalence and mortality in obese and nonobese population

Hypertension

Diabetes mellitus

Gall-bladder disease

Coronary heart disease

Mortality

☐ Nonobese
■ Obese

Obesity can seriously increase the incidence of certain diseases in a population.

Obstruction

Obstruction (for respiratory obstruction, *see* First Aid, p.518) is a blockage of an internal structure.

Occlusion is the state of being closed. This may be normal, as in the occlusion of the small gaps, called fontanelles, in the skull of a baby that occurs at about the age of eighteen months. An occlusion may also be abnormal, for example, when it is caused by an obstruction. Occlusion also refers to the way in which the teeth of the upper and the lower jaw fit together when the jaws are closed.

See also MALOCCLUSION.

Occult blood is blood that is present in such small amounts that it can be detected only by careful analysis. For example, minor bleeding in the intestines may not produce any obvious change in the faeces, but a simple chemical test on the faeces can detect the occult (hidden) blood.

Occupational hazards are any aspects of a person's work that may cause a disorder. Many occupations or ways of life carry the risk of particular diseases or disorders. For relevant information, *see* ACTINOMYCOSIS; ALCOHOLISM; ANTHRAX; ASBESTOSIS; ASPERGILLOSIS; BENDS; BRUCELLOSIS; BYSSINOSIS; CANCER; DEAFNESS; DERMATITIS; DUPUYTREN'S CONTRACTURE; HEATSTROKE; LEPTOSPIROSIS; MINAMATA DISEASE; PNEUMOCONIOSIS; PSITTACOSIS; RADIATION; RAYNAUD'S PHENOMENON; RINGWORM; STRESS; TUBERCULOSIS.

Occupational therapy is any activity, either physical or mental, that is performed to promote a patient's recovery. Occupational therapy, under the supervision of a registered therapist, is an integral part of treatment and rehabilitation. It can help by teaching a person skills and, in conjunction with physiotherapy, helping to restore muscles and joints that are damaged or wasted.

Odontitis is inflammation of the teeth. *See* PERIODONTITIS.

Oedema is a localized or general swelling caused by the build-up of fluid within body tissues. Excess fluid may be a result of (1) poor circulation of the blood; (2) a failure of the lymphatic system to disperse the fluid; (3) various diseases and disorders; or (4) a combination of factors.

Other causes of oedema include salt retention caused by disease of the heart or kidneys, or a reduction in the amount of protein in the blood, which may occur as a result of cirrhosis, chronic nephritis, or toxaemia of pregnancy (eclampsia). Localized oedema may result from injury or infection.

Q: How is oedema treated?

A: The treatment depends on the underlying cause of the oedema. Diuretic drugs, which make the kidneys eliminate excess salt and water, often produce an immediate improvement. Oedema caused by varicose veins and pregnancy can be prevented by wearing elastic stockings. Oedema of the ankles, from any cause, may be helped by lying down with the feet raised.

See also ANKLES, SWOLLEN.

Oedipus complex is a psychoanalytical term for the sexual love of a son for his mother, often accompanied by feelings of jealousy toward the father. The female counterpart is the Electra complex. *See* COMPLEX.

Oesophageal speech is a method of producing viable speech, after the surgical removal of the voice box (larynx), by vibrating air in the oesophagus instead.

Oesophagus, also known as the gullet, is a muscular tube about 25cm (10 inches) long that extends from the pharynx at the back of the throat to the stomach. In the neck, the oesophagus lies behind the trachea, and enters the thorax behind the aorta and heart to join the top of the stomach.

The oesophagus conveys food and drink from the pharynx to the stomach. This is achieved partly by gravity and partly by peristalsis (rhythmical waves of muscular contractions). When a person breathes in, air is directed to the larynx and the trachea. At the same time, however, saliva is able to run down the oesophagus. Where the oesophagus and the stomach join, there is a ring of muscle (the lower oesophageal sphincter) that prevents the stomach contents from passing back up the oesophagus.

See also ACHALASIA; DYSPHAGIA; HEARTBURN; HIATUS HERNIA.

Oestrogen is the collective name for several female sex hormones produced mainly by the ovaries but also by the adrenal glands.

At the onset of puberty, oestrogens stimulate the development of pubic hair and of secondary female sex characteristics, such as rounded hips and breasts. Oestrogens also play an essential part in the hormonal control of menstruation, being partly responsible (with progesterone) for the cyclical changes in the lining of the womb.

Oestrogens have a number of medical uses. For example, synthetic oestrogens are a component of most types of contraceptive pill, and are also used in the treatment of menstrual disorders and in hormone replacement therapy (HRT) at menopause.

In men, synthetic oestrogens are used in the treatment of cancer of the prostate gland.

See also HORMONES.

Olecranon is the part of the bone of the forearm (ulna) that sticks out at the back of the elbow. With the bone of the upper arm (humerus), the olecranon forms part of the elbow joint. *See* ELBOW.

Olfactory means relating to the sense of smell.

Oliguria is the excretion of abnormally small amounts of urine. It may occur as the result of a high fever, poisoning, or SHOCK, or it may accompany excessive fluid loss from sweating, vomiting, or diarrhoea. Oliguria may also be a symptom of a kidney disorder such as NEPHRITIS, PYELONEPHRITIS, or URAEMIA. If oliguria is persistent, a doctor must be consulted.

Omentum is a loose fold of the membrane (peritoneum) that hangs from the stomach and covers the front of the intestines. It protects the intestines and helps to seal any damage to the intestinal wall, so helping to prevent infection.

Onchocerciasis is the infestation with the parasitic worm *Onchocerca volvulus*. It occurs in regions of Africa, Mexico, and South America. The larvae of the worms are transmitted by the bite of infected black flies of the genus *Simulium*.

Oncology is the study of tumours. It involves the development of improved surgical techniques, radiotherapy, and chemotherapy for the treatment of malignancies.

Onychia is inflammation of the nail bed. *See* PARONYCHIA.

Onychogryposis is a deformity of the nails in which they become thickened and curve inward. It occurs most commonly on the nail of the big toe as a result of pressure from ill-fitting shoes. Onychogryposis may also be caused by repeated injury to the nail bed, or by fungal infections, such as RINGWORM.

Oophorectomy is the surgical removal of an ovary. It is usually performed when there is a cyst or a tumour in the ovary. It may also be necessary if a fertilized ovum has become implanted on the ovary (*see* ECTOPIC PREGNANCY). If there is a benign cyst in the ovary, a partial oophorectomy may be performed.

When a woman over 45 years of age has a HYSTERECTOMY, both ovaries are usually removed; this is called a bilateral oophorectomy. A bilateral oophorectomy may also be performed as part of the treatment for breast cancer.

Oophoritis is inflammation of an ovary. It may be caused by mumps, or other virus organisms. It may be secondarily related to SALPINGITIS, or an infection in the pelvis, such as appendicitis. The symptoms of oophoritis are pain as well as excessive menstruation. Most patients respond to treatment with antibiotics; severe cases may require surgery.

Ophthalmia is any inflammation of the eye. Ophthalmia neonatorum affects newborns; the conjunctivae are contaminated during birth, usually because the mother has gonorrhoea. Early treatment with antibiotic drugs avoids the onset of blindness.

Sympathetic ophthalmia is inflammation of one eye as a reaction to injury of the other eye. This disorder is rare, and it can usually be treated with drugs.

Electric ophthalmia is caused by prolonged exposure to intense light. Symptoms are pain, sensitivity to light, and excessive watering of the eyes.

See also CONJUNCTIVITIS; EYE DISORDERS; TRACHOMA.

Ophthalmic describes anything pertaining to the eye.

Ophthalmoplegia is paralysis of some or all of the muscles of the eye. It may affect one or both eyes, and may come on gradually or occur suddenly. External ophthalmoplegia is paralysis of the muscles on the outside of the eye that control movement of the eyeball. Internal ophthalmoplegia makes the pupil dilated and immobile.

Q: What causes ophthalmoplegia?

A: Ophthalmoplegia may occur temporarily with migraine or the muscle disorder myasthenia gravis. It may also occur in an advanced or acute stage of thiamine (vitamin B$_1$) deficiency; or with polyneuritis, particularly when associated with diabetes mellitus. It can also be caused by pressure on nerves that supply the optic muscles, whether from an aneurysm, brain tumour, or brain infection such as meningitis. Ophthalmoplegia can also occur with multiple sclerosis. External ophthalmoplegia is a result of hyperthyroidism (thyrotoxicosis); fatty tissues in the eye socket swell and press on the eyeball, which makes the eye bulge outward and eventually paralyzes the eye muscles.

Q: What are the symptoms of ophthalmoplegia?

A: Ophthalmoplegia in one eye causes double vision (diplopia), because the affected eye is immobile while the other eye is free to move. Internal ophthalmoplegia impairs vision because the pupil is unable to react to variations in the amount of light reaching the eye, and the lens is unable to adjust to focus at different distances.

Q: How is ophthalmoplegia treated?

A: The cause of the condition must be found and treated. However, if only one eye is affected, temporary relief from the distress of double vision can be obtained by wearing a patch that covers the paralyzed eye.

Ophthalmoscope

Ophthalmoscope is an instrument for examining the interior of the eye. It has lenses, a mirror, and a light that shines a bright beam through the patient's pupil. Using an ophthalmoscope, a doctor can examine the retina, optic nerve, and the eye's network of blood vessels, in the diagnosis of specific eye disorders and some physical conditions.

Opiate is any drug that contains opium or one of its constituents, morphine or codeine.

Opisthotonus is a severe form of body spasm in which the back, head, and legs arch backward. It is a symptom of strychnine poisoning and severe forms of TETANUS.

Opium is the dried secretion from the unripe seed pods of the opium poppy (*Papaver somniferum*). It has a bitter taste and a characteristic smell. Opium contains more than twenty alkaloid drugs, including MORPHINE, CODEINE, and papaverine. The effects of opium are similar to those of morphine and, like morphine, it produces physical dependence. Heroin is a semisynthetic derivative of opium. The medical use of opium and its constituents morphine and codeine, is strictly controlled by law.

See also DRUG ADDICTION.

Optic describes anything concerned with the eye or vision.

Oral describes anything pertaining to the mouth.

Oral cholecystogram is an X-ray examination of the gall bladder. It is used to diagnose gallstones and chronic inflammation of the gall bladder (cholecystitis). The patient is given a fat-free meal on the evening before an examination, and is then deprived of solid food. The following morning, the patient swallows an iodine-containing compound. Several hours later, a series of X-rays are taken of the gall bladder. The iodine compound becomes concentrated in the gall bladder and makes abnormalities such as gallstones visible on X-rays. The patient is then given a fatty meal, and more X-rays are taken. Absorption of fats from the meal causes the gall bladder to contract, and permits the bile ducts to become visible.

An oral cholecystogram gives a definite result in most cases. However, if the gall bladder and the bile ducts cannot be seen on the X-rays, an intravenous cholecystogram may be necessary.

Oral contraception. *See* CONTRACEPTION.

Oral surgery is surgery performed on the mouth. It may be performed by a dental surgeon to treat diseased or impacted teeth, gum disorders, or disorders of the underlying bone. Oral surgery is sometimes necessary in the treatment of a MALOCCLUSION.

An otolaryngologist, who specializes in disorders of the ear, nose, and throat, may perform oral surgery to treat cancer of the jaw, mouth, or tongue. Some disorders of the salivary glands, such as tumours or stones, may also require oral surgery. Fractures of the jaw and face usually require surgery.

Orbit is the bony socket that surrounds and protects the eye. It is considerably larger than the eye, the space being filled with loose fat so that the eye is free to move. Six muscles that move the eye are attached to the orbit at one end, and to the outer coat of the eyeball at the other. There is a hole at the back of the orbit through which the optic nerve and blood vessels pass.

See also EYE.

Orchidectomy is the surgical removal of a testicle. It may be necessary if there is a tumour of the testicle, or if the testicle has become twisted, as may occur with an undescended testicle (*see* CRYPTORCHIDISM). The removed testicle may be replaced with a synthetic substitute for cosmetic purposes.

Orchiopexy is surgical fixation of an undescended testicle in its correct place in the scrotum. In some forms of this operation, the testicle and the scrotum are temporarily attached to the inner side of the thigh.

Orchitis is inflammation of the testicles. It occurs most commonly as a complication of MUMPS, but it may also be caused by injury to the testicles, or by the spread of infection from elsewhere in the body, such as occurs in EPIDIDYMITIS. One or both testicles may become enlarged and extremely painful. Fever, nausea, and vomiting may also occur. These symptoms may be relieved by the

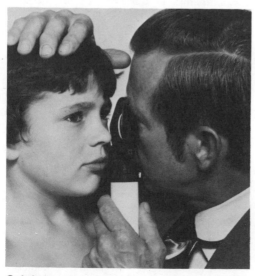

Ophthalmoscope enables a doctor to examine the interior of the eyes.

application of ice packs and the use of painkillers. The scrotum should also be placed on a cotton wool pad, which should be supported by adhesive tape stretched between the thighs. The inflammation usually subsides within a few days.

Orgasm is a pleasurable sexual climax. In men it is accompanied by the ejaculation of semen and by rhythmic contractions of muscles in the genital area. In women, orgasm is accompanied by contractions of the vagina.

An orgasm does not necessarily always occur during sexual intercourse, but continual failure to attain orgasm is, in most cases, caused by psychological factors.

Ornithosis. *See* PSITTACOSIS.

Orthodontics is the branch of dentistry that is concerned with the prevention and correction of abnormally positioned teeth. Orthodontic treatment is usually performed during childhood, when the jaw is still developing and when the gradual restraint of certain teeth can prevent development of a MALOCCLUSION.

Orthopaedics is a specialty of medical science concerned with the treatment of disorders of bones and joints. Orthopaedic surgery is the surgical prevention or correction of bone deformities. Orthopaedics also includes the study and treatment of rheumatic disorders and disorders of muscles or nerves that may aggravate or cause orthopaedic conditions.

Orthopnea is breathlessness that occurs in any position other than standing or sitting upright. The term commonly means difficulty in breathing when lying down. *See* BREATHLESSNESS.

Orthoptics is a technique used to correct defects in the muscles that control the alignment of the eyes. It involves a set of eye exercises to co-ordinate the movements of the two eyes. Orthoptic training is beneficial in the treatment of strabismus (squint).

Ossicle is any small bone. The term usually refers to one of the three small bones in the middle ear: the malleus, incus, or stapes. *See* EAR.

Ossification is the formation of bone. It occurs normally during the development of a foetus, when bone is formed from cartilage. It continues during childhood, and the final stage in bone formation, the ossification of the growing ends of bone, occurs during adolescence.

Abnormal ossification may develop within tissues that have been damaged, particularly in muscles, ligaments, and sometimes tendons. Bone formation may occasionally occur in a frozen shoulder (a form of tendinitis) in the muscle of the shoulder blade, but is more frequent in metabolic disorders associated with raised CALCIUM levels in the blood.

Osteitis is inflammation of bone that involves the marrow. It causes periostitis, a swelling and local tenderness of the periosteum, the membrane that surrounds the bone. For practical purposes, osteitis and osteomyelitis can be considered to have the same causes and treatment. *See* OSTEOMYELITIS.

Osteitis deformans. *See* PAGET'S DISEASE OF BONE.

A talk about Osteoarthritis

Osteoarthritis is a chronic disorder involving the joints. It is a degenerative change in the joints and should properly be called osteoarthrosis. It is not caused by inflammation. The degenerative changes take place because of the rubbing of the joint surfaces, causing a wearing away and disintegration of the tissues.

There is usually some additional factor that speeds up this process. The factors include unusual stresses on the joint, such as those resulting from obesity or bow-legs; disorders that damage the joint cartilage, such as rheumatoid arthritis and osteochondritis (bone and cartilage inflammation); or damage to the joint surfaces from a fracture or torn cartilage. Other factors are disorders of the joint, such as congenital dislocation of the hip, and the slowing down of the normal repair processes that take place in old age.

Q: Which joints are most likely to be affected by osteoarthritis?

A: The joints that carry the body's weight are most likely to develop osteo-

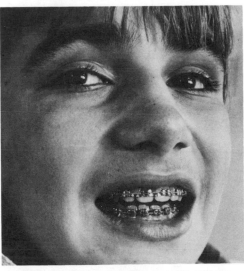

Orthodontic disorders can be treated with the use of highly specialized teeth braces.

Osteoarthritis

arthritis. For example, repeated injuries to an athlete's hips, knees, or ankles are likely to result in osteoarthritis in those joints in later life. Repeated attacks of gout or of septic arthritis can also cause osteoarthritis.

Q: *What happens to the joint in osteoarthritis?*

A: The slippery cartilage that lines the joint surface is gradually worn away, exposing the underlying bone. The bone becomes smooth and its edges become rough, with small areas of bony formation, known as osteophytes. The surrounding ligaments and membranes also become thickened because of the recurrent slight strains that occur in an osteoarthritic joint.

Q: *What are the symptoms of osteoarthritis?*

A: There is gradually increasing pain, with restriction of movement. The amount of pain varies from time to time; additional strains or unexpected movements make the condition worse. In most joints, this process is accompanied by a grating that can sometimes be heard and usually felt.

Q: *How is osteoarthritis diagnosed?*

A: A doctor makes the diagnosis after an examination of the joint is confirmed by X-rays. Swellings adjacent to the end joints of the fingers (Heberden's nodes) are common.

Q: *What is the treatment for osteoarthritis?*

A: Osteoarthritis is increasingly common with age, and treatment is directed toward improving general health. This includes encouraging weight loss if the patient is overweight, and teaching

exercises designed to strengthen surrounding muscles and maintain movement of the joint when it is not bearing weight. The emphasis should be on either resting without strain (not too much walking or standing), or on taking exercise without strain. Hot pads often give relief if a joint has become acutely painful. If necessary, canes, crutches, or walking frames can be used.

Morale can be maintained with encouragement from the doctor. During the initial stages, aspirin or some other painkilling drug may be prescribed. Various antirheumatic drugs, such as indomethacin and ibuprofen, may be used.

Q: *Does surgery help in osteoarthritis?*

A: Yes. There are many surgical procedures that are helpful in the treatment of osteoarthritis. Arthrodesis, an operation to fix the joint in one position, can be done to prevent further pain. The ankle is often fixed in this way.

Other operations include removing some of the membranes around the joint or forming a new joint, as is done in treatment for hallux valgus deformities.

In recent years total replacement of a joint has become possible by the insertion of a plastic and metal artificial joint. This has been done successfully in finger joints, hip joints, and knee joints.

Osteoarthropathy is any disease of the joints and bones. Usually the joints become damaged as a result of some other disorder. For example, nerves in the joints, which normally give a sense of position and are responsible for the sensation of pain, may be affected by inflammation (peripheral neuritis).

Common causes of such conditions include tabes dorsalis (damage to the lower spinal cord); neuritis associated with diabetes mellitus; and syringomyelia, another spinal cord disease. Repeated damage results in a thickening or enlargement of the joints, instability of movement, and osteoarthritis of the joint.

Chronic hypertrophic pulmonary osteoarthropathy is the medical term for CLUBBING of the fingers and toes in persons with chronic lung or heart disease.

Osteoarthrosis. *See* OSTEOARTHRITIS.

Osteochondritis is inflammation of bone and cartilage; in most cases, it leads to degeneration of these tissues (osteochondrosis). There are two forms of the disorder, osteochondritis dissecans and osteochondritis deformans juvenilis. Their causes are not known.

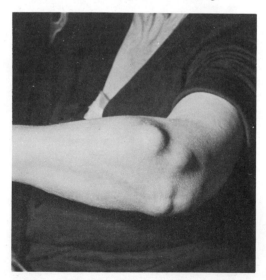

Osteoarthritis gradually destroys the cartilage of the joint, producing overgrowths of bone.

Q: *What are the symptoms of osteochondritis dissecans and how is it treated?*

A: The disorder usually affects young adults, who have recurrent attacks of mild pain, usually in the knee joint. Fluid in the area may increase, followed by sudden and recurrent locking of the joint.

What probably happens is that the blood supply to the local bone and cartilage is affected and causes a piece of cartilage and underlying bone to break off and move into the joint. This loose fragment causes the sudden locking and resulting pain.

The condition is usually diagnosed late. Bone and cartilage may heal if the joint is kept in a cast for eight to ten weeks. But an operation to remove the fragment is the best form of treatment.

Q: *What are the symptoms of osteochondritis deformans juvenilis and how is it treated?*

A: This disorder, also known as PERTHES' DISEASE, occurs in children. It usually affects the thoracic spine, the top of the thigh-bone (femur), the wrist, and the foot. The bone becomes softened and may easily be deformed by pressure or accident. The usual symptom is pain over the bone, and the damage can be seen on an X-ray. The disorder is relatively harmless, but may ultimately lead to osteoarthritis of the joint.

If the condition is diagnosed early, the joint can be rested in a cast so that further deformity does not occur. This is particularly important when the condition affects the hip joint.

Osteoclastoma is a bone tumour that is usually benign (noncancerous), although it invades the tissues surrounding the bone. This disorder commonly affects young adults and involves the bones on either side of the knee joint. There is pain with the swelling of the bone, and possibly fractures.

Treatment is the removal of the tumour by surgery, even if the surrounding joint and tissue have to be destroyed. Radiotherapy is used for treatment of areas such as the spine that are difficult to reach by normal surgical techniques. *See* OSTEOSARCOMA.

Osteogenesis imperfecta, or fragilitas ossium, is an inherited disorder in which the bones are abnormally brittle and may break easily, often causing deformities. The condition may be associated with a blue coloration of the whites of the eyes and with chronic, progressive deafness (otosclerosis).

A child with osteogenesis imperfecta may die in early life. Otherwise, there is a tendency for slight improvement with age.

Osteology is the study of the structure and function of bones. It also involves the study of all the diseases and disorders that affect bones.

Osteoma is a benign (noncancerous) tumour of bone. It usually forms on the skull or long bones. Most osteomas cause local thickening of bone and do not produce any symptoms. They can be left alone or removed if they are unsightly or obstruct a blood vessel. But an osteoid osteoma, a rare benign tumour of bone, can cause severe and deep pain. It is treated by surgical removal of the tumour, which gives immediate relief from pain.

Osteomalacia is a softening of the bones in an adult, similar to rickets in children. In persons with osteomalacia, the basic structure of the bone remains unaltered.

Q: *What are the symptoms of osteomalacia?*

A: Common symptoms are aching and painful bones, as well as fractures. Softened bones may also bend under the weight of the body.

Q: *What causes osteomalacia?*

A: Osteomalacia is also called adult rickets because it usually results from a lack of vitamin D and calcium in the diet. Other causes include kidney failure and intestinal disorders. *See* RICKETS.

Q: *How is osteomalacia diagnosed and treated?*

A: Diagnosis depends on bone X-rays and blood tests to determine calcium and phosphorus levels. The possibility of conditions with similar symptoms, such as osteoporosis, hyperparathyroidism, and Cushing's syndrome, must first be eliminated.

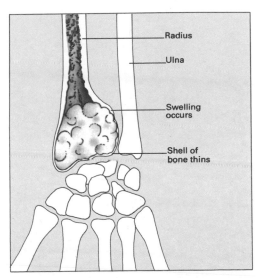

Osteoclastoma is a benign tumour of giant cells within the bone marrow causing swelling.

Osteomyelitis

Osteomyelitis, or osteitis, is inflammation of bone, including the marrow. It is usually caused by a bacterial infection.

There are two kinds of osteomyelitis: acute and chronic. Children most commonly suffer from acute osteomyelitis. Chronic osteomyelitis usually follows an acute attack and rarely occurs on its own. It can, however, be caused by tuberculosis.

Q: *Why does acute osteomyelitis occur?*

A: In acute osteomyelitis, bacteria may be carried by the bloodstream from another area of infection to the bone. It may be the result of a septic tooth, a boil, or an ear infection. It can also reach the bone through an injury such as an open fracture. There is frequently a history of recent minor injury or knocks to the bone. The growing end of the bone is the area most frequently infected.

Q: *What are the symptoms of acute osteomyelitis?*

A: Children may have several days of fever and general illness before suffering from local bone pain. But in both adults and children bone involvement is followed by a sudden increase in temperature, sometimes with vomiting, and local tenderness of the bone with painful movement of nearby joints. Swelling occurs and the skin becomes red.

Q: *How is acute osteomyelitis diagnosed and treated?*

A: X-rays seldom help diagnosis in the early stages, but a white blood cell count shows the type of response the body is making to acute infection, helping a doctor to diagnose osteomyelitis and begin treatment immediately. Massive doses of antibiotics, usually one of the penicillin drugs, are given for at least two months and the bone is immobilized in a splint. Careful assessment by an orthopaedic surgeon or doctor is necessary to ensure that an abscess has not formed. If an abscess is found, antibiotics are given and surgery performed to remove the abscess. If pus has formed, it is sometimes necessary to drain the bone by drilling holes in it.

Q: *What are the symptoms and treatment of chronic osteomyelitis?*

A: The usual symptom is pain and a discharge of pus. The bone abscess usually discharges through the skin, although sometimes pain and swelling occur over the bone and the patient has a mild fever. An X-ray confirms the diagnosis, and surgery is performed to remove any fragments of dead bone that can encourage continued infection. Complete cleansing of the area is more important than the use of antibiotics.

Brodie's abscess is a form of chronic osteomyelitis that occurs without a previous acute attack. The main symptom is deep, intense bone pain. The treatment is the same as for any other form of chronic osteomyelitis.

Q: *What other forms of osteomyelitis may occur?*

A: Tuberculosis may spread to bone, producing a "cold" abscess in which there is swelling without heat or redness to the skin, but with local pain. The patient usually experiences a slight fever, loss of weight, and general malaise. The diagnosis is confirmed by a combination of X-rays, blood tests, a Mantoux test (a test for tuberculosis infection), and the examination of pus from the abscess.

Treatment consists of antituberculous drugs, splinting of the bone, and an operation to remove the abscess.

It is important that a search be carried out for other possible areas of tubercular infection, especially in the lungs and kidneys. People who have had contact with the patient, particularly children, must be examined to prevent spread of the disorder.

Osteopathy is a system of medical treatment developed by the American physician Dr Andrew Taylor Still (1828–1917). Dr Still taught that the body is able to deal with any disorder provided any underlying defect in its structure is corrected. These defects are diagnosed in a conventional manner, if necessary

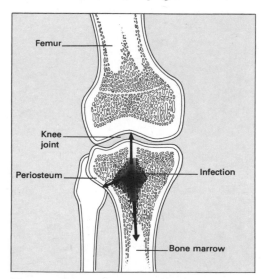

Osteomyelitis is an infection of the bone marrow that can spread to the periosteum.

Femur

Knee joint

Periosteum

Infection

Bone marrow

by the various tests and examinations used in conventional medical practice. The defects are treated by both manipulation of the spine and other bones and by conventional medical and surgical techniques to correct the underlying structural problem. For example, the relief of pressure on nerves can improve muscle tone and relieve pain in many cases.

Q: *How do osteopaths help their patients?*

A: An osteopath can sometimes help a patient suffering from a functional disorder for which orthodox medicine has proved less effective. The osteopath makes a careful assessment of the patient's condition, finally arriving at a diagnosis on which to base treatment. X-rays help to locate any abnormality, especially if it is in the spine.

Treatment of spinal disorders consists of a combination of manipulation and encouraging movement of the spine by gently turning the body or pulling it in certain directions. The osteopath is skilled in the art of manipulating the vertebrae of the spine by sensitive finger pressure. Similar methods are used in the treatment of other parts of the body.

Q: *What conditions respond to osteopathy?*

A: The main value of osteopathy is in the treatment of orthopaedic and rheumatic disorders, but it can be used to treat a much wider range of functional disorders. Many people consult an osteopath only for treatment of backache, sciatica, or shoulder pain caused by osteoarthrosis in the neck. However, osteopaths may treat many conditions from headache to painful periods (dysmenorrhoea) in which muscle spasm is, in part, a cause.

Q: *Can osteopathy prevent the development of certain conditions?*

A: Yes. Osteopathy can, in some cases, prevent the recurrence of backache or sciatica, because the treatment keeps the spine in the correct alignment. An osteopath may also notice minor faults before symptoms have developed and can often prevent the occurrence of a disorder by manipulation.

Osteoporosis is a disorder in which both calcium salts and bone fabric are lost. It is different from OSTEOMALACIA, in which only calcium is lost from the bone.

Q: *What are the symptoms of osteoporosis?*

A: There may be no symptoms. But the individual may lose height because of a collapse of the vertebrae and suffer from increasing kyphosis (bending forward of the spine). There may also be a vague, generalized backache because the vertebrae, in becoming thinner, tend to compress the surrounding nerves. Bones fracture more easily, causing more acute and severe pain. Such severe pain is caused by a compression fracture of one of the vertebrae, commonly in the midspine. Other bones, such as the hip, may fracture more easily than usual in the elderly.

Q: *What causes osteoporosis?*

A: The cause of osteoporosis is not precisely known, but it is probably caused by some kind of hormonal imbalance. It occurs most commonly in the elderly and more often in women than in men. The disorder may accompany Cushing's syndrome (overactivity of the adrenal glands) or hyperparathyroidism (overactivity of the parathyroid glands), or occur following prolonged bed rest.

Q: *How is osteoporosis diagnosed and treated?*

A: The diagnosis is usually made on the basis of the physical appearance of the patient and using X-rays to reveal that the bones are less dense than normal.

In most cases, treatment is not necessary because osteoporosis is part of the normal aging process. However, if there is severe pain, a back brace or support of some kind may have to be worn until the pain subsides.

Osteoporosis that is rapidly progressive may have to be treated with doses of vitamin D and additional calcium to help maintain bone formation and strength. Anabolic hormones, derived from male sex hormones, may help maintain the

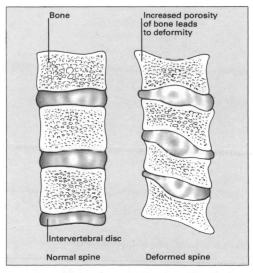

Osteoporosis weakens the bone and leads to deformities mainly in weight-bearing bones.

Osteosarcoma

bone structure. Women may be given female sex hormones, and this treatment has been shown to prevent further osteoporosis. But oestrogen treatment may have adverse effects on menstruation and cause the breasts to swell and ache.

Osteosarcoma is a malignant (cancerous) bone tumour that usually arises on either side of the knee joint or on the upper end of the armbone. The disorder is most common in the first twenty years of life, but may occur at any age with PAGET'S DISEASE OF BONE, in which the bones become thickened and soft.

Q: *What are the symptoms of osteosarcoma?*

A: There is local pain and swelling with an increased sensation of warmth, similar to that accompanying osteomyelitis (infection and inflammation of bone).

Q: *How is an osteosarcoma treated?*

A: Intensive radiotherapy is usually attempted first. If this fails, amputation of the affected limb must be considered. This operation is followed by chemotherapy to combat the spread of the tumour to the lungs and other tissues. These modern forms of treatment have improved life expectancy considerably. In the past, osteosarcoma was generally fatal.

    See also OSTEOMA.

Osteotomy is an operation in which a bone is cut, enabling a surgeon to reposition it. An osteotomy may be performed to lengthen or shorten a leg, or to correct bowed or bent legs. It may also be done to reset a fracture.

An osteotomy may be carried out in hip operations to alter the position of the thigh-

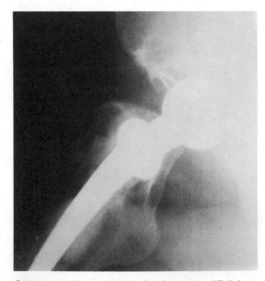

Osteotomy is required to implant an artificial hip joint (white) into the thigh-bone.

bone, and can be of help in the treatment of osteoarthritis of the hip. But total replacement of the hip joint with an artificial joint is often more effective.

Otalgia. *See* EARACHE.

Otic preparations are substances used in the treatment of external OTITIS and as an aid in removing wax (cerumen) from the ear.

A talk about Otitis

Otitis is inflammation of the ear. Inflammation of the outer ear is called otitis externa; inflammation of the middle ear is otitis media; and inflammation of the inner ear is called LABYRINTHITIS. Infection of the external ear flap (pinna) may be caused by otitis externa or by any skin disorder.

Q: *What are the symptoms of otitis externa?*

A: The symptoms include itching, pain in the ear, a slight discharge, and deafness. Occasionally the infection is localized and a boil forms. This condition is called furunculosis.

Q: *What causes otitis externa?*

A: It is often caused by a combination of bacterial and fungal infections. Such infections may result from scratching the ear; from swimming; or from excessive sweating. Otitis externa is more common in people with ECZEMA, and in those with diabetes mellitus.

Q: *How is otitis externa treated?*

A: The dead skin, pus, and wax should be removed by a doctor. Antibiotics and antifungal preparations may be prescribed to treat the infection. In some cases, it may be necessary to pack special dressings into the ear until the infection is cured.

Q: *How can otitis externa be prevented?*

A: The ears should be kept dry by wearing earplugs when swimming. A doctor may also advise the use of alcohol ear drops after swimming. The ears should not be scratched.

Q: *What are the symptoms of otitis media?*

A: The main symptoms are severe earache, deafness, and fever. There is an accumulation of pus in the middle ear that may build up to such an extent that the eardrum ruptures, thereby releasing the pus and relieving the earache. Young children may also have diarrhoea, abdominal pain, and vomiting.

Q: *What causes otitis media?*

A: It is most commonly caused by the spread of infection from the back of the nose, along the Eustachian tube, and into the middle ear. This may occur with the common cold; tonsillitis; or any infection that affects the upper part of the respiratory system, such as influenza, measles, or whooping cough. Less commonly, otitis media may be caused by sudden pressure changes (*see* BAROTRAUMA) or by an infection such as SINUSITIS. It may also occur after a TONSILLECTOMY or following rupture of the eardrum.

As a result of infection, there is increasing secretion from the membranes that line the middle ear. These secretions block the Eustachian tube and cause an increase in pressure, resulting in earache.

Q: *How is otitis media treated?*

A: In the early stages of otitis media, before the eardrum has burst, antibiotics are usually effective. A doctor may also prescribe painkillers, and nose drops to relieve the congestion at the lower end of the Eustachian tube. Antihistamine, taken in the form of tablets, may help to relieve blockage. Rarely, it may be necessary to perforate the eardrum surgically (*see* MYRINGOTOMY).

If the eardrum has ruptured and is discharging pus, the ear should, in addition, be kept clean and dry until the eardrum has healed.

Q: *Can otitis media cause any complications?*

A: Yes. The infection may spread to the mastoid bone, causing mastoiditis. Occasionally, treatment kills the infection but the pus may be unable to escape because the Eustachian tube is blocked. Such obstructions may be caused by enlarged adenoids and may result in continued deafness. In adults this condition may be treated by passing a tube into the nose and blowing clear the Eustachian tube. In children it is usually treated with a myringotomy and the insertion of a drainage tube. If the obstruction is not treated, permanent deafness may result.

Q: *What precautions should be taken in connection with otitis media?*

A: Any minor respiratory infection may result in otitis media, particularly in children, whose adenoids and tonsils may become swollen. To prevent this from happening, antihistamines may be prescribed at the first signs of a cold or throughout the winter. If these are ineffective, a doctor may recommend that the adenoids be removed surgically.

A child who is recovering from otitis media should not be allowed to swim until a doctor has given permission. It is also advisable to have the child's

hearing tested after the condition has been treated to make sure that there is no residual deafness resulting from GLUE EAR.

Otolaryngology. *See* OTORHINOLARYNGOLOGY.

Otology is the study of the ear.

Otomycosis is a fungal infection of the outer ear. The condition may be associated with monoliasis (thrush) or aspergillosis, a mould infection. It is a form of otitis externa, and is common following swimming or working in hot, humid conditions. *See* OTITIS.

Otorhinolaryngology is the study of the ear, nose, and throat, including their functions and their disorders.

Otorrhoea is a discharge from the ear. It may be caused by inflammation of the external ear (otitis externa), or a perforated eardrum. Any ear discharge should be reported to a doctor. *See* OTITIS.

Otosclerosis is a disorder of the middle ear that leads to progressive deafness. It is one of the main causes of deafness in young adults. Otosclerosis is caused by the gradual build-up of extra bony tissue around one of the small bones (the stapes) in the middle ear. As a result, the stapes cannot vibrate, thus preventing the transmission of sound from the eardrum to the inner ear. In some persons with otosclerosis, there is a family history of deafness. Otosclerosis usually affects one ear before the other, but eventually both ears become affected. *See* DEAFNESS.

Q: *What are the symptoms of otosclerosis?*

A: The major symptom is progressive

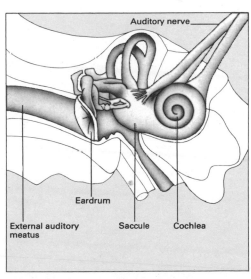

Auditory nerve

Eardrum

External auditory meatus

Saccule

Cochlea

Otitis can affect any part of the ear, producing inflammation, swelling, and pain.

deafness. There may also be noises in the ear (tinnitus), and the whites of the eyes may be slightly blue in some patients. The symptoms often become worse during pregnancy.

Q: *How is otosclerosis treated?*

A: Surgery is usually the most effective treatment. Fenestration, which is an operation to make an artificial opening into the inner ear, has largely been replaced by stapedectomy, in which the stapes bone is replaced by a synthetic substitute. This operation usually restores normal hearing. However, the patient should avoid exposure to loud noises because the sound vibrations may damage the artificial stapes.

Otoscope is an instrument for examining the ear. It provides a light source that enables the ear canal and the eardrum to be inspected.

Ovariectomy. *See* OOPHORECTOMY.

Ovaritis. *See* OOPHORITIS.

Ovary is a female organ that produces eggs and sex hormones. The two ovaries, each about the size of a walnut, lie on each side of, and usually slightly behind, the womb (uterus). They are attached to the womb and the inner walls of the abdomen by ligaments, which give them a mobility that many other internal organs do not have. This mobility may allow one or both ovaries to take up a slightly different position.

The surface of each ovary is covered by a thick layer of connective tissue called the tunica albuginea. Inside, the ovary is composed of many thousands of cells that have the potential to form ova (eggs) and a firm

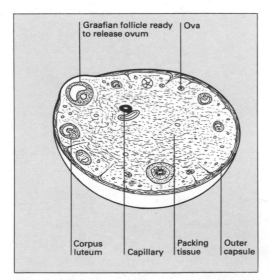

Graafian follicle ready to release ovum | Ova

Corpus luteum | Capillary | Packing tissue | Outer capsule

Ovary has hundreds of ova, one of which is released during each menstrual cycle.

structure of connective tissue. Before puberty, the ovaries are small and soft. After menopause they shrivel in size.

The ends of the FALLOPIAN TUBES, with their long, finger-like extensions, overhang the ovaries. In a woman of childbearing age, they collect an ovum (egg) when one is released every month.

Q: *How many eggs does an ovary produce?*

A: The ovaries usually produce one mature egg each month throughout the fertile life of a woman, beginning at menarche (the start of menstrual periods) and ending at menopause. During this time, the ovarian tissue is under regular rhythmical control by hormones from the PITUITARY GLAND at the base of the brain. *See* MENSTRUATION; OVULATION.

Q: *What disorders can affect an ovary?*

A: Inflammation of the ovaries, called OOPHORITIS, usually accompanies SALPINGITIS (infection of the fallopian tubes), but may result on its own from MUMPS.

Tumours of the ovary are usually CYSTS and most frequently occur in women over thirty-five years of age. About 95 per cent of these tumours are benign (noncancerous). In a younger woman, a follicle may sometimes develop into a cyst and be discovered during gynaecological examination. It is usually worth waiting to see if the cyst is still present after menstruation.

Q: *What symptoms may an ovarian tumour or cyst cause?*

A: Frequently there are no symptoms, unless the tumour has grown so large that it causes abdominal swelling or presses on the bladder to cause frequent passing of urine.

Ovarian tumours are commonly discovered during a routine gynaecological examination. They seldom cause pain unless they twist or are malignant (cancerous) and the cancer has already spread to involve adjacent tissues. *See* CANCER.

Cysts can be caused by an imbalance of the hormones from the pituitary gland, so that the ovary is subjected to a constant abnormal stimulus. This may produce a condition in which there is INFERTILITY, infrequent menstruation, and an abnormal growth of body hair (Stein-Leventhal syndrome).

Q: *How is a ovarian tumour treated?*

A: A laparoscopy, an examination of the inside of the abdomen with a lighted tube, X-ray, ultrasound scanning, and sometimes exploratory surgery may be done to confirm the presence of an ovarian tumour. Such examinations may confirm that the tumour is neither a FIBROID nor a swelling of a fallopian tube that sometimes follows salpingitis.

If an ovarian tumour is found, the ovary is generally totally or partially removed (*see* OOPHORECTOMY).

Q: *Can ovarian tumours or cysts produce complications?*

A: Yes. A cyst may occur in early pregnancy because of an increase in the size of the corpus luteum and this may occasionally remain, causing problems of obstruction later in pregnancy.

A tumour can cause the ovary to twist on its ligaments, resulting in severe abdominal pain. There may also be abdominal pain if the cyst ruptures or there is bleeding into the cyst.

Overweight and underweight. *See* WEIGHT PROBLEMS.

Ovulation is the release of a mature OVUM (egg) from an OVARY. It occurs about every four weeks in the middle of the menstrual cycle, approximately fourteen days before the next menstrual period. After ovulation, the ovum passes along a fallopian tube to the womb.

The development of an ovum is under hormonal control. Follicle-stimulating hormone (FSH) from the pituitary gland stimulates the ovum to mature within the ovary. On approximately the fourteenth day of the menstrual cycle there is a sudden increase in the amount of luteinizing hormone (LH), and ovulation occurs.

See also MENSTRUATION.

Ovum is a mature female reproductive cell, also known as an egg. Ova are formed in the ovaries, pass down the fallopian tubes, and enter the womb. Usually, one ovum matures each month, although not necessarily in alternate ovaries. If a SPERM fertilizes the ovum, it develops into an EMBRYO. If the ovum is not fertilized, it degenerates and passes out of the body at MENSTRUATION.

Oxycephalic describes the shape of a skull in which the top part appears unusually high and pointed. A newborn baby's head is often slightly pointed because of the moulding of the skull during childbirth, but it returns to a normal shape within a few weeks.

An oxycephalic skull may also occur as a form of congenital anomaly, which can be associated with syndactyly (webbing of the fingers). The anomaly is caused by the skull bones joining together earlier than normal, but it can be corrected surgically to prevent the possible development of mental retardation or blindness.

Oxygen is an odourless, colourless gas that makes up about twenty per cent of normal air. It is an essential component for respiration in animals and plants. *See* OXYGEN THERAPY; RESPIRATION.

Oxygen tent is a pliable, plastic sheet that is held by a frame above and around a patient's bed and is tucked in below the mattress to produce an enclosed atmosphere. Humidified oxygen is blown into the tent; the patient can then move freely in an atmosphere containing a much higher proportion of oxygen than normal.

The patient can be fed through openings in the side that can be sealed, and medical treatment, such as intravenous transfusions, can be given without difficulty.

Oxygen therapy is the administration of oxygen to patients. Oxygen gas is supplied from a high-pressure cylinder that has a valve to allow the release of oxygen at low pressure.

Q: *What disorders are treated using oxygen therapy?*

A: Any condition that causes decreased transfer of oxygen to the blood in the lungs may be helped by oxygen therapy. These conditions include heart failure; reduced circulation, as occurs in acute shock and a heart attack; pneumonia; and chronic bronchitis with emphysema. Oxygen is often given to newborn babies to assist their respiration in the first few minutes after birth.

Q: *How is oxygen therapy given?*

A: Oxygen is most commonly given through a mask that fits over the patient's nose and face. An alternative and more

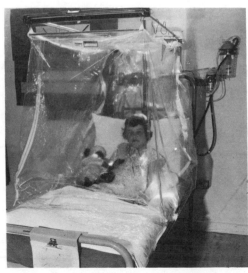

Oxygen tent is an airtight chamber with a raised oxygen composition maintained inside.

Oxyhaemoglobin

comfortable way is to administer oxygen through small plastic tubes inserted into each nostril and held in place by a lightweight apparatus like a pair of spectacles. A patient who requires oxygen therapy for some period of time is generally enclosed in an OXYGEN TENT.

Hyperbaric or high-pressure oxygen therapy is administered in centres that have a special chamber in which oxygen pressure can be increased to about three times normal. It is used in the treatment of gas gangrene and carbon monoxide poisoning, and in some radiotherapy treatments for cancer.

Q: Are there any other situations in which oxygen is used?

A: Yes. Oxygen is administered routinely in most operations as an aid to anaesthesia. It enables the anaesthetist to give a larger dose of an anaesthetic gas, such as nitrous oxide, without the risk of anoxia (lack of oxygen).

Q: Are there hazards in using oxygen?

A: Under medical control there are few hazards. Retrolental fibroplasia, which causes blindness in premature infants, is produced by high oxygen concentration. Also oxygen toxicity is a hazard for both adults and children when a high concentration of oxygen prevents the correct ventilation of the lungs.

Oxyhaemoglobin is a combination of haemoglobin (the red colouring matter in blood) and oxygen. Haemoglobin combines with oxygen in the lungs, and the resultant oxyhaemoglobin carries oxygen to the tissues. Oxyhaemoglobin gives the bright red colour

to arterial blood.

Oxytocin is a hormone that is produced by the HYPOTHALAMUS in the brain and is stored in the rear lobe of the PITUITARY GLAND. It stimulates the womb to contract during childbirth, and also stimulates the breasts to produce milk (lactation). A baby sucking at the nipple causes oxytocin to be released reflexly, which in turn increases lactation.

Oxytocin can be synthesized. Synthetic oxytocin may be given intravenously to induce labour. This is usually done only when labour is unusually slow, and administration of the drug is carefully supervised by an obstetrician. Induction of labour by this method is usually a safe procedure if carried out by an experienced obstetrician. Rarely, however, labour may not begin, or, if too much oxytocin is given, the contractions of the womb may be too strong and may endanger the baby.

Oxyuriasis is infestation with a type of threadworm (Enterobius vermicularis), that thrives in the large intestine. See WORMS.

P

Pacemaker is the area of the heart, called the sinoatrial node, that starts the rhythmical contraction of the heart by an electrical impulse.

See also CARDIAC PACEMAKER.

Paediatrics is the branch of medicine that is concerned with the growth, development, and diseases of children.

Paget's disease of bone, or osteitis deformans, is a bone disorder of unknown cause in which there is a slow progressive thickening of several bones, most often the pelvis, the lower limbs, and the skull. Elderly people are most commonly affected. Most forms of therapy are ineffective, but the condition is seldom severe enough to need treatment.

Q: What are the symptoms of Paget's disease?

A: There may be thickening of the skull, and the leg bones may bend because of gradual softening as well as thickening. Pain may be noticed in the legs. The diagnosis commonly is made during a routine examination of an elderly person, or from the X-ray investigation of some other condition.

Q: Are there any complications of Paget's disease?

A: Yes. Bones affected by Paget's disease fracture more easily than others and, rarely, form osteosarcomas.

See also BONE DISORDERS; HYPERPARA-

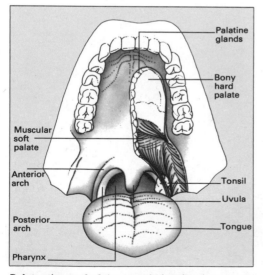

Palate, the roof of the mouth, has hard parts at the front and is soft at the back.

THYROIDISM; LEONTIASIS; MYELOMA; OSTEO-POROSIS; OSTEOSARCOMA.

Paget's disease of the nipple is a rare type of cancer of the mammary ducts. It begins superficially in the ducts, causing the nipple to become red and crust-like. If the condition is discovered and treated before it penetrates beyond the ducts, the survival rate is very high. The treatment is the same as for other types of breast cancer. *See* CANCER.

Pain is a sensation of physical or mental anguish or suffering caused by aggravation of the sensory nerves. The body is seldom able to adjust to pain stimuli, and pain is usually a symptom of inflammation or pressure.

Many pains can be relieved with commercial preparations. However, if a pain persists a doctor should be consulted. Even the most severe pains can be treated with strong ANALGESICS (painkilling drugs).

See also ANAESTHETICS; CORDOTOMY; COLIC; HEADACHE; HYPERAESTHESIA; HYPESTHESIA; MIGRAINE; PHANTOM LIMB; TIC DOULOUREUX.

Painkilling drugs. *See* ANALGESICS.

Palate is the roof of the mouth. It consists of two parts. The front part, the hard palate, is made up of the base of the two upper jawbones (maxillae) and the palatal bones of the skull. The back part, the soft palate, is fleshy and, at its midline, forms a small projection (the uvula). The soft palate consists of muscle. The whole of the palate is covered with a mucous membrane.

See also CLEFT PALATE.

Paleness. *See* PALLOR.

Palliative is a drug or a treatment that relieves the symptoms of a condition without producing a cure.

Pallor, or paleness, is a lack of normal skin colour. It may result from fatigue, cold, low blood pressure, or constriction of the blood vessels in the skin. Pallor may also be a symptom of various disorders such as ANAEMIA, CUSHING'S SYNDROME, and HYPOTHYROIDISM. The pallor of those who are ill is usually caused by the loss of the slight skin pigmentation that normally comes from exposure to the wind and the sun.

See also ALBINO.

Palm is the front part of the hand that extends from the wrist to the bases of the fingers. *See* HAND.

Palpation is a diagnostic method in which the hands are used to make an examination. Self-palpation of the breasts is recommended to women as a method of detecting a lump in the breast while it is still in the early stages of development and, therefore, easier to treat.

Palpitation is a rapid, violent, regular or irregular heartbeat. Palpitations are most commonly caused by anxiety, fear, excessive smoking, or by drinking too much coffee. They may also be caused by heart disease, anaemia, and hyperthyroidism.

See also HEART DISEASE.

Palsy. *See* BELL'S PALSY; CEREBRAL PALSY; PARALYSIS; PARKINSON'S DISEASE.

Pancreas is a large, soft, and irregular gland about 12-15 cm (5–6 inches) long that lies on the back wall of the abdomen, behind the stomach, and extends horizontally from the duodenum to the spleen. The area next to the duodenum is thicker than the rest and commonly is called the head. This is joined to the main part, the body, before reaching the thinner part, the tail, adjacent to the spleen. The pancreas has a large blood supply, mainly from the splenic artery, as well as many nerves from the autonomic nervous system.

Two ducts, the main pancreatic and accessory pancreatic ducts, join together and leave the head of the pancreas to join with the common bile duct just before it penetrates the duodenal wall, forming the ampulla of Vater, protruding into the duodenum.

Q: What are the functions of the pancreas?

A: The main part of the gland produces enzymes essential for digestion. Also lying within the structure of the pancreas are many microscopic areas, the ISLETS OF LANGERHANS, which are part of an endocrine gland manufacturing the hormones insulin and glucagon.

Pancreatic juice contains enzymes, activated by intestinal juice, that digest proteins, carbohydrates, and fats. The pancreatic enzymes trypsin and chymo-

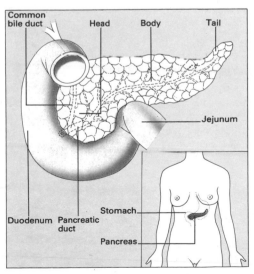

Pancreas is the gland that releases the essential hormone insulin into the blood.

Pancreatic cystic fibrosis

trypsin digest protein; amylase digests starches and other carbohydrates; and lipase changes fats into glycerol and fatty acids. Pancreatic juices are produced partly by nervous stimulation, but mainly as a reaction to hormone secretion in the upper part of the small intestine activated by food from the stomach.

See also CAT SCANNER; CYSTIC FIBROSIS; DIABETES MELLITUS; GLUCAGON; INSULIN.

Pancreatic cystic fibrosis is an inherited disorder that affects the pancreas, lungs, and sweat glands. *See* CYSTIC FIBROSIS.

Pancreatin is a preparation made from the pancreatic enzymes of animals. Pancreatin tablets are prescribed for patients who are unable to digest food properly because of a deficiency in natural pancreatic secretions, which may be caused by disorders of the pancreas, for example, CYSTIC FIBROSIS and PANCREATITIS.

Pancreatitis is an inflammation of the pancreas. It may be acute or chronic.

Q: What are the symptoms of acute pancreatitis?

A: Severe upper abdominal pain, often accompanied by backache, vomiting and fever with the onset of shock are the usual symptoms. The pain may continue for several days, or even weeks, before gradually decreasing. Concentration of the enzyme amylase is frequently increased in the blood and this, accompanied by a high white blood cell count, usually suggests acute pancreatitis.

Q: What causes acute pancreatitis?

A: The cause is often unknown, but it is commonly associated with drinking excessive alcohol. Attacks may also be associated with infection of the gall bladder and bile ducts (cholecystitis). Acute pancreatitis also can be associated with the passage of a gallstone into the duodenum, causing a temporary blockage of the pancreatic duct and back pressure of the enzymes. Damage is caused to the pancreatic cells, and an acute inflammation is set up. This may occur after abdominal surgery, particularly on the stomach or gall bladder. Virus infections, particularly mumps, may start an attack.

Q: How is acute pancreatitis treated?

A: Urgent hospitalization is necessary to confirm the diagnosis.

Treatment includes intravenous infusions, evacuation of the stomach, and large doses of painkilling drugs until the condition improves. Disturbances in the salts, particularly calcium, is probable, so calcium may be added to the infusion. Insulin may have to be given if there is an acute onset of diabetes mellitus. Antibiotics may be administered if there is evidence of bacterial infection.

Acute pancreatitis may recur as further acute attacks or as chronic pancreatitis. It can also be fatal.

Q: What are the symptoms of chronic pancreatitis?

A: The main symptoms are either intermittent or continuous upper abdominal pain of varying intensity and often accompanied by backache. During the moments when pain is most severe, there may be nausea and vomiting. Continued symptoms, caused by increasing damage to the pancreas, reduce the output of the digestive enzymes. This may result in the malabsorption of food, with excessive fat in the faeces (steatorrhoea). Some patients develop diabetes mellitus.

Q: What causes chronic pancreatitis?

A: Chronic pancreatitis may occur as a milder form of acute pancreatitis for the same reasons. But it is also associated with alcoholism, chronic cholecystitis or, less commonly, cancer in the pancreatic duct.

Q: How is chronic pancreatitis treated?

A: Treatment may include removal of the gall bladder (cholecystectomy) if gallstones are thought to be the cause. But, most importantly, the patient must avoid drinking alcohol. Abstention usually is followed by loss of pain and improvement in general health. A low fat diet may be necessary, and PANCREATIN may be given to help digestion. Vitamin

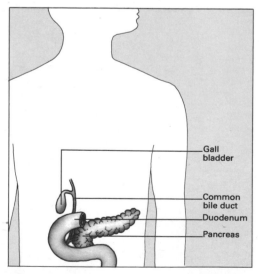

Gall bladder

Common bile duct

Duodenum

Pancreas

Pancreatitis is often associated with infection of the gall bladder.

supplements, especially of folic acid and vitamins A, D, B$_{12}$, and K, are particularly important if malabsorption is taking place.

Pandemic describes any disease, such as malaria, that affects many people over a large region or continent. *See also* EPIDEMIC.

Panophthalmitis is an inflammation of the entire eye. It can be a complication of any serious eye disorder, such as choroiditis, or result from infection following an eye injury. Panophthalmitis requires immediate treatment, or blindness may result.

Papilla is a small protuberance from the surface of a tissue. Papillae occur in many parts of the body. They are particularly numerous on the surface of the tongue, where specialized papillae contain the taste buds.

Papilloedema is an eye disorder in which the optic nerve is swollen and inflamed at the point where it joins the eye. The causes include: (1) any condition, such as a tumour, aneurysm (swelling of an artery) or subarachnoid haemorrhage, that causes an increase of pressure within the skull; or (2) certain medical conditions such as a sudden dangerously high blood pressure, meningitis or lead poisoning. Treatment of papilloedema is directed at the cause.

Papilloma is a benign (noncancerous) tumour of the skin, mucous membranes, or glandular ducts. Small papillomas may occur in the ducts of the breast and cause bleeding from the nipple. Chronic laryngitis may cause papillomas to grow on the vocal cords. In some people, multiple papillomas occur on the skin around the neck and armpits.

See also WART.

Pap test, or Papanicolaou test, is a procedure carried out for the early detection and diagnosis of cancer cells in the cervix of the womb. *See* CANCER; CERVICAL SMEAR.

Papule is a small, solid, raised spot on the skin. *See* RASH.

Paracentesis is a minor surgical procedure in which a needle is passed into a body cavity to remove fluid. It is usually performed under a local anaesthetic for diagnostic purposes, or to remove excess fluid.

Paracetamol is a mild pain-relieving (analgesic) and fever-reducing (antipyretic) drug. Its effects are similar to those of aspirin, although paracetamol is less effective in treating inflammation and rheumatic conditions. It does not produce some of the undesirable side effects that aspirin may cause, such as internal bleeding, but an overdose can cause liver damage, and kidney damage may result from prolonged large doses. Paracetamol should therefore not be used by patients with a disorder of the liver or kidneys.

Paraesthesia is a sensation, such as a tingling or disordered sensation of heat and cold that occurs without an apparent cause. It may be caused by nerve damage, either from pressure or NEURITIS, or by stroke in which part of the brain is damaged.

Paragonimiasis is infestation with small parasitic flukes of the genus *Paragonimus,* which form cysts in the lungs. Humans become infested by eating raw or undercooked crabs that contain larval flukes. When in human beings, the larval flukes usually migrate to the lungs by penetrating the intestine and the diaphragm. In the lungs the larval flukes grow into mature adults and produce eggs. Some of the larval flukes may mature in other parts of the body, such as the abdomen or the brain.

Q: *What are the symptoms of paragonimiasis?*

A: The major symptoms include persistent spitting of blood, breathlessness, and chest pains. There may also be clubbing of the fingers.

Q: *How is paragonimiasis treated?*

A: Treatment with drugs that kill the flukes is effective in most cases, but surgery may be needed to remove some of the adult flukes.

Paralysis is the temporary or permanent loss of the ability to move either a limb or the whole body, usually also accompanied by a loss of sensation. Paralysis is generally the result of muscle or nerve disturbance.

Q: *How does nerve disturbance cause paralysis?*

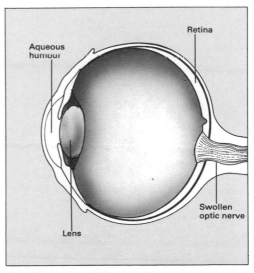

Papilloedema is swelling and inflammation of the optic nerve where it enters the eyeball.

Paralysis agitans

A: Usually paralysis is caused by damage to a peripheral (surface) nerve or to the central nervous system. The results of damage to a peripheral nerve are different from those due to damage to the central nervous system, brain, and spinal cord. Weakness may be caused by muscle disease.

Damage to a peripheral nerve causes complete loss of ability to move that muscle, or muscles, and consequent wasting away. Damage to the central nervous system produces weakness or loss of use of a group of muscles, such as those of an arm or leg, but without wasting away. The affected muscles may make the limb feel stiff, if it is forcibly moved, because of an increased tone. This is known as spasticity.

Q: How is paralysis treated?

A: Treatment depends on the cause and can be started only when a doctor and a neurologist have made a diagnosis.

Physiotherapy can be employed to train muscles that can still move and to maintain a full range of movement of joints, as well as to prevent stiffness. This may be helped by the use of electrical equipment, such as shortwave diathermy (high-frequency heat treatment) and hydrotherapy pools.

Paralysis of speech may require speech therapy, but if swallowing is involved a tracheotomy may be necessary in order to insert a tube into the windpipe.

Peripheral nerve injuries can be helped by nerve transplants, orthopaedic opera-

tions to immobilize a joint (arthrodesis), or the transplant of the tendon of a working muscle to aid paralyzed muscles.

See also BABINSKI'S REFLEX; BULBAR PARALYSIS; CEREBRAL HAEMORRHAGE; CEREBRAL PALSY; DYSARTHRIA; DYSPHAGIA; EXTRADURAL HAEMATOMA; HEMIPARESIS; MENINGIOMA; MOTOR NEURON DISEASE; MULTIPLE SCLEROSIS; MUSCLE; MYASTHENIA GRAVIS; NEUROLOGICAL DISORDERS; NEUROMA; PALSY; POLIOMYELITIS; POLYNEURITIS; STROKE; SUB-ARACHNOID HAEMORRHAGE; SYRINGOMYELIA.

Paralysis agitans. *See* PARKINSON'S DISEASE.

Paralytic ileus is a form of intestinal obstruction caused by paralysis of the muscles of the intestinal wall. It is a failure of the normal muscular contractions (peristalsis) that pass food along inside the intestine. The abdomen becomes swollen, and this condition results in symptoms of constipation, abdominal pain, and vomiting.

Q: What conditions produce a paralytic ileus?

A: A paralytic ileus most commonly occurs as a result of disturbance to nerves and tissue unavoidable in an abdominal operation. But it can also occur with peritonitis and severe chemical upsets, such as those coinciding with kidney failure, diabetic coma, and extreme loss of body potassium salts accompanying diarrhoea or associated with an operation. It may also be the result of disturbance to the autonomic nervous system associated with an injury to the spine; of drugs used to prevent spasm; or of treatment for high blood pressure.

Q: How is a paralytic ileus treated?

A: Hospitalization is necessary. The patient's stomach is kept empty with a tube to prevent further vomiting and is given intravenous fluids to supply necessary salts, water, and glucose. After two to three days, peristalsis restarts and the patient can be allowed to sip fluid before returning to a normal diet within the next three or four days.

See also ILEUS.

Paranoia. *See* MENTAL ILLNESS.

Paraphimosis is a condition in which the foreskin of the penis is retracted and cannot be returned to its normal position. It occurs when the foreskin is inflamed (*see* BALANITIS) so that the normal circulation of blood is constricted. As a result, the bulbous end of the penis (glans penis) becomes swollen and painful.

Q: How is paraphimosis treated?

A: With the patient under a general anaesthetic, the foreskin usually can be pulled back into position quite easily.

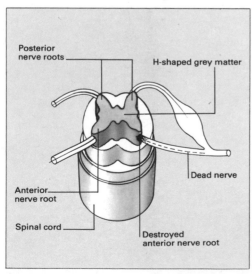

Paralysis may result from the destruction of anterior nerve roots in the spinal cord.

However, it is probably best if the surgeon performs a circumcision to prevent the condition from recurring.

See also PHIMOSIS.

Paraplegia is paralysis of the lower half of the body. It is usually caused by injury, damage, or disease of the spinal cord. *See* PARALYSIS.

Paraquat is an extremely poisonous herbicide. If it is swallowed, emergency medical treatment is needed to prevent damage to the heart, lungs, and kidneys, which may be fatal.

Parasite is any organism that lives at the expense of another (host) organism. Ectoparasites, such as lice, fleas, and mites, live on the outside of their hosts. Endoparasites, such as flukes and intestinal worms, live within their hosts. Some parasites carry, or themselves cause, diseases.

See also ENTAMOEBA HISTOLYTICA; FLUKES; GIARDIASIS; WORMS.

Parasympathetic nervous system is one of the two divisions of the AUTONOMIC NERVOUS SYSTEM; the other division is the SYMPATHETIC NERVOUS SYSTEM. Parasympathetic nerve fibres occur in some of the cranial nerves of the brain, and in the sacral nerves of the lower end of the spinal cord. Parasympathetic nerves connect with many parts of the body, including the eyes, the internal organs, and the intestines. The effects of the parasympathetic nervous system include constriction of the pupils, slowing of the heart rate, contraction of the bladder, increasing the rate of digestion, and constriction of the bronchi.

See also VASOMOTOR RHINITIS.

Parathormone is the hormone produced by the parathyroid glands. It controls the level of calcium in the blood and, indirectly, reduces the level of phosphate. It works by releasing calcium from the bones, increasing calcium absorption from food in the intestine, and reducing calcium excretion by the kidneys. At the same time, the excretion of phosphate from the body is also increased. The rise in the calcium level reduces the secretion of parathormone. This "feedback" mechanism has the effect of maintaining a constant level of calcium in the blood.

Parathyroid glands secrete PARATHORMONE, which controls the level of calcium in the blood. The four parathyroid glands are embedded, two on each side, in the thyroid gland tissue situated in the lower part of the front of the neck.

Q: Can anything go wrong with the parathyroid glands?

A: Yes. Lack of parathormone (hypoparathyroidism) often occurs if the parathyroid glands are accidentally damaged or removed during a partial THYROIDECTOMY. More rarely, the parathyroid glands

fail to secrete parathormone, or there may be resistance of the body tissues to the stimulating action of parathormone. Excessive secretion of parathormone (hyperparathyroidism) may also occur for no obvious reason.

Q: What are the symptoms of hypoparathyroidism?

A: Lack of parathormone (hypoparathyroidism) leads to an abnormally low level of calcium in the blood (hypocalcaemia), the major symptom of which is TETANY. This is a condition in which there is twitching and spasm of the muscles. *See* CALCIUM.

Q: What are the symptoms of hyperparathyroidism?

A: Excess production of parathormone (hyperparathyroidism) leads to a high level of calcium in the blood, and a serious drainage of calcium from the bones. Symptoms include weakness, nausea, and constipation. These may be accompanied by thirst and the frequent passing of urine.

Kidney stones (nephrolithiasis) are a common complication, and bone disorders with the formation of cysts may develop if the condition is not treated.

Q: How is hyperparathyroidism treated?

A: After a careful assessment and diagnosis has been made by a doctor, a surgeon may be asked to operate and remove the parathyroid gland.

Paratyphoid is a form of enteric fever that is caused by certain bacteria of the genus *Salmonella*. For symptoms and treatment of

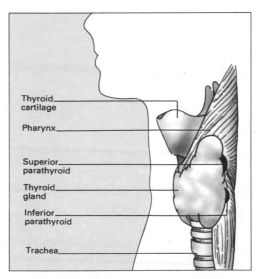

Thyroid cartilage

Pharynx

Superior parathyroid

Thyroid gland

Inferior parathyroid

Trachea

Parathyroid glands are embedded within the tissue of the thyroid gland in the throat.

Paresis

paratyphoid, *see* TYPHOID FEVER.

Paresis is weakness of the muscles. It may be caused by damage to the central nervous system. *See* PARALYSIS.

Parietal describes the two parietal bones which form the roof and sides of the skull. Parietal also describes the wall of a body cavity; for example, the parietal pleura is the membrane that lines the chest wall.

Parkinson's disease is a chronic disorder of the nervous system characterized by tremors, slow movements, and generalized body stiffness. It occurs most commonly in the middle-aged and elderly. Parkinson's disease does not affect mental faculties, although these may appear to be impaired if the patient's speech is affected. The disease is also known as paralysis agitans or shaking palsy, and is named after the English physician James Parkinson (1755–1824). Parkinsonism is the term that denotes the symptoms of Parkinson's disease.

The cause of Parkinson's disease itself often is not known, although parkinsonism may be caused by several factors. In some patients, parkinsonism is thought to be caused by arteriosclerosis, in which there is degeneration of the brain cells that control body movements. Parkinsonism also may be caused by encephalitis; a brain tumour; brain damage; or poisoning, either from drugs such as reserpine, or from chemicals such as manganese and carbon monoxide.

Q: *What are the symptoms of Parkinson's disease?*

A: The onset of symptoms usually is gradual and their progress is slow. The initial

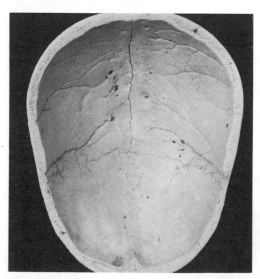

Parietal bones are the two bones that form the sides and roof of part of the skull.

symptoms include an occasional trembling of one hand and increasing clumsiness of the same arm. As the disorder progresses, both sides of the body become affected, movements become slow and stiff, and the patient may drool. The face assumes a blank and mask-like expression, with the eyes fixed and unblinking, because of rigid face muscles. Speech may also be impaired.

In the later stages there may be continual hand tremors with "pill rolling" movement of the fingers, the arms may be held in a bent position, and the body may be bent forward in a permanent stoop. The patient also may walk slowly with shuffling steps, and then start to run to prevent falling forward. This characteristic gait is called festination. The patient's handwriting may become small and illegible, and speech may become so slurred as to be unintelligible.

Q: *How is Parkinson's disease treated?*

A: There is as yet no cure, but the symptoms can be controlled in many cases. Drug treatment with levodopa (L-dopa), particularly when combined with carbidopa, can control the symptoms in some patients and enable them to resume a normal life for several years. Some patients respond to treatment with the drug amantadine, either by itself or combined with L-dopa.

If treatment with L-dopa or amantadine is ineffective, atropine-like drugs may be used. However, these tend to cause adverse side effects, such as constipation, a dry mouth, and retention of urine.

Occasionally, the surgical destruction of a small area of the brain may alleviate the symptoms. Such surgery usually is effective against the tremors.

Paronychia is inflammation of the skin that surrounds a nail. The affected area becomes red and swollen, and may discharge pus. Acute paronychia may be caused by a bacterial infection, often with staphylococcus, or by a viral infection, usually with the herpes simplex virus. Chronic paronychia occurs most commonly in those who have their hands in water for long periods of time. It is usually caused by monilia, which is a fungal infection. Chronic paronychia may damage the nail bed, which may result in distorted, ridged nails.

Q: *How is paronychia treated?*

A: The treatment of acute paronychia usually involves a combination of antibiotics and minor surgery, in which the inflamed area is drained of pus.

Paronychia that is caused by a viral infection usually responds to treatment with antiviral drugs that are applied directly onto the affected area. Chronic paronychia may be treated with anti-fungal creams. It is advisable to keep the hands dry by wearing rubber gloves when the hands are in water.

Parotid gland. *See* SALIVARY GLANDS.

Parotitis is an inflammation of the parotid glands, the salivary glands in the neck, in front of the ears. It is most commonly caused by MUMPS, but may occur with any virus infection of the salivary glands. It also can be caused by a bacterial infection resulting from a stone in the salivary duct (sialolithiasis) or by mouth infections (stomatitis), particularly in elderly people who are seriously ill and dehydrated. *See* SALIVARY GLANDS.

Paroxysm is a sudden increase in severity of the symptoms of a disease. The term also is used to denote a sudden spasm or convulsion.

Paroxysmal tachycardia is a sudden increase in the heart rate, for no obvious reason, to 150-200 beats a minute. The average rate during an attack is around 180. A large quantity of urine may be passed afterwards.

Q: What causes paroxysmal tachycardia?

A: Frequently the cause is not known, but the origin seems to be a sudden increase in the number of electrical stimuli starting the atrium of the heart, producing a rapid, regular contraction of the ventricles. This may occur in young people without any sign of heart disease, but arteriosclerosis is usually the cause in elderly people.

Q: How is paroxysmal tachycardia treated?

A: An acute attack should be treated by a doctor, but hospitalization may be necessary. Recurrent attacks may require treatment with drugs, and some patients are taught to hold their breath while trying to breathe out. This may stop an attack.

See also TACHYCARDIA.

Parrot fever. *See* PSITTACOSIS.

Parturition is another word for childbirth. *See* PREGNANCY AND CHILDBIRTH.

Patch test is a skin test that is used to identify the specific cause of an allergy. A small amount of the suspected causative agent (allergen) is applied to the skin and covered with adhesive tape, which is removed after two days. If the skin is red and swollen, the patient is allergic to the substance that was applied.

Patella, or kneecap, is a small, disc-shaped bone about 5cm (2 inches) in diameter that lies in the tendon of the quadriceps femoris muscle in front of the knee joint. The inner

surface that forms the front of the knee joint is covered by cartilage.

Q: What disorders can affect the patella?

A: Softening of the cartilage (chondro-malacia) may occur in young adults, causing an aching pain deep in the knee, which is made worse by walking. This usually heals without treatment.

Recurrent dislocation of the patella usually starts in adolescence when the individual keeps the knee slightly bent for too long and the patella slips sideways, causing severe pain and an inability to straighten the leg. The patella usually can be relocated without a general anaesthetic. Recurring dislocations can be cured by surgically repositioning the tendon.

The tendon of the patella also can rupture, usually because of some violent exercise, and requires surgery to stitch it back into place. In the same way, a fracture of the patella may occur. Treatment depends partly on the severity of the fracture and partly on the age of the patient.

See also KNEE PROBLEMS.

Pathogen is any organism or substance that can cause a disease.

Pathognomonic describes anything that is typical of a particular disease. *See* SYMPTOMS.

Pathology is the study of the changes that occur in the body as the result of a disorder, with particular reference to the underlying cause.

PCP. *See* PHENCYCLIDINE.

Pectoral refers to the chest.

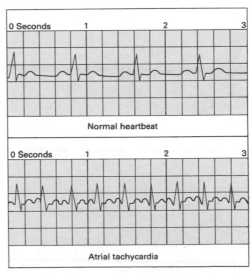

Paroxysmal tachycardia can increase a normal heartbeat of 80 to 180 beats per minute.

Pediculosis

Pediculosis is an infestation with lice. *See* LICE.

Pellagra is a deficiency disease that is caused by a lack of niacin (nicotinic acid), one of the vitamin B complex. Pellagra most commonly occurs in those whose staple diet is corn. Pellagra also may result from alcoholism; CIRRHOSIS of the liver; and malabsorption of food, which is often caused by chronic diarrhoea.

Q: What are the symptoms of pellagra?

A: Initial symptoms include a smooth, red tongue, a sore mouth, and ulceration of the inside of the cheeks. The skin on the neck, chest, and back of the hands may become brown and scaly. Often there is nausea, vomiting, and diarrhoea. There may also be insomnia, depression, confusion, and rapid changes of mood.

Q: How is pellagra treated?

A: Pellagra is treated by giving a balancing diet with niacin supplements.

Pelvimetry is measurement of the dimensions of the pelvis, either by physical examination or by X-rays or by both. Pelvimetry is used to determine whether the pelvis is wide enough for normal childbirth.

Pelvis is a basin-shaped cavity. There are two such cavities in the body. The pelvis of the kidney collects urine and funnels it into the ureter, the tube that leads to the bladder (*see* KIDNEY). But the term pelvis usually refers to bones in the lower part of the body that support the spine and connect to the legs at the hip joints.

The pelvis consists of two hip-bones, each composed of the pubis, ilium, and the ischium. These join in front of the pubic bone (symphysis pubis) and are attached at the back to the sacrum by the two sacroiliac joints. The coccyx, a small bone at the lower end of the spinal column, is attached to the sacrum.

The wide wings of the two hip-bones form the upper extremities of the pelvis and are known as the false pelvis. They sweep down to a narrower part called the true pelvis.

A female's pelvis is wider than a male's, and the entrance to the true pelvis is usually circular in shape. This allows childbirth to take place with ease.

Q: What structures does the pelvis contain?

A: The side walls of the pelvis contain muscles that help movement of the thighs. The bottom of the pelvis is made up of ligaments and muscles (the pelvic floor) that support the bladder and rectum and, in a female, the vagina and womb. The false pelvis supports the large and small intestine, which intertwine above the contents of the true pelvis.

Pemphigus is the general name for a variety of skin diseases characterized by successive outbreaks of large, fluid-filled blisters. It can result from a type of IMPETIGO caused by a staphylococcal infection.

In adults there are two rare forms of pemphigus that may be a form of AUTOIMMUNE DISEASE. They produce blisters in the mouth and on exposed mucous membrane, as well as on the skin.

It is difficult to distinguish between pemphigus and a similar disorder called pemphigoid, which occurs mainly in the elderly and produces itching of the skin followed by blistering.

Q: How are pemphigus and pemphigoid treated?

A: Pemphigus due to impetigo is treated with antibiotics, but the general treatment of other forms of pemphigus and pemphigoid is with corticosteroids to relieve and control the symptoms. Both diseases are, at present, incurable.

Penicillin is one of a group of antibiotics that once were extracted from moulds of the genus *Penicillium,* but now are synthesized. The basic penicillin is called penicillin G.

Over-use of penicillins can result in their becoming ineffective because of the development of resistant bacterial strains. But, penicillin G is still effective against many of the common bacterial infections, and it can be modified to produce a number of more effective penicillins, such as ampicillin, amoxycillin, and cloxacillin. Some of these derivatives are effective against a wider range of organisms than is penicillin G, and some

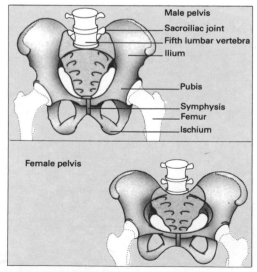

Male pelvis
Sacroiliac joint
Fifth lumbar vertebra
Ilium
Pubis
Symphysis
Femur
Ischium

Female pelvis

Pelvis of a woman is wider than a man's and the opening is shaped for easy childbirth.

are effective against bacteria that have developed a resistance to penicillin G.

Q: *How do penicillins work?*

A: The penicillins work mainly by killing bacteria while the bacteria are multiplying, but penicillins also inhibit the growth of bacteria to some extent.

Q: *Can the penicillins produce adverse side effects?*

A: Yes. All of the penicillins carry the risk of producing allergic reactions. However, these usually do not occur until a patient has had several courses of penicillin treatment. An allergic reaction may produce skin rashes, swelling of the throat, fever, and swelling of the joints. Rarely, ANAPHYLAXIS may occur, which may be fatal.

People who are allergic to one type of penicillin are allergic to all types, and usually to a similar group of antibiotics, the cephalosporins. Such people should warn their doctors so that other antibiotics are prescribed instead.

Penis is the male organ used for passing urine and for sexual intercourse. It is cylindrical in shape and is attached by its base to the front and sides of the pubic arch.

Q: *How is the penis constructed?*

A: The urethra, the tube for the passage of urine or semen, is surrounded by special tissue and ends in an external swelling called the glans. It lies on top of two tubular and honeycomb-like areas of erectile tissue. The glans at the end of the penis is particularly sensitive and, in an uncircumcised penis, is covered by a protective FORESKIN.

Q: *How does the penis function as a sexual organ?*

A: The erectile tissue becomes distended with blood, thus making the penis erect and hard. The blood is unable to drain out through the veins due to their being temporarily closed by special muscles. An erection results from physical or psychological sexual stimulation, and it enables the male to insert the erect penis into the female's vagina during sexual intercourse. It is at the stage of greatest sexual excitement (orgasm) that the semen is released into the vagina.

An erection ceases when the veins open so that the blood is able to flow back into the general circulation of the body.

Q: *What disorders can affect the penis?*

A: Inflammation of the glans (balanitis) may cause narrowing of the foreskin (phimosis) or cause it to act in a constrictive manner if it is pulled back (paraphimosis). *See* BALANITIS.

Venereal diseases, such as the chancre of syphilis or chancroid, form ulcers or cause infections of the urethra (urethritis). *See* GONORRHOEA; NONSPECIFIC URETHRITIS.

Small cysts (sebaceous cysts) may form on the skin of the penis and occasionally cancer can occur. On rare occasions, erections may be prolonged and painful (priapism).

Q: *How is cancer of the penis recognized and treated?*

A: Cancer of the penis occurs most commonly in elderly males who have not been circumcised and whose low standard of personal hygiene has caused repeated mild attacks of balanitis. A small ulcer that bleeds easily is the first sign that cancer may be present.

Cancer of the penis is treated either by amputating the end of the penis, or by radiotherapy.

See also CIRCUMCISION.

Pep pills are drugs that contain amphetamine. They produce a feeling of well-being and excitement, but are addictive. *See* AMPHETAMINES; DRUG ADDICTION; METHAMPHETAMINE; STIMULANTS.

Pepsin is an enzyme that starts the digestion of proteins in the stomach by breaking down the large protein molecules into smaller molecules, called peptides. In the small intestine, the peptides are further broken down by other enzymes into molecules (amino acids) that are small enough to be used by the body.

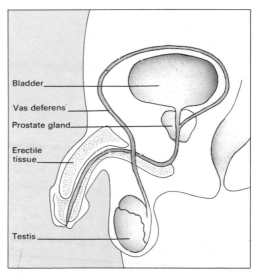

Penis is the outlet both for urine and, during sexual intercourse, for semen.

Peptic ulcer

Peptic ulcer is an eroded area in the stomach (when it is called a gastric ulcer) or in the first part of the duodenum (a duodenal ulcer). Peptic ulcers are caused by the combined action of pepsin and hydrochloric acid in the digestive juices of the stomach. They are more common in men than in women.

Q: *Why do peptic ulcers occur?*

A: Acute peptic ulcers occur suddenly, and usually are the result of an excess of alcohol, aspirin, or other drugs.

Sometimes they are called "stress ulcers," because they are considered to be related to periods of intense stress, such as those occurring with shock, severe burns, or accidents. This form of peptic ulcer heals rapidly.

Chronic peptic ulcers develop slowly and for a variety of reasons. It seems likely that there is an alteration in the normal protective action of the mucus and its underlying cells that prevents digestive juices from digesting the stomach itself. Why this occurs is often not known, but it is possible that continued anxiety and smoking in an individual with an inherited tendency to form ulcers can cause a peptic ulcer. The condition is made worse by certain drugs.

Q: *Can peptic ulcers occur in places other than the stomach and duodenum?*

A: Yes. Acid-secreting cells in a MECKEL'S DIVERTICULUM can become active, sometimes producing a peptic ulcer.

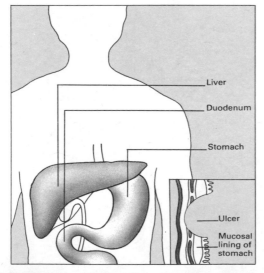

Peptic ulcer may affect the mucosal lining of the stomach, or occur in the duodenum.

Liver

Duodenum

Stomach

Ulcer

Mucosal lining of stomach

Peptic ulceration also may develop in the small intestine after a gastroenterostomy has been performed for a peptic ulcer. Or an ulcer may form in the lower end of the oesophagus (gullet) in a patient with a HIATUS HERNIA.

Q: *How is a peptic ulcer diagnosed?*

A: A barium meal test (*see* BARIUM) is the usual way of diagnosing a peptic ulcer; it reveals an ulcer, if it is present, in more than 90 per cent of patients. Endoscopy, using a FIBRESCOPE, can be done and a biopsy (sample of tissue for analysis) taken to exclude the possibility of cancer if this is suspected or if an ulcer is taking a long time to heal. The duodenum can also be examined, and this may detect an ulcer not revealed by a barium X-ray.

Q: *What are the symptoms of a peptic ulcer?*

A: Pain in the abdomen is the most common symptom of a peptic ulcer, but its frequency varies. There may be long periods when the ulcer is active and symptoms are present, followed by several months during which there are no symptoms.

The pain of peptic ulcer usually is high in the abdomen and often is described as a gnawing, deep ache accompanied by a feeling of hunger or nausea. It is relieved by taking bland food, milk, or ANTACID drugs, but is made worse by alcohol and by fried or spicy foods.

Pain from duodenal ulcer starts about two hours after a meal and is relieved by antacids or more food. The pain commonly wakens the patient in the night, and the symptoms go on for several weeks before gradually disappearing.

A gastric ulcer may be aggravated by eating, because of the sudden production of acid in the stomach, although the pain seldom wakens the patient. Pain may be relieved by vomiting.

These are the typical symptoms, but there is a great variation. In the elderly, pain may persist without relief from food or anticids.

Q: *How is a peptic ulcer treated?*

A: Most patients can be treated at home. Frequent small meals and snacks keep the stomach full, helping to absorb the acid.

For many years, a variety of strict diets, usually containing bland foods and milk, were used; the patient was advised to avoid coffee, tea and cola drinks. But these regimens are no longer essential: modern medical treatment is effective and patients have far fewer restrictions upon what they eat and drink. Fried foods are often blamed for ulcer pain because they increase the secretion of acid by the stomach. Some drinks, particularly alcohol, aggravate the symptoms.

Smoking should be prohibited. Any drugs that are known to aggravate peptic ulceration should, if possible, be stopped. Antacids and drugs to prevent gastric secretion and reduce the speed of emptying the stomach also are effective. Cimetidine reduces gastric secretion and produces rapid relief of symptoms with healing of the ulcer. Carbenoxolone, another type of drug, gives rapid improvement of symptoms. Tranquillizers are sometimes used to reduce stress and tension, and sleeping pills given to ensure a good night's sleep.

Hospitalization is rarely necessary; the pain, in most patients, is usually relieved by the use of drugs and bed rest at home. Admission to hospital is needed only if the family doctor or the specialist considers that complications such as pyloric stenosis, bleeding, or ulceration into the pancreas, causing continuous pain, is occurring.

Surgery (vagotomy or partial GAS-TRECTOMY) may be performed if the ulcer produces complications.

Q: *Can complications occur with a peptic ulcer?*

A: Yes. One complication of peptic ulcer is pyloric stenosis, an obstruction of the exit of the stomach. Pyloric stenosis results from a combination of scarring at the exit of the stomach or first part of the duodenum and inflammation produced by an active ulcer. Vomiting of large volumes of fluid, often with food from the previous day, is a common symptom. In severer cases, a partial gastrectomy is needed (*see* PYLORIC STENOSIS).

Bleeding is a common complication of peptic ulcer and the patient may vomit blood (haematemesis) or produce the dark black stools of melaena. Sudden massive blood loss causes weakness and fainting, and all patients who experience this symptom should be hospitalized. Blood transfusion, bed rest, and antacid drugs form the initial stage of treatment but, if the bleeding continues, emergency surgery may be necessary.

Another complication of a peptic ulcer is continuous pain. Pain may be constant and severe, often producing intense backache, if the ulcer penetrates through the stomach wall to involve the pancreas or liver. Medicinal treatment seldom is effective and surgery must be performed.

A peptic ulcer may perforate, suddenly producing severe, intense abdominal pain, often spreading to the shoulders and sometimes accompanied by vomiting. It is a form of PERITONITIS and requires immediate surgery.

Percussion is a diagnostic procedure in which a doctor places a finger over the part of the body to be examined and taps it sharply with a finger of the other hand. The sound and sensation felt enables a doctor to determine the size, position, and consistency of underlying body structures.

Physiotherapists may use a slightly different technique of percussion to vibrate the underlying tissues. This technique can help to free excessive mucus, so that it can be coughed up by the patient.

Perforation is a hole that is made in a part of the body, or the process of making such a hole as part of a surgical procedure.

Perfusion is a technique in which fluid is passed through a blood vessel or a part of the body, either for investigating or for treating a disorder. Occasionally, the terms perfusion and infusion are used interchangeably.

Perfusion may be used in the treatment of some types of cancer, such as cancer of the liver. A special CATHETER is passed along an artery to the area involved, and cancer-killing (cytoxic) drugs are perfused through the catheter. This technique allows a high concentration of a drug to be introduced to a localized area.

Periarteritis nodosa. *See* POLYARTERITIS NODOSA.

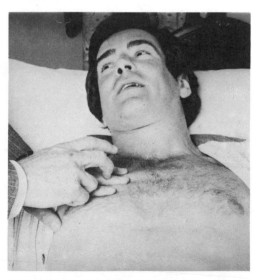

Percussion is a procedure commonly used in examinations of the heart and lungs.

Pericarditis

Pericarditis is an inflammation of the membranous sac that surrounds the heart (pericardium). A wide variety of disorders may cause pericarditis. It may be associated with RHEUMATOID ARTHRITIS, systemic LUPUS ERYTHEMATOSUS, and URAEMIA. It also may occur as a complication of cancer of adjacent structures, such as the lungs or oesophagus. Usually however, pericarditis occurs without an apparent cause.

Q: What are the symptoms of pericarditis and how is it treated?

A: In most cases, there is pain in the centre of the chest, which may vary in intensity and which may be worsened by movement or coughing. Other common symptoms of pericarditis include fever, breathlessness, coughing, and a rapid pulse rate. The treatment of pericarditis is directed toward the underlying cause. In the early stages of the disorder, painkillers are usually prescribed. Antibiotics may be necessary if pericarditis is caused by an infection. Various other treatments may be necessary if complications develop.

Q: Can pericarditis cause complications?

A: Yes. The most common complication is an accumulation of fluid in the pericardium. This causes pressure on the heart and a rapid pulse rate. One type of pericarditis, called constrictive pericarditis, causes scarring and thickening of the pericardium. This may result in progressive heart failure, with increasing breathlessness, enlargement of the liver, and OEDEMA.

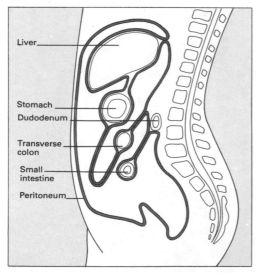

Liver

Stomach
Dudodenum

Transverse colon

Small intestine

Peritoneum

Peritoneum allows movement of the internal organs within its lubricated folds.

Pericardium is the bag-like structure that surrounds the heart. It consists of two layers, between which is a small amount of fluid. This fluid enables the heart to beat almost without friction. The inner layer of the pericardium is soft and membranous. The outer layer is thicker and fibrous, and helps to protect the heart.

Perimetry is a method of examining the area the eye can see (visual field) when it is focused on a central point. This point is marked in the middle of a blank screen. A small light or disc is moved inward from many points on the edge of the screen, and the point where the patient first sees it is charted.

Perinephric describes any tissues that surround the kidney.

Perineum is the area between the anus and the lower edge of the pubis at the front of the pelvis. In a female, it includes the opening of the vagina and the surrounding vulva, as well as the firm fibrous tissue area between the back of the vagina and the anal opening. In a male, the area is composed of the fibrous tissue behind the bag of skin that contains the testicles (scrotum). The tissue of the perineum heals easily. This is particularly important in a woman following childbirth, when the tissues may be damaged or deliberately cut (episiotomy) to enable the baby's head to pass through.

Periodontitis is a gum condition in which the mucous membrane, gums, and underlying bone become thin, and the teeth become loose. It usually follows an infection of the gums (GINGIVITIS).

Q: What are the symptoms of periodontitis?

A: Apart from loose teeth, the gums are swollen and there is often a discharge of pus from around one or more of the teeth. The breath smells foul (halitosis).

Q: How is the condition treated?

A: Skilled dental care is needed to remove the tartar from the teeth and treat the gingivitis. Improved oral hygiene, with regular brushing of the teeth, is necessary to avoid a recurrence of the condition.

Period pain. *See* DYSMENORRHOEA.

Periods. *See* MENSTRUATION.

Periosteum is a thin, fibrous membrane that covers the entire surface of the bones, except at the joints. It consists of a dense outer layer that contains nerves and blood vessels, and an inner layer which contains cells that help to form new bone. The periosteum plays an essential part in bone nutrition and healing.

Periostitis is an inflammation of the membrane that covers the bones (periosteum). It may occur after a bone fracture when the healing break becomes infected. It is usually caused by an infection of the bone, such as OSTEOMYELITIS; or, rarely, by SYPHILIS.

Peripheral means situated at the outer part of an organ or structure.

Peristalsis is a series of involuntary muscle contractions that move food along the intestines. In the stomach, peristalsis produces a churning action aiding digestion. Occasionally, reverse peristalsis may occur, causing vomiting.

Peritoneum is the membrane that lines the abdominal cavity and surrounds the abdominal organs, such as the intestines, liver, spleen, womb, and bladder. In some places it forms the MESENTERY, which supports the intestines. The peritoneum also secretes a fluid that lubricates the abdominal organs.

Peritonitis is an inflammation of the peritoneum, the membrane that lines the abdominal cavity. It usually accompanies an infection but, rarely, it may occur with conditions such as rheumatoid arthritis and disseminated lupus erythematosus.

Q: What causes peritonitis?

A: Peritonitis most commonly is caused by infection of an abdominal organ, such as appendicitis, cholecystitis, or diverticulitis, or following perforation of a peptic ulcer or inflamed appendix. It may be associated with SALPINGITIS or following an abdominal operation.

Q: What are the symptoms of peritonitis?

A: The chief symptom is severe generalized abdominal pain, in which the patient wants to lie still and may complain of aching shoulders caused by referred pain from an irritated diaphragm. Usually there is a fever and a rapid pulse rate. Vomiting often occurs as the result of the onset of a PARALYTIC ILEUS.

Q: How is peritonitis treated?

A: The patient is hospitalized and treatment is started with intravenous fluids, and antibiotics given in the infusion. Emptying of the stomach through a nasogastric tube is usually needed.

A surgical operation is required if a cause such as appendicitis or ruptured peptic ulcer is found.

Q: Are there any possible complications of peritonitis?

A: Yes. If treatment is not started immediately, death may result.

An abscess may form in the pelvis, particularly following salpingitis, or under the diaphragm (subphrenic abscess). Both may require surgical draining after the initial stage of peritonitis has settled.

Tuberculous peritonitis always develops because of tuberculosis elsewhere in the body. It may begin like acute peritonitis, but the onset is usually more gradual, with an increasing amount of fluid (similar to ascites). It requires antituberculous treatment.

Peritonsillar abscess. *See* QUINSY.

Pernicious anaemia, or Addison's anaemia, is a condition that results from a failure of the body to absorb vitamin B_{12}. It occurs because of a deficiency of a special substance (called an intrinsic factor) secreted by the stomach. The intrinsic factor normally combines with the extrinsic factor, vitamin B_{12}, to form a substance that can be absorbed by the body.

Q: What are the symptoms of pernicious anaemia?

A: The symptoms commonly are the combination of a slow onset of ANAEMIA, with tiredness, slight breathlessness, and a sore, red tongue. There may be symptoms of peripheral neuritis as well as loss of position sense and a slight staggering gait. Depression and mental disturbances suggestive of paranoia also may occur.

Q: How is pernicious anaemia treated?

A: Once the diagnosis has been made, treatment with injections of vitamin B_{12} produces a cure. The injections have to be continued on a monthly basis for the rest of the patient's life.

Patients with pernicious anaemia have a much greater chance of developing cancer of the stomach, and so a barium meal X-ray or gastroscopy (examination of the stomach) should be performed on all patients at the onset of treatment and repeated at regular intervals.

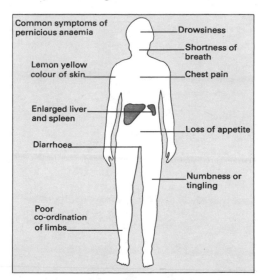

Common symptoms of pernicious anaemia

Drowsiness

Shortness of breath

Lemon yellow colour of skin

Chest pain

Enlarged liver and spleen

Loss of appetite

Diarrhoea

Numbness or tingling

Poor co-ordination of limbs

Pernicious anaemia results in a variety of symptoms affecting the whole body.

Peroneal

Peroneal means concerning the FIBULA bone in the lower leg, or the outer side of the leg next to the fibula. For example, the peroneal muscles are attached to the fibula.

Personality disorders are disorders of personal, social, and sexual relationships that are characterized by the individual's lack of awareness of the effects of his or her behaviour on others.

Q: How do personality disorders occur?

A: Personality disorders develop in childhood and later life, and become apparent in the abnormal ways in which a person reacts to other people. The person is usually unaware that his or her behaviour is abnormal, and attributes conflicts of temperament to faults in the other person. This causes feelings of frustration and often anxiety, and the development of a rigid personality unable to adapt to or learn from others.

Q: What are the different kinds of personality disorders?

A: Psychopathic personalities are concerned only with the achievement of their desires, and commonly respond with deceit or physical aggression if these desires are frustrated. Punishment has no deterrent effect. Alcoholism, sexual deviation, and violent criminal activity may occur.

Paranoid personalities have delusions about other people's feelings, and often interpret casual remarks as criticism of themselves. Obsessive personalities are highly conscientious and perfectionist, but also intolerant of others and mentally inflexible. Hysterical personalities constantly seek attention and affection, and make impossible emotional demands in personal relationships.

There are many other forms of personality disorders, many of which are difficult to cope with but do not necessarily prevent a person from playing a part in normal social life.

Q: How are personality disorders treated?

A: Treatment is difficult and is often not effective. Benefits may result from a relationship with a mature, affectionate person who can be firm and understanding. Group therapy may enable an individual to realize the destructive effects of the behaviour of other people with similar problems.

See also MENTAL ILLNESS.

Perspiration is the production of sweat by the sweat glands. The main constituents of sweat are water, sodium chloride (common salt), urea, lactic acid, and potassium salts.

In cold weather, perspiration is minimal. In extreme heat, about 1.5 litres (3 pints) of sweat per hour may be lost. Persons who have become acclimatized to heat may lose up to 4 litres (8.5 pints) per hour; it takes about six weeks to become acclimatized. During this period, the sweat glands gradually increase the amount of sweat, and decrease the amount of salts in the sweat, thereby preserving salts in the body.

Q: How do the sweat glands work?

A: A sweat gland consists of a coiled structure that lies deep within the skin, and a duct that passes through the skin layers to the surface. The coiled structure is well supplied with blood by capillaries. It absorbs fluid from the capillaries and surrounding cells and passes this to the surface through the duct. Some of the salts are reabsorbed in the duct, but when sweating is profuse, large amounts of salts may be lost.

The sweat glands are controlled by the AUTONOMIC NERVOUS SYSTEM. This is connected to the hypothalamus in the brain, which is part of the body's heat-regulating mechanism. Sweating also is influenced by the hormones ADRENALINE and NORADRENALINE, which can cause the cold sweats of fear.

Q: What are the functions of perspiration?

A: The main function of perspiration is to cool the body by evaporation. The other function of perspiration is the elimination of waste products, such as urea.

Q: What conditions may affect perspiration?

A: Perspiration may cease completely in the final stages of heatstroke. This is caused

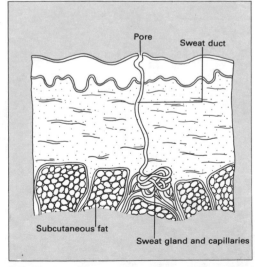

Pore

Sweat duct

Subcutaneous fat

Sweat gland and capillaries

Perspiration is produced by sweat glands in the skin and is secreted through the pores.

by a breakdown of the body's heat-regulating mechanism. Without emergency treatment, it may be fatal.

Increased sweating may occur with fever, irrespective of its cause, and in conditions that raise the metabolic rate, such as HYPERTHYROIDISM. CYSTIC FIBROSIS causes an excessive concentration of sodium chloride in the sweat.

Some people sweat excessively, particularly from the soles of the feet, palms of the hands, and the armpits. This condition is known as hyperhidrosis, and may be aggravated by stress. Bromhidrosis is a condition in which the sweat has an unpleasant odour. This is caused by the breakdown of a mixture of sweat and dead skin cells by bacteria.

Perthes' disease is a chronic disorder (osteochondritis) of the head of the femur (the ball part of the ball-and-socket hip joint), which degenerates because of an inadequate blood supply to the developing bone. The cause of the disorder is not known. It is most common in boys aged between five and ten years old, and usually affects only one of the hip joints. At this age the bone is not fully developed.

Q: *What are the symptoms of Perthes' disease?*

A: Movement of the affected joint may be limited, resulting in a limp. There may also be pain in the thigh and groin.

Q: *How is Perthes' disease treated?*

A: Most forms of treatment involve reducing the pressure on the affected hip. A weight-relieving caliper is often advised but may have to be worn for about two years. In some cases femoral osteotomy is performed. Children with the disease may develop osteoarthritis of the hip during adult life.

Pertussis. *See* WHOOPING COUGH.

Pes cavus is a condition in which the arches of the feet are abnormally high. In most cases there is no obvious cause, or it may be inherited. Other causes that have been identified include various muscular and neurological disorders, such as spina bifida or poliomyelitis in early infancy.

Q: *What are the symptoms of pes cavus?*

A: There are often no symptoms. However, pes cavus causes the weight of the body to be borne on the front part of the feet. The weakness of the small muscles of the foot leads to clawing of the toes and formation of calluses over the heads of the metatarsals, and corns on the toes.

Q: *How is pes cavus treated?*

A: Most cases require treatment by a chiropodist and the wearing of pads under the metatarsal heads. If these

measures fail, surgery may be necessary.

Pes planus. *See* FLATFOOT.

Pessary is a soluble tablet that dissolves at body temperature. It is inserted into the vagina to treat local vaginal infections or, occasionally, as a method of contraception.

A pessary is also a mechanical apparatus used to support the womb when prolapse is occurring.

Petechia is a small red spot in the skin that is caused by a minute haemorrhage of a blood capillary. Petechiae may be caused by blood clotting defects; coughing, particularly in whooping cough; disorders of the blood vessels; or bacterial ENDOCARDITIS. They may also appear in certain fevers, such as TYPHUS.

Pethidine is the international, nonproprietary name for a synthetic painkiller with similar effects and uses as MORPHINE. Pethidine has less sedating action than morphine, and has no cough-suppressant effects; it is also less constipating than morphine. Like morphine, pethidine is addictive.

The main use of pethidine is as a painkiller. It may also be used in the treatment of colic caused by gallstones or kidney stones, because of its antispasmodic effect. Pethidine may be combined with other drugs, such as antihistamines, as a form of pre-anaesthetic medication.

Q: *Can pethidine produce adverse side effects?*

A: Yes. Pethidine may cause dizziness, drowsiness, sweating, nausea, vomiting, and a dry mouth. Occasionally, it may also cause retention of urine, palpitations, and convulsions.

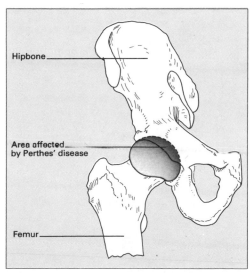

Hipbone

Area affected by Perthes' disease

Femur

Perthes' disease disrupts the blood supply to the epiphysis of the femur, causing distortion.

Petit mal

Petit mal is a mild form of epileptic attack in which there is a momentary loss of awareness, but no convulsions. *See* EPILEPSY.

Petroleum jelly is used in medicine to prevent dressings from sticking to the skin, and as a base for various ointments.

Pets and disease. The fur and feathers of many species of pet, particularly cats, may cause an ALLERGY. Animal fleas may live temporarily on man but do not cause more irritation than the occasional bite. Anyone handling animals should be immunized against TETANUS, as any animal bite may become infected with tetanus. Warm-blooded animals may carry RABIES.

There are many diseases that may be caused in humans by different varieties of pets. Birds may cause PSITTACOSIS and an allergic lung disease known as bird fancier's lung. Cats may cause CATSCRATCH FEVER, rabies, TOXOCARIASIS, and TOXOPLASMOSIS. Dogs may cause a rare form of LEPTOSPIROSIS, rabies, a HYDATID CYST, toxocariasis, and toxoplasmosis. Tortoises or terrapins may cause SALMONELLA.

Peyer's patch is a collection of lymph nodules that occur mainly in the ileum of the small intestine. *See* LYMPHATIC SYSTEM.

Phaeochromocytoma is a tumour of the central part (medulla) of the adrenal glands. The adrenal gland medulla secretes the hormones ADRENALINE and NORADRENALINE. A phaeochromocytoma causes excessive amounts of these hormones to be produced.

Q: What are the symptoms of a phaeochromocytoma?

A: The excessive amounts of adrenaline and noradrenaline cause attacks of palpitations, nausea, and severe headaches. These may be accompanied by a feeling of great anxiety. The patient also may be pale and sweating, the pulse may be rapid, and the blood pressure may be high. These attacks may occur at any time or they may be triggered by emotional stress, a change of posture, or pressure on the abdomen.

It may be necessary to perform urine tests and to take X-rays for the diagnosis of a phaeochromocytoma. This is because there are usually no indications of the condition, apart from high blood pressure, unless the patient is examined during an attack.

Q: How is a phaeochromocytoma treated?

A: The tumour is removed surgically only after the patient's hormone levels have been controlled with drugs.

Phalanx is the term given to any one of the bones of the fingers or toes. The thumbs and big toes each have two phalanges; the other fingers and toes each have three.

Phallus is another term for the PENIS.

Phantom limb is the illusion that a limb is still present after it has been amputated. It is a common symptom following an amputation, but usually disappears within a few months. Treatment with tranquillizers and antidepressant drugs may be needed.

Pharmacology is the study and research of drugs, their chemistry, effect on the body, and dosage.

Pharmacopoeia is an authorized book on drugs that contains information on their preparation, effect, dosages, and legal requirements of purity, strength, and quality.

Pharyngectomy is an operation to remove the pharynx, usually to treat cancer (*see* PHARYNX). The operation involves not only the removal of the pharynx (the larynx is also usually removed at the same time), but also its reconstruction using other tissues. This is a complex and highly skilled technique which often requires several operations to complete.

Pharyngitis is an inflammation of the pharynx. It is one of the most common of all disorders. Usually it comes on suddenly (acute pharyngitis), although some people have a persistent form of the disorder (chronic pharyngitis) which may be caused by smoking, drinking, persistent breathing through the mouth, or POSTNASAL DRIP. The symptoms of pharyngitis include a sore throat and discomfort or pain on swallowing.

Q: What causes acute pharyngitis?

A: Acute pharyngitis is most commonly caused by a common cold virus.

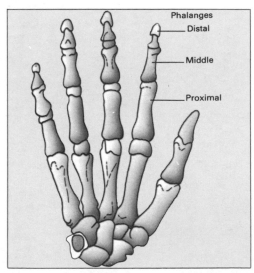

Phalanges
— Distal

— Middle

— Proximal

Phalanx is any of the fourteen small bones that form the phalanges of the fingers.

However, the cause can be the streptococcus bacterium, in which case the infection is known as a "strep throat". The condition is sometimes associated with inflammation of the larynx (laryngitis), inflammation of the mouth (stomatitis), glandular fever, tonsillitis, or nasal conditions, such as sinusitis. In rare cases, diphtheria or leukaemia may be the cause.

Q: Are there any particular problems associated with acute pharyngitis?

A: No, apart from those associated with any infection of the back of the throat and nose, such as laryngitis and otitis media (inflammation of the middle ear).

Q: Why do some people continually suffer from a chronic sore throat and discomfort on swallowing?

A: Chronic pharyngitis, like chronic laryngitis, may occur in those who smoke too many cigarettes or drink too much alcohol. It may also be caused by POSTNASAL DRIP resulting from chronic nasal inflammation. However, often a definite cause cannot be found.

The condition can often be cleared up by improved oral hygiene, giving up smoking, and through the use of antiseptic gargles. If the chronic inflammation is caused by respiratory tract allergies, the sore throat may clear up when the allergies are properly controlled.

Pharynx is the part of the throat situated behind the arch at the back of the mouth, and which connects together the mouth, nose, and larynx. It includes (1) the nasopharynx, the space just above the soft palate which joins up with the back of the nose and which contains the adenoids and openings of the Eustachian tubes; (2) the tonsils and the back of the tongue; and (3) the back of the throat.

Q: What conditions may affect the pharynx?

A: Infection may cause inflammation (PHARYNGITIS). Infections include glandular fever, tonsillitis, and adenoid problems. More rarely, Vincent's angina, syphilis, or diphtheria may cause inflammation, and occasionally it may result from cancer.

Phencyclidine, or **PCP,** is an anaesthetic drug that commonly is used in veterinary medicine. It was originally made as an anaesthetic for humans but was considered unsuitable because of its adverse side effects, such as hallucinations and agitation.

See also DRUG ADDICTION.

Phenobarbitone is a barbiturate drug (*see* BARBITURATES). Its main uses are as an anticonvulsant in the treatment of epilepsy and as a tranquillizer.

Patients undergoing long-term treatment can become tolerant to phenobarbitone. Care must be taken when withdrawing its use, particularly with epileptics. It should be prescribed with caution for the elderly, and for persons with cirrhosis of the liver or kidney disease. Combining alcohol or an antihistamine with phenobarbitone is hazardous and may produce a powerful and dangerous sedative, possibly leading to coma, respiratory failure, or death.

Phenol is another name for carbolic acid. *See* CARBOLIC ACID.

Phenylketonuria (PKU) is an inherited congenital anomaly that causes the accumulation of the substance phenylalanine in the blood. Normally an enzyme breaks down phenylalanine into amino acids. In about one in 10,000 people, this enzyme is missing. The chief symptoms are gradual mental deterioration, accompanied by irritability, vomiting, and convulsions. However, about one week after birth, when the baby has had protein in the diet, the heel is pricked and a PKU test (Guthrie test) performed. If phenylalanine is detected, further blood tests are taken. A special phenylalanine-free diet must be maintained throughout the child's growing life. Regular blood tests are made. In adulthood it may be possible to revert to a normal diet, except during pregnancy.

Phimosis is a condition in which the foreskin of the penis is so tight that it cannot be pulled back over the tip of the penis (glans).

Q: What problems occur with phimosis?

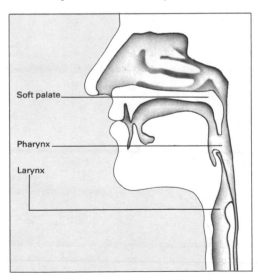

Soft palate

Pharynx

Larynx

Pharynx serves as a passageway for air from the nasal cavity to the larynx.

Phlebitis

A: During urination, the foreskin can be seen to bulge. The stream of urine is narrow and comes out slowly. In serious cases, the back pressure of the urine may damage the kidneys (hydronephrosis).

Q: *What causes phimosis?*

A: (1) It may occur following repeated infections (*see* BALANITIS). (2) At birth, the foreskin and tip of the penis are joined together. Separation of the two parts occurs gradually during the first few years of a child's life. Repeated attempts to forcibly pull back the foreskin before it is ready may cause phimosis where none had existed before.

Q: *What is the treatment for phimosis?*

A: The condition usually is corrected by circumcision. *See* CIRCUMCISION.

Phlebitis is an inflammation of a vein. *See* VENOUS THROMBOSIS.

Phlebolith is a chalky deposit in a vein. It results from a blood clot (thrombus) that has been present for so long that it has become calcified. It seldom causes symptoms as it usually occurs in abdominal veins. It does not usually require treatment.

Phlebothrombosis. *See* VENOUS THROMBOSIS.

Phlebotomus is a genus of bloodsucking flies. Some species transmit infections to humans; for example, *Phlebotomus sergenti* is one of the species that transmits LEISHMANIASIS.

Phlebotomy, or venesection, is the cutting of a vein.

Phlegm is thick MUCUS that is secreted by the mucous membranes of the nose, throat, or bronchial tubes.

Phlyctenule is a small blister that occurs most commonly on the conjunctiva of the eye. Symptoms include redness, swelling, pain, and sensitivity to bright lights (photophobia). Phlyctenules are common in children, and are thought to be an allergic reaction to an infection elsewhere in the body. Locally applied corticosteroid preparations and antibiotics are usually prescribed.

Phobia. *See* MENTAL ILLNESS.

Phonocardiogram is a graphic recording of heart sounds that is obtained using several microphones placed on the chest.

Photophobia is an abnormal sensitivity to bright light. It is a symptom of migraine, high fever, measles and German measles, and will occur with any form of acute brain infection, such as meningitis or encephalitis. Photophobia may accompany any infection of the eye. It is a common problem in albinos.

Phthirus pubis is the scientific name for the crab louse. It mainly infests the hair of the pubic region, but may also be found in the armpits, eyebrows, and eyelashes.

See also LICE.

Phthisis is a medical term for wasting. *See* WASTING.

Physiology is the study of the physical and chemical workings of animals and plants. It is closely associated with anatomy.

Physiotherapy describes the various techniques used by a specialist (a physiotherapist) for the relief of pain; improvement of joint and muscle function; and repairing, through training, damaged parts of the body.

See also DIATHERMY; ULTRASOUND TECHNIQUES.

Pica is the generally harmless desire to eat substances not considered food, such as coal, earth, and dried paint. Some pregnant women suffer from pica.

PID is an abbreviation for prolapsed intervertebral disc, commonly known as a slipped disc. *See* SLIPPED DISC.

Pigeon breast is a prominence of the breastbone (sternum), thought to be caused by a congenital abnormality, or respiratory illnesses in children. It does not require treatment.

Pigeon toed (toeing in) describes the condition in which a person walks with the feet turned inward. Most infants begin walking in this way because it aids balance. If there is no improvement after six months, a doctor should be consulted.

Piles. *See* HAEMORRHOIDS.

"Pill," the. *See* CONTRACEPTION.

Pilonidal sinus is a small duct containing dead hairs that sometimes forms a dermoid cyst. If such a cyst becomes infected, it must be removed surgically. Pilonidal sinuses are most commonly found over the sacrum above

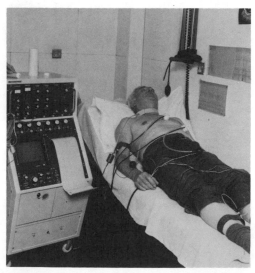

Phonocardiogram is a record of the sounds that the heart produces as it beats.

the anus; young hairy males are most commonly affected.

Q: How is an infected pilonidal sinus treated?

A: The infection is allowed to subside. The infected tissue often requires surgical drainage and ultimately removal of the sinus tissue. This eliminates the cause of the recurrent infection.

Pimple, or spot, is a small skin eruption containing pus. Pimples can occur anywhere on the body but are most common on the face. *See* ACNE.

Pineal body is a small structure that is situated in the centre of the brain. Its function is not known. Rarely, a tumour forms in the pineal body and may cause the early onset of puberty in boys.

Pink disease, or acrodynia, is a disorder caused by mercury compounds in baby teething powder, now withdrawn from the market. *See* MERCURY.

Pink eye is a form of conjunctivitis, usually caused by bacterial or viral infections. *See* CONJUNCTIVITIS.

Pinna is the visible external part of the ear. It consists of skin over cartilage. *See* EAR.

Pins and needles is a sensation of tingling related to a nerve disorder. *See* TINGLING.

Pinta is a chronic skin infection that is caused by a spiral-shaped bacterium called *Treponema carateum,* which is similar to the bacterium that causes syphilis and yaws. Pinta is transmitted by physical contact. After an incubation period of between one and three weeks, a small nodule appears on the skin. This gradually enlarges and becomes surrounded by other nodules. The lymph glands in the affected area also may swell. After about a year, blue patches develop, usually on the face and the limbs. These patches gradually fade, leaving scars. Pinta can be cured with penicillin.

Pinworm is a small, parasitic nematode worm that infests the intestine. Some authorities use the term to refer to the worm *Enterobius vermicularis* (*see* OXYURIASIS), and some to refer to the worm *Strongyloides stercoralis* (*see* STRONGYLOIDES).

Pituitary gland, or hypophysis, is a small gland about the size of a pea, situated at the base of the brain. It is connected by a short stalk to the hypothalamus, which helps regulate body temperature, blood pressure, fluid balance, weight, and appetite. The gland is protected by a circle of bone, called the pituitary fossa, in the centre of the skull just behind the point at which the two optic nerves join.

The pituitary gland is made up of two parts, the anterior or front lobe and the posterior or rear lobe.

Q: How does the pituitary anterior lobe function?

A: This is the most important of the glands that secrete hormones directly into the bloodstream. It produces hormones that stimulate other endocrine glands to manufacture their individual hormones. The level of these hormones is carefully regulated by special areas in the hypothalamus that are sensitive to the blood level of a variety of hormones and accordingly regulate the pituitary gland, sending chemical messages down the connecting stalk.

Q: What hormones does the anterior pituitary lobe produce?

A: The anterior lobe produces a number of hormones. They are: thyroid stimulating hormones (TSH) to control the production of the thyroid gland hormones, THYROXINE and triiodothyronine; adrenocorticotropic hormone (ACTH) to stimulate the cortex of the adrenal gland to produce hydrocortisone and other CORTICOSTEROIDS; follicle-stimulating hormone (FSH) and luteinizing hormone (LH) that control the testes and ovaries; growth hormone (GH) that maintains normal growth until adult life; and PROLACTIN, which helps lactation.

Q: How does the posterior lobe of the pituitary gland function?

A: The hypothalamus produces the two hormones oxytocin and vasopressin (antidiuretic hormone). These are stored in the cells of the pituitary's posterior lobe. The production of these hormones

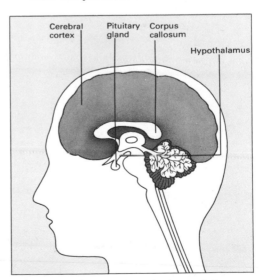

Pituitary gland, attached to the base of the brain, controls many endocrine secretions.

Pityriasis rosea

is carefully monitored by the same kind of "feedback" system that works in the anterior pituitary lobe.

Q: *What do vasopressin and oxytocin control?*

A: Vasopressin controls the excretion of water by the kidneys. An increase in vasopressin causes an increased reabsorption of water by the kidney tubules. A lack of vasopressin results in diabetes insipidus. Oxytocin stimulates the pregnant uterus to contract.

See also ACROMEGALY; ADDISON'S DISEASE; CUSHING'S SYNDROME; DWARFISM; GIGANTISM; HYPOPITUITARISM; HYPOTHYROIDISM; INFERTILITY.

Pityriasis rosea is a skin condition that starts with a slightly oval, pink, scaly area on the skin about an inch in diameter. It develops into a rash on the trunk, but rarely on the face. It causes mild itching, and the rash persists for six to eight weeks when it disappears spontaneously. The cause is unknown.

PKU. *See* PHENYLKETONURIA.

Placebo is a harmless substance without any medicinal effect. Although placebos are chemically inactive, many patients feel better after taking them.

Placenta is the specialized organ formed by a fertilized ovum (embryo) after it has attached itself to the lining of the womb. After the first few weeks of pregnancy it acts as an endocrine gland secreting chorionic gonadotropin to maintain the pregnancy.

The disc-shaped placenta is made up of twenty to forty smaller areas, called cotyledons. One side of the placenta is connected to the wall of the mother's womb; the other side is connected with the membrane containing the amniotic fluid that surrounds the embryo or foetus. The umbilical cord provides a direct link between the placenta and the developing baby, because it contains blood vessels that connect the centre of the placenta to the abdomen of the foetus.

By the time the fully developed foetus is ready to be born, the placenta weighs about one pound, and measures nine to ten inches across. The placenta is expelled shortly after the birth of the baby as part of the afterbirth.

Q: *How does the placenta work?*

A: The mother's blood flows through the uterine wall and an exchange of the substances that the foetus needs (such as food and oxygen) and those that have to be excreted (such as carbon dioxide and urea) takes place between the placenta and the uterine wall through a thin film of cells. Thus, there is no direct contact between the foetal and maternal blood circulations.

Q: *What abnormalities can affect the placenta?*

A: The umbilical cord may be attached to one side of the placenta, instead of to its centre. Or one or more of the cotyledons may lie apart from the main body of the placenta. There also can be abnormalities of the cord, or of the shape of the placenta. Sometimes, the placenta is situated in front of the foetus so that the exit from the womb is partly or completely blocked. This is known as a placenta praevia, and it is a serious complication of pregnancy. In most cases of placenta praevia it is necessary to perform a Caesarean section (*see* CAESAREAN SECTION).

Q: *Does the placenta have any other functions?*

A: Yes. Early in pregnancy, it produces the hormone called chorionic gonadotropin, which it also makes together with increasing amounts of oestrogen and progesterone to maintain pregnancy after the third month, when the ovaries cease to make the major contribution of these hormones.

Q: *Are there any conditions that may damage the placenta?*

A: Yes. Conditions in the mother such as high blood pressure, chronic nephritis, diabetes mellitus, and pre-eclampsia (toxaemia of pregnancy) damage the blood vessels and reduce the efficiency of the placenta. This increases the risk of intrauterine death of the foetus, and reduces the rate at which the foetus grows.

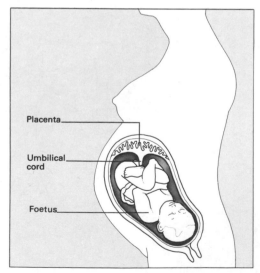

Placenta

Umbilical cord

Foetus

Placenta reaches full maturity by the 34th week of pregnancy, then slowly degenerates.

Recent research has shown that smoking also damages the placenta, resulting in smaller-than-average babies who have a greater chance of early death.

Q: What happens to the placenta before and during normal labour?

A: There is some deterioration in the way the placenta functions during the last two weeks of pregnancy. This probably is a factor in causing the onset of labour.

Once labour has started, the mother's blood supply to the placenta stops during contractions of the womb, and returns when the muscles relax. During the final minutes of labour, the restricted blood flow probably causes a slight increase in the carbon dioxide level in the foetal bloodstream. This acts as an additional stimulus for the baby to start breathing through the lungs immediately after birth.

The placenta is delivered in the third stage of labour. It should be examined to make sure that it is complete. If a piece of placenta is left in the womb, it can cause a postpartum haemorrhage. *See* LABOUR.

Plague (bubonic plague; black death) is a severe, potentially fatal infection that is caused by the bacterium *Yersinia pestis* (also called *Pasteurella pestis*). It occurs primarily in wild rodents but can be transmitted to humans. There are two main forms of plague that affect humans: bubonic plague, which results from the bite of an infected animal flea; and pneumonic plague, which results from inhaling droplets breathed by infected people. Both forms of plague are now rare.

Q: What are the symptoms of bubonic plague?

A: After a variable incubation period, which is usually between two and five days, there is a sudden onset of repeated shivering attacks, and the patient's body temperature rises to over (40°C) 104°F. The lymph glands become swollen and painful (buboes), and the patient may become delirious. The death rate in untreated patients is more than fifty per cent, with most deaths occurring within about five days.

Q: What are the symptoms of pneumonic plague?

A: After an incubation period of about two days there is a sudden onset of high fever; chills; and headache. There also may be increasing breathlessness, and coughing with foamy, bloodstained sputum. Most untreated patients die within about two days.

Q: How is plague treated?

A: Immediate treatment can be life-saving. Both forms of plague are treated with large doses of antibiotics, such as tetracycline, streptomycin, or chloramphenicol. The patient must be isolated to prevent the spread of infection. Prompt treatment usually improves the symptoms rapidly and enables most patients to survive the infection.

Q: How can plague be prevented?

A: Prevention is based on rodent control and the use of insect repellents to reduce the number of fleas. All people travelling to India or southeast Asia should be immunized against plague. Anybody who has been in contact with an infected person should be treated with antibiotics immediately.

Plantar reflex is the movement of the big toe when the outer side of the sole is stroked, causing it to point down. This reflex indicates that the nervous system is reacting normally. The opposite response is called the Babinski reflex, a pointing up of the big toe when the outer side of the sole is stroked. The lack of a plantar reflex and the presence of the Babinski reflex indicates a disorder of the nervous system, though this abnormal response is often seen in healthy infants under two years old.

Plantar wart (verruca) is a contagious wart. *See* WART.

Plaque has two medical meanings. (1) As a skin complaint, it is a group of eruptions that form a plate or patch on top of the skin. (2) Plaque as a dental disorder is an accumulation of hard material on the teeth that can

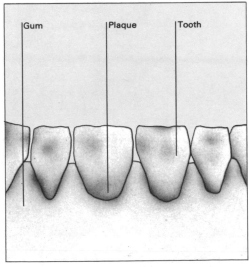

Plaque accumulates on teeth that are not cleaned regularly, and causes gum disorders.

Plasma

cause gum disorders, such as GINGIVITIS and PYORRHOEA.

Plasma is the fluid part of the blood in which the blood cells and the platelets are suspended. It consists of water in which many chemicals are dissolved, including proteins, salts, sugars, nitrogenous wastes, and carbon dioxide. Plasma is different from SERUM, which is the fluid that remains when blood has clotted; serum is plasma without fibrinogen and the other components of a blood clot.

Plasma is the main medium for the transportation of substances throughout the body. It carries nutritive substances to the body structures and removes their waste products. Plasma also makes possible chemical communication within the body by transporting hormones.

Plasma may be given by transfusion to patients who have lost serum through burns. It also may be used to treat shock, or disorders in which protein is lost from the body, such as ASCITES and NEPHROSIS.

See also PLASMA FRACTIONS.

Plasma fractions are the different proteins that can be extracted from the blood plasma and used to treat various disorders. For example, gamma globulin can give temporary protection against some diseases, such as measles; antihaemophilic globulin may be used to prevent bleeding in haemophiliacs; and albumin may be used in the treatment of NEPHROSIS and liver CIRRHOSIS.

Plasmodium is a genus of PROTOZOA, certain species of which cause MALARIA. The species that are known to cause malaria are *Plas-*

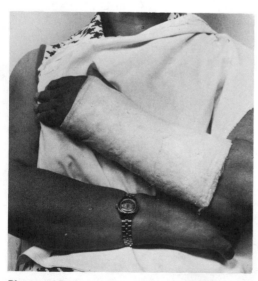

Plaster of Paris is a gypsum cement used to make a stiff bandage to immobilize limbs.

modium falciparum; Plasmodium malariae; Plasmodium ovale; and *Plasmodium vivax.* These parasitic microorganisms are carried by the Anopheles mosquito and infect the red blood cells in humans.

Plaster of Paris is a form of gypsum which, when mixed with water, forms a paste that hardens rapidly. It can be applied in cotton bandages and used to immobilize fractured limbs.

Plastic surgery is a special treatment concerned with restoring and restructuring damaged surface features. If the treatment is carried out merely to improve the patient's appearance, it is known as cosmetic surgery.

Platelet is a minute particle that is suspended in the blood plasma. Platelets also are known as thrombocytes. They are formed by the fragmentation of large cells in the bone marrow. Platelets play an essential part in the clotting of blood.

Plating is the application of bacteria to a culture medium in a shallow dish. Plating also refers to a surgical technique in which a metal plate is screwed onto a fractured bone.

Pleura is the membrane that surrounds each lung and lines the internal surface of the chest cavity. There are two pleurae, one around each lung. Each pleura consists of two layers: the parietal layer, which lines the chest cavity; and the visceral layer, which covers the surface of the lung. The space between the layers is known as the pleural cavity. It contains a small amount of fluid that lubricates the two layers, thereby facilitating the movements of the lung during breathing.

See also EMPYEMA; HAEMOTHORAX; PARACENTESIS; PLEURISY; PNEUMOTHORAX.

Pleurisy is an inflammation of the pleura. Most commonly it is caused by infection of the pleura or of the underlying lung, as may occur with PNEUMONIA. Pleurisy also may be caused by a pulmonary INFARCTION; an injury that penetrates the pleura; the spread of disease from elsewhere in the body, such as cancer; or as a complication of a generalized disease, such as kidney failure (*see* URAEMIA).

Q: What are the symptoms of pleurisy?

A: The onset is usually sudden, with localized pain near the area of inflammation that may be aggravated by breathing, coughing, or movement. If the part of the pleura that covers the diaphragm is affected, the pain may be referred to the shoulder on that side. There may also be rapid, shallow breathing and, if pleurisy is caused by infection, the patient may have a fever.

As the condition develops, the pain usually ceases because fluid forms in the pleural cavity and separates the inflamed surfaces of the pleura. If a large amount of fluid forms (pleural effusion), the underlying lung may collapse, causing breathlessness.

Q: *How is pleurisy treated?*

A: Treatment is directed toward the underlying cause. Initially, painkillers may be given and, if the patient has a fever, antibiotics may be prescribed. When a definite diagnosis has been made, the appropriate treatment can be given, such as anticoagulants for a pulmonary infarction.

Q: *Can pleurisy cause complications?*

A: Yes. Injury to the pleura or lung cancer may cause bleeding into the pleural cavity (haemothorax). Pleurisy that is caused by infection may result in an accumulation of pus in the pleural cavity (EMPYEMA). This may require antibiotic treatment or surgical drainage. Pleural effusions that are caused by cancer tend to recur. They may need treatment with cytotoxic drugs.

Pleurodynia is a sharp pain in the muscles of the chest wall that is similar to, but which is not caused by, pleurisy. Pleurodynia may be caused by FIBROSITIS.

Pleurodynia, epidemic, commonly known as Bornholm disease or Devil's grip, is an infection caused by one of the Coxsackie viruses. Children are most susceptible to the disease, especially in the summer and autumn.

The symptoms include pain in the region of the diaphragm, fever, headache, nausea, general discomfort and tenderness and swelling of the muscles. The illness lasts two to seven days and is followed by tiredness and depression that may persist for several weeks.

A doctor usually recommends that the patient is given strong painkilling drugs, confined to bed, and encouraged to drink plenty of fluids.

Plexus is a network of nerves, veins, or arteries. The solar plexus is a collection of nerves that lies behind the stomach.

Plumbism. *See* LEAD POISONING.

Pneumoconiosis is a general term for any lung disorder that is caused by the inhalation of dust particles. It is an occupational disorder. There are three main types of pneumoconiosis: (1) simple pneumoconiosis results from the deposition of inert dust in the lungs and is apparently harmless (for example, iron, tin, and carbon dust do not seem to cause any adverse effects); (2) irritant dusts, such as silica and asbestos, can cause silicosis or asbestosis, and these diseases cause scarring and gradual destruction of the lung tissue; (3) organic dusts may

cause a form of allergic reaction. For example, byssinosis is caused by cotton fibre dust.

Q: *What are the symptoms of pneumoconiosis?*

A: Simple pneumoconiosis seldom produces any symptoms. Coal dust, however, may cause scarring and destruction of lung tissue similar to that caused by silica and asbestos.

Pneumoconiosis that results from irritant dusts may cause increasing breathlessness, coughing, and spitting of blood. Asbestosis may lead to lung cancer.

The main symptom of pneumoconiosis that is caused by organic dusts is asthma. In some cases this may be complicated with bronchitis.

Q: *How is pneumoconiosis treated?*

A: There is no cure for this condition. It is essential that a person change jobs at the first suspicion of pneumoconiosis. It is impossible to remove the dust particles once they have reached the lungs, and lung deterioration is likely to continue for some time after a person has stopped inhaling the dust. Dust suppression and regular medical examinations are essential.

Pneumonectomy is the surgical removal of a lung. A partial pneumonectomy, which also is known as a lobectomy, is the removal of a section of a lung. A pneumonectomy most commonly is performed in the treatment of lung cancer. A partial pneumonectomy may be necessary in some cases of TUBERCULOSIS; BRONCHIECTASIS; or a lung abscess.

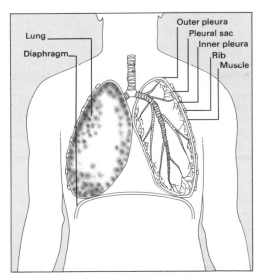

Pleura is a membrane that folds around the lungs and lines the inside of the thorax.

Pneumonia

Pneumonia is infection lungs by bacteria, viruses, or fungi. In rare cases, it may be aggravated by inhaled matter or worm infestations. If infection spreads down the bronchioles, it is known as bronchopneumonia. If only one lobe of the lung is involved, it is called lobar pneumonia.

Q: What kinds of infection cause pneumonia?

A: The common bacterial infections include *Hemophilus influenzae*, pneumococcus, and haemolytic streptococcus. Mycobacterium tuberculosis is now rare in Western countries. Antibiotic resistant staphylococcus is particularly dangerous and must be treated in a hospital.

In bacterial pneumonia, viruses include influenzas, chickenpox, measles, and Coxsackie. Similar pneumonia infections are produced by *Mycoplasma pneumoniae* and psittacosis. Fungal pneumonia may be caused by *Histoplasma capsulatum, Coccidiodes immitis*, or blastomycosis.

Q: What are the symptoms of pneumonia?

A: In bacterial pneumonia, the patient develops the symptoms of a cold followed by a sudden shivering attack, sputum that is often bloody, and a high fever (40°C; 104°F) with rapid respiration and pulse rate. The patient often feels pain due to pleurisy. Vomiting and diarrhoea may occur; confusion is common.

In other forms of pneumonia, especially among elderly patients, the symptoms develop slowly with clear evidence of bronchitis and a worsening cough, often with bloodstained sputum. Headache, muscle aches, and cyanosis

(blue tinged lips because of poorly oxygenated blood) are common. Progress depends on the individual's resistance to the type of infection. In elderly or weak patients death may occur. Children or babies show few symptoms suggesting a chest infection. But the child obviously is ill, and may collapse.

Q: How is pneumonia diagnosed and treated?

A: Diagnosis follows a doctor's examination and, usually, a chest X-ray. A specimen of the sputum is examined and cultured to identify the infective organism. Sometimes a white bood cell count may help to determine whether the infection is caused by bacteria or by a virus.

Antibiotics are used in the treatment of bacterial and fungal infections.

Breathing exercises and percussion to shake the chest wall encourage the patient to cough up sputum. If the sputum is thick and sticky, steam inhalations may also help. A seriously ill patient may need oxygen therapy. Painkilling drugs are prescribed if the patient has pleurisy.

Most patients suffering from mild forms of pneumonia can be treated at home with rest, antibiotics, and breathing exercises.

See also PLEURISY.

Pneumonitis is an inflammation of the lungs. It may be a symptom of several diseases, such as PNEUMONIA and PNEUMOCONIOSIS.

Pneumothorax is a condition in which there is air in the pleural cavity, the space between the lungs and the chest wall. It prevents the normal expansion of the lungs, thereby impairing breathing.

Q: What causes a pneumothorax?

A: The most common cause of a pneumothorax is a penetrating injury of the chest wall. This is known as a traumatic pneumothorax. Rarely, injury may cause a life-threatening form of traumatic pneumothorax in which a flap of tissue acts as a valve that allows air to be drawn into the chest, but not to be blown out again. The pressure within the chest rises rapidly and causes both lungs to collapse. This condition is known as a tension pneumothorax.

A spontaneous pneumothorax is caused by air leaking from the lungs. This may be the result of an underlying disorder, such as EMPHYSEMA, or by a congenital weakness of the lungs.

Q: What are the symptoms of a pneumothorax?

A: The symptoms of a pneumothorax vary greatly. A traumatic pneumothorax is

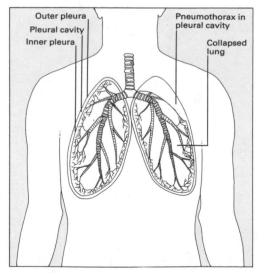

Outer pleura
Pleural cavity
Inner pleura

Pneumothorax in pleural cavity

Collapsed lung

Pneumothorax is air in the pleural cavity that can cause a lung to collapse.

always serious, because of damage to the chest wall. The main symptoms are breathlessness and pain. A tension pneumothorax causes extreme breathing difficulty, and may be rapidly fatal.

The symptoms of a spontaneous pneumothorax range from slight breath-lessness on exertion to the sudden onset of severe chest pains and extreme breathing difficulty.

Q: *How is a pneumothorax treated?*

A: A patient with a traumatic pneumothorax requires hospitalization so that the air in the pleural cavity can be removed by insertion of a needle into the chest wall. Then the injury is treated. A tension pneumothorax requires emergency medical treatment; the rapid removal of air from the pleural cavity may be life-saving.

Most patients with a small, spon-taneous pneumothorax do not require treatment because the air is gradually reabsorbed. Occasionally, the condition may recur, in which case surgery may be necessary.

Pock is an old word for a pustule, a small elevation of the skin filled with pus or lymph.

Pockmarks are small scars left after the healing of pustules. They may occur if any spot becomes infected and leaves a scar, such as may result in chickenpox if the spots are scratched. *See* PUSTULE.

Podagra. *See* GOUT.

Poisoning (for EMERGENCY treatment, *see* First Aid, p.562) is the taking into the body by eating, inhaling, injecting, or absorbing through the skin any substance that damages or prevents the normal working of the body.

Poker back, a rigid, slightly bent spine, is probably the result of the rheumatic disorder ANKYLOSING SPONDYLITIS.

Polio. *See* POLIOMYELITIS.

Polioencephalitis is an inflammation of the grey matter of the brain. It may be caused by encephalitis. It also may occur as a complica-tion of vitamin B_1 deficiency (BERI-BERI), when it produces acute mental disturbances similar to those of KORSAKOFF'S SYNDROME.

See also ENCEPHALITIS.

Poliomyelitis, also called infantile paralysis, is an infection of the nervous system caused by one of the three polio viruses. It occurs throughout the world. The disease is common in the summer months in temperate climates, and all year round in the tropics. Epidemics can occur, but the risk of an epidemic is lessened by improved sanitation and immuni-zation of children with oral vaccine.

Q: *How long does poliomyelitis take to develop and what are its symptoms?*

A: There is an incubation period of three days or more, followed by feverish illness. A sore throat and headaches develop over a period of one to two (and occasionally five) days. Most people recover after this stage without further symptoms. Ten per cent, however, suddenly develop severe headaches, fever, muscle pains, and neck stiffness, suggestive of meningitis. There is a tingling sensation in the limbs, and increased weakness and paralysis.

Throat and respiratory poliomyelitis may be fatal. Many patients suffering from paralysis during the illness regain most, or all, movement in time, but in severe cases paralysis may remain.

Q: *How is poliomyelitis treated?*

A: Mild cases require bed rest. Severe cases need isolation and complete rest, with slight sedation and painkilling drugs. With respiratory paralysis, artificial respirators and a TRACHEOSTOMY are necessary. A physiotherapist regularly moves the patient's joints to prevent stiffness. Extra fluids are given to prevent dehydration. The patient may have to be fed through a tube into the stomach, and a catheter is needed if the bladder is paralyzed.

Poliomyelitis is much easier to prevent than to treat. Infants should be given three doses of oral Sabin live attenuated virus vaccine (OPV), with boosters at five years, and when recommended by a doctor.

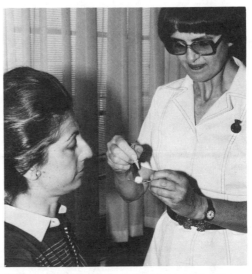

Poliomyelitis vaccine can be given orally on a lump of sugar.

Pollen

Epidemic poliomyelitis is unlikely in vaccinated communities.

Pollen is the powderlike substance produced by male flowers which fertilizes other plants.

Polyarteritis nodosa is a rare, potentially fatal inflammation of the small arteries. It often results in arterial thrombosis and death of the surrounding tissue. The cause of polyarteritis nodosa is not known. However, in some cases the onset of the disorder may be associated with bacterial infection or with certain drugs, such as sulphonamide. Polyarteritis nodosa usually occurs in persons between the ages of 25 and 50 years, and is more common in men than in women.

Q: *What are the symptoms of polyarteritis nodosa?*

A: The symptoms of this disorder are extremely variable. The most common symptoms include fever, recurrent abdominal pain, weight loss, peripheral neuritis, asthma, hypertension, oedema, and fatigue. The muscles and joints may ache, and nodules and ulcers may appear on the skin. The kidneys also may be affected, causing high blood pressure, swelling of the ankles, and, ultimately, kidney failure.

Q: *How is polyarteritis nodosa treated?*

A: There is, as yet, no cure for this disorder, which is fatal in most cases. However, the symptoms can be controlled and the life can be prolonged by treatment with large doses of CORTICOSTEROIDS. In some cases, parts of the intestine may die, resulting in PERITONITIS. Such cases usually require surgery.

Polyarthritis is any form of arthritis that affects several joints at the same time. *See* OSTEOARTHRITIS; RHEUMATOID ARTHRITIS.

Polycystic kidney is a congenital anomaly of the kidney in which some of its tissue fails to join up with the drainage tubules for urine. It leads to the formation of cysts that contain urine. Polycystic kidney may occur in several members of a family. A kidney transplant is the only treatment.

Polycythaemia is an excess of red cells in the blood. Polycythaemia vera is a rare disease of the part of the bone marrow that produces red blood cells. The number of red cells and the total volume of blood increases gradually over several years. The cause of polycythaemia vera is not known. The disorder cannot be cured but, by removing blood regularly from the veins (phlebotomy) and treatment with radioactive phosphorus, life can be prolonged.

Polydactylism is a congenital abnormality in which there are extra fingers and toes.

Polymorph is an abbreviation of polymorphonuclear leucocyte, a type of WHITE BLOOD CELL.

Polymyalgia rheumatica is an uncommon form of rheumatism that affects the elderly, usually those over sixty years of age. It is more common in women than in men. Polymyalgia rheumatica is characterized by pain and stiffness in the neck, shoulders, and back. There also may be a persistent headache. Patients often feel unwell, but rarely are seriously ill. The cause of the condition is unknown, but it is thought to result from a type of arterial inflammation. If the arteries in the eye become inflamed, the patient may suddenly become blind.

Treatment with corticosteroid drugs often is rapidly effective and must usually be continued for several months.

Polyneuritis is damage or inflammation of the nerves. Damage to one nerve (mononeuritis) or to several nerves in more than one area (mononeuritis multiplex) are closely related disorders.

Polyneuritis may be caused by injury; viral infection; toxic poisoning; industrial poisoning; vitamin B_{12} deficiency; alcoholism; diabetes mellitus; or cancer, most commonly of the lung. Symptoms may be mild, producing tingling or altered sensation in the affected area, or severe, affecting respiration. In most cases of polyneuritis, patients make a complete and spontaneous recovery, although some may require physiotherapy or corticosteroid treatment.

See also FRIEDREICH'S ATAXIA.

Polyp is a growth or tumour on a mucous membrane. It grows on a short stalk. Polyps are usually benign (noncancerous). They may occur anywhere in the body, but are most common in the nose, the cervix of the womb, within the uterine cavity, and in the rectum.

Polyps within the colon or large intestine may become malignant. A condition in which there are many intestinal polyps (familial polyposis) commonly develops into cancer.

Polyuria is the frequent passing of large amounts of urine. It is a typical symptom of diabetes and kidney disease, such as chronic NEPHRITIS.

See also DIABETES MELLITUS.

Pompholyx is a type of eczema that produces highly irritating blisters on the hands and feet. The cause is unknown. The condition lasts for one to two weeks, but commonly recurs.

The blisters break into small open sores that gradually heal. Treatment with soothing corticosteroid creams reduces the irritation until natural healing takes place. It is important to keep the area clean and dry to prevent secondary infection.

Pore is a minute opening in the skin which allows matter to pass through. *See* SKIN.

Porphyria is a group of congenital disorders of the metabolism or regulation of the body.

Porphyria is characterized by excessive secretions of porphyrins in the blood or liver. Porphyrins are nitrogen-containing organic compounds that are needed to unite with iron and the protein globin to form HAEMOGLOBIN.

There are two main types of porphyria: those that occur within the red blood cells, and those that involve the liver.

Q: What are the symptoms of porphyria in the red blood cells?

A: The symptoms occur most commonly in children, and may be very severe. They include blisters, red teeth, and purple or pink urine. If the skin is exposed to the sun, the blister formations may progress to a stage of scarring. The condition may be fatal, but in its mildest form the patient needs only to avoid sunlight.

Q: What are the symptoms of porphyria in the liver?

A: There may be severe abdominal pain, vomiting, and abdominal swelling. These may be accompanied by neurological disorders, such as epileptic seizures.

Q: How is porphyria treated?

A: Children with porphyria must avoid sunlight. In adults, the precipitating cause, usually drugs, must be discovered and avoided. Relatives of a person with porphyria should also be examined. Treatment with painkilling drugs may be necessary, and also dietary treatment.

Portacaval shunt is an artificially-produced junction between the hepatic portal vein and the inferior vena cava.

Portal vein is a vein that carries blood between two organs.

Port-wine stain, or port-wine mark, is a flat, purplish-red birthmark formed by abnormal blood vessels. *See* BIRTHMARK.

Postnasal drip is a discharge from the back of the nose down the back of the throat.

Q: What are the symptoms of postnasal drip?

A: One or both nostrils may be intermittently blocked. There may be a slight coughing of sputum as a result of the irritating effect of the discharge.

Q: How is postnasal drip treated?

A: Consult a doctor, because the treatment depends on diagnosing the cause. Continued use of nasal drops and sprays may only aggravate the condition, and for this reason they should not be used without medical supervision.
See also CATARRH.

Postpartum describes anything that occurs within six weeks after the birth of a baby.

Post-traumatic describes any medical condition that occurs as a result of or following an injury.

Postural drainage is a method used by physiotherapists and surgeons to position a patient so that gravity assists in the drainage of a congested area.

Pott's disease is tuberculosis of the spine. It mainly affects children and adults up to the age of forty. The disorder produces destruction of a vertebra by tuberculous osteitis (inflammation of the bone). Collapse of a vertebra results in the compression of the spinal cord and nerves. Pott's disease gives the individual the typical hunchback appearance of kyphosis. Paralysis may also occur.

Treatment includes curing the infection with antituberculosis drugs, relieving the spinal cord from pressure, removing any pus or bone, bed rest, adequate diet, and careful exercise.

See also KYPHOSIS.

Pott's fracture is a fracture of the ankle. The break usually involves the tibia (shin-bone) or fibula (the second of the two long bones in the lower leg), or both. The ankle joint often is dislocated, and the ligaments are torn.

Pott's fracture is a common injury. It is usually treated by manipulation into the correct position under general anaesthesia and immobilization of the ankle in a plaster cast for about six weeks. With severe fractures, the broken bones are operated on.

Poultice is a heated dressing that is applied to the skin to relieve congestion, inflammation, or pain, or to encourage a boil to discharge.

Poultices are seldom effective. They lose

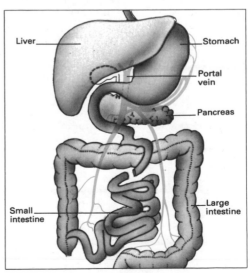

Portal vein receives the final products of digestion and transports them to the liver.

375

Prednisone

heat rapidly, damage the skin by making it moist, and may cause burns.

Prednisone and another corticosteroid drug, prednisolone, are synthetic preparations that have actions similar to the naturally occurring steroid hormone cortisol, which is formed by the adrenal glands.

Prolonged use of prednisone, like all corticosteroids, causes loss of calcium from the bones (osteoporosis), a tendency to develop diabetes mellitus, and the likelihood of developing a peptic ulcer. There is reduced resistance to infection, and the skin becomes thin and heals more slowly than normal.

Prolonged high dosage of prednisone may produce a typical moonface, acne, and an increase in body fat. If prednisone has been taken for a long period of time, the dosage must be reduced slowly so that the adrenal glands start producing cortisol again. *See* CORTICOSTEROIDS.

Pre-eclampsia is a condition that sometimes occurs late in pregnancy. Symptoms include: high blood pressure; swelling (oedema) of the legs, hands and, to a lesser extent, the face; and protein in the urine (albuminuria). It sometimes is called toxaemia of pregnancy, although there is no evidence to suggest that it is caused by a toxin. In fact, the cause of pre-eclampsia is not known. But the condition is more likely to occur in women who already have high blood pressure, who suffer from chronic nephritis, or who are expecting their first baby. Antenatal care is essential if pre-eclampsia is to be detected in its early stages.

Q: How is pre-eclampsia treated?

A: In the very early stages, the patient is instructed to take additional rest. She is advised not to lie on her back because this causes the womb to press on the blood vessels that supply it. She is given mild sedatives, and a strict diet plan emphasizing high protein and normal salt intake to prevent any further weight gain.

If these measures are not successful, the woman may be admitted to hospital, where she may be given drugs to reduce blood pressure. If these are not effective and tests show that the baby is not getting enough oxygen, labour is induced.

Q: What complications may occur with pre-eclampsia and how are they treated?

A: The most serious complication is ECLAMPSIA, in which convulsions and coma may occur in the woman. The more common complications are those that affect the foetus. The blood supply to the womb is reduced, and foetal growth is slowed. There is an increased likelihood of intrauterine death.

Prefrontal leucotomy. *See* LEUCOTOMY.

A talk about Pregnancy and childbirth

Pregnancy and childbirth. A normal pregnancy lasts about 265 days, although pregnancies naturally vary in duration.

Q: Can a woman always be sure that her estimated date of confinement is correct in the first place?

A: No. A woman whose periods have always been irregular is unlikely to reach an accurate date for delivery based on calculation. This is because the date of ovulation, and thus fertilization, probably occurred about two weeks before a period was due. It is possible for bleeding to occur during pregnancy, lasting one or two days. However, it may make a woman think she has menstruated and become pregnant a month later than was actually the case.

Q: What are the early symptoms of pregnancy?

A: Often, the earliest sign is the absence of a period (amenorrhoea). This may be accompanied by a feeling of heaviness in the breasts, slight nausea first thing in the mornings (morning sickness), and frequency of urination.

Q: What tests and examinations are carried out to confirm pregnancy?

A: A PREGNANCY TEST can be performed using a sample of urine, after the period has been overdue for eight days. If this is positive, it is relatively certain that the woman is pregnant. If the test is negative, it should be repeated in a week's time.

Once the period is more than three weeks overdue, a gentle vaginal examination usually reveals an enlargement of the womb. This, combined with other symptoms suggestive of pregnancy, may confirm pregnancy without a pregnancy test.

Q: How are the common problems of the first three months of pregnancy treated?

A: Morning sickness affects about fifty per cent of women. A doctor may prescribe antinauseant drugs to be taken at night. Eating biscuits before getting out of bed in the morning helps to control mild nausea. Breast tenderness is relieved by wearing a firm brassiere that gives good support. HYPEREMESIS gravidarum is a severe form of morning sickness.

Q: What information is required, and what examinations and tests are carried out by the obstetrician?

A: It is most important for the woman to

Pregnancy and childbirth

give the full history of any previous pregnancies or abortions she may have had.

She will also be asked about any illnesses or disorders she may have had. Chronic nephritis, diabetes mellitus, high blood pressure, and rheumatic valve disease of the heart all can cause problems during pregnancy. If there is a family history of diabetes mellitus, there is a possibility that the patient could develop mild diabetes while under the stress of pregnancy.

A complete physical examination includes weighing, breast examination, blood pressure test, urine test, cervical smear, and vaginal examination. At each subsequent visit blood pressure, weight, and urine are monitored, and the obstetrician checks the ankles for signs of oedema. The growth of the womb is checked each visit after the fourteenth week of pregnancy. The obstetrician can tell this by feeling the abdomen.

Finally, some laboratory tests are made on a sample of the woman's blood. These include a haemoglobin test to detect anaemia, and tests for blood group and Rhesus (Rh) factor and for signs of previous infections such as German measles (rubella).

The obstetrician usually discusses the findings of the examinations and tests with the patient to reassure her that the pregnancy is normal, and to emphasize the importance of regular antenatal examinations. At first these are generally given on a monthly basis, unless there is some abnormality present. But later in pregnancy the visits become more frequent, usually occurring every two weeks from the twenty-eighth week of pregnancy, and weekly from the thirty-sixth until delivery.

Q: *Should a woman in early pregnancy keep to a special diet and carry out routine exercise?*

A: Unless she suffers from a condition that demands special attention (such as obesity or diabetes mellitus), diet and exercise are dictated by common sense.

Q: *May sexual intercourse continue throughout pregnancy?*

A: Yes. In general, intercourse may take place as usual. If there is a history of spontaneous abortion, however, the obstetrician probably will advise avoiding intercourse during the first three months at around the time when a period would normally have occurred.

Q: *What tests and examinations may be carried out during the middle three months of pregnancy?*

A: Using ultrasonic equipment, the obstetrician usually can detect foetal life by the end of the second month of pregnancy. There is no danger for either the mother or foetus in this technique. Scans also detect potential problems and can accurately assess the progress of a pregnancy, in cases where there is doubt, after the fourth month.

Amniocentesis involves taking a sample of fluid from around the foetus by inserting a needle into the womb, under

	Days		
Jan.	1 2 3 4 5 6 7 8 9 10 11 12 13 14 15 16 17 18 19 20 21 22 23 24 25 26 27 28 29 30 31	Jan.	
Oct.	8 9 10 11 12 13 14 15 16 17 18 19 20 21 22 23 24 25 26 27 28 29 30 31 (1 2 3 4 5 6 7	Nov.	
Feb.	1 2 3 4 5 6 7 8 9 10 11 12 13 14 15 16 17 18 19 20 21 22 23 24 25 26 27 28	Feb.	
Nov.	8 9 10 11 12 13 14 15 16 17 18 19 20 21 22 23 24 25 26 27 28 29 30 (1 2 3 4 5	Dec.	
Mar.	1 2 3 4 5 6 7 8 9 10 11 12 13 14 15 16 17 18 19 20 21 22 23 24 25 26 27 28 29 30 31	Mar.	
Dec.	6 7 8 9 10 11 12 13 14 15 16 17 18 19 20 21 22 23 24 25 26 27 28 29 30 31 (1 2 3 4 5	Jan.	
April	1 2 3 4 5 6 7 8 9 10 11 12 13 14 15 16 17 18 19 20 21 22 23 24 25 26 27 28 29 30	April	
Jan.	6 7 8 9 10 11 12 13 14 15 16 17 18 19 20 21 22 23 24 25 26 27 28 29 30 31 (1 2 3 4	Feb.	
May	1 2 3 4 5 6 7 8 9 10 11 12 13 14 15 16 17 18 19 20 21 22 23 24 25 26 27 28 29 30 31	May	
Feb.	5 6 7 8 9 10 11 12 13 14 15 16 17 18 19 20 21 22 23 24 25 26 27 28 (1 2 3 4 5 6 7	Mar.	
June	1 2 3 4 5 6 7 8 9 10 11 12 13 14 15 16 17 18 19 20 21 22 23 24 25 26 27 28 29 30	June	
Mar.	8 9 10 11 12 13 14 15 16 17 18 19 20 21 22 23 24 25 26 27 28 29 30 31 (1 2 3 4 5 6	April	
July	1 2 3 4 5 6 7 8 9 10 11 12 13 14 15 16 17 18 19 20 21 22 23 24 25 26 27 28 29 30 31	July	
April	7 8 9 10 11 12 13 14 15 16 17 18 19 20 21 22 23 24 25 26 27 28 29 30 (1 2 3 4 5 6 7	May	
Aug.	1 2 3 4 5 6 7 8 9 10 11 12 13 14 15 16 17 18 19 20 21 22 23 24 25 26 27 28 29 30 31	Aug.	
May	8 9 10 11 12 13 14 15 16 17 18 19 20 21 22 23 24 25 26 27 28 29 30 31 (1 2 3 4 5 6 7	June	
Sept.	1 2 3 4 5 6 7 8 9 10 11 12 13 14 15 16 17 18 19 20 21 22 23 24 25 26 27 28 29 30	Sept.	
June	8 9 10 11 12 13 14 15 16 17 18 19 20 21 22 23 24 25 26 27 28 29 30 (1 2 3 4 5 6 7	July	
Oct.	1 2 3 4 5 6 7 8 9 10 11 12 13 14 15 16 17 18 19 20 21 22 23 24 25 26 27 28 29 30 31	Oct.	
July	8 9 10 11 12 13 14 15 16 17 18 19 20 21 22 23 24 25 26 27 28 29 30 31 (1 2 3 4 5 6 7	Aug.	
Nov.	1 2 3 4 5 6 7 8 9 10 11 12 13 14 15 16 17 18 19 20 21 22 23 24 25 26 27 28 29 30	Nov.	
Aug.	8 9 10 11 12 13 14 15 16 17 18 19 20 21 22 23 24 25 26 27 28 29 30 31 (1 2 3 4 5 6	Sept.	
Dec.	1 2 3 4 5 6 7 8 9 10 11 12 13 14 15 16 17 18 19 20 21 22 23 24 25 26 27 28 29 30 31	Dec.	
Sept.	7 8 9 10 11 12 13 14 15 16 17 18 19 20 21 22 23 24 25 26 27 28 29 30 (1 2 3 4 5 6 7	Oct.	

Estimated date of delivery can be calculated from the first day of the woman's last period.

Find the latter date (in light type) and the delivery date is below it (in heavy type).

Pregnancy and childbirth

local anaesthetic. This procedure may be carried out if there is any possibility of a congenital foetal abnormality, such as Down's syndrome. It also can detect developmental disorders of the nervous system, as well as other abnormalities.

Q: *What is "quickening," and at what stage can it be felt?*

A: Quickening describes the first movements of the foetus in the womb felt by the mother. A woman undergoing her first pregnancy usually feels it between the eighteenth and twentieth weeks. In subsequent pregnancies, however, when the mother is aware of what to expect, she may feel it about two weeks earlier.

Q: *What are the common problems of the latter half of pregnancy?*

A: Many minor problems may affect a woman as pregnancy progresses, although few are serious.

(1) *Backache.* This is extremely common because the ligaments that normally hold the joints in place are affected by hormones which cause them to become more stretched and relaxed.

The woman is advised to wear low-heeled shoes and to place a firm board under her mattress (or under her side of it). Muscle strengthening exercises and instruction on how to hold the body properly help to relieve backache. Occasionally, it is necessary to wear a lumbar support corset.

(2) *Headaches.* A common symptom, these may be associated with fatigue and the additional stress and anxiety placed

upon a woman during pregnancy. They are generally not serious and seldom need more than simple treatment.

(3) *Constipation.* This is a common complaint throughout pregnancy, caused by the production of the hormone progesterone. This hormone has a relaxing effect on the intestinal tract. The condition is often improved by adding increased bulk to the diet, such as bran and fresh vegetables, as well as by drinking additional fluids.

(4) *Increased frequency of urination.* This occurs not only in the early days of pregnancy, but also toward the end because of increased pressure on the bladder.

Painless increase in urination is seldom anything to worry about. If there is any discomfort, however, it should be reported to the obstetrician because urinary infections, such as CYSTITIS, can occur during pregnancy.

(5) *Heartburn.* The production of the hormone progesterone during pregnancy causes relaxation of the muscle at the lower end of the oesophagus (gullet). This allows the acid contents of the stomach to pass back into the oesophagus.

The symptoms can be improved by taking frequent small meals, and by avoiding a large meal before going to bed. ANTACID medicines often can help, as can raising the head and shoulders at night.

(6) *Ankle swelling.* This is a common symptom caused by the effect of

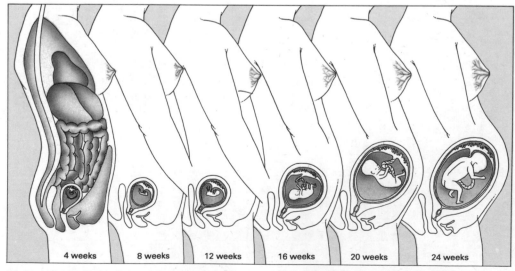

| 4 weeks | 8 weeks | 12 weeks | 16 weeks | 20 weeks | 24 weeks |

At 4 weeks the foetus's heart has developed, and by 8 weeks it has nearly all the organs.

After week 12 the mother's breasts enlarge, and the abdomen swells.

378

progesterone on the blood vessels, as well as by the pressure and weight of the pregnant womb on the veins that carry blood from the legs. Varicose veins may aggravate the condition.

To treat swollen ankles, the feet should be raised above the level of the pelvis as often as possible during the day, and the foot of the bed should be raised at night.

(7) *Varicose veins and haemorrhoids.* Varicose veins may occur as a result of increased pressure (improving after the birth). The enlarged womb presses on the veins of the pelvis and obstructs the blood flow from the legs to the heart. Haemorrhoids (piles) are a similar condition, usually caused by the pressure set up in the anal area by the straining action of constipation.

During pregnancy, women with varicose veins may wear elastic stockings to prevent aching. Haemorrhoids can be relieved with ointments preventing constipation.

(8) *Insomnia.* Sleeplessness commonly occurs in the last few weeks of pregnancy. Insomnia may be caused by the large abdomen, backache, or vigorous foetal movements. If necessary, the obstetrician may prescribe a mild sedative.

(9) *Palpitations and sweating.* These symptoms are similar to those experienced during MENOPAUSE and are caused by the effects of the hormones on the mother's body during pregnancy. They are seldom severe.

Q: *What regimen of diet and exercise should be followed in the latter half of pregnancy?*

A: During the second half of pregnancy, the mother should pay particular attention to diet. The foetus requires increased nourishment, but the woman must avoid excessive weight gain.

First-class proteins (such as those in eggs, milk, fish, and meat), together with vegetable proteins, are particularly important.

Energy requirements are supplied mainly by carbohydrates in the diet. These should be adjusted to fit in with the protein and the small amount of fat that makes up the remainder of the diet.

Fresh fruit and vegetables are an essential part of the diet because they supply vitamins and the bulk that helps to prevent constipation. The obstetrician often prescribes small doses of supplementary vitamins and iron.

Milk contains protein, calcium, and phosphorus, the minerals responsible for bone formation. But milk is not essential as long as the diet includes meat and cheese.

Regular exercise is an essential part of maintaining good health. Routine antenatal exercises are an essential part of maintaining physical and psychological well-being.

Q: *When should a pregnant woman start attending antenatal classes?*

A: The timing depends on the recommendation of the individual obstetrician, but it is usual to defer antenatal classes until the last three months of

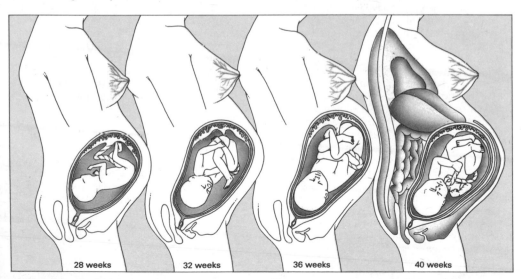

28 weeks   32 weeks   36 weeks   40 weeks

At 28 weeks the foetus usually settles in the womb with the head pointing down.

The womb continues to enlarge, until about two weeks before delivery it "lightens".

pregnancy. Usually a series of eight to twelve weekly classes are attended by the same group of prospective parents. They are told about the normal development of the foetus, the progress of pregnancy, and the stages of labour.

The class also is shown exercises to strengthen the back and pelvic muscles, as well as special methods of breathing which may be of assistance during the various stages of labour. The women are asked to practise these exercises at home.

At least one class is devoted to the care of the newborn baby: how to bathe and dress the baby, as well as how to change a nappy. Often a mother who has just had a baby returns to the class to demonstrate baby care, bringing her own infant with her.

It is usual, at some point during ante-natal classes, to discuss the problems that may arise in labour, and the kind of action that the obstetrician may take.

Q: *What is "lightening", and when can it be expected to occur?*

A: Lightening is the sensation of increased physical comfort that is experienced when the foetus has descended into the lower part of the womb, in the pelvic cavity, thus relieving pressure on the upper abdominal area. It usually occurs about the thirty-sixth week, but, in women who have had babies before, it may not occur until labour starts.

Q: *What special tests or examinations are carried out by the obstetrician during the last three months of pregnancy?*

A: Provided the pregnancy is developing normally, the only special tests needed are a reassessment of the level of haemoglobin in the blood to check for anaemia, a repetition of the antibody test for the Rh (rhesus) factor, and sometimes a test of the urine to ensure that there is no infection. The obstetrician usually performs an internal, gynaecological examination about the thirty-seventh week of pregnancy. This is done to assess the size of the pelvis to ensure that there is enough room for the foetus to be born.

Q: *Why may pregnancy end prematurely, and is this a problem?*

A: In many cases the cause of premature birth is not known. Factors that may contribute to prematurity include pre-eclampsia, twins, and antepartum haemorrhage. If premature rupture of the membranes occurs, without the onset of labour, it usually is advisable to keep the woman resting in bed until at least the thirty-fourth week of pregnancy, when labour may be induced.

The main problem of premature labour is that it produces an immature baby who will require specialized care.

Q: *What are the problems associated with prolonged pregnancy?*

A: There is a gradual deterioration in the placenta toward the end of pregnancy. Even at forty-two weeks, however, the placenta may be capable of providing a mature foetus with all the nourishment it needs. But there is a greater likelihood of foetal death occurring, so the obstetrician may induce labour if the woman is considered to be more than a week overdue, and if the circumstances are favourable for induction.

Q: *Is infection serious during pregnancy?*

A: German measles (rubella) is a serious infection when contracted by a woman in early pregnancy. It greatly increases the risk of congenital anomalies in the foetus. Infection with a type of herpes virus may be fatal to the foetus. Any infections should be reported to the obstetrician.

Q: *What is the onset of labour?*

A: During the final two or three weeks the woman may notice the occasional, irregular, but firm contraction of her womb. The abdomen hardens, but no discomfort is felt. If this is confused with the actual onset of labour, it is termed a false labour. Labour commences when regular, powerful contractions occur every twenty to thirty minutes accom-panied by a dull ache or pain in the lower abdomen and back.

Sometimes there is a "show" of blood and mucus from the vagina as the plug of mucus which blocks the cervix during pregnancy breaks apart and the cervix starts to open.

Rupture of the membranes (bag of waters), followed by a rush of clear fluid from the vagina, may occasionally be the first sign of labour.

As soon as the contractions are oc-curring every ten to fifteen minutes, or the membranes have ruptured, the patient should go to the hospital. She should take a suitcase that has already been packed with some clothing for the baby, and a dressing gown, nightdress, and nursing brassiere, as well as toilet articles for the mother.

Q: *What occurs during labour, and how can the mother help?*

A: Labour is divided into three stages. The first stage continues, with regular con-tractions of increasing frequency, until the cervix of the womb is fully open (dilated). The second stage includes the passage of the baby through the pelvis, until it is delivered. The third stage is the expulsion of the placenta and membranes from the womb.

The first stage of labour varies greatly in duration, but commonly takes between five and ten hours. It is shorter in women who have previously had a baby.

At first, contractions may occur only every twenty to thirty minutes, each one lasting for ten to fifteen seconds. As the contractions become more frequent and longer in duration, the cervix progressively dilates. It is during these contractions that the breathing methods, learned in the antenatal classes, are useful. Usually during this first stage of labour, the membranes rupture.

Eventually the contractions occur every two to three minutes, and the woman feels the urge to push. This sensation may be accompanied by a dull, deep backache. This is the beginning of the second stage of labour. The second stage is one of hard, physical effort with contractions coming every one to two minutes, and each one lasting at least thirty seconds. The second stage seldom continues longer than two hours, and is frequently over in less than an hour. Before it commences, the obstetrician usually carries out a careful, sterile gynaecological examination to ensure that the cervix is fully dilated, and to assess the position of the foetal head.

During the second stage of labour the foetal head is pushed further down into the pelvis. When it reaches the pelvic floor, the back of the head turns round to the front of the pelvis. The foetus's chin is pressed down onto its chest. As the foetus extends the head from this bent position upward, the mother's vulva is extended and stretched open. The head is "crowned" at the moment when the vulva is stretched round the greatest circumference of the foetal head.

During this stage, the mother can help by taking a deep breath prior to the contraction, and forcibly trying to expel the baby through the pelvis by "bearing down" during the contraction. It is most comfortable if she can keep her knees bent, and her head and shoulders raised. This exercise and position is taught in the antenatal and natural childbirth classes.

As the foetal head is crowned, the obstetrician may decide to cut the skin at the back of the vulva (episiotomy) so that the foetal head can be delivered more easily, and to ensure that the vagina does not tear. A neat cut is easier to repair than a ragged laceration. Once the head comes through, the rest of the body follows quite rapidly.

Just after being born, the baby's mouth is sucked clear of mucus so that breathing can take place easily, and the eyes are cleaned. The umbilical cord is clamped, tied and cut, and the baby is wrapped in a towel. The baby often is handed to the mother so that she can enjoy her first moments with her child.

The third stage of labour usually is over within thirty minutes. Contraction of the womb is helped by an injection of ergometrine given to the mother as the baby is delivered. There is slight vaginal bleeding as the obstetrician gently manoeuvres the placenta out of the womb. All that is required of the mother at this stage is a final, gentle push.

While waiting for the placenta to be expelled, the obstetrician may inject a local anaesthetic, stitch up the episiotomy, and repair any minor damage to the vagina that has occurred during delivery of the baby.

Q: *What can the woman's partner do to help during labour?*

A: During the first stage of labour, which may last some hours, he can accompany his partner while she walks up and down in her room or the corridor of the hospital. During contractions, he can apply gentle pressure with his hands to her back and remind her to breathe

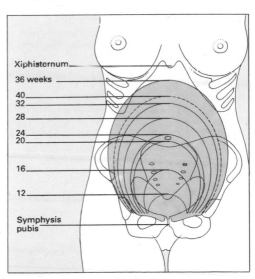

Xiphisternum

36 weeks

40
32

28

24
20

16

12

Symphysis pubis

The womb rises steadily during pregnancy, reaching its greatest height at week 36.

correctly. In the second stage, while in the delivery room, he can provide encouragement to his partner. He also can help to support her neck and legs when she is trying to expel the foetus.

Q: *How can pain be reduced during labour?*

A: Painkilling drugs can be given during labour if requested. Inhalation of a special gas or an epidural anaesthetic causes only slight discomfort, and allows the woman to remain conscious throughout labour. A skilled anaesthetist is required to give the epidural injection.

Occasionally, quite severe headaches may occur for two or three days after delivery. From time to time, general anaesthesia is needed during labour.

Q: *What can the obstetrician do if labour is not normal?*

A: Sometimes the obstetrician decides, before labour commences, that a normal delivery would be too risky. This may occur with a placenta praevia, abnormalities of the pelvis or, sometimes, if the woman has previously had a Caesarean operation. In such cases, the obstetrician performs a Caesarean operation just before the baby is due.

Sometimes, problems occur once labour has already started, such as foetal distress, or prolonged labour. To deal with these problems the obstetrician either performs a Caesarean, if labour still is in the first stage, or helps the delivery by carefully applying forceps around the baby's head. In this way, the baby is gently, firmly, and steadily pulled out. A MALPRESENTATION requires repositioning of the baby's head by internal manipulation. This can be done either by the hand or, more usually, with a pair of special forceps.

Q: *Are there any dangers involved in the use of forceps?*

A: There is a slight chance that the foetus will be damaged or bruised as a result of pressure exerted by the forceps. The risks of foetal damage should be weighed against the risks of not using additional methods to help a difficult delivery.

Q: *How long is it necessary to stay in hospital?*

A: This depends on the obstetrician's advice as to whether both the mother and the baby are well enough to return home. If the pregnancy has been normal, the mother and child are well, and lactation is established, discharge from hospital can often take place within forty-eight hours of delivery.

Q: *What can the mother do to help in her physical recovery after labour?*

A: It is usual to allow twenty-four hours of rest after labour. The mother can help to get her figure back to normal with exercises to strengthen the muscles of the pelvis, abdomen, and back. Care should be taken not to do these too strenuously at first. The ligaments of the joints are still soft, and excessive exercise could cause joint strains.

Q: *Why is it sometimes necessary to induce labour artificially, and how is it done?*

A: Labour is induced if either the health or life of the mother or foetus is at risk. It may be recommended for a variety of reasons: pre-eclampsia; a pregnancy that has continued for more than a week or ten days past the expected date of delivery; a placenta praevia in which the placenta is obstructing the passage of delivery; a maternal problem such as diabetes mellitus; or rhesus incompatibility of the blood, which could lead to haemolytic disease of the newborn.

Labour is usually induced by artificially rupturing the membranes that surround the baby (amniotomy). Intravenous oxytocin may be given to help the uterus contract. Occasionally, drugs alone, by mouth or by injection, bring on labour. The procedure is carefully monitored, and an induced labour should follow the pattern of a normal labour.

Q: *Are there any things that a woman should avoid during pregnancy and the puerperium?*

A: Yes. All drugs, including aspirin, must be avoided during early pregnancy unless they have been prescribed by a doctor. This is primarily to reduce the chances of congenital malformation in the foetus. There also is evidence that drugs, such as marijuana, heroin, and cocaine, can cause problems in babies soon after they are born. Drug addiction must be stopped before labour takes place.

Mothers who smoke cigarettes are more likely to go into premature labour than those who do not. Their babies also tend to be born smaller than average, greatly increasing the chances of the baby dying.

Some drugs may adversely affect the mother. For example, many commonly used drugs aggravate the symptoms of heartburn during the latter months of pregnancy and should be avoided.

Pregnancy test is a urine test to confirm whether or not a woman is pregnant. It is about 95 per cent accurate in women whose periods are two to three weeks overdue. Most tests will not produce a reliable result until the period is at least eight days overdue.

Premature birth describes any birth before the thirty-seventh week of pregnancy or a baby whose birth weight is less than 5.5lb (2.5kg). About two thirds of premature births occur before the thirty-sixth week of pregnancy. Low birth weight does not necessarily result from a short pregnancy: it may be a result of reduced intra-uterine growth during the full length of pregnancy, caused by conditions such as pre-eclampsia.

Some premature babies are perfectly healthy and well-developed. Those who are not fully developed are placed in an incubator, and require the specialist care of a hospital. This may include frequent feeding by spoon or dropper if the baby is unable to suck, and injections of vitamin K to prevent bleeding.

Premedication is a drug or combination of drugs that is given to a patient before a general anaesthetic. It produces a state of mild drowsiness and dries the secretions in the mouth and the bronchi, the main airways to the lungs.

Premenstrual tension, or syndrome, consists of various symptoms that, in some women, occur regularly for several days before each menstrual period. Symptoms vary in severity and include irritability, depression, fatigue, headaches, breast tenderness, and a feeling of abdominal swelling. There may also be running nose, asthma, migraine, and backache. Premenstrual tension can also make women anxious, intolerant, and prone to accidents.

Q: What causes premenstrual tension?

A: The cause is thought to be a hormonal disturbance, accompanied by retention of water within the body tissues.

Q: Can premenstrual tension aggravate any other problems?

A: Yes. Depression, from causes other than premenstrual tension, tends to be increased. Women who suffer from epilepsy may have convulsions only during this time. Any marital problems may be made worse if the wife's irritability is increased.

Q: What treatments can help premenstrual tension?

A: A doctor may prescribe a diuretic (water-removing) drug. This is often quite effective and may also be combined with medication to help depression. Tranquillizers help to combat irritability, but make fatigue worse.

If these simple treatments are not successful, hormone preparations of progesterone sometimes give relief from the symptoms. In some cases, a doctor may prescribe the contraceptive pill.

Q: Do many women suffer from premenstrual tension?

A: Yes. At least one in ten women has the symptoms in a severe form, and a further two in ten have them to a lesser extent. Many other women experience some of the symptoms from time to time. Premenstrual tension becomes more common with increasing age, and the more pregnancies a woman has had. It disappears after the menopause.

Premolar is a bicuspid tooth, which is well adapted for grinding food. There are two pairs of premolars in each jaw, located between the canine teeth and the molars.

Prenatal. *See* ANTENATAL.

Prepatellar bursitis, commonly called housemaid's knee, is an inflammation of the bursa in front of the kneecap. *See* BURSITIS.

Prepuce. *See* FORESKIN.

Presbyopia is longsightedness that occurs as a normal process of aging. As a person becomes older, the lens of the eye loses its elasticity so that the muscles that adjust it become less effective. Distant vision remains unaltered, but the ability of the eye to focus on close objects is impaired. Spectacles usually correct the condition.

Presenile dementia is a degenerative process of the brain that results in loss of memory and inability to care for oneself. It begins before the onset of old age. *See* ALZHEIMER'S DISEASE.

Presentation is an obstetric term used to indi-

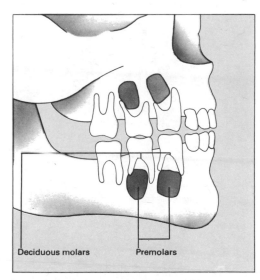

Deciduous molars   Premolars

Premolars begin to form at about the age of 2, and are complete at about the age of 6.

Priapism

cate which part of a foetus is positioned lowest in the womb, just above the cervix. The position of the baby's body is called the "lie".

The normal presentation is occipital, meaning that the back of the head is just above the cervix. *See* MALPRESENTATION; PREGNANCY AND CHILDBIRTH.

Priapism is a persistent, painful erection of the penis without sexual stimulus. It is caused by blockage of the veins in the penis. It is sometimes caused by local infection, leukaemia, or sickle cell anaemia. Sometimes, blood can be extracted from the penis. Anticoagulant drugs also may help.

Prickly heat, or miliaria, is an intensely irritating, fine red rash. The irritation is caused by the body's inability to produce sweat because the sweat glands have become blocked by dead skin cells.

Calamine lotion may give some relief, and light cotton clothing should be worn.

Primapara is the medical term for a woman who has had one pregnancy lasting at least twenty-eight weeks, producing a baby or twins, either stillborn or alive. *See* MULTIPARA.

Procaine hydrochloride is one of the safest and least toxic local anaesthetics. However, excessive amounts of procaine or an allergy to it may be associated with lowered blood pressure and possibly fatal cardiac arrest.

Procidentia. *See* PROLAPSE.

Proctalgia is pain in the anal region without obvious cause. Proctalgia fugax is an intermittent pain in the anal region, commonly occurring at night.

Proctitis is inflammation of the rectum and

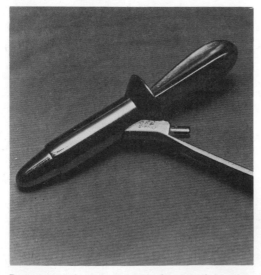

Proctoscope is an instrument for examining the rectum to detect certain disorders.

anus. The main symptoms are pain in the rectal region and a frequent desire to pass faeces. Defecation is painful and may be accompanied by diarrhoea and the passing of blood and mucus. This often is followed by tenesmus (spasm of the local muscles) and pain. The symptoms may be controlled with antispasm and painkilling drugs. But hospitalization may be necessary for thorough investigations to be carried out.

Proctology is a medical specialty concerned with disorders of the anus and rectum.

Proctoscope is a metal or plastic tubular ENDOSCOPE, often containing a light, that is used to examine the rectum.

Prodromal means any early, minor symptom or sign of disease that occurs before the onset of the actual condition.

Progesterone is a female sex hormone produced by the corpus luteum in an ovary during the second half of the menstrual cycle. It prepares the lining of the womb for the reception of a fertilized ovum (egg). Preparations called progestogens have similar effects to progesterone and are used in some contraceptive pills.

See also MENSTRUATION; OESTROGEN.

Progressive muscular atrophy is a form of MOTOR NEURON DISEASE in which there is increasing wasting of the muscles resulting from degeneration of the spinal cord. The exact cause of the condition is unknown. There are several similar conditions occurring at different ages which are characterized by muscular weakness that worsens gradually over several years. There is no treatment.

Prolactin is a hormone that is produced by the front lobe of the PITUITARY GLAND in women. It stimulates the glands in the breasts (mammary glands), thereby starting milk production (lactation) at the end of pregnancy and sustaining it after childbirth. Prolactin has this effect only when certain hormones, such as OESTROGEN, PROGESTERONE, and OXYTOCIN, are also present.

Prolapse is an abnormal, downward displacement of a part of the body. Examples include prolapse of the rectum, in which the membranes that line the rectum protrude through the anus; and prolapse of the womb (uterus), in which the supporting ligaments become so weak that the womb is displaced into the vagina. Prolapse of the rectum is relatively uncommon, and may be the result of an underlying disorder or a congenital abnormality.

Q: How is prolapse of the rectum treated?

A: This seldom is a problem when it occurs in infants, providing a doctor is consulted. By applying gentle pressure to the protruding tissue, it generally can be pushed back inside, and the condition usually is self curing in a matter of weeks.

In the elderly, prolapse of the rectum is a more serious matter. If it recurs frequently, or if it is not possible to push it back, an operation may have to be done to remove the prolapsed tissues. Alternatively, a circle of wire or nylon can be placed around the anus to tighten the opening.

Q: *Why does prolapse of the womb occur?*

A: The cause is a gradual slackening of the ligaments that support the walls of the vagina and the womb. This usually happens because the ligaments are stretched during childbirth; they also become weakened after menopause because of lack of hormone production. Although prolapse of the vagina may occur without prolapse of the womb, the two usually occur together.

Q: *What are the symptoms of prolapse of the womb?*

A: The main symptom is a sensation of "something falling out of the vagina." This is sometimes accompanied by a deep ache in the lower abdomen. If the prolapse is severe, the neck of the womb (cervix) sticks out of the vagina, between the labia; this is known as a procidentia.

Other symptoms include incontinence of urine on coughing, laughing, or lifting weights (stress incontinence); and, occasionally, difficulty in defecating. The prolapse may be accompanied by a vaginal discharge.

Q: *How is a prolapse of the womb treated?*

A: The best treatment is a surgical operation to shorten the ligaments that support the womb, and to stitch the top of the vagina back into a secure position. This operation usually is accompanied by removal of part of the cervix.

If an operation cannot be performed, a plastic ring (pessary) can be inserted into the vagina to hold the womb in place.

Q: *Is there any way in which a woman can prevent a prolapse of the womb from occurring?*

A: Yes. Care during childbirth is essential so that the second stage of labour does not last too long (*see* PREGNANCY AND CHILDBIRTH). After childbirth, the woman should strengthen the muscles and ligaments surrounding the womb by doing postnatal exercises, as recommended by a physiotherapist.

Prone is the position of the body when lying face downward.

Prophylactic is any agent that is used to prevent disease, for example, immunization in childhood or the use of antimalarial drugs.

The term prophylactic also describes any chemical or physical device used to reduce the risk of contracting a venereal disease.

Proptosis is a forward bulge, especially of the eye. It is the main feature of EXOPHTHALMOS, but it also may occur if there is a tumour in the eye or in the eye socket.

Prostaglandins are a group of hormone-like substances found in most body tissues. They affect PERISTALSIS, the blood vessels, the bronchial tubes, and the uterus.

Prostatectomy is an operation to remove the prostate gland. This may sometimes be done through the penis (transurethral prostatectomy), or in an abdominal operation. Prostatectomy always results in sterility.

See also PROSTATOMEGALY.

Prostate gland is a walnut-sized organ that is part of the male urogenital system. It lies beneath the bladder and surrounds the urethra, the tube that carries urine from the bladder. The prostate gland produces secretions that maintain the vitality of SPERM.

Prostate problems generally cause difficulties with urination, because the prostate gland surrounds the urethra (the tube that carries urine from the bladder). A gradual enlargement of the prostate gland (benign prostatomegaly) normally occurs with increasing age. But enlargement also may be caused by cancer of the prostate. Inflammation of the prostate (prostatitis), caused by an infection, tends to occur in younger men.

Q: *What symptoms occur with prostate problems?*

A: The symptoms caused by benign

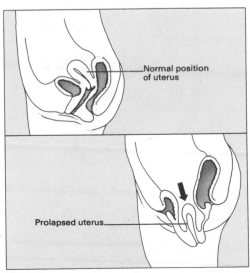

Prolapse (severe) of the uterus occurs when the muscles in the pelvic floor give way.

Normal position of uterus

Prolapsed uterus

Prostatic hypertrophy

prostatomegaly, prostatitis, and cancer are all similar. There is increased frequency of passing urine, combined with a feeling that the bladder is not empty, even immediately after urination. Sometimes there is extreme urgency as well as slight discomfort on passing urine (dysuria) or, alternatively, the patient is unable to pass urine even when he has the opportunity. Usually he has to urinate several times at night (nocturia), and occasionally there is blood in the urine (haematuria).

Sometimes the patient cannot pass urine at all. This may occur gradually over a matter of a few weeks (chronic retention), with backflow of excess urine leading to kidney failure (uraemia). Or it may occur suddenly, as a painful acute retention of urine. Any form of retention needs urgent treatment.

Q: How are prostate problems treated?

A: Treatment depends on the cause. *See* PROSTATITIS; PROSTATOMEGALY.

Prostatic hypertrophy is enlargement of the prostate gland. *See* PROSTATOMEGALY.

Prostatitis is inflammation of the prostate gland. It may occur as the result of a venereal disease, nonspecific urethritis, or infection spreading from the intestine, or it may develop after an examination of the inside of the bladder (cystoscopy).

Prostatitis causes symptoms similar to those of other prostate problems. Painful and frequent passing of urine (dysuria) is a common symptom if the infection is acute.

Prolonged treatment with antibiotics may

be necessary, and the patient usually is advised to avoid sexual intercourse until the infection is cured.

Prostatomegaly is an increase in the size of the prostate gland. It normally occurs in men over the age of fifty years and slowly, but steadily, develops so as to cause the minor symptoms of prostate problems. This condition is known as benign prostatomegaly and often needs no treatment. But if the symptoms become severe or are caused by cancer, medical treatment is necessary.

Q: Can complications arise from benign prostatomegaly?

A: Yes. Complications arise from back pressure of the urine and poor drainage from the bladder. These may result in (1) retention of urine, and bleeding from a dilated vein, which causes blood in the urine (haematuria); (2) urinary infection and the formation of bladder stones (calculi) due to incomplete emptying of the bladder; and (3) damage to the kidney, causing hydronephrosis and uraemia.

Q: How is benign prostatomegaly treated?

A: Surgical removal of the prostate gland (prostatectomy) is the only way of curing the symptoms. Occasionally it may be necessary to reduce the pressure caused by retention of urine by catheterizing the patient for a few days before the operation.

Q: What is the treatment for prostatomegaly caused by cancer?

A: In the early stages of the disorder, an operation to remove the prostate gland often cures the condition. In later stages, particularly if the man is elderly and the cancer has spread, treatment with female hormones (oestrogens) or removal of the testes is often effective. It can prevent further spread and development for many years, as well as reduce the size of the gland and lessen the symptoms.

Prosthesis is the medical term for the replacement of any part of the body by an artificial substitute. Some external prostheses are used for purely cosmetic reasons. *See* REPLACEMENT SURGERY.

Prostration is a dangerous state of physical and mental exhaustion that occurs as a result of excessive fatigue, heatstroke, or illness.

The victim should be placed in the recovery position (*see* First Aid, p.573) and someone should remain with him or her until professional medical help arrives. It is essential to find the cause of prostration so that appropriate treatment can be given.

Protein is one of a class of complex nitrogenous compounds that are built up from

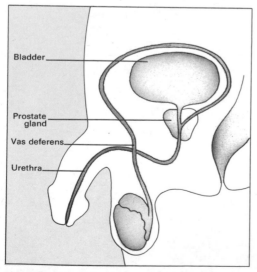

Prostate gland often becomes enlarged in men past middle age, and impedes urination.

Bladder

Prostate gland

Vas deferens

Urethra

simpler amino acids. Proteins are an essential part of the fabric of every living cell in the body.

Human proteins are formed in the liver from amino acids derived from the digestion of protein-containing foods (such as meat and fish). The principal proteins produced in the liver are albumin and globulin, which pass in the bloodstream to various cells, which can make their own complex proteins from them.

Proteins are formed from about twenty different amino acids, and the body is able to synthesize most of these. A total of eight essential amino acids cannot be made by the body, and so they must be obtained from the diet. Complex proteins, such as the red blood pigment haemoglobin, may contain minerals. Other important proteins include the enzymes that are necessary for the normal metabolic activities of the body.

See also AMINO ACID.

Prothrombin is a protein substance that is an essential factor in the clotting of blood. When bleeding takes place, soluble prothrombin is changed by a series of reactions into the insoluble protein thrombin. Anticoagulant drugs depress the formation of prothrombin in the liver and reduce the ability of the blood to clot.

Protozoa are the simplest single-celled organisms to be classified as animal. Some species can cause infectious diseases. *See* AMOEBIC DYSENTERY; MALARIA; SLEEPING SICKNESS.

Proximal describes a part of the body that is closer than some other part to a central point. The part that is farther away is referred to as being distal.

Prurigo is a skin condition in a patient who has been suffering from severe itching (pruritus). Small, firm lumps appear on areas of the skin associated with crusting and sometimes obvious scratch marks.

Pruritus. *See* ITCHING.

Pseudocyesis is the medical term for a false pregnancy.

Pseudomonas is a group of bacteria. *Pseudomonas aeruginosa* can infect human beings, causing pneumonia, endocarditis, or urinary infections. Treatment of pseudomonas infections is often difficult. Few antibiotics are capable of killing the bacteria.

Psittacosis, also called ornithosis and parrot fever, is a rare form of pneumonia caused by a microorganism (*Chlamydia psittaci*) carried by birds. It is usually caught by inhaling dust from faeces or feathers of infected birds. The disorder is infectious and can be transmitted from one person to another by means of airborne droplets (produced by coughing).

Q: What are the symptoms of psittacosis?

A: The infection usually takes between one and three weeks to develop and may begin suddenly or slowly as an influenza-like illness with fever, aching muscles, and malaise accompanied by a cough. The cough produces a small amount of sputum that may become bloodstained as the illness progresses.

Without treatment, the illness lasts for about two weeks with a gradual improvement followed by a further month of malaise, weakness, and often mild depression.

Usually the disorder is fairly mild, but occasionally it can be severe and even fatal in the elderly, if untreated.

Q: How is psittacosis treated?

A: The tetracycline group of antibiotics are usually used in treatment, producing a rapid improvement within two days. The patient should be kept isolated in bed until the fever has subsided. Strong cough mixtures, oxygen, and other forms of treatment for pneumonia may be needed.

Psoriasis is a chronic skin condition that is found in about one per cent of the population. The cause is unknown, but heredity probably is the most important factor; children of an affected parent have a one in four chance of developing the condition. Psoriasis may appear for the first time soon after a streptococcal throat infection. The condition usually occurs in persons between the ages of ten and twenty-five and, although it may disappear for short periods of time, long periods of freedom from it are rare.

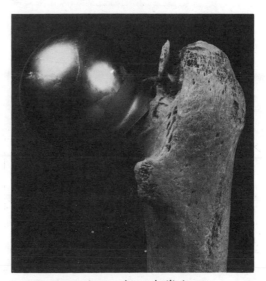

Prosthesis can be used to substitute an artificial part for the head of a femur.

Psychedelic

Q: *What are the symptoms of psoriasis?*

A: A typical lesion of psoriasis is an oval, slightly raised area covered with dry, silvery scales overlying a red area of skin. The size, extent, and distribution of the lesions varies considerably. They may be scattered all over the body, including the scalp, or there may be only one or two rather large lesions, with normal skin elsewhere on the body. The pattern of distribution may be influenced by hormonal changes that occur at puberty, at menopause, or during pregnancy.

Some drugs, such as chloroquine, aggravate the condition. The lesions can join together into extensive areas of scaling skin. Lesions on the scalp do not affect hair growth, and it is unusual for the lesions anywhere on the body to cause more than the mildest irritation.

The condition is often improved by sunlight, and it is noticeable that psoriasis is more common in temperate regions than in the tropics.

Q: *Are there any complications with psoriasis?*

A: Yes. In about a quarter of the patients, the fingernails become pitted, ridged, or discoloured. The nails also may break much more easily than normal.

A form of arthritis sometimes occurs in patients suffering from psoriasis. Any joint may be affected, but commonly it is those of the fingers and lower spine. This produces a condition similar to a mild form of rheumatoid arthritis.

Q: *What is the treatment for psoriasis?*

A: Most doctors start by prescribing a simple course of ointments, such as those containing coal tar and salicylic acid. If these prove ineffective, the drug dithranol may help, but dithranol may stain the skin brown and cause allergies. Psoriasis of the scalp may be treated with various shampoos and creams to separate the scaly skin from the hair.

For more severe cases, corticosteroid creams are applied under a layer of polythene at night. This treatment generally is successful for a short time. The use of cytotoxic drugs is sometimes advisable in patients who have extensive and severe psoriasis. This treatment should be given only under the close supervision of a dermatologist.

Ultraviolet light is of benefit to patients with psoriasis, and treatments involving sunlight, or artificial ultraviolet light, produce an improvement. Recently a new form of treatment has been instituted using psoralens, drugs that increase the skin's sensitivity to light. The administration of psoralens is followed by courses of exposure to ultraviolet light (PUVA treatment).

Many patients with psoriasis become extremely depressed by their condition. It is therefore important for the doctor to keep up their morale because of the social anxieties created by this condition.

Psychedelic describes a mental condition that involves visual hallucinations and an abnormal intensification of feelings, usually induced by drugs such as lysergic acid diethylamide (LSD) or mescalin. *See* DRUG ADDICTION.

Psychiatry is the medical specialty that deals with mental illness, also called psychiatric illness.

Psychoanalysis is a method of treating mental illness devised by Sigmund Freud. An alternative method of treatment based on similar theories of human behaviour was devised by Carl Jung, and is known as analytical psychology.

Psychology is the study of behaviour. Human psychology attempts to measure development, change, normality and abnormality. A psychologist, who is not necessarily a doctor, is trained to make these comparative assessments.

There are various subspecialties within the field of psychology. Educational psychologists assess the mental, social and emotional development, and intelligence, especially applied to education. Clinical psychologists are trained in psychotherapy and assess those with mental illnesses.

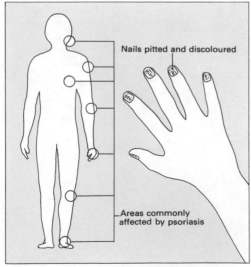

Nails pitted and discoloured

Areas commonly affected by psoriasis

Psoriasis is a skin condition that commonly affects certain parts of the body.

Psychomotor seizure is a form of convulsion, usually caused by temporal lobe epilepsy. *See* EPILEPSY.

Psychoneurosis is a mental disorder that has mental but not physical symptoms, unlike a psychosomatic disorder. Psychoneurosis is an ill-defined term, however, and is often used interchangeably with NEUROSIS.

Psychopathy is a form of personality disorder in which there is emotional instability without a specific mental disorder. Psychopathic behaviour is amoral and antisocial, with a lack of concern for the welfare of others. *See* MENTAL ILLNESS.

Psychopharmacology is the study of the effects of drugs on the mind.

Psychosis is a mental disorder in which paranoia, persistent delusions, hallucinations, and a loss of contact with reality are prominent features.

Psychosomatic disorders are illnesses in which emotions and mental disturbances are thought to produce or aggravate physical symptoms. Symptoms produced by over-activity of the sympathetic nervous system include sweating and palpitations, fainting and nausea, and some skin conditions. Stress and anxiety may cause or aggravate asthma, migraine, and peptic or duodenal ulcers.

Psychotherapy. *See* MENTAL ILLNESS.

Ptomaine poisoning is an old term for a type of food poisoning that was thought to be caused by the bacterial decomposition of proteins forming ptomaine (a poison). It was later discovered that the digestive processes usually destroy ptomaine before poisoning can occur.

Ptosis is the dropping or drooping of an organ such as the stomach (gastroptosis), kidney (nephroptosis) or, especially, the eyelid. Stretched ligaments, obesity, or lack of muscle tone are responsible for most ptoses. *See* HORNER'S SYNDROME.

Q: Can ptosis be treated?

A: Abdominal ptoses can sometimes be treated by wearing a surgical belt which helps to strengthen the abdominal muscles. Ptosis of the eyelid improves with treatment of the underlying cause. In some cases, a special contact lens can be worn to hold up the drooping lid.

Puberty is the period between childhood and adolescence when hormonal body changes produce development of the secondary sexual characteristics. *See* ADOLESCENCE.

Pubis, also called the pubic bone or os pubis, is the smallest of the three bones at the lowest part of the front of the pelvis. The three bones, including the ischium and ilium, together form the innominate bone. The midline joint, made up of strong ligaments and a disc of fibrocartilage, is known as the pubic symphysis. Toward the end of pregnancy, the cartilage in a woman's pubic symphysis softens to allow the pelvis to widen for childbirth.

Puerperal fever, also called childbirth fever, is any fever causing a temperature of 38°C (100.4°F) or over that lasts for more than twenty-four hours within the first ten days after a woman has had a baby.

Puerperal fever resulting from streptococcal infection of the womb used to be a common cause of maternal death after childbirth. Now, puerperal fever is rare because of high standards of hygiene in maternity wards.

Q: What causes puerperal fever?

A: The most common causes are influenza; tonsillitis, and infections of the urinary and genital tracts. In a few cases, fever results from a breast infection that occurs during lactation.

Q: How is puerperal fever diagnosed and treated?

A: After a careful examination, an obstetrician uses a swab to take a sample from the vagina and submits this, and a specimen of urine, for bacteriological tests. A blood test to detect anaemia, and whether white blood cells show reaction to bacterial infection is taken. The patient is occasionally isolated to prevent the spread of infection to other patients.

Once the tests have been made, treatment with antibiotic drugs usually lasts for at least a week, or until the patient's condition improves.

Puerperium is the recovery time after the

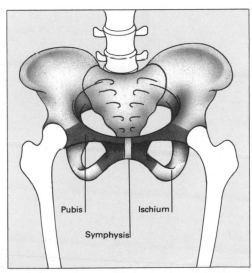

Pubis, a bone at the front of the pelvis, protects the urinogenital internal organs.

Puerperium

delivery of a baby. This period is generally considered to end with the obstetrician's postnatal examination at about six weeks.

Q: *What particular care should a mother take during puerperium?*

A: During puerperium, a healthy mother and baby have to deal with each other, for the first time, as individuals. If the woman has never been a mother before, she is naturally anxious about handling, washing, and feeding the baby. It is during this time that nurses can help to build up her confidence by showing her how to do things in the correct way, and by reassuring her that the baby's crying is not necessarily caused by hunger or pain. The reassurance helps a great deal toward the woman's recovery.

During the first twenty-four hours, it is often advisable to rest in bed. After this time, however, the woman is encouraged to get up and walk around. This helps to prevent deep vein thrombosis.

Routine care includes observations of the lochia (vaginal discharge) as well as vulval swabbing with antiseptic solutions to keep the area clean and to help the healing of any lacerations or cuts. If there are any stitches in the perineum, these may cause discomfort, and a rubber ring is more comfortable when sitting.

There may be problems with passing urine in the first twenty-four hours, caused by swelling around the urethra (exit tube from the bladder) as a result of labour. Occasionally, it is necessary to pass a catheter into the bladder in order to release the urine. It is usually necessary to give laxatives to produce normal working of the bowels.

A transient depression, in which tears mix with laughter, commonly occurs a few days after delivery. These are known as the "blues" and usually pass within twenty-four to forty-eight hours. They result from the combination of excitement, fatigue, and anxiety that is mixed with the happiness of having a baby.

Q: *Are there any serious conditions that may develop during the puerperium?*

A: Yes. Occasionally a woman who has had pre-eclampsia develops the more serious condition of eclampsia. This can usually be prevented by careful obstetric care.

PUERPERAL FEVER occurs in about two per cent of women during the ten days after delivery.

Depression may occasionally become increasingly severe and, in five to ten per cent of women, may require medical treatment. Increasing fatigue and a feeling of futility, combined with despair at her own inadequacy in dealing with the baby are sufficient symptoms for the mother or her family to discuss the matter with the doctor. Occasionally, a true psychotic illness occurs that requires admission to hospital.

A postpartum haemorrhage is a serious complication that may result from infection of the genital tract or retention of part of the placenta in the womb. This needs urgent treatment in the hospital.

Q: *What physical changes take place in the mother during the puerperium?*

A: During this time, lactation begins and the mother's body undergoes considerable change. First, a large amount of body fluid is lost, followed by a gradual tightening of the ligaments and tendons that have become softened by the effect of hormones during pregnancy. The womb gradually becomes smaller and produces less lochia, which also changes in colour. The mother notices that she is returning to her original weight and shape.

Q: *May sexual intercourse be resumed during the puerperium?*

A: Deep sexual intercourse must not be resumed within the first month of the puerperium to avoid the possibility of introducing infection into the womb. Contraception should consist of the sheath and contraceptive creams until the postnatal examination by the obstetrician, when some other form of contraception may be recommended.

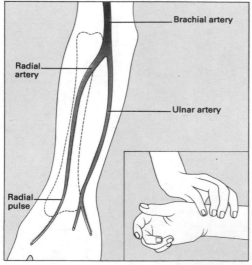

Pulse can be felt by depressing the radial artery onto the radius bone just above the wrist.

390

Pulled muscle is a common term for a muscle that has been slightly damaged by a sudden rupture of fibres within the muscle tissue.

The pulled muscle causes pain and stiffness that gradually improves over a number of days. Treatment with painkilling drugs, heat and massage, and exercises that fully stretch the muscle help to prevent it from tearing again when it is used.

Pulmonary describes anything having to do with the lungs. *See* LUNG.

Pulmonary function tests. *See* LUNG FUNCTION TESTS.

Pulpitis is inflammation of the pulp of a tooth, usually caused by infection of the central cavity. *See* TOOTHACHE.

Pulse is the rhythmical expansion and contraction of an artery that can be felt near the surface of the body. The rate and regularity of the pulse is an indication of the pumping action of the heart and varies with age and activity. The pulse rate of a young baby is about 110 beats per minute; for a resting adult it is about seventy beats per minute. A trained athlete at the extreme of physical effort may have a pulse rate of up to 180 beats per minute, with a resting pulse rate of less than sixty beats per minute.

Irregularities of the pulse may occur in even a healthy young person when the rate varies slightly with breathing (sinus arrhythmia) or occasionally misses a beat.

Ectopic beat (missed beat) occurs more frequently in persons who smoke or those who have some underlying form of heart disease. Rapid pulse rates are known as TACHYCARDIA and slow pulse rates as BRADYCARDIA. Totally irregular pulse rates are usually caused by atrial FIBRILLATION.

Q: Where is the best place to feel the pulse?

A: The most convenient place to feel for the pulse is over the radial artery just before it passes into the wrist. This pulse may be detected by gently pressing down onto the tissues about 2.5cm (1 inch) above the base of the thumb. An alternative place is just in front of the ear, where the temporal artery passes to the forehead.

Patients who have collapsed from shock or undergone cardiac arrest do not have detectable pulses in these places. The only place that a pulse can be felt is over the carotid artery where it passes up the neck alongside the Adam's apple.

Punch drunk is an imprecise term used to describe a form of chronic brain damage usually caused by repeated minor injuries to the head. The repeated damage produces multiple concussions, minor haemorrhages, and loss of brain substance that results in a gradual physical and mental deterioration.

Q: What symptoms are shown by a person who is punch drunk?

A: The condition develops gradually with slurring speech, staggering gait, and dementia. There is a lack of tolerance to alcohol and outbursts of aggression occur.

PUO is an abbreviation of pyrexia (fever) of unknown origin. The term is commonly used by doctors when a patient has had an undiagnosed fever for longer than a week.

Pupil is the circular opening in the centre of the coloured area (iris) of the eye. Light passes through the pupil to the back of the eye (retina). The pupil contracts in bright light and when the eye is focusing on a near object. It dilates in dim light, when the eye is focusing on a distant object, and at times of excitement or emotion. The ability of the pupil to change size is known as the pupil reflex. The size of the pupil is controlled by muscles in the iris, which are supplied by nerves in the autonomic nervous system. An abnormal pupil reflex can indicate a neurological disorder.

Q: What can go wrong with the pupil?

A: Disorders that affect the iris, such as IRITIS, can make the pupil irregular in shape. If iritis causes the iris to stick to the lens, pupil reflex is absent.
Constriction of the pupil may be caused by old age, over-sensitivity to light (PHOTOPHOBIA), HORNER'S SYNDROME, or drugs. Dilation of the pupil may be caused by blindness or poor sight, GLAUCOMA, paralysis of the nerve that controls eye movements (oculomotor

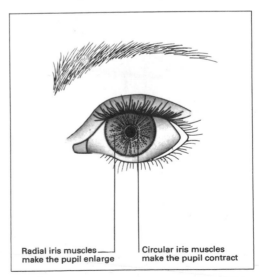

Radial iris muscles make the pupil enlarge | Circular iris muscles make the pupil contract

Pupil of the eye becomes larger or smaller as the iris muscles relax and contract.

Pupil reflex

nerve paralysis), or drugs, such as cocaine. ARGYLL-ROBERTSON PUPIL is failure of the pupil to adjust to the intensity of light but a normal pupil reaction, when focusing. ADIE'S SYNDROME is a congenital anomaly in which one pupil adjusts more slowly than the other.

Q: How are pupil disorders treated?

A: Most disorders of the pupil improve with treatment of the underlying cause. Miotic drugs, such as pilocarpine, constrict the pupil; mydriatic drugs, such as atropine and homatropine, act as pupil dilators.

Pupil reflex is the constriction of the pupil of the eye in response to light. *See* PUPIL.

Purgative is any substance that increases bowel movement. *See* LAXATIVES.

Purpura is a skin discoloration caused by bleeding (haemorrhage) into the skin. A small haemorrhage is called a petechia and a large one, as in a bruise, is called an ecchymosis. Purpura may result from fragility of the blood vessels or a blood disorder.

Q: What causes fragility of the blood vessels?

A: Fragility of the blood vessels usually is inherited, although it seldom is serious. In a more serious inherited form of the disorder, there are obvious abnormalities of the blood vessels in the lips, mouth, and fingers, a condition known as inherited telangiectasia.

Prolonged treatment with drugs such as aspirin and cortisone may also result in purpura. Scurvy (caused by lack of vitamin C) is another disorder that causes purpura. A rare, but serious, cause of purpura is an allergy (Henoch-Schönlein

purpura), which may follow a streptococcal infection that damages the blood vessels.

Q: What defects of blood clotting cause purpura?

A: Various clotting defects can cause purpura. They include haemophilia, THROMBOCYTOPENIA (deficiency of platelets in the blood that help coagulation), and liver disorders in which the level of prothrombin (a protein necessary for blood clotting) is lowered. Drugs also may cause clotting defects. Examples include heparin or warfarin (used in the treatment of thrombosis) and phenylbutazone (used in the treatment of rheumatoid or arthritic disorders).

Q: What are the symptoms of purpura and how are they treated?

A: There may be purple or reddish spots on the skin. Other symptoms may vary from very minor bleeding under the skin to major areas of bruising and haemorrhage into tissues, such as the pleural membranes surrounding the lungs, the back of the eye, or the intestines. Repeated bleeding may cause anaemia.

Treatment of purpura must depend on the accurate diagnosis of the cause. Serious conditions, such as allergic purpura, need urgent hospitalization, with specialized investigation and care.

Purulent. *See* PUS.

Pus is the thick liquid produced by inflammation in abscesses and other infected areas. It contains white blood cells, cellular debris, and fluid. The white blood cells gather in the area to fight infection; the fluid drains from the damaged tissue.

Pustule is a small, pus-containing area just under the skin.

Pyelitis is an infection of the pelvis of the kidney. *See* PYELONEPHRITIS.

Pyelogram is an X-ray of the kidneys made using special iodine-containing dyes, which are opaque to X-rays. There are two main methods of obtaining a pyelogram: intravenous pyelography (IVP) and retrograde pyelography. In retrograde pyelography, a small tube is inserted into one or both of the ureters using a cytoscope (*see* CYTOSCOPY). The dye is then forced along the tube to the kidneys.

See also INTRAVENOUS PYELOGRAM.

Pyelonephritis is an inflammation of the kidney and the renal pelvis, which is the hollow cone into which urine flows from the kidney. The onset of pyelonephritis may be sudden (acute pyelonephritis) or gradual (chronic pyelonephritis).

Acute pyelonephritis usually is caused by

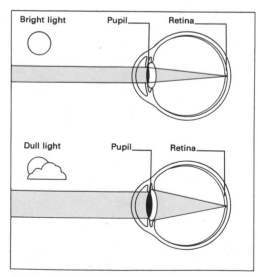

Pupil reflex automatically regulates the amount of light entering the lens of the eye.

the spread of infection from the bladder. Occasionally, it may be caused by the spread of infection through the bloodstream. Chronic pyelonephritis causes destruction and scarring of the kidney tissue as a result of an untreated bacterial infection. Both forms of pyelonephritis are associated with an obstruction to the flow of urine.

Q: *What are the symptoms of acute pyelonephritis?*

A: Usually, there is a sudden onset of pain in the lower back, fever with chills, nausea, and vomiting. Urination may be painful (DYSURIA) and more frequent than usual.

Q: *How is acute pyelonephritis treated?*

A: Acute pyelonephritis is treated with antibiotics and an increased fluid intake. Surgery may be necessary if an obstruction is present.

Occasionally, the treatment eliminates the symptoms without destroying the infection. Such a symptomless infection is rare in men.

Q: *What are the symptoms of chronic pyelonephritis?*

A: The disorder progresses over several years with recurrent attacks of acute pyelonephritis. Usually, there are no symptoms between attacks. Chronic pyelonephritis may cause HIGH BLOOD PRESSURE, and eventually kidney failure with URAEMIA and a large output of urine.

Q: *How is chronic pyelonephritis treated?*

A: Treatment involves removal of any obstruction, which may require surgery and a prolonged course of antibiotics. Treatment for high blood pressure and uraemia also may be necessary.

Pyemia is a serious condition in which septicaemia (blood poisoning) occurs from a pus-forming area and produces multiple abscesses throughout the body.

Q: *What are the symptoms of pyemia?*

A: The symptoms of pyemia are violent shivering because of sudden chill with high rises in temperature, followed by sweating. Frequently, jaundice develops, as well as abscesses in various areas of the body, such as the liver, lungs, and kidneys.

Q: *How is pyemia treated?*

A: The development of pyemia requires urgent hospitalization with full investigations to find the cause. Large doses of antibiotics must be given for some weeks to ensure recovery. Abscesses may have to be lanced.

Pyloric stenosis is a narrowing of the exit (pylorus) from the stomach to the duodenum that causes a partial obstruction. It also is known as pyloric obstruction.

Q: *What causes pyloric stenosis?*

A: Congenital hypertrophic pyloric stenosis occurs in about one in 500 babies and is four times more frequent in boys than girls. It is a genetic disorder.

Pyloric stenosis in adults is caused by spasm or scarring of the pyloric muscle. This is commonly associated with a peptic ulcer, often because of the scarring from repeated ulceration.

Q: *What are the symptoms of congenital hypertrophic pyloric stenosis?*

A: The symptoms usually start in the second week of life with occasional vomiting after feeds. Within a few days, there is vomiting after every feed. It is termed projectile vomiting, because the milk is ejected out of the mouth with a characteristic violence. The baby is constipated and hungry and rapidly becomes dehydrated if the vomiting continues.

Q: *How is congenital hypertrophic pyloric stenosis treated?*

A: The usual treatment is an operation that is performed after the baby has been given intravenous fluids to correct any dehydration and to replace salts that may have been lost. The thickened muscle around the pylorus is cut to prevent it from going into spasm.

Q: *What are the symptoms of pyloric stenosis in an adult?*

A: Vomiting may occur with any peptic ulcer, but in pyloric stenosis large quantities of fluid are brought up. A partial obstruction is indicated if the

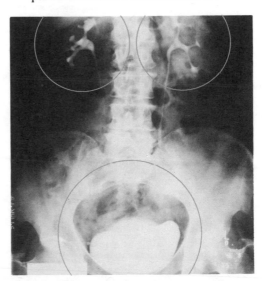

Pyelogram is an X-ray of the kidneys taken after injection of an iodine compound.

Pyloroplasty

vomit contains food eaten six to twelve hours previously.

The patient may complain of a feeling of fullness and, if vomiting is frequent, there will be a loss of weight and sometimes dehydration. Once suspected, the stomach is emptied and a barium meal X-ray taken. A gastroscopy, an examination of the inside of the stomach, helps to confirm the diagnosis.

Q: How is the adult form of pyloric stenosis treated?

A: Because it is not always certain whether the stenosis is caused by spasm or scarring, a trial of medical treatment with antispasm drugs, as well as treatment for peptic ulcers, is given. The course may be continued if the symptoms improve and frequent small meals can be eaten. If the symptoms remain, a surgeon will operate to remove part of the stomach (partial GASTRECTOMY) or to create a new opening from the stomach to the intestine (GASTROENTEROSTOMY).

Pyloroplasty is an operation to relieve the obstruction of PYLORIC STENOSIS by cutting through the pyloric muscle.

Pylorospasm is a spasm of the pyloric muscle at the exit from the stomach, causing the symptoms of PYLORIC STENOSIS.

Pylorus is the narrow exit from the stomach into the duodenum. It contains a circular muscle called a sphincter. The pyloric sphincter helps to control the gradual emptying of the stomach.

Pyogenic is any condition that produces PUS.

Pyorrhoea is a discharge of pus from any part of the body, such as from a boil. The term most commonly is applied to a discharge of pus from the gums.

Pyrexia. *See* FEVER.

Pyridoxine (vitamin B_6) is essential to the body for the formation of proteins from amino acids. It is found in many foods, particularly eggs, cereals, meat, and fish. Pregnant women and those taking contraceptive pills need more vitamin B_6 than usual.

Pyrogen is any substance that produces a fever.

Pyrosis. *See* HEARTBURN.

Q

Q fever is an infectious disease, caused by the microorganism *Coxiella burneti,* a variety of RICKETTSIA. Q fever commonly occurs in sheep and cattle. Humans usually become infected by inhaling droplets from the milk, urine, or faeces of infected animals. The placenta of infected animals is particularly infectious. Rarely, the infection is transmitted by a tick bite, or from handling wild animals.

Q: What are the symptoms of Q fever?

A: After an incubation period of between nine and twenty-eight days, there is a sudden onset of fever, severe headache, shivering, muscle pains and, often, chest pains. A dry cough may develop after about a week. The fever may rise to about 40°C (104°F), and usually lasts for one to three weeks. Complications, such as PNEUMONIA and ENDOCARDITIS, also may develop. Despite the severity of the disease, death is rare, even in untreated patients.

Q: How is Q fever treated?

A: The disease is treated with antibiotics, usually tetracycline. A vaccine against Q fever has been developed, but it is still being tested.

Quadriceps is a muscle with four heads. The term usually is applied to the quadriceps femoris, the large muscle in front of the thighbone. It consists of a group of four muscles that share a common lower tendon. This tendon surrounds the kneecap (patella) and is attached to the front of the tibia (shinbone). Contraction of the quadriceps femoris straightens the lower leg.

Quadriplegia is paralysis of all four limbs. *See* PARALYSIS.

Quarantine is a period of isolation from public contact after exposure to an infectious disease so that the infection does not spread. The length of the quarantine period varies

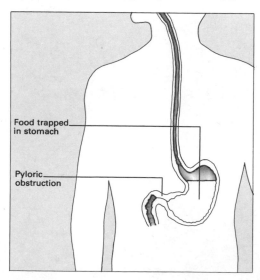

Food trapped in stomach

Pyloric obstruction

Pyloric stenosis is thickening in the wall of the pylorus causing intestinal obstruction.

according to the incubation period of the infection. For example, the incubation period of mumps varies between ten and twenty-eight days. The quarantine period is twenty-eight days after the time of the last (not first) contact with an infected person.

Total isolation of potentially infected persons is not always necessary. It is often sufficient for them to be restricted in their movements or to be under medical supervision. If symptoms appear, total isolation may become necessary.

Quickening is the term used to describe a mother's awareness of her unborn baby's first movements. It usually occurs between the eighteenth and twentieth weeks of pregnancy but in subsequent pregnancies it usually occurs about two weeks earlier. *See* PREGNANCY AND CHILDBIRTH.

Quick's test is a blood test performed to measure the amount of prothrombin, an essential factor in the blood clotting process. Quick's test is used to monitor the effects of ANTICOAGULANT drugs.

Quinine is a bitter, white, crystalline alkaloid substance obtained from the bark of the cinchona tree. It is effective against MALARIA, but has largely been replaced by synthetic antimalarial drugs. However, it is still used to treat malaria in areas where strains of malaria have developed that are resistant to the synthetic drugs.

Quinine also is used to treat night cramps in the elderly.

Excessive doses of quinine may cause headaches, vomiting, noises in the ears (tinnitus), and visual disturbances which may result in blindness. This collection of symptoms is known as cinchonism.

Quinsy, known medically as peritonsillar abscess, is an infection of the tissue around the tonsils. It is usually caused by the spread of infection from TONSILLITIS.

Q: What are the symptoms of quinsy?

A: The symptoms include fever, severe pain on swallowing, even of saliva, and difficulty in opening the mouth (trismus). The patient's breath smells foul, and there may be earache (otalgia).

Q: How is quinsy treated?

A: Treatment with antibiotics usually is effective in the early stages of the infection. However, if the symptoms are severe, a surgical incision of the abscess may be necessary. This allows the pus to drain, and usually gives immediate relief. Quinsy tends to recur and a doctor may recommend that the tonsils be surgically removed (TONSILLECTOMY). This operation should be performed about four weeks after the abscess has healed.

Rabbit fever is an infectious disorder that is transmitted by the bite of an infected blood-sucking insect or tick. It is known medically as tularaemia. *See* TULARAEMIA.

A talk about Rabies

Rabies, also known as hydrophobia, is a virus infection transmitted to man and certain other mammals by the saliva of an infected animal. Infection is through a bite (usually from a dog) or by skin or mucous membrane contact with infected saliva. The incubation period of the disorder can be as short as two weeks or as long as a year; the usual time is one to two months. Death invariably follows within a week of developing symptoms. Anti-rabies injections usually prevent symptoms occurring if they are given as soon as possible contact has occurred.

Immunization is available for people who are particularly at risk. Because of strict control of the import of animals, rabies does not occur in the U.K.

Q: How can you tell if an animal has rabies?

A: The animal, including a wild animal, behaves abnormally, often without fear of humans. At first it is extremely agitated and vicious, but later this is followed by gradual paralysis which makes it move slowly.

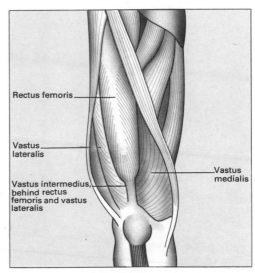

Quadriceps femoris is the strong muscle in the thigh with ligament attachments.

Rectus femoris

Vastus lateralis

Vastus intermedius, behind rectus femoris and vastus lateralis

Vastus medialis

Radiation

Q: *What are the symptoms of rabies in humans?*

A: The first symptoms are fever, depression, and increasing restlessness turning into uncontrollable excitement. There is agitation in which painful spasms of the throat muscles occur, accompanied by excessive saliva which froths and flows down the chin. Drinking even a sip of water produces spasms of the swallowing muscles, followed by saliva flow, hence the name hydrophobia (meaning fear of water).

Q: *How is rabies treated?*

A: The bite must be thoroughly cleaned, as this may prevent the spread of the virus. A person who has been in contact with rabies is given an injection of gamma globulin, which gives temporary protection until a series of rabies vaccine injections can be given.

  Treatment of the symptoms involves complete isolation of the patient. Doctors and nurses must be immunized before contact with the patient. The patient is sedated, and mechanical artificial respiration is used to help control the symptoms. However, once the symptoms begin to appear, recovery is extremely rare.

Radiation is any form of electromagnetic energy wave such as heat, light, or X-rays, or any stream of ions (electrically charged atoms or molecules) or subatomic particles. The earth is exposed to radiation from the sun's rays and from radioactive materials in the earth itself, much of which is harmless,

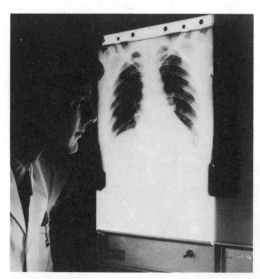

Radiology is a branch of medicine dealing with the understanding of X-ray photographs.

low level radiation. Damage to human tissue and cell formation may be caused by high energy radiation. Low energy radiation scarcely penetrates the skin. A very high dosage of radiation causes RADIATION SICKNESS.

Q: *How is radiation used in medicine?*

A: The use of X-rays in radiology, including the use of isotopes such as radioactive dyes as tracers, is a normal diagnostic procedure in hospitals. Radiotherapy is a method of treatment that employs an intense source of radiation, as in cancer treatment.

  Ultraviolet light is used to treat certain skin diseases, such as acne and psoriasis. Physiotherapists use infra-red heat and shortwave diathermy to treat rheumatic and muscular disorders.

Radiation sickness is an illness caused by over-exposure to ionizing RADIATION from radioactive substances, such as radium and uranium, or from X-rays. The symptoms depend mainly on the total dosage of radiation and the duration of exposure. Acute radiation sickness results from the absorption of a high dose of radiation over a short time. Delayed radiation sickness results from repeated or prolonged exposure to low doses of radiation. Adequate precautions can prevent the danger of radiation sickness in persons who might be exposed to the dangers of radiation in their work.

Q: *What are the symptoms of acute radiation sickness?*

A: The initial symptoms usually appear within a few hours of exposure and they include nausea, vomiting, diarrhoea, and burns. At a later stage there may be conjunctivitis, loss of hair, disorientation, a staggering gait, and convulsions. Anaemia and a severe, often fatal form of gastroenteritis also may develop. The body's immune system may be affected, thereby making the person vulnerable to infection.

  Radiation may damage the foetus in a pregnant woman. This may result in a natural abortion, or the foetus may suffer from any of a variety of congenital defects, such as mental retardation or skull damage.

Q: *What are the symptoms of delayed radiation sickness?*

A: There may be cataracts, HYPOTHYROIDISM, and a reduction in fertility. People who have been exposed to low levels of radiation for a long time have an increased likelihood of developing cancer and leukaemia. Such effects may not become apparent for several years.

Radiculitis is a form of NEURITIS in which

there is inflammation of the spinal nerves in the spinal canal.

See also SLIPPED DISC.

Radiography is the use of radiation, usually X-rays, for studying the internal structures of the body as an aid to diagnosis. The X-rays are recorded on photographic plates, or they may be projected "live" on a fluoroscope or a television screen so that a doctor can study the movement of various structures within the body.

See also RADIOTHERAPY.

Radiology is the study of the techniques used in RADIOGRAPHY and RADIOTHERAPY, both of which require a degree of specialization.

Radiotherapy is the treatment of disorders using RADIATION. The machinery used is similar to X-ray equipment, but contains a source of high energy radiation, such as radium or a radioactive isotope of cobalt. An injection of a radioactive isotope, such as iodine, is another technique of radiotherapy.

Q: What conditions can be treated by radiotherapy, and is the treatment effective?

A: Conditions treated vary from rodent ulcers to cancer anywhere in the body. It is often used in conjunction with surgery, or cytotoxic drugs, so there is a higher degree of success than if one form of treatment is used alone.

Radium is a rare, naturally occurring radioactive element. It produces alpha, beta, and gamma rays, which can be used in RADIOTHERAPY.

Radius is the outer of the two bones of the forearm; it forms part of the elbow joint and the wrist joint. It rotates round the other forearm bone, the ULNA, allowing the hand to rotate at the wrist.

See also COLLES' FRACTURE.

Rale is the abnormal sound heard by a doctor when listening to air passing into or out of a diseased lung. The rattling rale produced when there is a partial blockage of an air passage is called a rhonchus.

Ranula is a small cyst under the tongue, commonly caused by the blockage of a salivary duct. Although not serious, a ranula should be examined and treated by a doctor.

Rash is a temporary discoloration or eruption of the skin, usually caused by an infection or an ALLERGY.

Rauwolfia is a drug obtained from the dried roots of the oriental shrub *Rauwolfia serpentina*. It contains a number of alkaloids, formerly used to treat high blood pressure.

Raynaud's phenomenon is an intermittent spasm of small arteries, usually in the fingers and toes, occurring in bad weather. It is most frequent in young women. It usually occurs without obvious cause, but may occasionally be caused by pressure on the nerves supplying the arteries, rare blood disorders, or SCLERODERMA. The fingers become white and numb and then, as circulation improves, swollen, painful, and blue-red in colour. In severe cases gangrene and ulceration of the fingertips may occur. Treatment with drugs to dilate the blood vessels is often effective. If known, the cause itself is treated.

See also ACROCYANOSIS; CHILBLAINS.

RBC is an abbreviation for red blood cell. *See* RED BLOOD CELL.

Recessive is a term used to describe certain genes in HEREDITY. It is the opposite of DOMINANT.

Rectal fissure, also known as anal fissure, is a tear in the mucous membranes that line the anus. It may extend into the lower part of the rectum, and commonly accompanies CONSTIPATION. *See* FISSURE.

Rectocele is a relaxation of the tissues that support the rectum so that it forms a type of hernia into the rear wall of the vagina. A rectocele occurs with PROLAPSE of the uterus. It may be accompanied by a similar prolapse of the front wall of the vagina, and may involve the bladder and urethra, causing stress incontinence (sudden loss of urine on straining). The symptoms and treatment are those associated with prolapse.

Rectum is the final portion of the large intestine, extending through the pelvis from the end of the colon to the anus. Situated in front of the sacrum and behind the bladder, the rectum is about 12cm (five inches) long. The upper part is covered by the peritoneum,

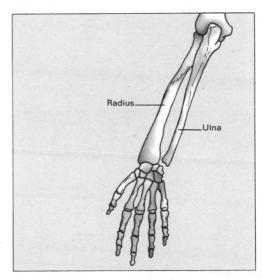

Radius is the outer bone of the forearm. It is shorter but stronger than the ulna.

Red blood cell (RBC)

the membrane that lines the abdominal cavity, and the lower part is supported by the muscles and ligaments of the pelvic floor.

The desire to defecate is caused by the feeling that occurs when faeces are passed from the colon into the rectum. Failure to defecate reduces the desire to do so, and chronic constipation may then develop.

Q: *What conditions can affect the rectum?*

A: Conditions that affect the rectum include infections such as amoebic dysentery, schistosomiasis, ulcerative colitis, and Crohn's disease of the rectum.

The rectum may undergo a prolapse, in which its internal mucous membranes become detached from the underlying wall and protrude from the anus. This usually corrects itself in infants, but in adults an operation probably is necessary.

Tumours of the rectum may be either benign (noncancerous) or malignant (cancerous). Such tumours are similar to those elsewhere in the colon, except that they produce bleeding, rectal pain, and spasmodic anal contractions. *See* CANCER.

Red blood cell (RBC), also called an erythrocyte, is one of the various types of cells in blood. An RBC is shaped like a biconcave disc and contains the red colouring matter haemoglobin. Its function is to transport oxygen from the lungs to the tissues in the form of oxyhaemoglobin. In the tissues, the oxygen is exchanged for carbon dioxide, which the blood carries back to the lungs, where it is exhaled.

Red blood cells are formed in the bone marrow contained in the ends of the long

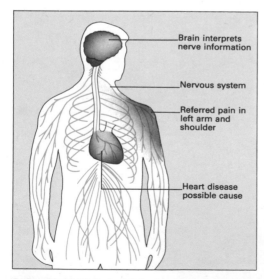

Referred pain is pain felt in an area away from the site of a disorder or previous injury.

bones, vertebrae, breast-bone, and pelvis bones.

Underproduction of RBCs causes ANAEMIA, and overproduction POLYCYTHAEMIA. Some kinds of anaemia may be the result of abnormal formation of blood cells, such as THALASSAEMIA and SICKLE CELL ANAEMIA.

See also BLOOD; HAEMOGLOBIN.

Red eye is a condition in which there are brilliant red patches across the white of the eye. Occasionally the entire white of the eye is involved. Red eye is usually painless and is caused by bleeding under the conjunctiva (a subconjunctival haemorrhage). A subconjunctival haemorrhage may occur following a minor injury to the eye or following vigorous nose blowing. Red eye also may occur in more serious conditions, such as PINK EYE, IRITIS, and GLAUCOMA.

Referred pain is felt in one part of the body (usually on the surface), although the place of origin is elsewhere in the body.

Reflex is an involuntary muscular response to a stimulus, also known as a reflex action. The automatic muscular response is triggered by a nerve pathway between the point of stimulation and the responding muscle, without the involvement of the brain. For example, a person who touches something hot immediately recoils and pulls his or her hand away from the source of heat, even before the brain registers pain. A more commonly known example is the knee jerk reflex, produced in a test that is part of a doctor's basic examination of the nervous system (*see* KNEE JERK).

A conditioned reflex is any reflex not inborn or inherited. For example, a soldier can be trained to fall flat at the first sound of gunfire.

Refractory means failing to respond, or responding slowly, to treatment.

Regional ileitis. *See* CROHN'S DISEASE.

Regression, in medicine, is a return to an earlier stage of a disorder (which could be favourable or unfavourable). Biologically, filial regression is a return to the normal or average in inherited conditions. Psychologically, regression is a return to an earlier type of behaviour, such as childish behaviour.

Regurgitation is a backflow of fluid. The term usually applies to the passing back of food from the stomach to the mouth, usually because of eating too quickly with insufficient chewing. Various disorders of the oesophagus also can cause regurgitation.

Regurgitation also describes the backflow of blood in the heart, caused by damage or diseased heart valves and sometimes leading to heart failure.

Reiter's disease, or Reiter's syndrome, is

thought to be a form of venereal disease, a combination of NONSPECIFIC URETHRITIS (NSU), conjunctivitis, and arthritis. It sometimes follows a period of diarrhoea or, more commonly, a urethral discharge. The disorder is more common among young men than among women.

Relapse is the return of the symptoms of a disorder after an apparent recovery.

Relapsing fever, also known as recurrent fever or tick fever, are diseases carried by ticks or lice. The patient has a high fever for about ten days, then the temperature returns to normal. However, a relapse follows in a day or two. This pattern is repeated until immunity is built up by the patient.

Q: What causes relapsing fever?

A: The disorder is caused by a spirochaete organism (*Borrelia duttoni*) which can be transmitted from infected animals to humans by ticks. The ticks commonly are found in West Africa, the western U.S.A., and various other tropical and sub-tropical regions of the world.

Q: What are the symptoms of relapsing fever?

A: After an incubation period of seven days, the patient has shivering attacks, headache, high fever, rapid heartbeat, vomiting, muscle and joint pain and, possibly, a rose coloured skin rash. Delirium may occur. The fever rises to a peak during the following five to ten days and then suddenly falls.

After a short period of a day or two, a relapse occurs, often accompanied by jaundice, and the pattern of symptoms is repeated. Most patients respond to treatment with antibiotic drugs.

Relaxant is any agent that causes mental or physical relaxation when tension is present because of a mental or physical disorder. Physiotherapy often includes relaxation exercises, as do most antenatal classes. A simple hot bath also can relax tense muscles.

Special groups of drugs can be prescribed, usually with painkillers, to relax muscles after an injury or an operation. During surgery, similar drugs are used to produce complete muscle paralysis, which helps the surgeon while operating.

Remission is a period, during the course of an illness, during which a patient's symptoms become less severe or may even disappear completely.

Renal refers to anything having to do with, or shaped like, a kidney. *See* KIDNEY.

Renal calculus is a stone in the kidney. *See* CALCULUS; NEPHROLITHIASIS.

Renin is a hormone that is released by the kidney to maintain normal blood pressure if it should fall. *See* KIDNEY.

Rennin is an enzyme, produced in a baby's stomach, which curdles milk and aids in its digestion.

Replacement surgery, also known as spare-part surgery, concerns the replacement of diseased or damaged parts of the body with natural or artificial substitutes. Materials used range from plastic and metal to donated human tissue, so that many parts of the body, such as arteries, tendons, joints, and the cornea of the eye can receive some form of surgery. *See* TRANSPLANT SURGERY.

Reportable diseases are those which, in most countries or states, must be reported to the community health officer, who can then take action to control the spread of disease. *See* INFECTIOUS DISEASES.

Repression is a psychiatric term used to describe the transfer of unpleasant memories from the conscious to the unconscious mind. It can affect a person's attitude to situations in later life that force him or her to confront the past memory. Examples of repression related situations include a fear of heights (acrophobia) and a fear of strangers (xenophobia).

Resection is the removal of a part of an organ or a bone. Usually, it means that the remaining undamaged sections are joined together. *See* SUBMUCOUS RESECTION.

Reserpine is the principal alkaloid obtained from the root of the rauwolfia plant. *See* RAUWOLFIA.

Resolution has two medical meanings: (1) the ability of the eye to distinguish between two separate but close objects; and (2) a return to normal, or an improvement, of any

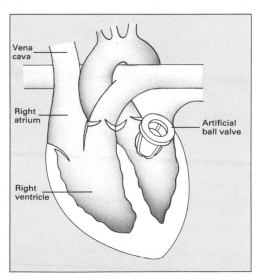

Replacement surgery may be performed to replace a damaged heart valve.

399

Respiration

inflammatory condition, such as a boil.

Respiration, or breathing, is the process by which oxygen from the air is exchanged for carbon dioxide from the body cells. The physical process of breathing involves the inspiration of air into the lungs, from where oxygen is carried by the blood to the tissues. Here it is exchanged for carbon dioxide, a waste product. *See* LUNG DISORDERS; LUNG.

Respirator is an apparatus used to purify the air a person inhales. It may be a simple gauze mask or a complex piece of machinery which extracts dusts and gases from all the air in a building.

An artificial respirator is also a machine that is used in medicine to aid or maintain breathing. It commonly is used during general anaesthesia when the patient's breathing muscles have been paralyzed by muscle-relaxant drugs.

See also ARTIFICIAL RESPIRATION.

Respiratory disorders. *See* LUNG DISORDERS.

Respiratory distress syndrome is a lung disorder of the newborn, particularly of premature babies. Other predisposing factors include poorly controlled diabetes mellitus in the mother and maternal haemorrhage before the onset of labour. The second baby of a twin birth is liable to have respiratory distress syndrome.

Q: What causes respiratory distress syndrome?

A: The condition may be caused by a failure in the foetus of the immature lung to produce a substance that prevents the lung from collapsing once air has been inhaled immediately after birth. In a premature baby, areas of the lung may remain collapsed. These areas become inflamed, producing an abnormal membrane. Provided the baby can survive a few days, the necessary substance that keeps the lungs open is produced and the baby survives.

Q: What are the symptoms of respiratory distress syndrome?

A: Usually the symptoms begin immediately after birth, although they may not be apparent for two or three hours. Symptoms include rapid breathing, often with an expiratory grunt, a bluish tinge to the skin (cyanosis) and, sometimes, respiratory arrest.

Q: How is respiratory distress syndrome treated?

A: Treatment is carried out in a neonatal special care unit or a neonatal intensive care unit, depending on the severity of the condition. Mild cases may be treated with just supplemental oxygen; severe cases may be treated with mechanical ventilation.

Respiratory stimulants are drugs or other substances used to stimulate the physical action of breathing.

Respiratory stimulants may be used in the respiratory failure that occurs during barbiturate or other forms of poisoning.

Restless legs is a common complaint of the elderly in which there is a feeling of general discomfort that compels a person to move his or her legs, sometimes almost involuntarily, when sitting at rest or lying down.

The condition may be associated with iron deficiency anaemia, varicose veins, or polyneuritis. It may follow a partial gastrectomy. Tranquillizers (such as the phenothiazines) used in the treatment of mental illness may also be a factor. Treatment with muscle relaxant drugs is sometimes effective.

Resuscitation is any one of various methods used to restore breathing and heart action. *See* First Aid, p.518.

See also ARTIFICIAL RESPIRATION; CARDIAC MASSAGE.

Retention is the inability to pass urine. The term also is used for a method of keeping false teeth in their correct position, and it is a psychological term meaning the ability to retain past memories.

Q: What causes urinary retention?

A: Retention may result if normal sensations from the bladder are disturbed by anaesthetic or painkilling drugs. Antispasm drugs and antidepressants also may cause retention.

Physical causes of retention include nervous disorders such as polyneuritis,

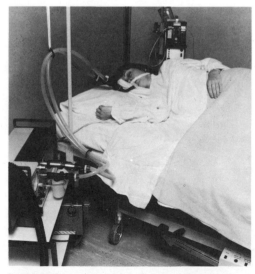

Respirator is used to help a patient breathe – most commonly during surgery.

multiple sclerosis, and the effects of a stroke. Bladder disorders, prostate problems, stricture (narrowing) of the urethra, or pregnancy also can cause sudden retention. Gradual retention when a person has a full bladder results in overflow INCONTINENCE. Treatment is directed at the cause.

Retina is the light-sensitive area at the back of the eyeball. It consists of a layer of cells called rods and cones. Rod cells are sensitive to various intensities of light, and cone cells are sensitive to colour. *See* DETACHED RETINA; EYE; RETINITIS.

Retinitis is inflammation of the retina, the light-sensitive surface inside the back of the eye. Retinitis is a symptom of a wide variety of conditions, including tuberculosis, kidney disease, arteriosclerosis, syphilis, eclampsia, leukaemia, congenital toxoplasmosis, hypertension, diabetes mellitus, and some diseases of the brain. Retinitis also may be caused by damage to the retina through excessive exposure to light (photoretinitis). Other forms of retinitis, such as RETINITIS PIGMENTOSA and retinitis proliferans, may be caused by an inherited disorder or by scarring following repeated retinal haemorrhages.

Retinitis pigmentosa is a degenerative condition of the retina of unknown cause (*see* RETINITIS). Degeneration of the light-sensitive rod cells in the retina occurs first, and night blindness is generally the first symptom. This usually begins in early adult life. The colour sensitive cone cells become involved more gradually, daytime vision deteriorates, and the field of vision is reduced from the edges inwards (telescopic vision). Although the cause of retinitis pigmentosa is unknown, it shows a hereditary tendency and is often associated with other congenital anomalies.

Q: How is retinitis pigmentosa treated?

A: There is as yet no treatment for the condition.

Retrobulbar neuritis is an inflammation of the part of the optic nerve that is within the eye socket. It may be caused by the spread of infection from the sinuses; bleeding into the nerve from an injury; a generalized illness, such as MULTIPLE SCLEROSIS or DIABETES MELLITUS; or infections of the nervous system, such as POLYNEURITIS and ENCEPHALITIS. Often, however, there is no apparent cause for the condition.

Q: What are the symptoms of retrobulbar neuritis?

A: The main symptoms are a rapid and progressive loss of vision; pain when the eye is moved; and a headache. The condition usually affects only one eye. There may be a spontaneous, almost complete recovery. However, further attacks are common.

Q: How is retrobulbar neuritis treated?

A: An eye specialist should be consulted to diagnose and treat the cause. Sometimes, retrobulbar neuritis is treated with corticosteroid drugs. Smoking is usually forbidden.

Retrograde amnesia is a loss of memory for events that occurred before a trauma, such as a head injury. *See* AMNESIA.

Retroversion is a backward displacement of an organ. The term most often is applied to the womb (uterus).

See also PROLAPSE.

Rhesus factor. *See* RH FACTOR.

Rheumatic diseases stem from a wide group of disorders. They include various forms of arthritis and various inflammatory disorders of muscles and ligaments. Symptoms of most rheumatic diseases include muscle stiffness, aching and, sometimes, joint pain. Continued discomfort requires medical investigation.

Q: How are rheumatic diseases treated?

A: Drugs based on aspirin are used when the complaint is mild. Various antirheumatic drugs also may be prescribed. Sometimes, in extremely painful cases, a local anaesthetic and a corticosteroid drug are injected directly into the area of pain to relieve the immediate local symptoms.

Heat, hydrotherapy, shortwave diathermy, ultrasonic treatment and joint exercises are often given by physiotherapists as short-term relief.

The following table lists rheumatic disorders and related diseases; each has a

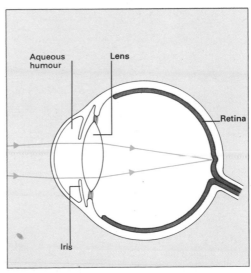

Retina receives light stimuli through the iris and lens, and transmits the image to the brain.

Rheumatic fever

separate article in the A-Z section of this book.

Rheumatic type	Related disease
Arthritis	
(a) Unknown cause	ANKYLOSING SPONDYLITIS
	OSTEOARTHROPATHY
	PSORIASIS
	REITER'S DISEASE
	RHEUMATOID ARTHRITIS
	SPONDYLITIS
	STILL'S DISEASE
(b) Osteoarthritis	OSTEOARTHRITIS
(c) Infective arthritis	PYELONEPHRITIS
(d) Metabolic arthritis	ACROMEGALY
	GOUT
	HAEMOCHROMATOSIS
	HAEMOPHILIA
	HYPERPARA-THYROIDISM
	HYPOTHYROIDISM
	OSTEOMALACIA
	SCURVY
	SICKLE CELL ANAEMIA
(e) Cartilage disorders	CHONDROMALACIA
	MENISCUS
	OSTEOCHONDRITIS
	SLIPPED DISC
Generalized diseases often involving joints	CROHN'S DISEASE
	SARCOIDOSIS
	ULCERATIVE COLITIS
Rheumatic fever	RHEUMATIC FEVER

Rheumatic type	Related disease
Disorders of connective tissue	ALLERGY (particularly to drugs)
	LUPUS ERYTHEMATOSUS
	POLYARTERITIS NODOSA
	POLYMYALGIA RHEUMATICA
	SCLERODERMA
Rheumatism	BACKACHE
	BURSITIS
	CAPSULITIS
	CARPAL TUNNEL SYNDROME
	FEVER
	FIBROSITIS
	MYALGIA
	MYOSITIS
	POLYNEURITIS
	TENDINITIS
	TORTICOLLIS
Miscellaneous	PARKINSON'S DISEASE
	various psychological disorders

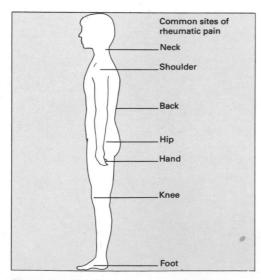

Rheumatic disease most commonly affects muscles and joints of the body.

Common sites of rheumatic pain
Neck
Shoulder
Back
Hip
Hand
Knee
Foot

A talk about Rheumatic fever

Rheumatic fever is a form of allergic reaction by the body to a particular kind of streptococcal infection. The infection usually occurs with tonsillitis. Rheumatic fever causes damage to the body's tissues, and this damage is most serious when it involves the tissues of the heart. Fever-related damage can also involve the central nervous system, the joints, skin, and subcutaneous tissues.

Rheumatic fever most commonly occurs in children between the ages of five and fifteen years, but it may also affect young adults.

Q: *What are the symptoms of rheumatic fever?*

A: Usually the patient has tonsillitis or a severe sore throat. This may have improved by the time the symptoms of rheumatic fever appear, which is usually about two weeks later. The most common symptom of rheumatic fever is a form of arthritis in which the joints become tender, swollen, and red.

Typically, as the swelling of one joint seems to settle, another joint becomes swollen and inflamed. The patient appears unwell, flushed, and has a moderate fever.

Less commonly, symptoms of

breathlessness, fever, or mid-chest pain due to underlying rheumatic pericarditis cause the patient to consult a doctor. It is then that the doctor, when examining the heart, detects the abnormal murmurs produced by inflammation of the heart valves.

Another possible symptom is CHOREA. It is caused by inflammation of the brain, which causes the victim to twist and turn the limbs involuntarily, become clumsy and irritable, and have facial contortions. The sufferer also may grunt and have difficulty in speaking normally.

Q: *What other symptoms may occur with rheumatic fever?*

A: Painless nodules may develop under the skin, particularly over the surface of the large joints, such as the knee and elbow. Transient rashes are also common, but seldom last for more than a day or two.

Abdominal pains are a common occurrence in young children and are probably caused by a combination of a swollen liver, slight heart failure, and inflammation of the lymph glands behind the peritoneum, the membrane that lines the abdominal cavity.

Q: *What is the progress of rheumatic fever?*

A: Usually the fever and joint pains subside within two or three weeks. A patient with chorea may take some months before losing all the symptoms. Skin rashes usually disappear by the end of the fever, and any nodules around the joints gradually become smaller and disappear in a matter of weeks.

The only permanent damage that can be caused by rheumatic fever is to the heart valves. Any pericarditis or rheumatic myocarditis disappears, but scarring occurs on the lining of the heart (endocardium) causing distortion of the heart valves, and eventually resulting in VALVULAR DISEASE of the heart.

However, at least half of all patients who develop the cardiac form of rheumatic fever make a recovery without any valve damage.

Q: *How is rheumatic fever treated?*

A: The most effective and still the basic form of therapy is aspirin. In patients with arthritis, the inflamed joints are rested, often in splints padded with cotton. Corticosteroid drugs are usually prescribed if aspirin is found to be ineffective. Bed rest is essential for those patients with heart involvement until the acute stages of the illness have passed.

It is essential that all patients with rheumatic fever are given antibiotics, preferably penicillin, to kill any residual streptococcal infection.

Q: *For how long should rheumatic fever be treated?*

A: Because the diagnosis usually is made while the patient is in hospital, treatment is started immediately and the patient allowed to return home only when symptoms have improved to such a degree that relatively normal activity can take place. Continued treatment with aspirin is necessary for some weeks or months. Antibiotic treatment should be continued for some years.

Any patient who has had rheumatic fever, particularly if the heart has been involved, must have antibiotics for any dental surgery.

Q: *Can a patient have a second attack of rheumatic fever?*

A: Yes. At present a second attack of rheumatic fever is extremely unusual because the continued daily use of antibiotics prevents further streptococcal infections. Some doctors recommend the use of antibiotics at the onset of any acute throat infection occurring in anyone who has had rheumatic fever. This may further reduce the chances of another attack.

Rheumatism is a general term for any condition that is characterized by stiffness and pain in the muscles and joints. *See* RHEUMATIC DISEASES.

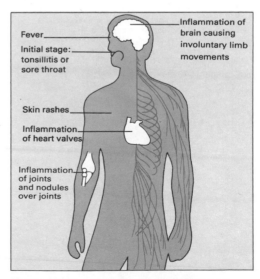

Fever

Initial stage: tonsillitis or sore throat

Skin rashes

Inflammation of heart valves

Inflammation of joints and nodules over joints

Inflammation of brain causing involuntary limb movements

Rheumatic fever begins with a throat infection but progressively causes other symptoms.

Rheumatoid arthritis

A talk about Rheumatoid arthritis

Rheumatoid arthritis is a common disorder of the joints, usually symmetrically involving the body. There is a loss of the joint surface and degeneration because of inflammation of the surrounding tissues. The cause is not known, but it is a common condition affecting one per cent of the population. It is more common in women than in men, and usually affects people between the ages of thirty and forty.

Q: *What are the symptoms of rheumatoid arthritis?*

A: The small joints of the hands and feet usually are involved, but larger joints also may become stiff and swollen, with the corresponding joints on both sides of the body being affected. The stiffness and swelling tend to be worse in the mornings or after exercise, and there may also be tenderness. Frequently, nodules can be felt over joints or bones where they are near the skin surface. The patient frequently feels unwell and easily becomes fatigued. The onset may be sudden (acute) or gradual (chronic).

The joints become deformed, partly because of damage to the surrounding tissues and partly because of shortening of the tendons. Patients with an acute onset of the disorder are obviously ill, with a fever and considerable joint pain. Those with a milder form of rheumatoid arthritis complain more of stiffness and lethargy.

Synovial membrane	Inflammation of synovial membrane	Synovial membrane calcifies
Cartilage	Erosion of cartilage	
Bone		Fusion of the bones
Normal joint	Early stage	Advanced stage

Rheumatoid arthritis begins with inflammation that eventually leads to calcification.

Q: *How is rheumatoid arthritis treated?*

A: Bed rest in hospital often produces an improvement in the acute form of rheumatoid arthritis while treatment is begun. Treatment can be started at home for less severely ill patients.

Drug treatment for rheumatoid arthritis consists mainly of adequate dosage of aspirin or aspirin-like drugs. If these do not seem successful, some of the newer antirheumatic drugs can be used; however, such drugs do not seem to have many major benefits in comparison to aspirin. In severe forms of rheumatoid arthritis, indomethacin or phenylbutazone may be prescribed. Other forms of drug treatment include injections of gold salts, d-penicillamine, and chloroquine.

Use of corticosteroid drugs results in dramatic improvement in the symptoms of rheumatoid arthritis. But their use has to be closely controlled, because they may have to be taken for many years, with an increasing likelihood of adverse effects, without preventing the gradual progress of the underlying disorder.

Diet should be normal and the patient should have frequent nutritious meals and take additional vitamins. Splints may be worn during the day or only at night if one or two joints are more severely affected than the others. Physiotherapy using gentle movements and exercises helps to maintain a full range of movement of the joints until the disorder naturally improves.

Q: *Do many patients become disabled?*

A: Most patients with rheumatoid arthritis make a complete recovery. But about thirty per cent are left with some disability, and a further ten per cent progress to a severely disabling form of rheumatoid arthritis, regardless of the treatment.

Q: *What other forms of treatment are there for rheumatoid arthritis?*

A: Various forms of orthopaedic surgery may be performed on joints that have become seriously deformed but in which the active disease has ceased. Minor operations to relieve adhesions or to remove the synovial membrane (which lines the capsule of a joint and secretes lubricating fluid) may produce considerable improvement. Dramatic progress in replacement surgery now enables surgeons to insert plastic joints in fingers and to carry out total joint replacement in the hips and knees.

However, many patients cannot benefit from these procedures, and may have to rely on specially designed appliances and equipment that can make everyday life easier.

Rh factor (rhesus factor) is the basis of the Rh system of blood groups, which is independent of the ABO system. The Rh factor was first discovered in the blood of the rhesus monkey.

Eighty-five per cent of the population is Rh positive. People without the Rh factor are Rh negative. If Rh positive blood is transfused into an Rh negative person, rhesus antibodies (agglutinins) are formed. There is no adverse reaction the first time this occurs. But subsequent transfusions of Rh positive blood will result in a transfusion reaction in which the red blood cells of the Rh positive person are destroyed. For this reason, it is essential that blood is grouped for A, B, O, and Rh factors before a transfusion is carried out.

Haemolytic disease of the newborn results from the incompatability of an Rh positive foetus and an Rh negative mother. *See* BLOOD GROUPS; BLOOD TRANSFUSION; HAEMOLYTIC DISEASE OF THE NEWBORN.

Rhinitis is inflammation of the mucous membrane that lines the nose, producing a watery discharge. It may be caused by an infection, such as the COMMON COLD; by an allergy, such as HAY FEVER; or the cause may be unknown, for example as with VASOMOTOR RHINITIS. Persistent inflammation may result in gross swelling of the mucous membrane and the formation of a POLYP.

Rhinophyma is a form of ROSACEA in which there is swelling of the sebaceous (grease-producing) glands in the nose, which becomes large, red, and misshapen. Antibiotics given at an early stage may be effective. In severe cases, plastic surgery may help.

Rhinoplasty is plastic surgery of the nose to correct its shape. *See* DEVIATED NASAL SEPTUM; SUBMUCOUS RESECTION.

Rhinorrhoea is the medical term for a thin, watery discharge from the nose. *See* RUNNING NOSE.

Rhonchus. *See* RALE.

Rhythm method is a method of contraception which depends for its effectiveness on abstaining from sexual intercourse for that part of a woman's menstrual cycle during which she is fertile (*see* OVULATION). *See* CONTRACEPTION.

Rib is one of the twelve pairs of thin, curved bones that form the wall of the chest and surround the lungs and heart. The movement of the rib-cage and the diaphragm controls the flow of air into and out of the lungs.

The ribs are joined at the back to the thoracic vertebrae of the spine. The upper seven pairs are called the true ribs, because they are connected in front to the breastbone (sternum). The remaining five pairs of ribs are called the false ribs. The eighth, ninth, and tenth pairs of ribs are connected to the breastbone by cartilage.

Q: What is a cervical rib?

A: It is a rare additional rib, joined to the seventh cervical vertebra in the neck. A cervical rib may cause pressure on the nerves and blood vessels serving the arm, and produce symptoms of neuralgia or Raynaud's phenomenon. Surgical removal of the rib cures the symptoms.

Q: Can the ribs be broken?

A: Yes. A fracture is the most common injury to a rib. It is most likely to occur in the middle ribs. Although painful, a broken rib is seldom serious. The usual treatment is to give the patient painkilling drugs, but sometimes a surgeon will inject the area of the fracture with a local anaesthetic.

A complete fracture sometimes pierces the chest wall. This causes air to collect in the chest cavity (pneumothorax) or allows bloody fluid to accumulate (haemothorax). Hospital treatment and surgery are necessary if either condition occurs.

Riboflavin, or vitamin B_2, is a water-soluble vitamin of the B complex group. It is found in many foods, particularly beef, fish, liver, kidney, leafy green vegetables, milk, and milk products, such as cheese.

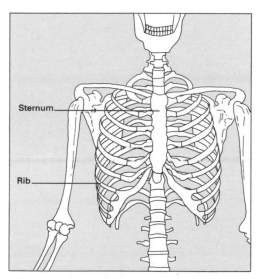

Rib is one of twenty-four bones forming a cage for the chest cavity.

Rickets

Riboflavin is essential for the production of energy in the body. Deficiency results in eye disorders, forms of dermatitis, and cheilosis (in which there are small sores at the corners of the mouth).

Rickets is a bone disease of children that is caused by a lack of vitamin D. Vitamin D deficiency in adults causes OSTEOMALACIA. Vitamin D is formed in the skin when it is exposed to sunlight. It also may be obtained from some foods, such as fish and eggs. Lack of vitamin D affects the kidneys and disrupts the calcium and phosphorus metabolism in the body. This in turn affects the deposition of calcium in the bones, resulting in deformity (*see* CALCIUM).

Q: *What are the symptoms of rickets?*

A: Infants with rickets are sometimes restless, grow more slowly than normal, and do not crawl or walk until older than usual. If the condition continues, the ends of the long bones become enlarged. When the infant starts to walk, the legs may bend, resulting in either bow-legs or knock-knees. The chest also may be deformed, producing a pigeon breast, and small knobs may develop on the ends of the ribs. Occasionally, there may be spasms (tetany) due to the low level of calcium in the body.

Q: *How is rickets treated?*

A: Rickets is treated by giving a concentrated supply of vitamin D in addition to an adequate diet. Calcium supplements may also be prescribed to help to restore the normal calcium metabolism. Any deformities usually disappear if the

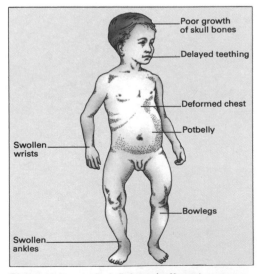

Rickets (vitamin D deficiency) affects bone formation, producing a variety of symptoms.

Poor growth of skull bones

Delayed teething

Deformed chest

Potbelly

Swollen wrists

Bowlegs

Swollen ankles

condition is treated in the early stages.

Rickettsia is a group of microorganisms that have characteristics of both bacteria and viruses. Rickettsia cause many diseases and usually are transmitted by parasites, such as fleas, lice, mites, and ticks. Rickettsial diseases tend to be of sudden onset and produce various symptoms, which are usually the result of blockage of the blood vessels by the rickettsia.

There are four main groups of rickettsial disease: the TYPHUS group; the spotted fever group, including ROCKY MOUNTAIN SPOTTED FEVER; Q FEVER; and trench fever, which is transmitted by lice and causes an illness that is similar to a mild form of Rocky Mountain spotted fever.

Rigor is a sudden attack of shivering with a high fever, followed by excessive perspiration. It is most commonly associated with the onset of an acute infectious illness, such as malaria or pneumonia.

Rigor mortis is the stiffening of the body after it dies. It may last for several hours before the body becomes relaxed again.

Ringing ears denotes a disorder of the ear. It is medically known as tinnitus. See TINNITUS.

Ringworm is an infection of the skin caused by a fungus from the group called dermatophytes. The three main types of these fungi are *Epidermophyton, Microsporum*, and *Trichophyton*. Typically they produce raised reddened rings or scaling of the skin as they feed on the dead skin tissue (epidermis), and affect the live tissue underneath.

Q: *What areas of the body are likely to be affected by ringworm?*

A: The feet may pick up the fungi *Trichophyton* in public places such as swimming pools or changing rooms. This form of the infection is known as ATHLETE'S FOOT (tinea pedis). Sometimes a secondary infection develops, causing CELLULITIS. The toenails develop a gnarled, thickened appearance if they become infected with tinea.

Ringworm of the nails (tinea unguium) is commonly caused by either the *Epidermophyton* or *Trichophyton* fungi. Jock itch (Dhobie itch) is a skin infection by the fungi *Epidermophyton* caused by a combination of tight underwear, obesity, and hot weather. Ringworm of the scalp (tinea capitis) usually is caused by the fungi *Microsporum*, and sometimes a variety of *Trichophyton*.

Q: *How is ringworm treated?*

A: A number of antifungal creams can be used to treat ringworm of the body, athlete's foot, and jock itch.

Ringworm is a contagious disease,

especially among children, so patients should avoid contact with other individuals wherever possible. Athlete's foot is extremely common and patients should not walk barefoot.

Rinne's test is a hearing test in which a vibrating tuning fork is placed alternately with its prongs near the auditory canal of the ear (air conduction), then with its base on the bone behind the ear (bone conduction). Normally the sound is heard for some time longer when the tuning fork is placed by the auditory canal. This is a positive result. In conductive deafness, the sound is heard longer through the bone. This is a negative result.

See also DEAFNESS.

Rio Grande fever is a local name for brucellosis. *See* BRUCELLOSIS.

Rocky Mountain spotted fever is an infectious rickettsial disease caused by the microorganism *Rickettsia rickettsii*, which is transmitted by ticks. It occurs in the western states of the U.S.A. and also in South America.

Q: What are the symptoms of Rocky Mountain spotted fever?

A: After an incubation period of about a week there is the sudden onset of a severe headache, muscle pains, and a high fever. Within four days, a rash appears on the arms and legs, and spreads rapidly to the rest of the body. Areas of the rash may coalesce and ulcerate. A dry, unproductive cough also may develop. In severe cases, the patient becomes delirious or comatose. The fever lasts between two and three weeks.

If untreated, various complications may develop, such as pneumonia, brain damage, and heart damage.

Q: How is Rocky Mountain spotted fever treated?

A: Immediate treatment with antibiotics, such as tetracycline, usually produces a rapid improvement. Hospitalization may be necessary in severe cases.

A vaccine against Rocky Mountain spotted fever is available.

Rodent ulcer is a form of skin cancer, sometimes called a basal cell carcinoma. It usually appears on the face, tip of the nose, eyelids, or ears. Although it is classified as a cancer, it spreads only by local ulceration and not by metastasis (spread of malignancy through the blood and lymph). Most patients are over the age of fifty.

At first a rodent ulcer appears as a small, pearl-like nodule which slowly grows and ulcerates in the centre to form a small scab. Early treatment produces a cure rate of over ninety-five per cent.

Romberg's sign is the inability to maintain balance when the feet are together and the eyes are shut. If the sense of balance is disturbed, as may occur with TABES DORSALIS, the person sways and may fall.

Rosacea, also called acne rosacea, is a skin inflammation associated with disorders of the sebaceous (oil secreting) glands in the skin. It usually affects the forehead, cheeks, nose, and chin.

Q: What are the symptoms of rosacea?

A: The chief symptom is frequent flushing of the skin, with residual redness. The sebaceous glands produce acne-like lumps, giving the skin a rough reddish appearance. Sometimes, there are also symptoms of seborrhoeic dermatitis with scurf on the scalp, and inflammation of the eyelids.

Q: How is rosacea treated?

A: Tetracycline drugs and other broad-spectrum antibiotics usually are effective. Corticosteroid creams should not be used for any length of time because they may damage the skin. Solutions containing sulphur may be beneficial.

See also RHINOPHYMA; SEBORRHOEA.

Roseola (roseola infantum), also known as exanthema subitum, is a disease of young children. The cause is not known, but it is thought to be a viral infection.

Q: What are the symptoms of roseola infantum?

A: After an incubation period of between four and seven days, there is the sudden onset of high fever, which may reach

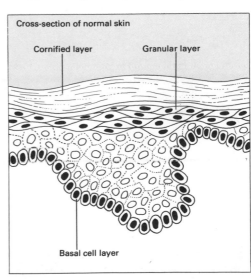

Cross-section of normal skin

Cornified layer   Granular layer

Basal cell layer

Rodent ulcer is a malignant growth that begins in the basal cells, usually on the face.

Roundworms

40.5°C (105°F). The fever usually lasts for three or four days, and may cause convulsions. The fever then disappears suddenly, and a pink rash appears. This occurs mainly on the body, but the limbs and face also may be mildly affected. The rash usually disappears within two days.

Q: How is roseola infantum treated?

A: Treatment is directed towards alleviating the symptoms. Aspirin or paracetamol may be prescribed to reduce the fever, and a doctor may also advise that the child is sponged with tepid water.

Anticonvulsant drugs may be given if the child has previously had convulsions.

Roundworms, also called nematode worms, are a group of parasitic worms. Members of this group that parasitize humans are found in most parts of the world. In some areas, usually those with poor sanitation, up to 90 per cent of the population may be infested. Roundworm infestations include ascariasis, enterobiasis, ankylostomiasis, strongyloidiasis, and trichuriasis.

Ascariasis is infestation of the small intestine with the giant intestinal roundworm (*Ascaris lumbricoides*). The adult worm produces eggs that pass out in the faeces. The infestation is transmitted by eating food that is contaminated by these eggs. When the eggs are swallowed, they develop into the adult ascaris worm. Ascariasis seldom causes symptoms. In some cases, there may be abdominal pain; fever; and coughing. Rarely, worms may block the bile or pancreatic ducts, causing jaundice or pancreatitis. The appendix may also become blocked. Treat-

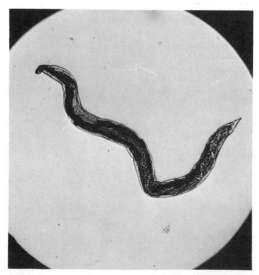

Roundworms: the eggs or larvae develop into adult worms in the intestine.

ment with drugs is usually effective.

Enterobiasis and strongyloidiasis are infestations with *Enterobius vermicularis* and *Strongyloides stercoralis* respectively. These roundworms are commonly known as pinworms, seat worms or threadworms. The life cycles of both worms are similar. The adult worms infest the large intestine and the female emerges from the anus to lay eggs on the skin. The worms are spread either by direct contact between contaminated hands and the mouth, or by eating contaminated food. Treatment with piperazine, thiabendazole, or smilar drugs is usually effective. A doctor may advise treatment for the whole family.

Ankylostomiasis is infestation with hookworms (*Ankylostoma duodenale* and *Necator americanus*). The adult worms live in the intestines and discharge eggs in the faeces. The eggs develop into larvae in the soil, then penetrate the skin and travel in the blood to the lungs and then into the intestine, where they develop into adults, attach themselves to the intestinal wall and suck blood. Ankylostomiasis may cause a skin rash; a cough; anaemia from loss of blood; and occasionally, abdominal pain. In children, infestation with a large number of worms may cause malnourishment, which may affect the child's growth. Treatment with bephenium hydroxymaphthoate or thiabendazole is usually effective. Anaemia may be treated with iron tablets.

Trichuriasis is infestation with the whipworm (*Trichuris trichiura*), which lives in the intestine. It is caught by eating food infected with eggs, or larvae that have developed in moist soil. Trichuriasis may not produce any symptoms. Occasionally, there may be abdominal pain and bloodstained diarrhoea. In children, prolapse of the rectum may occur. Trichuriasis is often difficult to cure, but drugs, such as mebendazole, may be effective.

See also OXYURIASIS; STRONGYLOIDES; TRICHURIASIS.

Rubella is the medical term for German measles. *See* GERMAN MEASLES.

Rubeola is the medical term for measles. *See* MEASLES.

Running nose is a discharge from one or both nostrils. It results from any condition that causes inflammation of the lining of the nose (rhinitis). The most common cause is the COMMON COLD, although it also may be caused by an ALLERGY or SINUSITIS. A running nose following a head injury may be a sign of a fractured skull in which the cerebrospinal fluid leaks into the nose. The fluid may then become infected, and the condition can result in MENINGITIS.

Q: How is a running nose treated?

A: Decongestant nasal drops and sprays may relieve a running nose, but they should not be used for more than about three days. Antihistamines may also help by reducing the amount of mucus produced. A doctor should be consulted if a running nose persists for more than three or four days.

See also CATARRH; NOSEBLEED; RHINITIS.

Rupture is the bursting of an organ or tissue, such as an inflamed appendix. It also is a common term for a hernia. *See* HERNIA.

Ryle's tube is a thin rubber tube that is used to administer test meals and to empty the stomach after surgical operations. It is one of the many types of naso-gastric tubes. It may be inserted through the nose or through the mouth. One end of the tube is slightly enlarged so that it can be swallowed easily.

S

Sabin's vaccine is a vaccine against POLIO-MYELITIS. It is a preparation of one or a combination of the three poliomyelitis viruses, which have been modified so that they confer immunity without causing any symptoms. Sabin's vaccine is taken orally and is considered to be the most effective form of poliomyelitis immunization.

Sacroiliac is the area of the body related to the sacroiliac joint that connects with the two large ilium bones on each side of the sacrum at the base of the spine. Strong ligaments surround the joint; these can become strained, causing backache and pain related to the movement of the joint. Inflammation of the sacroiliac joint is a symptom of ANKYLOSING SPONDYLITIS and other RHEUMATIC DISEASES of the joints.

Sacrum is a triangular bone that forms the rear part of the PELVIS. It binds the two hip bones together, and transmits the weight of the body from the spine to the pelvis.

The sacrum is made up of five sacral vertebrae, which are fused together to form a single bone. At the lower end it forms a joint with the coccyx. The upper end is joined to the fifth lumbar vertebra with an intervening disc. On each side are the SACROILIAC joints with the two ilium bones of the pelvis.

SPONDYLOLISTHESIS, a congenital condition in which the lumbar vertebra tends to slip forward onto the sacrum, may occur. The result can be chronic backache.

Sadism is a sexual practice by individuals who enjoy inflicting pain upon others.

In normal love play, sexual partners quite often inflict slight pain upon each other and this may form part of the mutual pleasure. But extreme forms of sexual activity in which sadism plays a part is considered to be abnormal.

See also MASOCHISM.

Safe period is the period during a woman's menstrual cycle when conception is least likely to occur. *See* CONTRACEPTION.

Saint Vitus's dance is another name for Sydenham's chorea. *See* CHOREA.

Salicylate is a salt of salicylic acid. The most common compound of salicylic acid is acetyl-salicylic acid (aspirin).

See also ASPIRIN.

Saline commonly refers to a solution containing salt (sodium chloride). Physiological saline is a solution of sodium chloride that is of the same concentration as the body fluids (isotonic). This solution may be given by intravenous infusion to replace salt that is lost either during surgery or as a result of shock.

Saliva is a watery, slightly alkaline fluid that is secreted by the three pairs of salivary glands in the mouth. Saliva helps to keep the mouth clean, aids speech, lubricates food, and makes taste possible (because the sensory nerves for taste respond only to dissolved substances). It contains various salts and the enzyme PTYALIN that begins the digestion of starch.

Salivary glands are located in the mouth. They produce saliva. The two parotid glands are in front of each ear; the two subman-

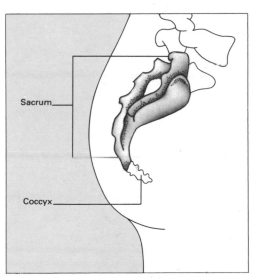

Sacrum is a triangle of five fused bones at the lower end of the spine, above the coccyx.

Salk vaccine

dibular glands are, like the two sublingual glands, situated mainly on the floor of the mouth beneath the tongue; and the small buccal glands are in the mucous membranes of the cheeks and lips. The salivary glands can be affected by viral infection (such as mumps), bacterial infection, stone formation (SIALOLITHIASIS), or cancer.

Salk vaccine is a vaccine against poliomyelitis. It contains three types of dead poliomyelitis virus. It has to be injected and has now been largely superseded by the orally administered SABIN'S VACCINE.

Salmonella is a genus of rod-shaped bacteria, some species of which can cause disease in humans. The most serious salmonella bacteria cause TYPHOID and PARATYPHOID fevers. Other salmonella infections may cause gastroenteritis, which may vary from a mild to a severe, and occasionally fatal, form of food poisoning.

Q: *What are the symptoms of salmonella gastroenteritis?*

A: The symptoms may vary from mild abdominal pain with occasional diarrhoea, to extremely severe vomiting and persistent diarrhoea. They usually occur within about two days of eating contaminated food. The severe form may result in shock due to fluid loss, requiring immediate hospitalization. In some cases, a fever develops, but this rarely lasts for more than about a day.

Occasionally, the infection may spread into the bloodstream (septicaemia) and cause localized abscesses in other parts of the body. Deaths from salmonella

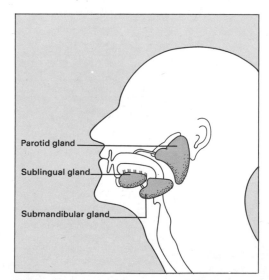

Salivary glands secrete saliva to moisten the mouth and help begin the digestion of food.

gastroenteritis are usually confined to the young, the elderly, and those who already have a serious underlying physical disorder.

Q: *How is salmonella gastroenteritis treated?*

A: Treatment is directed toward alleviating the symptoms and includes plenty of fluids, a bland diet, and antispasmodic drugs to relieve abdominal cramps. Generally, antibiotic drugs are not prescribed because they may prolong the course of the illness. However, antibiotics become necessary if the patient develops septicaemia.

If a large amount of fluid has been lost by vomiting and diarrhoea the patient may be given fluids intravenously to replace the lost fluid. If the patient has localized abscesses, surgery may also be necessary.

Salpingectomy is the surgical removal of a fallopian tube (oviduct). One tube may have to be removed because of an ECTOPIC PREGNANCY. Both tubes may have to be removed if continued abdominal pain occurs, because of chronic salpingitis (*see* SALPINGITIS). The operation also is performed as a means of sterilization. *See* STERILIZATION.

Salpingitis is inflammation of the fallopian tubes. It may affect only one tube, but usually both are involved. The surrounding tissues and the ovaries also may become infected and inflamed.

Salpingitis most commonly is caused by the spread of infection following sexual intercourse. A venereal disease such as gonorrhoea is one such infection. It may also occur following childbirth, an abortion, or sometimes after the insertion of an IUD (intrauterine device). Rarely, salpingitis occurs in young girls and adolescents as a result of tuberculosis.

Q: *What are the symptoms of salpingitis?*

A: Acute salpingitis occurs suddenly and produces severe abdominal pain; a purulent vaginal discharge; fever; and, occasionally, vomiting. Chronic salpingitis may occur after treatment for the acute form of the disease. With chronic salpingitis, there may be a dull abdominal ache, irregular and painful periods, and pain while having sexual intercourse. Many women also feel vaguely ill, with backache, fatigue, and weight loss.

Q: *How is salpingitis treated?*

A: Immediate treatment with antibiotics is nearly always successful in curing the infection. Severe cases may need surgical removal to avoid infertility.

Chronic salpingitis is difficult to treat because the fallopian tubes become scarred, inflamed, and blocked. A long course of antibiotics is usually prescribed, and the patient may also be advised to abstain from sexual intercourse for several weeks. The sexual partner of a woman with salpingitis should also be examined and, if necessary, treated.

Sandfly fever is a virus infection, with high temperature, transmitted by the sandfly (*Phlebotomus papatasii*) and similar species that are common around the Mediterranean and the Asian subcontinent in hot, dry weather.

Saphenous vein is one of the two long surface veins in the leg.

The great saphenous vein runs from the inner side of the ankle to the groin, where it dips down to join the femoral vein. The small saphenous vein runs from behind the outer part of the ankle to join the popliteal vein in the tissues behind the knee.

See also VARICOSE VEIN.

Sarcoidosis is a condition of unknown origin in which areas of scar tissue are formed in many parts of the body, most commonly in the lungs, liver, eyes, skin, and the lymphatic system. It is also known as sarcoid.

Q: What are the symptoms of sarcoidosis?

A: Frequently there are no symptoms at all. Diagnosis is often made from a routine chest X-ray or a physical examination in which the patient's lymph nodes are found to be enlarged. Some patients, however, have symptoms of fever, breathlessness, vague muscle aching, joint pains, and skin lesions (ERYTHEMA NODOSUM). The liver may become affected in a minor way and, rarely, cardiac involvement may result in heart failure.

Q: How is sarcoidosis treated?

A: The aim of treatment is to prevent further damage to body tissue. If the patient has no symptoms and there is no evidence of damage, regular examination is all that is necessary. Corticosteroid drug treatment may have to be given for patients with severe symptoms.

Sarcoma is a malignant (cancerous) tumour formed from connective tissue. The usual treatment for sarcoma is surgical removal, often followed by radiotherapy or, in the case of bone tumours (Ewing's sarcoma), by a combination of radiotherapy and multiple-drug chemotherapy. *See* TUMOUR.

Scab is a protective layer of dried serum and blood, usually discharged from a wound. The tissues beneath the scab, thus protected, are allowed to heal; the scab falls off when healing is complete.

Scabicides are drugs used in the treatment of scabies. Benzyl benzoate and gamma benzene hexachloride are commonly used scabicides. *See* SCABIES.

Scabies is a contagious skin infestation, caused by the itch mite *Sarcoptes scabiei*. The female mite burrows beneath the skin and lays eggs. These in turn produce larvae which mature and mate, and the females form tunnel-like nests. The victim's body suffers an allergic reaction to the mite in the form of an itching rash of the eczema type, which may be widespread. The mite burrows in the hands, fingers, wrists, pubic areas and, sometimes, the soles of the feet.

Q: What are the symptoms of scabies?

A: For the first month following contact, there are no symptoms. During this period, the eggs of the mite hatch and develop into adults. The female lays several eggs a day for several weeks, so that by the end of the month many more females have burrowed beneath the skin. A rash and intense itching then occur as an allergic reaction.

Q: How is scabies treated?

A: The patient takes a bath and is painted over the whole body surface (excluding the eyes, nose, and mouth) with SCABICIDES. This treatment is repeated twice at daily intervals. A doctor may prescribe antihistamine drugs to relieve the allergic reaction. Usually the patient's family has to be treated as well, because the infection spreads very easily.

Scald is a burn to skin or flesh by hot vapour or liquid. *See* First Aid, p.524.

Scalene node biopsy is a diagnostic proce-

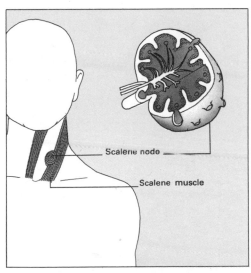

Scalene node, a lymph node in the neck, may be examined by a scalene node biopsy.

Scalp

dure. It is an operation to remove part or all of a lymph gland from behind the scalene muscles in the neck. The gland is then subject to microscopic examination.

Scalp is a part of the covering of the skull consisting of hair, skin, and underlying layers of muscle and fibrous tissue (fascia).

Scalpel is a knife with a short, thin blade used during a surgical operation.

Scaphoid is one of eight small bones in the WRIST. It is jointed to the radius bone in the forearm, and is one of the bones most likely to be fractured in a fall.

See also COLLES' FRACTURE.

Scapula, or shoulder blade, is one of a pair of flat triangular bones that, together with the upper bone of the arm (humerus), forms the SHOULDER joint. The ball-and-socket joint at the shoulder allows a wide range of movement, activated by muscles at the front and back of the chest wall, as well as those from the scapula.

Scar, known medically as cicatrix, is a healed wound, burn, or incision. It is composed of tough fibrous tissue.

Scar tissue inside the body seldom causes any problems. But adhesions (long strips of scar tissue) in the abdomen may distort the intestine and lead to intestinal obstruction.

Scar tissue on the skin may become abnormally thickened, raised, or red. This is known as a KELOID scar. Most unsightly scars can be removed or treated by PLASTIC SURGERY.

Scarlatina. See SCARLET FEVER.

Scarlet fever, or scarlatina, is an infectious disease caused by bacteria called group A beta haemolytic streptococci. It may develop

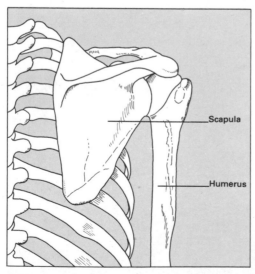

Scapula is a flat, triangular bone that forms the posterior part of the shoulder.

after a sore throat or acute tonsillitis. Scarlet fever can be spread by contaminated food or by infected droplets in the air.

The symptoms usually take from three to five days to appear. The patient is contagious while the bacteria are still in the nose and throat, which may be for two or three weeks. Some persons become carriers of the infection for several months.

Q: *What are the symptoms of scarlet fever?*

A: There is usually a sudden fever and a sore throat. There may also be vomiting, diarrhoea, and a severe headache. About two days after infection, a rash of small red spots appears, initially on the neck and chest but spreading rapidly to the rest of the body and limbs. Typically the face is flushed, with a pale area around the mouth. The surface of the tongue is coated with small red spots protruding from a milky white background. The rash usually lasts for three or four days, after which the other symptoms gradually disappear. Often the skin flakes off after an attack, and sometimes there is considerable, temporary loss of hair.

Q: *How is scarlet fever treated?*

A: Penicillin or other antibiotics are usually given for ten days. The full course recommended by a doctor must be completed to prevent complications, such as ear infections and pneumonia, from developing. Aspirin may also be prescribed to relieve the fever, headache, and sore throat.

Schick test is a method of testing immunity to diphtheria. A small amount of diphtheria toxin is injected into the skin. If immunity to diphtheria is not present, a small red inflamed area develops on the skin.

Schistosomiasis, also known as bilharzia, is a parasitic disease that occurs mostly in Africa, South America, and the Far East. It can be caught by swimming in infected water.

The worm responsible for schistosomiasis is a species of fluke (*Schistosoma*), which uses freshwater snails and humans as hosts.

The symptoms are fever, cough, muscle pains, and skin irritation, followed by blood in the urine or faeces.

Schistosomiasis is difficult to treat. Special drugs are available but can be given only by intravenous or intramuscular injection, and must be used with care because of their many toxic effects. Surgery may be needed if internal organs are severely scarred.

Schizoid is a psychological term that describes a personality type. Schizoid persons are often considered to be emotionally withdrawn, preferring to keep their feelings to themselves.

Some people believe that being schizoid is a personality disorder similar to SCHIZO-PHRENIA, but this is not necessarily so.

Schizophrenia, previously known as dementia praecox, is a complex group of related, but poorly defined, psychotic disorders. It occurs most commonly in young adults.

In schizophrenia, there is a disorganization of the thought processes so that abnormal emotional responses result. Logical thought is disrupted and socially unacceptable conclusions are reached. Normal life becomes complicated, and the patient enters a secret world of hallucinations and deluded thoughts, which may manifest itself as PARANOIA.

Often the individual who ultimately develops schizophrenia is shy, withdrawn, and finds difficulty in making friends. But such characteristics do not automatically imply that such a person is schizophrenic.

Hospitalization is needed for the acute form of schizophrenia. Prolonged drug treatment and sometimes ECT can control the disorder.

Sciatica is pain along the course of the sciatic nerve, which serves the buttock and the back of the thigh and leg. It is usually caused by pressure on the sciatic nerve which may be the result of a slipped disc; osteoarthritis of the spine; congenital anomalies of the spine, such as spondylolisthesis; or tumours of the spinal canal. *See* SLIPPED DISC.

Scirrhus is a hard, cancerous TUMOUR.

Sclera is the white, fibrous, outer coat of the eyeball. It forms the visible white of the eye, and surrounds the optic nerve at the back of the eyeball.

Scleroderma is an uncommon progressive disease that involves the fibrous tissue of the skin, joints, and internal organs, particularly the lungs, kidneys, and intestine. The cause of scleroderma is not known, but is thought to be a form of autoimmune disease. It is more common in women than men, and most cases occur during middle age.

Q: What are the symptoms of scleroderma?

A: The symptoms usually develop gradually. Initially, the fingers and toes become pale and painful when cold (RAYNAUD'S PHENOMENON). There may also be tightening and thinning of facial skin, difficulty in swallowing, pain in the joints, swelling of the hands, and muscle weakness. If the lungs or the heart are affected, PLEURISY, PERICARDITIS, or HEART FAILURE may occur.

Q: How is scleroderma treated?

A: There is no specific treatment. Scleroderma may occur in a mild form that is compatible with a long life, but it often causes early death because of the involve-ment of the internal organs. The symptoms can often be alleviated. Corticosteroid drugs may be prescribed to reduce the pain and swelling in the joints. Physiotherapy may help to preserve muscle strength.

Sclerosis is hardening of any body structure. *See also* ARTERIOSCLEROSIS; MULTIPLE SCLEROSIS.

Scolex is the head end of a tapeworm, by which the worm attaches itself to the intestinal wall using small hooks or suckers. *See* TAPEWORMS.

Scoliosis is a curvature of the spine to one side. It may be caused by an alteration in the position of the underlying bones or by a reaction of the spinal muscles, both of which make the spine temporarily change position.

Treatment depends on the cause.

See also KYPHOSIS; LORDOSIS; VON RECK-LINGHAUSEN'S DISEASE.

Scotoma is a loss of part of the field of vision, often experienced as a blind spot. Causes include a lesion within the eyeball, choroiditis, or haemorrhage. Migraine may cause flashes of light to be seen. Treatment depends on the cause.

Scrofula is an old term for tuberculosis of the lymph glands in the neck. It is often accompanied by ulceration of the overlying skin. *See* TUBERCULOSIS.

Scrotum is the bag of skin that contains the testicles, epididymides, and part of the spermatic cords. The skin of the scrotum contains muscles that can raise or lower the testicles, thereby keeping them at the optimum temperature for sperm production.

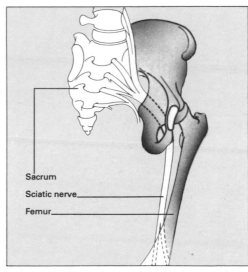

Sacrum

Sciatic nerve

Femur

Sciatica is pain anywhere along the path of the sciatic nerve that runs down the leg.

Scurvy

Any skin condition may affect the scrotum. The commonest disorders are a SEBACEOUS CYST and tinea cruris (*see* RINGWORM).

See also TESTIS.

Scurvy is a deficiency disease that is caused by a lack of vitamin C (ascorbic acid) in a person's diet. Vitamin C is essential for the maintenance of the normal structure of the connective tissues. Vitamin C deficiency results in weakening of the blood capillaries, with subsequent bleeding, and defects of the bones.

Unboiled tomato juice, orange juice, or fresh fruit can be taken regularly to prevent scurvy.

Q: What are the symptoms of scurvy?

A: Scurvy in infants may cause irritability, fever, loss of appetite, and failure to gain weight. The infant may keep his or her limbs motionless because of pain caused by bleeding under the periosteum (the tissue layer covering the bones). The infant may also be anaemic.

In adults, there may be a delay of between three and twelve months after the onset of severe vitamin C deficiency before any symptoms appear. Initially there may be lethargy, irritability, weight loss, and aching of the joints. As the disease develops, there may be bleeding under the skin, particularly under the nails; the gums swell and bleed; bruising may occur spontaneously; and wounds may not heal.

Q: How is scurvy treated?

A: Treatment involves the administration of large amounts of vitamin C until the

symptoms have disappeared. In addition to a balanced diet, vitamin C supplements may also be necessary for several months after the symptoms have disappeared.

Seasickness. *See* MOTION SICKNESS.

Sebaceous cyst, sometimes called a wen, is a swelling in the skin. It occurs when the duct of a sebaceous gland becomes blocked. The gland continues to produce waxy sebum, and becomes enlarged. Sebaceous cysts can occur on any hair-covered part of the body, but are most common on the scalp. They grow slowly, and only very rarely become malignant (cancerous).

See also CYST.

Sebaceous gland is a small gland in the skin. Sebaceous glands occur most commonly on the face, nose, scalp, over the shoulders, and in the genital area, but do not occur on the palms of the hands or on the soles of the feet. The glands produce SEBUM, a greasy secretion that conditions the skin.

Seborrhoea is a skin disorder caused by over-activity of the sebaceous glands. It results in dandruff (scaling of the skin of the scalp), often accompanied by blepharitis (scaling and redness of the eyelids) and slight greasiness of the face. In infants, the crusting of the scalp (cradle cap) is a form of seborrhoea. Seborrhoea is not serious, and tends to occur more in winter than in summer.

Q: How is seborrhoea treated?

A: Various commercial shampoos, some containing selenium, are available. These should be used two or three times a week. Scalp solutions containing corticosteroid drugs may be prescribed to control the condition until there is improvement. An infant's scalp needs only oiling and baby shampoo.

See also DANDRUFF.

Sebum is a thick, slightly greasy secretion that is produced by the SEBACEOUS GLANDS in the skin.

Secretion is the release of any substance produced by body cells. For example, hormones are secreted into the bloodstream, and saliva is secreted into the salivary ducts.

Sedatives are drugs that are used to reduce excitement or irritability. In small doses, they usually calm a patient; larger doses may produce sleep.

See also HYPNOTICS; TRANQUILLIZERS.

Sedimentation rate, or erythrocyte sedimentation rate (ESR), is a type of blood test. It is performed by placing blood containing an anticoagulant in a long, narrow glass tube and observing the speed at which the red blood cells settle and form a sediment at the bottom.

Faster sedimentation rates occur in the

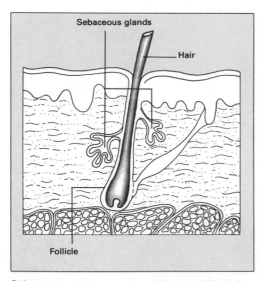

Sebaceous glands are situated around the hair shafts, which they lubricate with sebum.

presence of any serious infection, malignancy, or inflammatory disorder. The test does not diagnose any particular disorder, but indicates that one may be present.

Seizure is the sudden onset of a condition or illness. The term is, however, most commonly used to mean a convulsion of epilepsy, but can also refer to the rigor (shivering attack) that may accompany the start of an acute feverish illness, such as malaria. *See* CONVULSION; EPILEPSY.

Semen is the thick, creamy secretion produced by the male on ejaculation. It consists of sperm and the fluids secreted by the prostate gland and seminal vesicles. *See* SPERM.

Semicircular canal is one of the three fluid-filled tubes that form part of the inner ear. They are arranged at right angles to each other, one for each plane of movement. The canals are the body's organs of balance (*see* BALANCE). Disorders that affect the semicircular canals, such as LABYRINTHITIS and MÉNIÈRE'S DISEASE, usually cause vertigo and disturb the patient's sense of balance.

Seminal vesicles are two small pouch-like structures in which the SPERM of a male is stored. They are situated next to the prostate gland and at the end of the vas deferens. They produce secretions that keep the sperm active and alive.

Seminoma is the most common form of cancer of the testicle. It usually occurs in males between the ages of thirty and forty. *See* CANCER.

Senescence is the process of growing old. It usually refers to the later stages, when aging causes a failure of the normal functioning of the body.

Senility is, like senescence, the aging process of the body and mind, and is commonly associated with people of great age. Senility also involves a gradual deterioration of physical strength and co-ordination, accompanied by mental deterioration.

Sepsis is the presence in the body or bloodstream of disease-producing microorganisms, such as bacteria or viruses. It may result in abscesses throughout the body or blood poisoning. *See* ABSCESS; BLOOD POISONING; PUS.

Septal defect is a hole or some other defect in a septum or membranous wall dividing an organ or structure. Usually, the term refers to an anomaly present at birth in the septum between the two sides of the heart. *See* CONGENITAL HEART DISEASE.

The diagnosis may be confirmed, either in infancy or later in life, by passing a catheter (a pliable tube) into the heart and observing that it can pass through the septal defect into the other side of the heart. Septal defects of the heart may be accompanied by other congenital anomalies of the valves, and they are repaired by heart surgery.

Septic is any condition that produces pus, and is caused by sepsis. *See* PUS; SEPSIS.

Septicaemia is SEPSIS occurring in the blood. *See* BLOOD POISONING.

Septum is a thin layer of membranous tissue that forms a dividing wall between the two parts of an organ. There are septa between layers of muscle, between various parts of the brain, and between the two halves of the scrotum. Most commonly, the term refers to the division between the two halves of the heart, the atrial septum and the ventricular septum. A septum is also present between the two halves of the nose, formed partly by cartilage and partly by bone. *See* DEVIATED NASAL SEPTUM.

Serology is the study of SERUM and the investigation of IMMUNITY to disease.

Serum is the clear, watery fluid that remains after blood has clotted; it is blood plasma without the clotting components. Serum from persons or animals that are immune to a particular disease (antiserum) can be injected into a patient to confer temporary, passive IMMUNITY.

Q: Are there any possible dangers from the use of an antiserum?

A: Yes. Until recently, many antisera were prepared from animals, and these often produced an allergic reaction known as SERUM SICKNESS. Now, however, many antisera are prepared from humans, which greatly reduces the likelihood of producing serum sickness.

Serum sickness is a form of allergic reaction

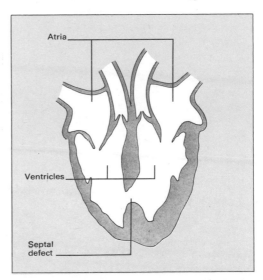

Septal defect is a weakness or hole in the wall that separates the two ventricles of the heart.

415

Sex hormones

that may occur one to two weeks after the injection of a serum. Many drugs, including penicillin, occasionally produce a condition indistinguishable from serum sickness.

Q: *What are the symptoms of serum sickness?*

A: A skin rash and intense irritation (urticaria) are usually the first signs. These are commonly accompanied by joint stiffness, swelling, and a mild fever that lasts several days. Frequently the lymph glands enlarge, particularly near the site of the injection, causing a generalized aching.

In severe forms of serum sickness, the heart muscles may be involved (myocarditis), and very rarely the kidneys are affected. Kidney involvement causes a form of nephritis, with ankle swelling and high blood pressure. Occasionally polyneuritis occurs, and recovery from this form of the disorder is seldom complete. However, most patients with serum sickness make a rapid and complete recovery within four weeks.

Q: *How is serum sickness treated?*

A: Treatment depends on the doctor. Injections of antihistamines followed by doses of antihistamines by mouth usually control the irritation and joint stiffness. If these measures fail, corticosteroid drugs may be given to decrease the symptoms. Drug treatment is usually continued until the symptoms cease. *See* ANAPHYLAXIS.

Sex hormones are the hormones produced by the gonads: the ovaries in females and the testicles (testes) in males. Their production is under the control of the pituitary gland at the base of the brain. The main hormones produced by the ovaries are oestrogens (*see* OESTROGEN) and PROGESTERONE; the testes produce TESTOSTERONE. Small amounts of sex hormones are also produced by the adrenal glands.

See also HORMONES.

Sexual intercourse, also known as coitus, is the physical act of sexual union between a man and woman. It begins with the insertion of the man's penis into the woman's vagina and the beginning of physical movements, partly voluntary and partly reflex. The act usually ends with the male orgasm and ejaculation of semen and may be accompanied by the female orgasm.

See also SEXUAL PROBLEMS.

Sexually transmitted diseases. *See* VENEREAL DISEASES.

A talk about Sexual problems

Sexual problems. There is some dispute as to what is normal in sexual experience and what is abnormal. Much depends on individual sexual development, which can be affected by various factors, including genetic inheritance.

Healthy sexuality depends on age, culture, individual desire, and physical and psychological attitudes to sex. Feelings of sexuality begin in infancy and develop along with physical, social, psychological, and instinctive characteristics, all of them unique to a particular individual.

Sexual problems may arise because of a physical disorder, or because of psychological disturbances during growth and development, or in a relationship with another person or persons. The causes are varied and complex.

Q: *What physical disorders cause sexual problems?*

A: Sexual precocity, a very rare form of early puberty and sexual development, can give rise to sexual problems. It is caused by hormone disorders in childhood. Some people are born as hermaphrodites, with a combination of the sexual characteristics of both sexes. There may also be other genetic anomalies that result in abnormal physical or sexual features. This makes it difficult for them to have a normal sex life (*see* HERMAPHRODITE).

Painful intercourse (DYSPAREUNIA) is a disorder that can be caused by a tight hymen, vaginitis (inflammation of the vagina), or salpingitis (inflammation of the fallopian tubes). After menopause, painful intercourse may occur because vaginal secretions dry up slightly.

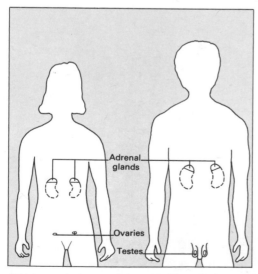

Sex hormones are produced by the ovaries, testes, and adrenal glands.

416

Painful intercourse in a man is often caused by balanitis, an infection of the end of the penis. Polyneuritis and diabetes mellitus can cause some men to fail to achieve an erection.

Q: *What psychological disorders cause sexual problems?*

A: Psychological disorders are the most common causes of sexual problems. They usually arise when there is difficulty in the relationship between the two people concerned. There is often a failure to understand each other's needs and desires, and this can become combined with feelings of guilt or anxiety that cause impotence in men and frigidity in women. Once sexual intercourse has failed, the symptoms tend to get worse.

Vaginismus is a severe form of frigidity in which the woman's vaginal muscles go into spasm, preventing penetration by the man's penis (*see* VAGINISMUS).

A common male problem is premature ejaculation, in which a man has an orgasm before the woman has become sexually satisfied. Thus, the man may feel he has failed, and the woman is left unsatisfied and frustrated.

Q: *How are frigidity, impotence, and premature ejaculation dealt with?*

A: The key to mutual pleasure is to relax and not to be overconcerned with orgasm. More time should be spent in pre-intercourse love play. Some women always fail to reach an orgasm, and this is usually because of psychological factors, such as the fear of becoming pregnant, or feelings of guilt or inferiority.

It is necessary for a man and a woman to have consideration for each other if impotence or frigidity are not to interfere with their sex life. Practice of gentle stimulation by the woman may help the man to control his orgasm. Giving a frigid woman gentle massage and sexual fore-play help the woman to experience sexual pleasure and even orgasm. *See* FRIGIDITY; IMPOTENCE.

Q: *What other sexual problems may have a psychological basis?*

A: Many sexual problems arise because of a failure in normal psychosexual develop-ment. Many variants of sexual behaviour are thought to develop from early childhood. Most people enjoy the touch of soft materials, such as fur, and these certainly encourage sexuality. But when a person is obsessed with materials such as rubber or leather, for example, and it is the sole source of sexual gratification (fetishism), it is a marked abnormality.

Some people, particularly men, remain at an infantile stage of sexuality. They are usually terrified of any form of physical sexual relationship with the opposite sex. But they still have a sex drive, and the only way they can get satisfaction is by frightening, as opposed to loving, the opposite sex. For example, some men get sexual gratification by indecently exposing themselves to unsuspecting women. Another form of retarded sexual development is paedophilia, in which loving and often sexual relationships develop between an adult and a child.

The problem of homosexuality is discussed elsewhere (*see* HOMOSEXUA-LITY). Everyone has some degree of homosexual feeling, but it may become increased to such an extent in some people that they appear entirely homosexual. But this also means that a few people fall in the centre of sexual feelings, halfway between homosexual and heterosexual.

Q: *How can such psychological causes of sexual problems be treated?*

A: It is important to discuss the problems with someone who has an understanding of sexual disorders, and who can offer reassurance. A couple who fear that they are in some way abnormal may be relieved to find that problems of this kind are fairly common and that they are relatively easy to treat.

Q: *Can problems resulting from a failure of psychosexual development be treated?*

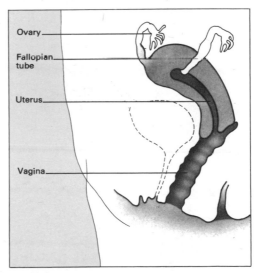

Ovary

Fallopian tube

Uterus

Vagina

Sexual problems in women may be caused by infection of the genitalia.

Sexual problems

A: It is often extremely difficult to treat developmental sexual problems because they have become deep-seated by the time of adulthood. They are unlikely to be detected early enough in adolescence for psychotherapy and psychoanalysis to have much effect. Sexual problems can cause great distress to the individual concerned, and various forms of treatment (including types of behaviour therapy, such as aversion therapy and hypnotherapy) are often unsuccessful. Treatment with female sex hormones can reduce the sex drive in men who have committed sex crimes, although there are certain risks to the patient.

Q: *Can excessive sex drive be a problem?*

A: Yes. Increased libido (sex drive) can be associated with psychotic disorders, such as manic-depressive illness and some personality disorders, as well as with psychotic illness. This can lead to violently antisocial behaviour, including rape. In most people, however, an increase in libido accompanies a feeling of well-being and is controlled by normal social constraints.

Promiscuity is not necessarily the result of an increase in libido, and it usually indicates that the individual has problems maintaining any form of secure relationship.

Q: *What sexual problems occur in adolescence?*

A: The sexual problems of adolescence usually centre on sexual ignorance, fear of venereal disease, and anxiety about sexual success. Masturbation is a common form of sexual outlet that may induce fears and anxieties (*see* MASTURBATION). Most adolescents also go through a homosexual phase, and may fear that the feeling is going to be permanent (*see* HOMOSEXUALITY). Such problems can be helped by discussion with parents, and by routine education about the basic biological facts of life.

Q: *What sexual problems occur in the elderly?*

A: Sexual intercourse may continue into old age provided the partners are healthy. The most common problems arise after an illness or operation; the break from regular sexual intercourse may be sufficient to stop it completely. This may not be a problem to the person who has had the illness, but it may create frustration in the healthy partner.

The best way to deal with this situation is frank discussion between the partners in the hope that either sexual intercourse will be resumed or the less fit partner will realize that some form of sexual stimulation is still necessary.

If regular intercourse has been maintained, there are seldom any problems, apart from a slight dryness of the vagina after menopause. Lubricant jellies or a cream containing oestrogens can be prescribed by a doctor.

Q: *Does any form of drug treatment help in treating sexual problems?*

A: Yes. There are drugs that reduce the sex drive, and they are sometimes used in the treatment of sexual deviants, such as paedophiles and psychopaths.

Depressed individuals can have their libido increased by antidepressant drugs. Small amounts of the male sex hormone testosterone are sometimes prescribed during menopause to increase a woman's sex drive. However, it is more usual for hormone replacement therapy to be used for some months during menopause.

Sheehan's syndrome is a rare condition in which there is a reduction in the production of pituitary hormones as a result of shock or bleeding following childbirth. This is caused by thrombosis of the blood vessels supplying the pituitary gland, which causes the tissues to die. Prolactin, the milk-stimulating hormone, is not produced, and breast-feeding cannot take place. See HYPOPITUITARISM; PITUITARY GLAND.

Shigella is a genus of rod-shaped bacteria that are closely related to SALMONELLA; they can cause diseases of the intestine, such as

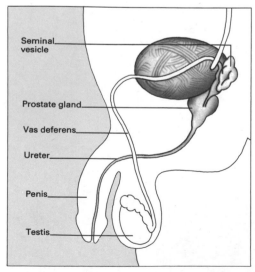

Seminal vesicle

Prostate gland

Vas deferens

Ureter

Penis

Testis

Sexual problems in men may be caused by infection of the genitalia.

bacillary dysentery (*see* DYSENTERY). The bacteria are spread by infected faeces, contaminated food, or flies.

Shingles, known medically as herpes zoster, is an acute inflammatory infection of part of the central nervous system that produces pain and blisters on the skin over the ends of nerves. It is most common in people over age 50 years, although it can occur in children. The virus *Varicella zoster,* which also causes chickenpox, is the infecting agent.

Q: What are the symptoms of shingles?

A: The patient feels unwell, often with a headache, and has a fever, chills, and sometimes pain in the area where the infection is occurring. After three to five days, a red rash appears, which rapidly develops into the clear blisters typical of shingles. As new blisters erupt, the old ones form pus and then scabs, which fall off between seven and ten days later. The blisters appear on the area supplied by the infected nerves, and may cover any part of the body. The chest is a common site. It is usual for the affected area to be sensitive to touch, and the patient often suffers severe pain. As the blisters heal, the central part of the affected area may be without sensation at all.

Q: How is shingles treated?

A: In most cases, the infection is not severe and can be treated with painkilling drugs and a soothing lotion, such as calamine lotion. Once the blisters heal, the patient often feels weak and tired, and needs a long convalescence. Extra vitamins should be added to the diet.

A special antiviral lotion can be applied to the painful area before the blisters appear to stop them spreading. Painkilling drugs during the acute phase of the disorder reduce the chance of prolonged pain (post-herpetic neuralgia), which is difficult to treat.

Shivering is an uncontrollable trembling caused by rapid, involuntary muscle contractions, which produce a large amount of heat. It may be a response to cold, emotional shock, or fear. Extremely severe shivering is known as RIGOR.

Shock (for EMERGENCY treatment, *see* First Aid, p.566) is separable into two categories: emotional shock and physical, or organic, shock.

Emotional shock, caused by any frightening experience, makes the patient feel faint, dizzy, and possibly confused.

Physical shock can be an immediate or a delayed reaction. It follows physical damage and loss of blood, such as from a severe injury, or electric shock. It also occurs after surgery. Finally, physical shock can occur as a form of ANAPHYLAXIS or following a heart attack.

Shock therapy is a form of treatment for certain types of mental illness. *See* ELECTROCONVULSIVE THERAPY.

Shortness of breath. *See* BREATHLESSNESS.

Shortsightedness (myopia) is a visual defect in which distant objects cannot be seen clearly. It occurs because light entering the eye is focused in front of the retina instead of on it. Distant objects are out of focus because either the lens of the eye is too curved (and bends the light rays too much), or the eyeball is too long, a condition that is usually inherited. Close objects can be seen sharply, and even in old age shortsighted people may be able to read easily without glasses.

Shortsightedness can be corrected by wearing spectacles with concave (converging) lenses. *See* SPECTACLES.

Shoulder is the junction of the arm and the trunk. The ball-and-socket shoulder joint is located between the humerus (upper arm bone) and scapula (shoulder blade). It is held in place by strong muscles and ligaments, and supported by the clavicle. The shoulder muscles control a wide range of movement.

Q: What disorders can affect the shoulder?

A: Dislocation of the shoulder joint is the most common complaint. It mainly results from weakness of the ligaments, although it is also common in certain contact sports. Repeated shoulder dislocation may need surgical treatment to tighten the ligaments.

The shoulder joint can be affected by

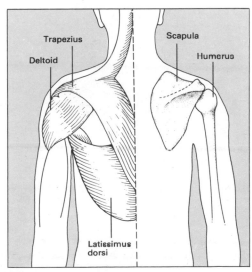

Shoulder joint between the humerus and the scapula is moved by strong muscles.

Trapezius

Deltoid

Scapula

Humerus

Latissimus dorsi

Shoulder blade

any JOINT DISORDERS, particularly rheumatoid arthritis.

Pain in the shoulder may be the result of inflammation of the shoulder membrane, ligaments, or tendon (FROZEN SHOULDER) although it may be a referred pain from such disorders as arthritis in the neck (spondylosis), pleurisy and angina pectoris.

Shoulder blade. *See* SCAPULA.

Shunt is an abnormal junction between two body passages that allows the contents of one to pass to the other, by-passing the normal channel. The term usually refers to a junction between two blood vessels, such as an arteriovenous shunt in which an artery is connected directly to a vein, so by-passing the capillary network.

Sialolithiasis is the presence of a stone (calculus) in the duct of a salivary gland. It prevents the escape of saliva, which accumulates in the affected gland and causes it to swell.

The stone is made of calcium salts, and can usually be detected by an X-ray. But, in some cases, a special radiopaque dye may have to be injected into the duct to reveal the presence of the stone.

Q: What are the symptoms of sialolithiasis?

A: Painful swelling of one salivary gland when eating. The swelling settles when the meal ends, only to begin again at the next meal.

Q: How is sialolithiasis treated?

A: In some cases the stone escapes spontaneously, and no treatment is required. Usually, a minor operation is necessary to remove the stone.

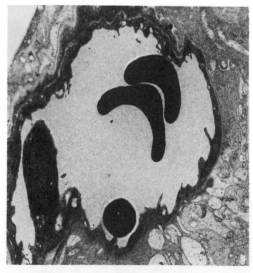

Sickle cell anaemia is characterized by the presence of deformed red blood cells.

Siamese twins are identical twins (which are formed from a single egg) that are still joined at birth, most commonly at the hip, chest, or head. Siamese twins are known medically as conjoined twins (*see* TWINS). They are extremely rare and often difficult to deliver so that a Caesarean operation is usually necessary.

The likelihood of both twins surviving a surgical separation is greater when only superficial tissues are shared.

Sickle cell anaemia is a hereditary form of ANAEMIA characterized by the presence of abnormal, sickle-shaped red blood cells. It occurs almost exclusively in black people. The abnormal cells are unable to pass easily through the capillary blood vessels, and this may lead to widespread thrombosis. They are also more fragile than normal blood cells, so they are easily destroyed by the buffeting in the circulation. This may lead to severe anaemia, which may be made worse by infection.

Q: How is sickle cell anaemia treated?

A: There is no curative treatment for the condition. Therapy is directed toward alleviating the symptoms as they arise. Blood transfusions are usually given only when the anaemia is severe enough to cause serious illness.

Siderosis, or haemosiderosis, is any condition causing excess iron in the tissues. It is usually caused by breathing in dust or fumes containing iron particles, hence its common name is welder's disease.

If siderosis affects the lungs, which is more common in young children, haemoptysis (the coughing up of blood) eventually can lead to death. If it occurs in the kidneys, it may lead to a condition similar to HAEMOCHROMATOSIS.

SIDS (sudden infant death syndrome), also known as cot death, is thought to be a respiratory disorder that usually affects infants under the age of six months.

Q: Are some babies more likely than others to succumb to SIDS?

A: Such deaths are more likely to occur in families living in crowded conditions, during the winter months, and in bottle-fed infants. SIDS is more common at night than in daytime. Boys of low birth weight succumb more often than do girls under similar conditions.

Q: What causes SIDS?

A: During sleep, the respiration of all infants is irregular, with brief periods when breathing stops completely. But if respiration stops for longer than 15 or 20 seconds, death can occur.

In most cases SIDS cannot be prevented, because obvious warning symptoms have not yet been discovered. In all cases of SIDS, it is the parents who suffer grief and shock, often blaming themselves. The family needs social and psychological support at this time. Help can be provided by the paediatrician, the family's doctor, and family counsellors. The family can also be helped by their religious adviser, or by contacting the Foundation for the Study of Infant Deaths, which can give immediate counselling and support.

Sigmoidoscopy is an examination of the S-shaped part of the colon (the sigmoid colon), the lower part of the colon that joins the rectum. It is performed using a sigmoidoscope, a lighted tube that can be inserted up to about ten inches beyond the anus.

Q: *Why is a sigmoidoscopy performed?*

A: A sigmoidoscopy may be done in a routine examination, to exclude any local disease or cancer of the rectum and sigmoid colon, or in the investigation of tropical diseases, such as amoebiasis and schistosomiasis, and in conditions such as ulcerative colitis and Crohn's disease.

A small piece of tissue (biopsy) may be taken. A sigmoidoscopy is commonly performed before a barium enema, or before the full length of the colon is examined with a flexible fibrescope (*see* BARIUM).

Silicosis is a form of pneumoconiosis caused by inhaling silica. It is an occupational hazard of coal miners, quarry workers, and stone workers, as well as anyone who is exposed to silica dust. The fine particles of silica cause scarring within the lungs, impairing lung function and causing increasing shortness of breath.

Over a period of years, a person with silicosis suffers frequent attacks of chronic BRONCHITIS that increase the development of the chronic pulmonary disorder emphysema. There is an increased incidence of tuberculosis and spontaneous pneumothorax, a collection of air in the pleural cavity. Death usually results from pneumonia or heart failure.

See also PNEUMOCONIOSIS.

Sinus is a cavity, usually filled with air or blood. There are many sinuses throughout the body. The term usually refers to the cavities in the bone behind the nose. These sinuses reduce the weight of the skull, and act as resonant chambers for the voice.

Sinus is also the medical term for a drainage channel formed from an abscess to the surface of the skin or to an internal organ.

See also SINUSITIS.

Sinusitis is inflammation of the mucous membranes that line the sinuses of the skull (the cavities within the skull bones that open into the nose). Acute sinusitis may be caused by a nasal infection (RHINITIS) in which the sinuses become blocked, or by the common cold, or any feverish respiratory illness, such as influenza. Sometimes, acute sinusitis may be caused by a dental abscess; a fracture of a bone in the face; or sudden pressure changes (*see* BAROTRAUMA). Chronic sinusitis may be caused by an allergy, such as hay fever; repeated attacks of acute sinusitis; or inadequate treatment of acute sinusitis combined with nasal obstruction, as may occur with a POLYP, a DEVIATED NASAL SEPTUM, or chronic dental infections.

Q: *What are the symptoms of sinusitis?*

A: The area over the affected sinus may be painful and tender, and there is usually a severe headache. The nose may be blocked on the affected side with a thick, sometimes bloodstained discharge causing the patient to breathe through the mouth. The patient may also have a fever, chills, and a sore throat.

Q: *How is sinusitis treated?*

A: Painkilling drugs may be used to relieve the pain. Decongestant nose drops and inhaled steam may help to open the sinuses and promote drainage of mucus that has accumulated within the affected sinus. A doctor may also prescribe antibiotics and advise bed rest.

In severe cases, surgery may be necessary to wash out the infected sinus. *See* CALDWELL-LUC OPERATION.

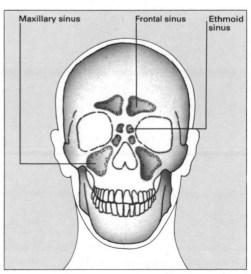

| Maxillary sinus | Frontal sinus | Ethmoid sinus |

Sinus is a cavity in bone. Eight of these are located in the bones of the face.

Skeleton

Skeleton is the bony framework of the body; it consists of about 206 bones. The bones can be classified into two groups: the axial skeleton and appendicular skeleton. The skeleton has three functions: it protects the internal organs; it supplies support for the substance of the body; and, through the action of muscles, it allows movements of the body.

Q: What is the axial skeleton?

A: The axial skeleton is the main supporting framework of the body. It consists of the skull, spine, and rib-cage. The spine consists of seven cervical, twelve thoracic, and five lumbar vertebrae. The five sacral vertebrae and the four bones of the coccyx at the base of the spine are joined together to make a solid bone at the back of the pelvis. The thorax is composed of twelve pairs of ribs, joined at the back to the thoracic vertebrae; the upper ten pairs are joined by cartilage at the front to the breastbone (sternum). Some people have an extra rib or an extra vertebra.

Q: What is the appendicular skeleton?

A: The appendicular skeleton consists of the limbs. The upper limbs are composed of the shoulder girdle, collar-bone, and shoulder blade, as well as the bones of the arms and hands.

The lower limbs consist of the pelvis, which is joined to the sacrum, and which provides support for the bones of the legs and feet.

Q: How does the skeleton protect the internal organs?

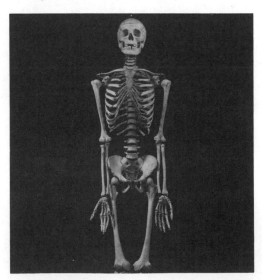

Skeleton is the framework to which muscles, ligaments, and other structures are attached.

A: The skull is the most protective part of the skeleton because it completely surounds the brain and the internal organs of the ear, and supplies a major form of protection for the eyes. The thorax (chest) protects the heart, lungs, liver, and spleen. The spine and pelvis help to protect the abdominal organs, such as the intestine, kidneys, bladder, and, in females, the womb.

Skin, known medically as integument, is the largest "organ" in the body, weighing about 3kg (7lbs) and covering about 1.7sq metres (18sq ft) in an adult. It is a waterproof covering, a defence against damage and infection, a regulator of body temperature, and a sensory organ.

Specialized areas of the skin constitute particular organs. For example, the female breast is composed of about twenty modified sweat glands and the nails are developed from a special layer of hard keratin (a tough protein substance) that grows over the outer skin at the ends of the fingers and toes.

Certain areas of the skin, such as the scalp, armpits, and pubic areas, are more thickly covered with hair than are others. A finer growth of hair covers the rest of the body, except for the soles of the feet and the palms of the hands.

Q: What is the structure of the skin?

A: The outer layer of the skin consists of dead cells that break away continually. They are formed as the underlying layer of living cells gradually grow outward to form the protective substance keratin. These two layers are known as the epidermis.

Beneath the epidermis is the dermis. It consists of supporting connective tissue surrounding blood and lymph vessels, sweat and sebaceous glands, nerve endings, and hair follicles. Fat storage cells lie beneath the dermis.

Skin complaints are not always easy to treat, and it is important that attempts at self-treatment do not make the condition worse and a doctor's diagnosis more difficult.

The symptoms of most skin complaints can be considered as various forms of lesion, dry or moist skin, or skin that itches. A combination of these symptoms is quite common.

Primary lesions should not cause difficulty unless they are blisters that break (as with chickenpox), when the skin should be kept clean, and a soothing lotion applied.

Dry skin is helped by moisturizing creams, and moist skin with calamine lotion. Itching is particularly distressing; clothes made from artificial fibres often aggravate the complaint. Antihistamine drugs are moderately effective, and a change to a natural fibres can help. If itching is severe, regular bathing gives relief. Sometimes a doctor may prescribe a local anaesthetic to help the patient over the worst of the symptoms.

Both corticosteroid and antibiotic creams should be used with caution and only on medical advice, because they can be dangerous if used for the wrong condition. Corticosteroids prevent the normal biological reaction to infection, thus an infection may spread. Antibiotics should be used only if the condition is a bacterial infection; used for any length of time, they can cause skin allergy.

Secondary lesions are caused by natural development of the disease, or because the patient interferes with the normal healing process by scratching the skin. This often leaves an ulcerated or eroded region.

Most individual skin disorders have separate articles in the A-Z section of this book. **Skin grafts** are layers of skin transferred surgically from one part of a patient's body to another part. Skin grafts are of two main types: (1) a full-thickness graft, which includes the underlying layer of fat and is usually employed for only small areas of skin; and (2) a Thiersch's, or split-skin graft, a thinner layer of skin taken from a healthy part of the patient's body.

For a full-thickness graft, surgeons leave one end of a flap of skin attached to the donor (healthy) area, and the free end attached to the area to be grafted. This allows the blood supply to continue while the graft and its blood supply is becoming established. When the graft has taken, the end still attached to the donor area may be removed and stitched to the recipient area. This is known as a pedicle graft.

In patients with severe burns, it may not be possible to take sufficient skin from donor areas of the patient's body. Temporary grafting, using skin from another person or even that of a pig, can give protection while the patient recovers from the burn.

See also GRAFT.

Skull. *See* CRANIUM.

Sleep. Little is known about why sleep is essential for good health. It seems that the central nervous system needs a regular period of rest from waking activities. But it is not known why about a third of every twenty-four hours has to be spent in this recovery phase. People who go without their normal amount of sleep lack concentration and may ultimately have hallucinations.

Normal sleep consists of two types. The first is known as slow-wave sleep because during it there is reduced electrical activity in the brain. It is also known as non-REM

(rapid eye movement) sleep, because the eyes do not move rapidly during this phase. During slow-wave sleep, there is a decrease in the basal metabolic rate, blood pressure, and respiratory rate so that the person lies still and is totally relaxed.

The second type of sleep is known as paradoxical or REM sleep, because of the rapid eye movement that takes place behind the closed eyelids. Also during this phase, dreaming takes place, the heartbeat and respiration become irregular, and there may be limb movement. An electroencephalogram shows electrical brain activity similar to that which occurs when a person is awake.

There is a period of normal wakefulness as a person falls asleep, followed by a state of relaxation that becomes light sleep, before the body enters the phase of slow-wave (non-REM) sleep. Slow-wave sleep initially lasts about two hours before the first episode of REM sleep begins. Sleep then alternates between periods of slow-wave and REM sleep lasting ten to twenty minutes and occurring every hour and a half until the patient awakes refreshed.

REM sleep is now known to be essential, because waking a person repeatedly at the beginning of each period of REM sleep produces depression, anxiety, and fatigue out of proportion to the amount of sleep that has been lost. Dreaming is a necessary part of normal sleep, and is also probably necessary for the well-being of the mind. Everyone dreams, even if he or she cannot remember the dreams on waking.

See also DREAMS; INSOMNIA; SLEEP PROBLEMS.

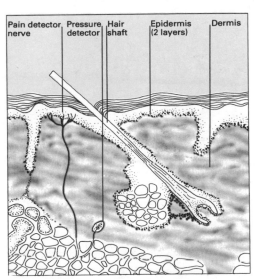

Skin is sensitive to a wide range of outside stimuli, including pressure and pain.

Sleeping sickness

Sleeping sickness, or African trypanosomiasis, is a disorder caused by protozoans called trypanosomes. They enter the blood of a human by the bite of an infected tsetse fly. Sleeping sickness occurs in tropical and subtropical regions of Africa where infected cattle and wild animals complete the disease's cycle by infecting the fly.

Sleeplessness. *See* INSOMNIA.

A talk about Sleep problems

Sleep problems. Insomnia (the inability to sleep) is the most common sleep problem and one that causes a lot of distress (*see* INSOMNIA). But other sleep problems commonly occur, particularly in children.

Q: What sleep problems occur in children?

A: Sleep problems may be associated with behaviour problems in children. For example, a child may refuse to settle down at night and may constantly get up or make excuses about some minor discomfort. Such children are often worried about something and need a set ritual, without overexcitement, at bedtime. Another problem is the young child, usually aged between three and five, who wakes in the early hours of the morning. A solution that can be tried by the parents is to stop afternoon naps and put the child to bed later in the evening. SLEEPWALKING and SLEEPTALKING are two problems that are common in childhood and tend to improve with the approach of puberty.

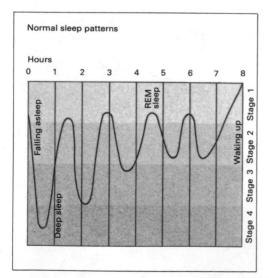

Sleep problems occur if the normal depth and rapid eye movement (REM) pattern is broken.

Q: Can excessive amounts of sleep be a serious symptom?

A: This is not usually a serious condition. Hypersomnia, as it is sometimes called, may develop after serious illnesses during the convalescent period. It may also be a factor in anaemia and depression, and sometimes occurs in adolescence as normal behaviour. Hypersomnia can, however, be a symptom of narcolepsy, a form of epilepsy in which the person suddenly falls asleep and may continue to sleep for hours and even days. It is more common in women than in men and may coincide with menstruation.

Sleep reversal, in which a person sleeps all day, is always a serious symptom when there is no obvious cause. It can happen in disorders such as Alzheimer's disease, encephalitis, and sleeping sickness.

Q: How can sleep problems be treated?

A: A full understanding of how the sleep disorder occurs is most important to the doctor, although diagnostic tests such as an electroencephalograph test may be of help. Drugs of the hypnotic and amphetamine group and, sometimes, one of the anti-depressant drugs can help to control some of the problems.

Q: Can the use of drugs create its own problems?

A: The amphetamine group of drugs is useful in treating many of the excessive sleep problems such as narcolepsy and hypersomnia. But amphetamines are addictive and so the doctor must take great care to ensure that excessive amounts of drugs are not being used.

A much greater problem is the use of sedative and hypnotic drugs in the treatment of insomnia. Although it is not known exactly how these drugs work, it seems that there is a reduction in the length and number of periods of REM sleep (*see* SLEEP) during their administration. This can cause mild depression for reasons that are not fully understood. When the drugs are stopped, sleep may be disturbed for ten to fourteen days. REM sleep increases, and the person feels that the insomnia is worse than before. After about two weeks, natural sleep patterns return.

Another problem with sleep-inducing drugs is the slight daytime sedation that may occur and reduce a person's speed of reaction. This is particularly relevant when driving a vehicle, using machinery or, most important of all, taking alcohol. Alcohol in combination with barbiturates, for example, is extremely dangerous and can be fatal.

See also BARBITURATES; DREAMS; MANIC-
DEPRESSIVE ILLNESS; NARCOLEPSY; SLEEP-
TALKING; SLEEPWALKING.

Sleeptalking is a common occurrence in children. It may consist of no more than a few
grunts or an occasional word, or it may be a
whole sentence. It is even possible to hold a
brief conversation with a sleeptalker. Sleeptalking is probably the result of a vivid dream
or a nightmare. *See* SLEEP PROBLEMS.

Sleepwalking, or somnambulism, is most
common between the ages of four and fourteen and more frequent in boys than girls. It
seldom lasts for more than about half an
hour, and is more likely to occur when the
child is sleeping in a strange room.

The individual may appear normal and can
perform complex movements, such as
opening and shutting doors and walking
down stairs. The eyes may be closed or open,
and may appear to be looking at something.

The sleepwalker may grunt or speak, but
returns to bed with no memory of the episode in the morning (*see* SLEEPTALKING).

*Q: Is it dangerous to wake someone who is
sleepwalking?*

A: No. However, it is better not to try
because the sleepwalker may be frightened to wake in a strange place. It is best
to attempt to lead the sleepwalker back
to bed.

Q: Why does sleepwalking occur?

A: The cause is not known. It is associated
with the dreaming stage of sleep, or with
underlying fears and anxieties.

See also SLEEP.

Slimming. *See* WEIGHT PROBLEMS.

Slipped disc, also known as a prolapsed
intervertebral disc, is a disorder of the spine.
The discs between the bones of the spine
(vertebrae) are composed of gristle-like
fibrous tissue with a soft centre. A disc can
rupture as a result of strain, allowing its soft
centre to pass through the ruptured outer
fibre. The soft tissue protrudes into and compresses the spinal canal, which contains the
spinal cord and nerves. Pressure on the spinal
nerves produces pain, felt either locally
(backache and lumbago) or as referred pain
in another part of the body, as in sciatica.
Muscle weakness; paralysis; and loss of
sensation is possible in severe cases.

In childhood and adolescence, the discs are
flexible and pliable, and so strain at this stage
is unlikely. The discs harden in later life, and
the soft centres gradually solidify. By the age
of forty-five or fifty, the centre is of the same
tough composition as the outer edge.

The discs of the neck (cervical region) and
those of the lower spine (lumbar region) are
the most likely to rupture because they are
the most mobile. A slipped disc in the
thoracic spine, behind the chest, can occur in
some people.

Q: What are the symptoms of a slipped disc?

A: In the neck, it is usually the result of a
twisting injury that develops into a stiff
neck. The pain is intense when the
patient tries to move or cough. Gradually
the pain spreads as the disc presses on the
nerves that affect one shoulder and arm.
Loss of sensation in the skin and muscle
weakness may develop because of nerve
damage. If the disc protrudes deeply into
the spinal cord, there is loss of sensation
or paralysis lower down the body. It may
cause disruption in the nerves controlling
walking, or cause difficulty in urinating.

The symptoms in the lower spine are
usually caused by a slipped disc either
between the fourth and fifth lumbar
vertebrae, or between the fifth lumbar
and first sacral vertebrae. There is severe
pain in the back, making it difficult for
the patient to move. The pain gradually
improves over a matter of days.

The back pain may be followed by
sciatica, with pain in one buttock, the
thigh, leg, and foot. A tingling sensation
is common, and is aggravated by
coughing, sneezing, or bending. The
patient limps, because of spasms in the
back muscles, and is unable to raise
the affected leg at right angles to the
body.

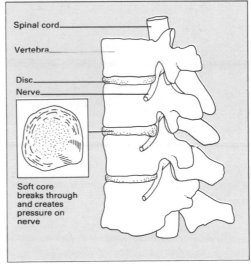

Spinal cord

Vertebra

Disc

Nerve

Soft core
breaks through
and creates
pressure on
nerve

Slipped disc is a section of intervertebral disc
that protrudes onto a nerve.

Smallpox

A slipped disc higher up in the lumbar region results in pain in the groin and in the front of the thigh.

Q: *How is a slipped disc treated?*

A: Painkilling drugs may be prescribed in mild cases; spinal manipulation may also help. A slipped disc in the neck usually involves immobilizing the neck with a stiff collar. This helps the patient sleep or to drive a car without too much pain. In addition, antirheumatic drugs, physiotherapy in the form of short-wave diathermy and massage, and, in severe cases, hospitalization and continuous TRACTION may be recommended.

A slipped disc in the lumbar region is treated with rest, painkillers, and antirheumatic drugs. Traction and a plaster-of-Paris jacket or a surgical corset that immobilizes the spine are commonly used for several months in severe cases. Occasionally, surgical removal of the disc may be necessary.

Q: *Are there any other disorders that have symptoms similar to those of a slipped disc?*

A: Osteoarthritis, tumours of the spinal cord, and secondary tumours of the vertebrae produce similar symptoms. Cervical rib trouble may produce disc-like pains down an arm.
Spondylolisthesis, in which one vertebra slips forward on another, and ankylosing spondylitis cause similar back pains.

Smallpox occurs in two forms, variola major or variola minor, and is a serious, infectious disease. It produces blisters which, after healing, leave scars. Death occurs in fifteen per cent of patients with variola major, but in only 0.2 per cent of variola minor (alastrim) cases. The disease is transmitted mainly by direct contact with a smallpox patient or by contact with contaminated clothing.

The World Health Organization has declared that, from 1st January 1980, the world is free of smallpox. However, some countries, particularly in Africa, still require travellers to be vaccinated against smallpox.

Q: *What are the symptoms of smallpox?*

A: After an incubation period of ten to fourteen days, the patient has a high fever, headache, chills, and often muscle pains and vomiting. These symptoms last for two to three days, resulting in shock, when a diffuse pink skin rash may occur.

After the second day small pink spots appear on the face and, within twenty-four hours, they cover the body. The spots become blisters filled with a clear fluid and, after three days, contain pus; the blisters then form into scabs. After eight to ten days, improvement begins and the scabs drop off, leaving small pitted areas where the blisters formed.

Q: *What is the treatment for smallpox?*

A: The first step is isolation of the patient and, sometimes, the medical staff giving treatment; the medical staff also must be vaccinated. Quarantine lasts for a period of two weeks from last contact with the infection. All of the patient's clothing and bed linen should be sterilized. Intra-venous fluids are given to maintain the level of body fluids; antiviral drugs can reduce the severity and the mortality rate in an epidemic.

Antibiotics should be used only if secondary infection occurs.

Q: *Can vaccination prevent smallpox?*

A: Yes. The vaccine against smallpox has been so successful that the disease has been officially eradicated.

Smear is a technique of preparing tissue for examination with a microscope. *See* CERVICAL SMEAR.

Smegma is a thick, greasy secretion produced by the sebaceous glands under the foreskin of the penis. In uncircumcised males it is thought to be a factor, if the glans (end of the penis) is not kept clean, in cancer of the penis.

Smell, sense of, is the ability to detect odours. The organ of smell consists of a group of sensitive cells situated in the upper part of the nasal cavity, which is connected to the brain by the olfactory nerve. The sense of smell is not well developed in humans. It is limited to the sensation of seven basic odours

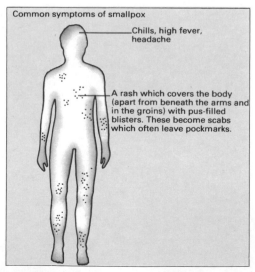

Common symptoms of smallpox

Chills, high fever, headache

A rash which covers the body (apart from beneath the arms and in the groins) with pus-filled blisters. These become scabs which often leave pockmarks.

Smallpox is an acute contagious disease with a variety of characteristic symptoms.

and their combinations. It is, however, an important contributory factor to the sense of taste (*see* TASTE). And like the sense of taste, it becomes less acute as a person becomes older.

Inflammation or blockage of the nasal passages, as with a common cold, dulls the sense of smell. The sense is also less acute in persons who smoke. A skull fracture can destroy the sense of smell completely (anosmia).

A talk about Smoking

Smoking of tobacco, in cigarettes, cigars, or a pipe, is a habit that meets many of the criteria that define an addiction. For some smokers, it provides a relief from anxiety and tension; but for others, it becomes a physical and psychological burden. Cigar and pipe smoking, although they present some hazards to health, are thought to be less dangerous than cigarette smoking.

Four times as many deaths are caused by cigarette smoking as by road accidents. Cigarette smoking damages the lungs, blood vessels and, to a lesser extent, other organs such as the heart.

Cancer of the lung is the most publicized hazard, and the peak of its incidence in men is just before retirement in the fifty-five to sixty-five age group (when one in seven deaths results from lung cancer). Two out of every five heavy smokers die before the age of sixty-five.

In women who smoke, the highest mortality rate occurs ten years earlier than in men, but only one death in twenty is caused by lung cancer.

Every cigarette that is smoked reduces the life expectancy by about ten minutes. A person of thirty-five who smokes a packet of cigarettes a day can expect to live at least five years less than a person of the same age who does not smoke.

People who smoke not only damage their own health, but also harm others. Studies have shown that people who have to live or work in smoky environments, although non-smokers themselves, have an increased risk of developing respiratory ailments.

Q: *What are the harmful substances in tobacco and what do they do?*

A: There are four main groups of dangerous substances in tobacco smoke. Nicotine is the substance that causes addiction. It stimulates the release of adrenaline and other substances in the body that cause an increase in pulse rate, rise in blood pressure, and narrowing of the blood vessels in the skin. Adrenaline also

causes an increase in fatty substances in the blood, and makes blood platelets (factors in blood clotting) stickier and therefore more likely to form blood clots.

Carbon monoxide is a poisonous gas produced by the incomplete burning of tobacco. In the lungs, it combines with haemoglobin in the blood and thus prevents the haemoglobin from carrying its full quota of oxygen through the circulation. It reduces a person's athletic ability, and also acts as a poison.

Various substances in tobacco irritate the lining of the bronchi, inducing spasm and increasing bronchial secretions. At the same time, these irritants damage cells that usually sweep the secretions out of the lungs. This increases the likelihood of developing bronchitis.

Cancer-producing substances are present in the tar in cigarette smoke.

Q: *Is there any way of reducing the dangers of cigarette smoking?*

A: Yes. Obviously, the best way of avoiding the dangers of cigarette smoking is to give up the habit. If this seems impossible, the smoker can use brands with low nicotine and tar content. Cigarettes, preferably with filters, should be smoked to a long and not a short stub. (The greatest concentration of tar and other irritants is in the stub of the cigarette.) Removing the cigarette from the mouth between puffs helps to reduce the amount of smoke that is inhaled.

Q: *What effect does smoking during pregnancy have on the baby?*

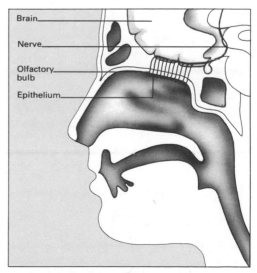

Smell stimuli entering the nose pass through the olfactory bulb up to the brain.

Brain

Nerve

Olfactory bulb

Epithelium

427

Snakebite

A: Babies born to mothers who smoke are 140-360 grams (5-13 ounces) lighter on average than those born to mothers who do not smoke. Also, pregnant women who smoke are more likely to have a miscarriage, a stillborn baby, or an infant that dies soon after birth. Twice as many premature babies are born to smoking mothers than to mothers who do not smoke. There is also evidence to suggest that by the age of eleven the children of mothers who smoked more than ten cigarettes a day during pregnancy are slightly shorter and slightly below the average in reading, mathematics, and general ability than are the children of nonsmoking mothers.

Q: *What are the effects of smoking on the lungs?*

A: There are two main effects of smoking on the lungs. Chronic bronchitis and, eventually, emphysema commonly occur in heavy smokers, and a morning cough, which clears the bronchi, is a common feature of all smokers. Early lung damage can be detected by pulmonary function tests before there is any obvious short-ness of breath.

Among people who smoke a packet of cigarettes a day, lung cancer occurs twenty times more frequently than in nonsmokers. The risk is increased in those who smoke high tar cigarettes, who inhale deeply, and who began smoking in adolescence.

Q: *Can smoking cause other cancers of the body?*

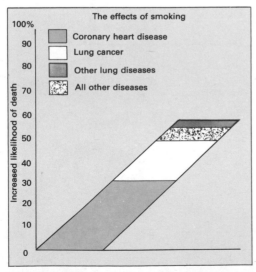

Smoking of tobacco increases the likelihood of death from various diseases by 57 per cent.

A: Yes. There are more cancers of the bladder and pancreas in smokers than in nonsmokers. Cancer of the mouth, tongue, larynx, and oesophagus are also more common in smokers of all kinds of tobacco, including pipe smokers and cigar smokers.

Q: *Can smoking affect the heart?*

A: Yes. Cigarette smoking increases the likelihood of ARTERIOSCLEROSIS, and there is twice the risk of CORONARY thrombosis than in those who do not smoke. The risk of developing other blood vessel disorders, such as BUERGER'S DISEASE, is also increased.

Q: *Are other diseases more likely to occur in smokers?*

A: Yes. Dental disorders, gingivitis, and other infections of the gums more commonly occur in smokers. Smokers are also more likely to develop tuberculosis, probably because the damaging effect of the irritants in tobacco lowers the resistance of the lungs.

Although smoking does not cause peptic ulcers, the continued habit prevents them from healing. Con-sequently, complications are more common and mortality from perforated ulcers is greater.

Q: *What are the benefits from stopping smoking?*

A: Within a few days or weeks there is an improvement in the sense of taste and smell, a gradual reduction in the amount of morning coughing, and less shortness of breath during exercise.

Although lung damage, such as that caused by chronic bronchitis and emphysema, cannot be reversed once it has occurred, it no longer gets worse.

However, the greatest long term benefit is the steady decrease in the chances of getting cancer. If a person who stops smoking cigarettes lives for ten years, his chance of developing lung cancer is no more than for someone who has never smoked.

Q: *How may a person stop smoking?*

A: For most people, stopping smoking is a goal that can be achieved only by gradual stages. First, only light a cigarette when there is a definite desire to smoke one. This should reduce the total amount of cigarettes smoked in a day, because it eliminates all the cigarettes that are smoked merely out of habit, and without positive intention. Next, decide when the next cigarette is to be smoked, and do not smoke until then. Each time you survive a period, of, say two or three hours without a cigarette, you will feel a definite sense of achievement. The gap between cigarettes can gradually be increased until you have reduced your total amount of cigarettes smoked in a day to about ten.

The next stage, in which you decide not to smoke until the following day, is the most difficult. For your first complete day without cigarettes, choose a day when you are constantly busy or physically active. After you have not smoked for two weeks your physical addiction to nicotine will have been cured, and any continued desire to smoke will be caused by nervous tension only.

Q: *Are there any other ways of stopping smoking?*

A: Yes. Often people decide that they cannot give up smoking on their own. Some doctors run smoking clinics or group therapy, or recommend aversion therapy as methods of giving up smoking. Some people may be helped by hypnosis. Injections of drugs similar to nicotine have been tried, but have not been successful.

Those who are unable to stop smoking should at least attempt to reduce smoking, or change to cigars or a pipe.

Snakebite. For EMERGENCY treatment, *see* First Aid, p.514. The only poisonous snake in the U.K. is the adder, which is not found in Ireland.

Snake venom is a complex protein substance that varies in its effect from species to species. Some venoms cause mainly tissue damage, others principally affect the nerves, and some cause destruction of blood cells and act as an anticoagulant. It is usually impossible to tell from the marks of a bite which species of snake has bitten a person. If possible, the snake should be killed, because this provides a positive identification, which is an important factor in treatment.

Sneezing is a sudden, involuntary, explosive expulsion of air resulting from irritation of the nose. A sneeze may project infected droplets 3 to 4 metres (10 to 12ft) so a sneeze should be blocked by a handkerchief or hand.

Snellen's chart is a chart of letters of decreasing size used to test a person's eyesight. *See also* SPECTACLES.

Snoring is noisy breathing during sleep that is caused by vibration of the soft palate. It usually occurs when the soft palate falls backward, thus partly blocking the nose, while sleeping on the back with the mouth open.

Snoring may be habitual, or it may result from an underlying condition that blocks the nose, such as swollen adenoids; mucus; a DEVIATED NASAL SEPTUM; or a nasal POLYP.

Snow blindness occurs when the eyes are directly exposed to intense ultraviolet light reflected off snow. It can also occur from exposure to arc welding flames, high-voltage electric sparks, and artificial sun lamps. The light causes severe eye pain and photophobia, a dislike of bright light. It may result in conjunctivitis, and sometimes inflammation of the retina.

Sodium is a metallic chemical element. Its salts, particularly the chloride, form the principal salts within the body. Most people get sufficient sodium in the food they eat.

Q: *What happens if the body's level of sodium is incorrect?*

A: Any condition that causes excessive loss of sodium from the body, such as severe vomiting and diarrhoea, kidney disease, a disorder of the adrenal glands (Addison's disease), or excessive use of diuretic drugs, produces signs of dehydration and shock.

Less commonly, lack of sodium occurs in the body fluids because of diabetes insipidus or excessive sweating. An excess may occur when a patient is recovering from acute kidney failure (when there is an imbalance of sodium and water). This may lead to symptoms of mental confusion, thirst, and high blood pressure.

Sodium bicarbonate is a white, odourless, crystalline powder that is used medically as an ANTACID to neutralize the stomach's acid

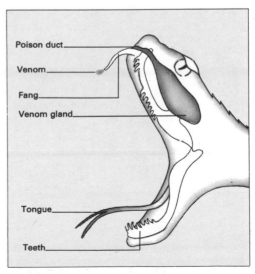

Poison duct

Venom

Fang

Venom gland

Tongue

Teeth

Snakebite may inject venom through a groove in the poison fang as the snake bites.

Soft sore

secretions and in weak solution as intravenous infusions in the treatment of certain disorders.

Soft sore. *See* CHANCROID.

Solar plexus. *See* PLEXUS.

Somatotype is a particular type of physique. For example, an ectomorph is tall and thin with poorly developed muscles; an endomorph is short and rounded; and a mesomorph is muscular and well-built.

Somnambulism. *See* SLEEPWALKING.

Sonne dysentery. *See* DYSENTERY.

Sonography. *See* ULTRASOUND TECHNIQUES.

Soporific is anything that causes drowsiness.

Sordes is a foul crust on the lips, teeth, and gums often found in patients with a fever.

Sore is any tender or painful lesion or ulcer on the skin, especially in the mouth or throat. *See* BEDSORE; MOUTH ULCER; SORE THROAT.

Sore throat is a symptom of many disorders, including the COMMON COLD, DIPHTHERIA, GLANDULAR FEVER; INFLUENZA, LARYNGITIS, MEASLES, PHARYNGITIS, QUINSY, and TONSILLITIS.

Temporary relief may be obtained by sucking medicated throat lozenges, and by taking aspirin or paracetamol. It is also advisable to stop smoking; to drink plenty of fluids; and to eat soft foods. A doctor should be consulted if a sore throat persists.

Spare part surgery is any form of surgery that uses artificial parts to replace diseased or injured parts of a patient's body. *See* REPLACEMENT SURGERY; TRANSPLANT SURGERY.

Spasm is a sudden involuntary contraction of a muscle or group of muscles, usually accompanied by pain and movement.

Spastic describes a condition in which a recurrent muscular contraction occurs. This condition is present in neurological disorders that affect the brain, such as those that follow a STROKE, or in CEREBRAL PALSY resulting from congenital brain damage.

Spastic colon. *See* MUCOUS COLITIS.

Spectacles, or eyeglasses, may be prescribed to correct visual defects. Recently, CONTACT LENSES have become a common alternative.

Common defects for which spectacles may be prescribed are ASTIGMATISM (distortion of the lens); hyperopia (LONGSIGHTEDNESS); myopia (SHORTSIGHTEDNESS); and PRESBYOPIA (loss of elasticity in the lens because of age). Glasses may also be required to correct a congenital disorder or a birth injury to the eyes.

Spectacles do not make the eyes lazy nor worsen a person's eyesight. But the eyes should be tested yearly.

Q: What types of spectacle lens are available?

A: As well as the usual concave or convex lenses (available in specified shapes and sizes under the National Health, subsidized), there are three main other types of lens. Dark lenses are used especially by albinos; by those with certain eye disorders in which light may cause pain; and in conditions of extremely bright light. Bifocals are glasses with divided lenses for each eye, correcting vision for both far and near objects. And trifocals correct vision for middle distance as well.

Some modern lenses are of variable darkness according to light intensity.

Speculum is an instrument used for examining the interior of the body, usually through one of the normal openings such as the ear, nose, rectum, or vagina.

Speech defects include any condition that results in a failure to speak normally. Most are first detected in childhood, when a baby fails to begin talking at the usual age.

Probably the most common cause of delayed speaking is some form of mental retardation. But hearing problems also cause difficulty in learning to speak. A rare cause of failure to speak is AUTISM.

Q: Are there any other conditions that may cause failure to develop normal speech?

A: Yes. Children with CEREBRAL PALSY or a CLEFT PALATE have difficulty in pronouncing words clearly.

Some children, who are in other ways normal and intelligent, develop a kind of word deafness. Sounds are not understood, although they are heard, and this results in disordered speech.

Stuttering or stammering, however,

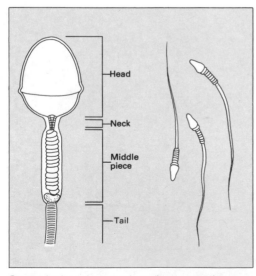

Sperm is the microscopic male gamete that fertilizes the female gamete, the ovum.

Head

Neck

Middle piece

Tail

may be the result of severe emotional disturbances.

Q: *When should a parent become concerned about speech defects in a child?*

A: A parent who notices that a baby is not reacting to sounds (by moving the eyes or head) between the ages of four and six months should discuss the matter with a doctor, because the infant may have a hearing problem. If an infant of eight to nine months is not able to repeat sounds, then a thorough assessment is needed.

The age at which a child learns to speak varies. But, on the average, a child of two-and-a-half should be able to understand simple speech and be speaking reasonably well.

Q: *How can speech defects in children be treated?*

A: Treatment of speech defects depends on the cause. Speech defects that are the result of deafness may be overcome by the use of a hearing aid or an operation. Lisping or stuttering can often be improved if the child is encouraged by the family to speak slowly and correctly. More complicated speech problems need help from a speech therapist. Autistic children require special training.

Q: *What speech disorders occur in adults?*

A: Once speech has been learned, the onset of deafness has no effect on the ability to speak, although speech may be louder than normal because the person cannot hear his or her own voice. Loss of speech (aphasia) may occur after any form of brain damage that involves the speech area of the brain. Recovery may be complete, or it may leave some degree of disability involving the use of incorrect words or phrases (dysphasia).

Extreme hoarseness may occur if the laryngeal muscles are partially paralyzed or destroyed. Dysarthria, speech that is correct but altered, may be the result of muscular or neurological disorders, such as Parkinson's disease.

Q: *How can speech defects in adults be treated?*

A: Treatment depends on the cause. Cancer of the larynx may require surgery. If necessary, the patient may be taught OESOPHAGEAL SPEECH. Drug treatment may help in neurological or muscular disorders. A speech therapist can help a patient with dysphasia after a stroke.

Sperm is the male sex cell, known also as a spermatozoon. It is produced in the testicles and ejaculated in SEMEN. After sexual intercourse, fertilization may occur if a sperm from the male combines with an ovum (egg) from the female. Both sperm and ovum each contain half the normal number of chromosomes that are required to form a single cell.

Infertility in men may be caused by an absence of sperm. One cause of this is a blockage of the vas deferens between the testicle and the prostate gland. Another cause is failure to produce sperm, or deficiency of healthy sperm.

Infection of the reproductive tract, epididymitis, and prostatitis cause defective sperm. Mumps causing orchitis may stop production of sperm. Other factors include obesity, smoking, drinking alcohol, and serious illness. Sperm production takes place only if the temperature of the testicles is two degrees below that of the rest of the body.

Spermatic cord consists of blood vessels; nerves; fibrous tissue; and the tube (VAS DEFERENS) that carries sperm from the EPIDIDYMIS of the TESTIS to the PROSTATE GLAND.

Spermatocele is a cyst in the epididymis and contains spermatic fluid. *See* CYST.

Spermicide is a substance that kills sperm. *See* CONTRACEPTION.

Sphincter is a ring of muscle that closes or constricts an opening or passage in the body when the muscle contracts.

Sphygmomanometer is an instrument that measures blood pressure. A rubber cuff is placed round the upper arm, or sometimes the thigh, and inflated with air to a pressure greater than that of the blood in the arteries. This temporarily stops the flow of blood. The air pressure is then gradually released while a stethoscope is used to listen for the sound of the pulse over the artery as the blood starts

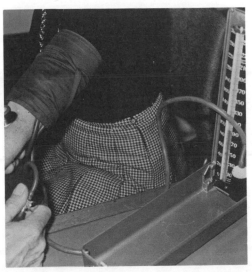

Sphygmomanometer is an instrument used to measure blood pressure.

Spina bifida

to flow again. When this sound is heard, the air pressure in the cuff equals the upper blood pressure, known as the systolic blood pressure. The pressure is further reduced in the cuff until the sounds disappear. This is known as the diastolic pressure. The blood pressure is expressed in millimetres of mercury. *See* BLOOD PRESSURE.

Spina bifida is a congenital anomaly of the spine in which one or more vertebral segments are not joined together. The defect may extend over a number of vertebrae, usually in the lumbar or sacral regions.

The disorder is classified as either spina bifida occulta, in which few signs define its presence; or spina bifida cystica, in which there is a protruding sac that contains either membranes (meningocele) or the spinal cord (myelocele) or both (myelomeningocele). Spina bifida is commonly associated with HYDROCEPHALUS. If the protruding sac is damaged, meningeal infection or death may result.

Spina bifida occulta seldom produces neurological symptoms. But in cases in which the spinal cord is involved, the patient's legs may be paralyzed and urinary and faecal incontinence is common, although congenital anomalies such as CLUBFOOT may be the only outward sign of the disorder.

Q: What is the treatment for spina bifida?

A: Only for meningocele and myelocele is an immediate operation required. In such cases, surgery is needed to cover the area with skin to prevent meningitis.

In paralyzed children with myelocele or myelomeningocele, a decision must be made by the specialists and the family whether or not to operate, since surgery usually cannot prevent lifelong disability. These conditions occur in only one out of eight hundred live births.

Q: Can spina bifida be detected in a foetus before birth?

A: Spina bifida can be detected by checking the mother's blood for a high level of alpha-feto protein. The disorder can also be detected by measuring the amount of this protein in the amniotic fluid surrounding the foetus (*see* AMNIOCENTESIS).

Spinal cord is the part of the central nervous system that extends along the spinal column from the base of the brain to the second lumbar vertebra in the small of the back. It is covered by the three membranes (pia, dura, and arachnoid) that make up the meninges and is bathed with cerebrospinal fluid.

The spinal cord is composed of 31 bundles of nerves, formed of sensory and motor fibres that carry impulses from the brain and relay messages from various parts of the body back to the brain. At the lower end of the spinal cord is the cauda equina, a fan-shaped network of nerves running in the spinal canal and supplying the lumbar, sacral, and coccygeal nerves that serve the lower part of the body.

See also NERVOUS SYSTEM.

Spinal curvature is any abnormal shape of the spine. A normal spine appears straight when viewed from the front, and from the side has an elongated double S-shape, with four curves.

Abnormal sideways curvature of the spine, when viewed from the front, is called SCOLIOSIS. LORDOSIS is an increased curvature of the lumbar spine, and KYPHOSIS is abnormal curvature of the thoracic spine.

Spinal fluid. *See* CEREBROSPINAL FLUID.

Spine, also called the spinal column or backbone, is a part of the axial skeleton (head and trunk). It is made up of seven cervical (neck) vertebrae; twelve thoracic (chest) vertebrae; five lumbar vertebrae; and the sacrum and coccyx.

The vertebrae are separated by tough, intervertebral discs of fibrocartilage and held together by ligaments. In addition, there are muscles that extend up and down, supporting the spine and the body, and producing movement. Some of these muscles extend up to the back and side of the skull to help to support the head.

Q: What disorders may affect the spine?

A: Many spinal disorders cause pain in the back (*see* BACKACHE). SPONDYLOLISTHESIS, a common cause of low back pain, affects

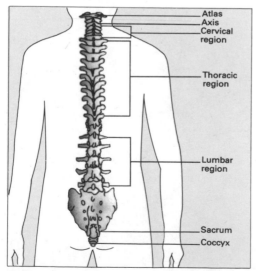

Atlas
Axis
Cervical region

Thoracic region

Lumbar region

Sacrum
Coccyx

Spine consists of thirty-three vertebrae that encase and protect the spinal cord and nerves.

the joint between the fifth lumbar vertebra and the sacrum. Fusion of the small joint between the sacrum and the coccyx can cause stiffness in this region, particularly in the elderly.

Congenital anomalies of the spine may include additional vertebrae, usually in the lumbar region; half vertebrae in the thoracic spine; fusing of the fifth lumbar vertebra with the sacrum; or the opposite effect, in which the first sacral vertebra is separated from the rest of the sacrum.

See also SLIPPED DISC; SPINA BIFIDA; SPINAL CURVATURE; VERTEBRA.

Spinal puncture. *See* ANKYLOSING SPONDYLITIS; BACKACHE; LUMBAR PUNCTURE.

Spinal tap. *See* LUMBAR PUNCTURE.

Spirochetes are spiral-shaped bacteria. *See* BACTERIA.

Spirometer is an apparatus used in lung function tests for measuring the volume of air that is breathed in and out. The patient breathes through a tube connected to the instrument, which produces a record on a moving strip of paper. *See* LUNG FUNCTION TESTS.

Splanchnic describes anything concerned with the intestines or internal organs, such as the liver and spleen.

Splay foot is another term for flatfoot (pes planus). *See* FLATFOOT.

Spleen is an abdominal organ that stores blood and plays a part in the body's immune system. It is about the size of a man's fist and varies in weight between 140 grams (5 oz) and 280 grams (10oz), depending on the amount of blood it contains. It lies in the upper left part of the abdominal cavity, above and behind the stomach, and is protected by the lower ribs. It has a large blood supply through the splenic artery.

The spleen is composed of sponge-like tissue (splenic pulp), consisting of white lymphoid tissue scattered throughout the reddish mass that makes up the basic substance of the spleen.

The white pulp produces lymphocytes (white blood cells), and the red pulp stores excess red blood cells and filters out any damaged cells, debris, and bacteria in the circulation.

Q: What disorders may affect the spleen?

A: The most common disorder is enlargement of the spleen, which may have various causes. It occurs in forms of chronic haemolytic ANAEMIA, such as sickle cell anaemia; malignant conditions of the lymphatic system, such as HODGKIN'S DISEASE, LEUKAEMIA and POLYCYTHAEMIA vera; in CIRRHOSIS of the liver, when there is an increase in venous pres-

sure; in various inflammatory diseases, such as mononucleosis, hepatitis, malaria, brucellosis and kala-azar; and in conditions such as SARCOIDOSIS.

If the spleen is damaged by injury, such as a blow to the abdomen in a motor accident, it can be removed in an adult with little or no effect on the patient's general health (*see* SPLENECTOMY).

Splenectomy is the surgical removal of the spleen. There may be various reasons for this operation, including rupture of the spleen; enlargement of the spleen, often accompanying cirrhosis of the liver; and varicose veins in the oesophagus that cause internal bleeding.

Splenic anaemia is a type of ANAEMIA associated with enlargement of the spleen. It is a form of Banti's disease, which combines anaemia, splenic enlargement, and haemorrhage, and is caused by cirrhosis of the liver.

Splenomegaly is enlargement of the spleen (*see* SPLEEN; SPLENECTOMY).

Splint is a device that is used to immobilize and support an injured part of the body, usually a fractured limb.

For EMERGENCY treatment, *see* First Aid, p.546.

Splinter is a slender piece of wood, metal, or similar material embedded in the layers of the skin. It can also be a fragment from a fractured bone.

If the splinter enters or is the cause of a wound, it may be difficult to find or remove. This should be done by a doctor.

For EMERGENCY treatment of splinters, *see* First Aid, p.589.

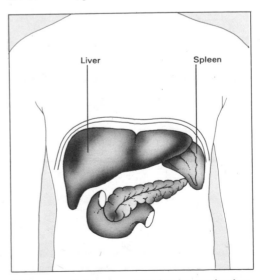

Spleen is mainly responsible for the production of white blood cells during adult life.

Spondylitis

Spondylitis is inflammation of the vertebrae. The most common form is ANKYLOSING SPONDYLITIS, which is a rheumatoid disorder. There are various possible causes, including tuberculosis of the vertebrae.

Symptoms of spondylitis include back pain, pain on movement, a stiff back, and occasionally fever. Diagnosis is confirmed by an X-ray, white blood cell count, and raised sedimentation rate (ESR). Treatment usually involves rest, spinal support, improvement of posture and therapy specifically directed at the cause of the inflammation. Occasionally surgery may be necessary to prevent pressure on the spinal cord or nerves.

Spondylolisthesis is a deformity of the spine in which one vertebra slides forward over the top of another. It can occur in the neck or, more commonly, in the lumbar spine.

Q: *What are the symptoms of spondylolisthesis?*

A: The main symptoms of spondylolisthesis in the neck are weakness and pain in the arms, caused by compression of the spinal cord. Later symptoms are paralysis in the lower part of the body, with disorders of the bowel and bladder.

Spondylolisthesis in the lumbar spine is one of the causes of backache and SCIATICA.

Q: *How is spondylolisthesis treated?*

A: Treatment of spondylolisthesis in the neck depends on the severity of the condition. Often, the initial treatment is traction, which can only be applied to a patient in bed. A metal frame is attached to the skull and weights are attached to stretch the neck. Following this treatment, a neck cast may be necessary. Sometimes an operation is required to correctly reposition the vertebrae.

There is no need to treat spondylolisthesis of the lumbar region unless the symptoms are severe. If they are, a surgical corset and muscle-strengthening exercises may be sufficient; in some cases, an operation is necessary.

See also SLIPPED DISC.

Spondylosis is osteoarthritis that affects the spine. It involves a degeneration of the joints, frequently accompanied by breakdown of the intervertebral discs (*see* SLIPPED DISC).

Spondylosis in the neck usually affects the lowest three vertebrae. It causes aching and stiffness in the back of the neck and a grating sound when turning the neck. The patient may also have a headache, and pain or muscle weakness in the arm. Spondylosis of the lower spine most commonly occurs in people who have done heavy manual labour or who have a history of either injury or degenerative changes following slipped disc or osteochondritis (inflammation of bone and cartilage). Backache with muscle spasm are the usual symptoms. The condition may cause pressure on local nerves resulting in pain in the legs or round the ribs.

Q: *Does spondylosis always produce symptoms?*

A: No. X-ray examination of the spine shows many of the characteristics of spondylosis in people as they get older, but symptoms may not occur. Symptoms may occur, however, if there is some minor injury to the spine, such as that caused by a fall or sudden twist.

Q: *How is spondylosis treated?*

A: Treatment depends on the severity of the symptoms. Aspirin or antirheumatic drugs are usually helpful, but sometimes temporary immobilization of the spine in a neck splint or spinal support is necessary. Physiotherapy, with heat, massage or manipulation may also be used.

Spore is the reproductive cell of a primitive organism, such as a fungus or bacterium. It is usually protected by a thick membrane, which makes it resistant to the effects of heat, chemicals, and dehydration. As a result, prolonged boiling or intense heat is usually required to kill spores.

Sports injuries are many and varied, depending on the physical demands of each individual sport and on the fitness, stamina, and strength of the athlete. Many of the injuries occur because of repeated movements or stresses on particular joints, bones and muscles. Training for a particular sport is

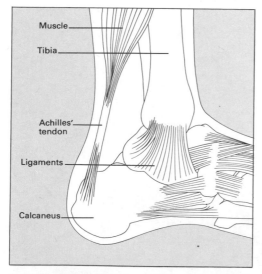

Muscle
Tibia
Achilles' tendon
Ligaments
Calcaneus

Rupture of the Achilles' tendon can occur if a person takes sudden exercise.

aimed at increasing the stamina and strength of the participant in line with the stresses to be met.

The first requirement before a person takes part in any sport is physical fitness. This requires the slow development of physical capacity in all areas, so that it is possible for the body to withstand the initial strain of training. Too much exercise too soon can produce muscle and ligament strain, inflamed tendons (tenosynovitis) inflamed bursae (bursitis), and stress fractures of bones.

Stamina implies an increase in reserve capacity, especially of the heart and the lungs. The heart has to pump blood at an increased rate, and the lungs have to take in oxygen more rapidly. Strength develops by building muscle power, a slow process of using muscles a little harder over a period of time. When an individual has developed to a required peak, he or she is less likely to suffer injury and, if injured, finds that increased fitness aids the healing process.

Sprain (for EMERGENCY treatment, *see* First Aid, p.592) is an injury to a joint in which some of the ligaments are severely stretched or even partly torn, producing swelling, pain, and tenderness. These symptoms disappear when the joint is rested.

Sprue is an intestinal disorder characterized by impaired absorption of food (particularly fats) in the small intestine. It is common in the tropics but also occurs in temperate countries, where it is known as idiopathic or nontropical sprue.

Q: What causes sprue?

A: There are many disorders that may cause sprue or the similar symptoms produced by malabsorption of food in the intestine. The disorders include COELIAC DISEASE, which may appear spontaneously at any age, or which may result from intestinal infections that are common in the tropics and which impair normal digestion. A different condition, the malabsorption syndrome, may produce identical symptoms. This may be the result of PANCREATITIS, in which there is insufficient secretion of the enzymes necessary for digestion, or of other factors that interfere with normal intestinal activity, for example, the metabolic disorder AMYLOIDOSIS; worm infestations; irradiation treatment; or operations in which part of the stomach or small intestine are removed.

Q: What are the symptoms of sprue?

A: The patient usually appears unwell, is underweight, and has a dry, pale skin. Soreness at the corners of the mouth (cheilosis) and a red tongue are present because of vitamin B deficiency. There may be clubbing of the fingers and swelling of the ankles (oedema); the abdomen may also swell. The patient may complain of weakness, fatigue, and frequent cramps in the muscles.

Bruising may occur easily, and diarrhoea, with large pale, fatty stools that float, may be an obvious feature.

Q: How is sprue treated?

A: Treatment depends on the cause. Coeliac disease is treated with a gluten-free diet and the avoidance of all wheat and rye protein. Tropical sprue is treated with vitamins and antibiotics.

Sputum is the material that is coughed up from the windpipe, bronchi, and lungs. A small amount of clear mucus is produced by the lungs each day, and this is swept through the windpipe (trachea) and over the larynx by the hair-like cells that keep the lungs free of dust and other particles. The amount of sputum increases in any minor respiratory infection.

Bloodstained sputum may be an indication of an underlying condition, such as severe infection or cancer. It requires prompt investigation.

Squint. *See* STRABISMUS.

Stammering. *See* STUTTERING.

Stapedectomy is an operation to remove the stapes (one of the small bones in the middle ear). The stapes is replaced with a plastic or metal equivalent, which transmits sounds to the round window of the inner ear.

A stapedectomy may be necessary in the treatment of DEAFNESS due to OTOSCLEROSIS.

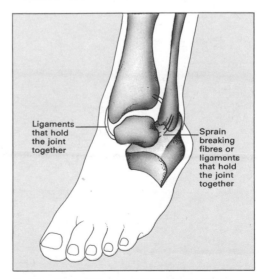

Ligaments that hold the joint together

Sprain breaking fibres or ligaments that hold the joint together

Sprain of the ankle is painful because the fibres and ligaments become stretched or torn.

Stapes

Stapes is one of the three small bones (ossicles) in the middle ear; it is shaped like a stirrup iron. The stapes transmits sound vibrations to the round window of the inner ear. See EAR; OTITIS; OTOSCLEROSIS.

Staphylococcus is one of a group of BACTERIA that grow in clumps and, on microscopic examination, appear like bunches of grapes. Staphylococci are extremely common microorganisms and cause boils and other forms of skin sepsis characterized by pus.

Some staphylococci have the ability to resist antibiotics; for this reason doctors take particular care when treating staphylococcal infections. Staphylococci may also contaminate food and cause FOOD POISONING.

Startle reflex, also known as Moro's reflex, is the reflex reaction in infants under the age of three months to sudden movement or loud noise. The startle reflex can be seen if a baby is gently lifted a short way from a bed or table and then released, or if the table is hit hard. The infant throws his or her arms outward and then moves them slowly inward in a grasping movement as the legs are stretched out. This is usually accompanied by a cry.

A symmetrical movement is an indication that the central nervous system is functioning normally. An asymmetrical movement, in which one arm or leg seems to lag behind the other, can be one indication that brain damage (cerebral palsy) may have occurred.

Starvation is the physical change that the human body undergoes if there is a long and continued lack of sufficient nutrition. Provided fluids are available, a person can usually survive complete starvation for six to eight weeks finally dying.

In infants, starvation may cause marasmus or kwashiorkor. See KWASHIORKOR; NUTRITIONAL DISORDERS.

Steatorrhoea is excessive fat in the faeces. It usually indicates a failure of fat absorption in the small intestine, and commonly occurs in SPRUE, but it may also accompany severe JAUNDICE.

Stenosis is a narrowing of a duct or tube within the body. It may develop in various places, such as at a heart valve (aortic or mitral stenosis); at the exit of the stomach from spasm of the muscle (pyloric stenosis); or in the duct of a salivary gland following infection or the passage of a small stone. Stenosis may also develop in the carotid artery or arteries of the leg, producing symptoms of reduced blood flow, such as transient minor strokes or intermittent claudication (see INTERMITTENT CLAUDICATION; STROKE).

Sterility is the inability to produce offspring. Sterility also refers to the stage of being free from living microorganisms, such as bacteria and viruses. See INFERTILITY; STERILIZATION.

Sterilization is any method by which various microorganisms, such as bacteria and viruses, are killed. Forms of sterilization include: boiling; dry heat; exposure to steam at high pressure; exposure to various gases or liquids; or exposure to radioactivity.

Sterilization is also the term used to describe an operation to make a man or woman infertile.

Q: How is a man sterilized?

A: A man can be sterilized by having a vasectomy, a simple operation that can be performed under a local anaesthetic, and which usually takes less than half an hour. Each vas deferens (the duct that carries sperm from the testicle) is cut and the ends tied off. For details, *see* VASECTOMY.

Q: How is a woman sterilized?

A: The corresponding procedure in a female is known technically as a tubal ligation. Each fallopian tube (the duct that carries eggs from an ovary to the womb) is cut and the ends tied. The operation is usually done under a general anaesthetic, and the woman may have to remain in hospital for four or five days. Nowadays many women are sterilized with a laparoscope (a type of ENDOSCOPE), and the tubes clipped or electrically burnt. This treatment requires only two days in hospital.

Q: Can sterilization be reversed in men or women?

A: Yes, but the chances of success are about 20% in women and 60% in men.

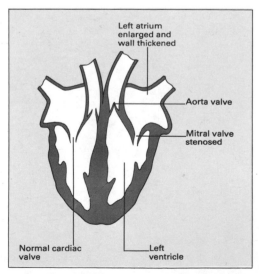

Left atrium enlarged and wall thickened

Aorta valve

Mitral valve stenosed

Normal cardiac valve

Left ventricle

Stenosis of a valve produces muscle thickening in the part of the heart behind it.

Q: *In what circumstances should a couple consider sterilization?*

A: A couple may consider sterilization if two or more children have been born with congenital anomalies (*see* GENETIC COUNSELLING). More usually, sterilization may be carried out for social reasons: for example, a woman aged over thirty who has already had children may dislike other forms of contraception, or find that they fail.

Sternum, or breast-bone, is a flat, dagger-shaped bone that forms the front part of the chest wall. It is about 17cm (7 inches) long in men and about 13cm (5 inches) long in women, and about 4cm (1.5 inches) across at its widest part.

The sternum is made up of three segments: the widest, top part (the manubrium), also known as the handle; the body of the sternum; and the tip (the xiphoid process or xiphisternum). In children the three parts of the sternum are jointed, but in adults they are fused to form one continuous bone.

Anomalies of the sternum may produce a protuberant, pigeon-chested appearance, or a sunken, funnel-chested appearance. These relatively common anomalies do not cause any major problems. *See* PIGEON CHEST.

Steroid is a class of chemical compounds. The term is commonly applied to the cortico-steroid hormones produced by the adrenal glands. Other steroids include the hormones progesterone, the oestrogen group, and testosterone, as well as bile salts and cholesterol. *See* CHOLESTEROL; CORTICOSTEROID.

Stethoscope is an instrument for listening to the internal sounds of the body.

Stevens-Johnson syndrome is a rare skin disorder in which there are painful blisters in the throat and mouth, the conjunctiva of the eyes, and the anal region. Other reddish nodules, and sometimes blisters, may appear on the arms and legs. Blisters in the throat may be so painful as to prevent swallowing. Treatment with corticosteroid drugs may be necessary.

Stiff neck involves either difficulty in moving the neck from its normal position, or an abnormality known medically as torticollis that forces the neck to remain in an unusual position.

Q: *What causes a stiff neck?*

A: The most common cause is a twisting or whiplash injury suffered from jerking the neck too hard, as in a car accident or in a sports injury. It may also occur after sleeping with the neck in an awkward position. In infancy, stiff neck may be caused by muscle spasm; in the elderly it is usually caused by spondylosis.

Q: *How is a stiff neck treated?*

A: Usually with painkilling drugs and, if inflammation is present, with anti-rheumatic drugs. Treatment depends on the cause. If the stiffness is caused by local injury then heat, massage, and traction may be required.

Diagnosis before treatment is important because the stiffness may result from a slipped disc or other abnormality in which manipulation may cause further damage or delay before correct diagnosis. *See* SLIPPED DISC.

Stiffness is a common symptom of disorders of the muscles and joints. It can be accompanied by aching pain. Aspirin will relieve the pain, as will massage. Recurrent morning stiffness is a characteristic of rheumatoid arthritis.

Stigma is any physical mark on the body characteristic of a disorder or an occupation, or any mark, spot, or wound that appears for no apparent physical or psychological reason.

Stillbirth is the birth of a dead foetus after twenty-eight weeks of pregnancy. It can result from various disorders, such as congenital anomalies in the foetus, haemolytic diseases of the newborn, placental insufficiency, or maternal disorders such as diabetes mellitus, anaemia, or heart disease.

See also MISCARRIAGE.

Still's disease is a juvenile form of RHEUMATOID ARTHRITIS. Initial symptoms include a sudden high fever, vague rashes that appear and disappear all over the body, and enlargement of the lymph glands and spleen. The fever may continue for several weeks

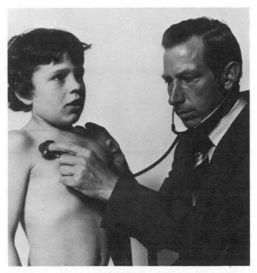

Stethoscope is used to listen to the heart beat, and to detect lung irregularities.

Stimulant

before any joint pain occurs, or the joints may become swollen and tender within a few days.

Aspirin-type drugs are usually prescribed until spontaneous improvement occurs, and corticosteroids may be given to treat severe cases.

Relapse is common, but eventually there is full recovery in most cases.

Stimulant is a drug or other agent that increases the activity of an organ or other part of the body.

See also AMPHETAMINES.

Sting is the damage and pain caused by contact with the poison from a plant or insect. For EMERGENCY treatment, *see* First Aid, p.514.

Stitch is a term popularly used to refer to a severe pain in the abdomen, usually under the rib-cage, that occurs with physical exertion. It is caused by a cramp in the muscles of the abdominal wall.

In surgical practice, the term stitch is equivalent to suture. *See* SUTURE.

Stokes-Adams attack is a form of heart block. The normal electrical impulses that regulate the heartbeat are blocked, and the heart first stops contracting and then continues at a much slower rate than normal. The rate may spontaneously return to normal. Stokes-Adams attacks are characterized by a sudden loss of consciousness, sometimes with immediate recovery, but often followed by a period of faintness, dizziness, and nausea when the patient tries to sit up. The length of these episodes may vary from periods as short as a few seconds

to a few minutes. Occasionally a complete heartblock may persist.

A mechanical pacemaker is the most effective form of treatment, although drug treatment may sometimes be used. Stokes-Adams attacks are most common in the elderly and are associated with coronary heart disease. *See* HEARTBLOCK; PACEMAKER.

Stomach is the muscular storage organ of the intestinal tract. It lies in the upper part of the abdomen, under the liver and below the left side of the diaphragm.

Food and liquid from the mouth enter the stomach from the oesophagus (gullet). The stomach can hold up to 1.5 litres (three pints) of fluid.

The three chief activities of the stomach are: contracting and squeezing the food it contains; digestion and sterilization of the food by the gastric secretions; and intermittent and gradual release of the contents into the duodenum so that digestion can continue. The stomach is also able to absorb some substances, such as alcohol, and this explains the rapid effect if drunk when the stomach is empty.

The stomach is composed of three layers of muscle covered with a membrane (the peritoneum). The inner surface is lined with mucosa that secrete gastric juices. The lower and narrow end of the stomach is formed of tough muscle fibre ending in the pyloric sphincter, which closes the exit to the duodenum.

See also DIGESTIVE SYSTEM.

Stomachache is a vague feeling of upper abdominal discomfort often accompanied by distention. It is one of the symptoms of IN-DIGESTION. *See* ABDOMINAL PAIN.

Stomach disorders. Relatively few disorders directly involve the stomach, but these include some of the most common complaints, such as gastroenteritis and peptic ulcers. Many disorders that primarily involve other parts of the body can also affect the stomach. *See* ABDOMINAL PAIN; BELCHING; BILIARY COLIC; BLOOD, VOMITING OF; CANCER; COLIC; DIARRHOEA; FLATULENCE; FOOD POISONING; GASTRITIS; GASTROENTERITIS; HYPERCHLORHYDRIA; HYPEREMESIS; INDIGESTION; LOSS OF APPETITE; MOTION SICKNESS; NAUSEA; PEPTIC ULCER; PYLORIC STENOSIS; PYLOROSPASM; VOMITING.

Stomatitis is inflammation of the mouth. It may be caused by a local disorder in the mouth, or it can occur as the result of generalized disease of the body.

A doctor or dentist should be consulted to obtain treatment for the cause of the problem. The mouth must be kept clean with mouthwashes, and any deposit must be clean-

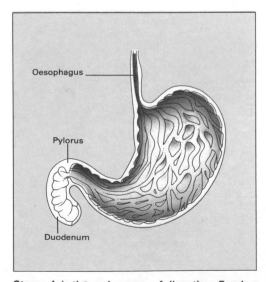

Oesophagus

Pylorus

Duodenum

Stomach is the main organ of digestion. Food enters it through the oesophagus.

ed off the teeth and lips. Dehydration may have reduced the amount of salivation, and plenty of fluids should be drunk.

Infection of the SALIVARY GLANDS may occur with stomatitis, and sometimes infected material may enter the lungs and cause PNEUMONIA.

Stone. *See* CALCULUS.

Stool is the common name for faeces. *See* FAECES.

Strabismus, also called a squint, is a condition in which the axes of the eyes are not parallel even when a person is looking at a distant object. It is usually the result of an imbalance in the movement of the two eyes. In convergent strabismus (cross-eye), the axes of the eyes converge; in divergent strabismus (lazy eye) they diverge.

Q: What symptoms may develop with strabismus?

A: If only the unaffected eye is used, the other eye may get worse and defective vision or blindness (amblyopia) may occur in that eye. Paralytic strabismus, caused by paralysis of an eye muscle, results in double vision (diplopia). This may be accompanied by giddiness, vertigo, and a tendency to incline the head to one side.

Q: What is the treatment for strabismus?

A: The most important aspect of treating strabismus is first to correct defective vision by wearing spectacles all the time. If this fails, a patch over the good eye or atropine drops to produce blurred vision ensures that the patient uses the eye with poor vision. Occasionally, eye exercises may be used to teach the patient to co-ordinate movements. If vision is equally good in both eyes, an operation may be performed to move the eye muscles, thereby positioning the eyes normally.

Strain is a term that is used to describe either an emotional or a physical disorder.

An emotional strain causes symptoms of fatigue, anxiety, and sometimes slight depression. This may result in irritability, difficulty in sleeping, and loss of weight.

Physical strain can cause tearing of muscle fibres, resulting in local pain and stiffness. It is different from a sprain, which is more serious, and may involve tearing of the ligaments around a joint. Rest, painkilling drugs, and physiotherapy with infrared heat treatment and gentle exercise help a physical strain to heal.

Strangulation is the constriction of a tube or passage within the body. It may result in partial or complete obstruction of the affected part. Strangulation is one of the causes of INTESTINAL OBSTRUCTION.

Strangury is extremely painful urination. It is most commonly caused by CYSTITIS (inflammation of the bladder) or by a stone (calculus) in the bladder.

Streptococcus is a genus of bacteria that appears to grow in straight strings or chains, as seen under a microscope. Many streptococci are harmless and are normally found in the body without causing any disorder. Some types, however, cause conditions such as sore throat and tonsillitis, scarlet fever, impetigo, erysipelas, rheumatic fever, acute nephritis, puerperal fever; others may infect wounds.

Q: Can streptococcal infections have complications?

A: Yes. Infection by streptococcus may be followed by an allergic reaction involving other tissues of the body. This can lead to disorders such as acute nephritis, rheumatic fever, chorea, and scarlet fever.

Q: How are streptococcal infections treated?

A: Almost all streptococcal infections respond to large doses of penicillin, and this treatment usually produces a cure if used for long enough.

A talk about Stress

Stress is a physical and psychological reaction to excessive stimulus. It is considered by some experts to be a psychological disorder caused by constant mental strain; but it is also a physiological response.

Physical stress on various parts of the body

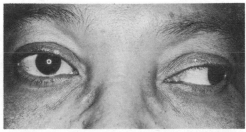

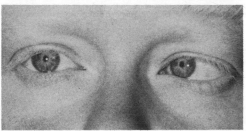

Strabismus is the misalignment of the axes of the eyes whichever way they look.

Stress incontinence

can cause damage. For example repeated minor injuries to a bone, such as one in the leg or foot of a runner, may cause a stress fracture in that bone.

Psychological stress, to a minor degree, is necessary for normal alertness and awareness, but excessive stress can have the opposite effect. The most common cause of psychological stress is fatigue, and a state of stress may be aggravated by a physical illness or by a mental disorder such as DEPRESSION.

Q: What are the symptoms of stress?

A: Symptoms of stress vary. Some people appear on the outside to be calm, but are inwardly in turmoil; others panic. Some people experience great discomfort in acute stress; they become hot and sweaty, have a rapid heartbeat, or even vomit or faint. Others may react with hysterical amnesia.

Q: What physical disorders can stress produce?

A: Disorders produced by stress vary greatly, but there are many disorders that can be triggered off or made worse by psychological stress, particularly when it is combined with anxiety or depression. Asthma and migraine are likely to occur more frequently with stress, and stress is a factor in causing peptic ulcer, irritable bowel syndrome, and ulcerative colitis.

In some people, the onset of hyperthyroidism (overactivity of the thyroid gland) is associated with a period of stress. Neurodermatitis, a skin condition accompanied by intense irritation,

is often a stress disorder, and hyperhidrosis, or excess sweating, is thought to be affected by stress.

Heavy, prolonged menstrual periods (menorrhagia) occur in some women as a result of continued stress, and may even lead to a cessation of periods (amenorrhoea) in younger women.

Q: How is stress treated?

A: A person who suspects that he or she is suffering from stress should consult a doctor. The doctor will be able to decide whether external stress is the main factor or whether the condition is caused by depression or a phobic anxiety state. The doctor will also be able to give medication or advice that may help to relieve the symptoms of stress.

Stress incontinence is the inability to prevent loss of urine during physical stress, such as coughing, laughing, or sudden movement. It may be caused by a structural abnormality, such as a PROLAPSE of the womb. In such cases, the womb may pull the bladder from its normal position, and weaken the muscle that closes the bladder.

Women who suffer from stress incontinence should consult a doctor in order to diagnose the cause.

Stricture is an abnormal narrowing of a duct or passage within the body. It may be caused by inflammation; injury, with subsequent scarring of the tissues; a muscle spasm; or pressure, as from a growth or tumour. Strictures may also be caused by a congenital anomaly, such as, HIRSCHSPRUNG'S DISEASE.

Stridor is a high pitched rasping sound produced by partial obstruction of the vocal cords. It is a common condition in children with croup. Stridor may also be produced by inflammation or tumours of the larynx or vocal cords.

A talk about a Stroke

Stroke (for EMERGENCY treatment, *see* p.554), also known as apoplexy, is a stoppage of the blood supply to part of the brain. The blockage can have one of three causes: (1) a blood clot, from somewhere else in the body (embolus), obstructing an artery; (2) clotting within an artery (cerebral thrombosis); or (3) the bursting of a blood vessel (cerebral haemorrhage). A stroke may be a relatively minor occurrence, and temporary strokes that are followed by complete recovery also occur.

Transient, temporary strokes may occur as

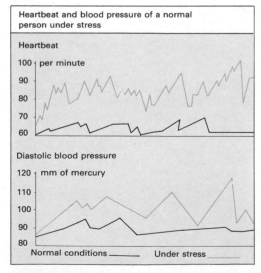

Heartbeat and blood pressure of a normal person under stress

Heartbeat

100 per minute
90
80
70
60

Diastolic blood pressure

120 mm of mercury
110
100
90
80

Normal conditions _____ Under stress _____

Stress can be measured in terms of specific physiological responses to external factors.

a result of disturbances in blood flow to the brain. This may be caused by constriction of the carotid and vertebral arteries in the neck by patches of arteriosclerosis in their walls. These constrictions reduce the blood supply so that a slight drop in blood pressure, from any cause, may produce a stroke. This is particularly likely to occur in an elderly person, and may be the result of illness, coronary thrombosis, or cardiac irregularities such as atrial fibrillation, as well as anaemia, sudden blood loss, or pressure on the neck from a tight collar. Temporary strokes may also occur from small emboli, usually blood clots, that form on the arteriosclerotic areas of the arteries, or sometimes from damaged heart valves that have been caused by sub-acute endocarditis. These small particles cause a momentary blockage of a small artery in the brain, which produces symptoms that disappear without loss of consciousness.

Q: What are the symptoms of a stroke?

A: The symptoms depend on the area of the brain that is involved. In an acute apoplectic stroke, breathing is difficult, and there is paralysis of part of the body, often affecting one whole side of the body, including the face, trunk, and one leg and arm. The skin feels clammy to the touch, and speech may be affected. Loss of consciousness may occur extremely rapidly, but occasionally a patient may remain conscious but confused. A temporary stroke may produce all the symptoms of a severe stroke, but the person usually recovers completely after a short time.

Q: What can be done to help someone who has a stroke?

A: An ambulance must be called immediately. Keep the patient quiet and warm (with a rug or blanket), either sitting up or lying down with the head and shoulders raised. An unconscious patient should be placed in the recovery position (*see* First Aid, p.573). The patient should not be moved until professional help arrives, unless it is essential. Do not give the patient anything to eat or drink. In most cases, the patient will be taken directly to hospital.

Q: What is the hospital treatment for stroke patients?

A: Careful nursing is necessary, including constant exercise of the limbs, to prevent stiffening or contraction of the muscles. Many routine actions (such as walking and sitting down) may have to be learned again. This is the task of a physiotherapist. A speech therapist may

help the patient to speak again. Recovery from a stroke is never quick because retraining, a long and slow process, may take several months.

It is rare that the cause of a stroke can be actively treated. Anticoagulants will make a cerebral haemorrhage worse, therefore they can only be given if the neurologist considers that a slowly progressing stroke is due to cerebral thrombosis. Occasionally a neurosurgeon will operate if an aneurysm has been found to be the cause of subarachnoid haemorrhage or, less commonly, to remove a large clot following a cerebral haemorrhage. Rarely, haemorrhage occurs underneath (subdural) or outside (epidural) the dural layers that surround the brain. These haemorrhages can be diagnosed by the appropriate neurological investigations and can be treated surgically.

Q: What are the patient's chances of making a full recovery from a stroke?

A: Each case must be judged on the severity of its symptoms. In the most severe cases, patients fail to regain consciousness at all and die shortly after an attack.

Many patients return to normal health, however, with only a slight speech defect and perhaps some awkwardness in walking or handling objects. In some cases, people are left paralysed on one side (hemiplegia) with a speech disorder (aphasia) and an inability to control bladder and bowel functions (incontinence).

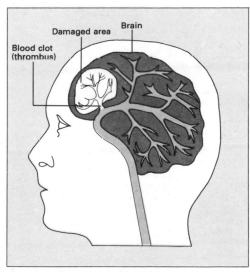

Stroke is caused by a blood clot that stops the blood supply to an area of the brain.

Strongyloides

Strongyloides is a genus of roundworms, one
species of which (*Strongyloides stercoralis*) is a
common intestinal parasite in people who
live in hot climates. Infestation with this
roundworm is called strongyloidiasis.

There may be no symptoms if the infestation is light. But migration of larvae through
the lungs usually produces a cough. Heavy
infestations may also cause abdominal pain,
vomiting, and diarrhoea. In most cases, drug
treatment with thiabendazole is effective. It is
advisable to have regular drug treatment in
areas where the parasite is common.

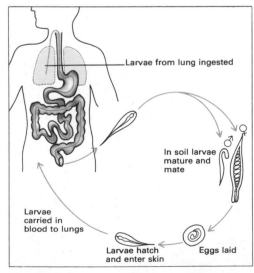

Larvae from lung ingested

In soil larvae
mature and
mate

Larvae
carried in
blood to lungs

Larvae hatch
and enter skin

Eggs laid

Strongyloides is a roundworm that enters the
bloodstream through the skin of the foot.

Strychnine is a poisonous alkaloid obtained
from the seeds of the tree *Nux vomica*.
Strychnine poisoning causes extreme activity
of the central nervous system, leading to
repeated muscle spasms that end in death
unless the victim's stomach is immediately
washed out, and an injection of muscle
relaxant drug given.

Stuffy nose is a common term for the blockage of one or both nostrils, resulting in difficulty in breathing. It is common in infections
that cause inflammation of the nose, but may
be caused by a POLYP or a DEVIATED NASAL
SEPTUM.

See also CATARRH.

Stupor is a state of semicoma, with suppression of the senses and of the normal thought
processes.

Stuttering, or stammering, is a speech disorder in which speech is faltering or hesitant,
and the initial sounds of words are repeated.
It usually starts between the ages of two and
five years, and is more common in boys than
in girls.

In many children, stuttering is caused by
psychological factors, and may be aggravated
by parental anxiety. If there is no sign of improvement after the child is seven years old,
or if the stuttering gets worse, a speech therapist should be consulted.

Stye, medically known as a hordeolum, is an
abscess of an eyelash hair follicle. It is caused
by a bacterial infection, and is commonly
associated with blepharitis (inflammation of
the eyelid).

The symptoms of a stye include swelling,
redness, and pain. But when the stye bursts,
there is relief from pain and an immediate
improvement.

Treatment is to bathe the stye with a cot-
tonwool swab soaked repeatedly in hot
water. Removing an affected eyelash sometimes helps to produce immediate discharge.

See also BLEPHARITIS.

Styptic is a substance such as alcohol, silver
nitrate, or alum, that stops bleeding by its
astringent action.

Subacute bacterial endocarditis is inflammation of the lining of the interior of the heart,
especially the heart valves. Severe inflammation of rapid onset is called acute bacterial
endocarditis. More usually, infection is of
slow onset, known as subacute bacterial
endocarditis. It is most likely to occur in
people whose heart valves are deformed or
damaged as a result of a congenital anomaly,
rheumatic fever, or following heart surgery.
People who inject themselves with opiates or
other drugs, risk infection from septicaemia
(blood poisoning), which may cause subacute
bacterial endocarditis.

Q: *What are the symptoms of subacute bacterial endocarditis?*

A: In the early stages, the patient may feel unwell, with occasional slight fever, and aching muscles and joints. The aching is commonly accompanied by tender spots in the fingertips and a particular kind of fine rash (petechiae).

    The patient becomes ill and weak as the disease progresses, with intermittent high fever and sometimes heart failure.

Q: *How is the disorder diagnosed and treated?*

A: A doctor may become suspicious if the patient has a heart murmur with a vague onset of intermittent fever. Blood samples, taken on several occasions, can be cultured to reveal the presence of bacteria. In such patients, the urine contains blood because of damage to the kidneys.

    Without treatment, the disease is fatal, but with antibiotics, about three-quarters of patients affected survive. The penicillin group of antibiotics are the most frequently used and are given by intravenous or intramuscular injection for four to six weeks. The patient usually starts to feel better within a week.

Subarachnoid haemorrhage is bleeding into the space between the membranes that surround the brain, in which cerebrospinal fluid circulates. It most commonly occurs in people between the ages of twenty-five and forty-five, and is caused by the bursting of a blood vessel that was abnormally weak at birth. In the older age group, subarachnoid haemorrhage may occur when arteriosclerosis causes damage to an artery, or it may be associated with a bleeding disorder.

Q: *What are the symptoms of a subarachnoid haemorrhage?*

A: Most patients have a sudden and severe headache. There is also a temporary or prolonged loss of consciousness. After the patient recovers consciousness, he or she is confused, may vomit, and may have convulsions. Temporary weakness of the muscles may follow, or complete paralysis of one side of the body, and the neck becomes stiff.

Q: *How is subarachnoid haemorrhage treated?*

A: About a third of all patients die from the initial haemorrhage, and a further fifteen to twenty per cent die within the next month. It is therefore necessary to find the area of bleeding as quickly as possible. Neurosurgery may prevent further bleeding.

Subclavian describes anything that lies beneath the clavicle (collar-bone).

Subconjunctival haemorrhage is bleeding between the conjunctiva (the thin, transparent membrane that covers the outside of the eye) and the sclera (the fibrous tissue that forms the white of the eye). A subconjunctival haemorrhage causes the white of the eye to become red. *See* RED EYE.

Subconscious describes mental activity that occurs beneath the levels of normal conscious awareness. Psychoanalysts define it as a level between the conscious and the unconscious.

Subcutaneous means beneath the skin and above the underlying layers of tissue, such as muscle. The subcutaneous layer contains fat and connective tissue, and varies in thickness in different parts of the body.

Subdural describes the space between the dura and arachnoid mater, two of the membranes that cover the brain.

    Haemorrhage into the subdural space may occur as the result of a head injury. In an acute haemorrhage, the patient is usually in coma and the bleeding results in extensive damage to the brain.

Sublingual gland is the smallest of the salivary glands. There are two sublingual glands located between the side of the tongue and the jawbone, one on each side of the face. *See* SALIVARY GLANDS.

Subluxation is a partial or incomplete dislocation. It may occur in a joint or in the lens of the eye. *See* DISLOCATION.

Submandibular gland is one of the salivary glands. There are two submandibular glands, one in each side of the mouth under the jawbone and below the back teeth. *See* SALIVARY GLANDS.

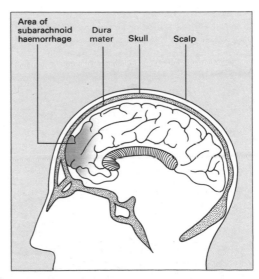

Area of
subarachnoid   Dura
haemorrhage   mater   Skull   Scalp

Subarachnoid haemorrhage into the tissues of the brain increases intercranial pressure.

Submucous resection

Submucous resection is a common operation on the nose, carried out under a general anaesthetic, to correct a DEVIATED NASAL SEPTUM. The operation removes the deformed part of the nasal septum (the cartilage and bone that divide the nostrils), allowing the two layers of mucous membrane to take up a straight position along the midline.

Subphrenic means beneath the diaphragm.

Succus entericus is the secretion of the glands that line the small intestine. It contains various enzymes essential for the digestion of food. *See* DIGESTIVE SYSTEM.

Sudden infant death syndrome. *See* SIDS.

Suffocation, or asphyxiation, is the result of blockage of the air passage, or a reduction or absence of oxygen in the air breathed in. For EMERGENCY treatment, *see* First Aid, p.518.

Brain damage occurs within five minutes if the condition is not treated, because of the shortage of oxygen. Treatment is to clear the airway, if it is obstructed, and give artificial respiration.

Sugar is a sweet-tasting carbohydrate that occurs in many foods. The sugar commonly used to sweeten food is sucrose. But there are many other sugars. They are either simple monosaccharides (such as dextrose, glucose, and fructose) or complex polysaccharides (such as sucrose and lactose).

Sugars are a good source of energy and can be broken down by the body to form glucose (blood sugar). Glucose can be reconstructed by the liver and body cells into various other forms of carbohydrates.

Excess intake of sugar causes obesity, and may be a contributory factor in arteriosclerosis.

See also CARBOHYDRATES; GLUCOSE; INSULIN.

A talk about Suicide

Suicide is the taking of one's own life. It is a common cause of death between the ages of twenty and forty, second only to accidents. Attempted suicide is responsible for about twenty per cent of all emergency hospital admissions.

Q: Why do people try to commit suicide?

A: The reasons are usually complex, and may be part of a wider personality disorder. There may be a history of antisocial behaviour, delinquency, alcoholism, poor school attendance, poor work record, depression, loneliness, or indications of problems with social relationships. Many people who attempt suicide do not really want to kill themselves at all. Their attempts are desperate acts to draw attention to their plight.

The major reason for suicide, however, is mental illness. An elderly or chronically ill person may take his or her life in a state of acute depression, misery, and pain. A person with a personality disorder, unable to cope with stress, depression, or a physical disorder, is a typical potential suicide.

Q: How can suicide be prevented?

A: Seek professional help, if it is thought that a person is likely to commit suicide. If there is time, seek help from the family doctor. Alternatively, there are many social or religious groups that specialize in helping the suicidal individual.

A doctor may suggest psychotherapy or prescribe antidepressant drugs. Seriously depressed people should, however, be hospitalized immediately for observation.

Q: What should be done if someone has already attempted suicide?

A: Get the suicide victim to hospital as quickly as possible. In the meantime, give appropriate first aid (*see* the First Aid section). Collect and keep any bottles, and look for a suicide note.

If a person telephones to say that he or she has attempted suicide, find out the exact location and address, keep the person talking, and get someone else to call for the police and other emergency aid. Continue talking until help arrives.

Deaths by suicide in England and Wales		
Male	Year	Female
2523	1969	1803
2271	1970	1669
2263	1971	1682
2198	1972	1572
2250	1973	1573
2280	1974	1619
2184	1975	1509
2330	1976	1486
2360	1977	1581
2436	1978	1586

Suicide attempts are more often successful by men than they are by women.

Sulpha drugs are drugs of several related

types that are used in the treatment of infection. Sulphonamide, which is an antibiotic, is an example of one type.

Possible side effects of sulpha drugs include nausea, diarrhoea, vomiting, skin rashes, and, very rarely, STEVENS-JOHNSON SYNDROME, although modern preparations have largely eradicated the likelihood of this happening.

Sulphones are a group of drugs used in the treatment of leprosy. These include dapsone and sulfoxone. Possible side effects include allergic dermatitis, loss of appetite, nausea, vomiting, and giddiness.

Sunburn occurs after exposure to ultraviolet light. For EMERGENCY treatment, *see* First Aid, p.594. Mild sunburn usually occurs a few hours after exposure as red skin that eventually peels away. Severe sunburn, however, results in extreme pain, swelling, and blistering a few days after excessive exposure, accompanied by fever, weakness, and symptoms suggestive of mild shock. The blisters are second-degree burns and may become infected.

Q: How is sunburn prevented?

A: Those who are vulnerable to sunburn, particularly those with fair skins, should sunbathe for only short periods. For example, twenty minutes in the morning and twenty minutes in the evening for the first few days. Sunburn lotions and creams, if used, should be regularly applied. Ultraviolet rays that are reflected off water, sand, or snow have particularly strong effects.

Q: Are there any long-term hazards of sunburn?

A: Yes. Constant exposure to sunlight damages the skin and causes wrinkles. It also alters skin structure, producing warty lumps called keratoses that may ultimately form rodent ulcers or cancer of the skin.

Sunstroke (for EMERGENCY treatment, *see* First Aid, p.567) is a form of heatstroke that is caused by overexposure to the sun. *See* HEATSTROKE.

Superfluous hair is an excessive growth of hair, or the presence of hair in an unusual place. *See* HIRSUTISM.

Supine describes the position of lying on the back with the face upward.

Suppository is a cone-shaped or cylindrical medication that is inserted into the rectum for therapeutic purposes. Suppositories usually consist of glycerin or cocoa butter that contain medication and liquefy at body temperature. Suppositories for insertion into the vagina are called pessaries. *See* PESSARY.

Suppuration is the formation and discharge of pus. It may occur when an abscess or a wound becomes infected with pyogenic (pus-forming) microorganisms.

See also PUS.

Suprapubic means above the pubic bone in the pelvis. The suprapubic region is the lowest area of the abdomen.

Suprarenal gland. *See* ADRENAL GLAND.

A talk about Surgery

Surgery is the branch of medicine that treats disorders by surgical operation. For example, a surgeon can remove a diseased part of the body, correct deformities, repair injuries, or carry out internal examinations.

There are many different specialties within surgery, but every surgeon is trained in certain basic techniques and skills before starting further specialized training.

Q: What are some of the common surgical specialties?

A: Some surgeons specialize in dealing with certain age groups, such as children (paediatric surgery); or particular conditions, such as cancer, when the surgeon is part of a team including other doctors and radiotherapists. Common specialties include abdominal surgery or surgery of the gastrointestinal tract; accident surgery or the immediate treatment on emergency hospital admission; cardiac surgery or treatment of heart conditions; and cosmetic surgery, which is really a subspecialty of plastic surgery. Other specialist areas include

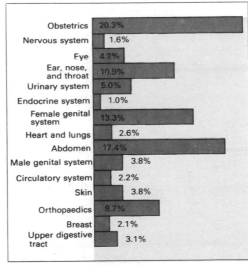

Specialty	Percentage
Obstetrics	20.3%
Nervous system	1.6%
Eye	4.2%
Ear, nose, and throat	10.9%
Urinary system	5.0%
Endocrine system	1.0%
Female genital system	13.3%
Heart and lungs	2.6%
Abdomen	17.4%
Male genital system	3.8%
Circulatory system	2.2%
Skin	3.8%
Orthopaedics	8.7%
Breast	2.1%
Upper digestive tract	3.1%

Surgery is used to treat many different kinds of conditions and disorders.

Surgery

dental surgery, which includes facio-maxillary surgery, used in the treatment of teeth and damage to facial bones; genitourinary surgery for treatment of urinary disorders and male genital problems; gynaecological surgery, treatment of disorders of the female reproductive system; and neurosurgery, treatment of the brain and nervous system.

There is also obstetric surgery, the specialty of dealing with childbirth; ophthalmic surgery, treatment of eye disorders; orthopaedic surgery, treatment of bone and joint disorders; otorhinolaryngological surgery (ENT), treatment of ear, nose, and throat disorders; and plastic surgery to reform and replace damaged tissues.

There are three other common specialities: rectal surgery, a subspecialty of abdominal surgery; thoracic surgery, treatment of the chest, particularly the lungs; and vascular surgery, treatment of the blood vessels.

Q: *Are there certain procedures that are used in all forms of surgery?*

A: Yes. The surgeon ensures that the patient is as fit as possible before an operation. Even in a serious accident or emergency, time spent in resuscitation gives the patient a better chance of recovery.

Asepsis (the absence of infection) is essential to prevent microorganisms from entering the patient's body. This is achieved by careful sterilization of all surgical instruments, and by all medical staff wearing masks and special sterile clothing. The patient's skin is sterilized with antiseptic fluid before an operation.

Q: *Are special surgery techniques necessary in some operations?*

A: Yes. Surgeons operating on the eye or ear may perform microsurgery, using a microscope. Eye surgeons may also use laser beams in the treatment of certain disorders. Cryosurgery, a freezing technique, can be used by eye surgeons as well as in surgery on other parts of the body. Cautery, or the use of heat or chemicals to destroy tissue, is another surgical technique. In replacement surgery, damaged body tissues, such as arthritic joints or damaged heart valves, may be replaced by artificial ones.

Avascular surgery is a technique used to prevent excessive bleeding in the limbs. This technique must be performed within a certain time to prevent tissue death. The patient is anaesthetized and the limb tightly bandaged, squeezing the blood out from the hand or foot upward, and then a tourniquet is left in place. This stops blood entering the limb and makes surgery simple and clean. The tourniquet must be released after about thirty minutes.

In heart surgery, special kinds of anaesthesia, which reduce the patient's body temperature, allow the heart to cease working and thus protect the brain from damage for longer than would normally happen. A heart-lung machine may be used while the heart is repaired or replaced.

Q: *Are there any risks in having an operation?*

A: Yes. There is always some risk in surgery, although the surgeon takes every precaution possible when operating. Risks include atelectasis (collapse of part of the lung because of the anaesthetic), postoperative pneumonia, or some rare or unexpected reaction to the anaesthetic drugs.

Immediately after the operation, the main danger is a sudden haemorrhage from the operated area, producing shock. A common problem in the immediate recovery period following all abdominal operations is paralytic ileus, or failure of the intestine to work. Continued paralytic ileus may result in abdominal swelling that opens the wound or the area of operation in the intestine. Breakdown or bursting of any wound may occur if the patient is ill or debilitated.

Lung infections, such as pneumonia,

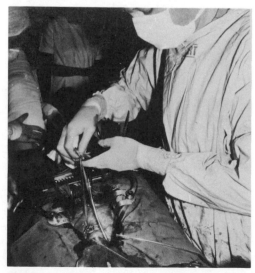

Surgery is a branch of medicine that deals with manual diagnosis, repair, or correction.

and urinary retention are common problems. But a problem that can occur suddenly and unexpectedly is a pulmonary embolus from a blood clot formed in a deep vein, usually in the legs or pelvis.

Wound infections may develop from the cause of the original operation, such as in appendicitis, or they sometimes occur, despite all precautions, during the operation.

Late complications of any operation may occur from the scar tissue or adhesions that are formed. In the abdomen, these may cause obstruction.

Q: *Do all operations have to be performed in a hospital?*

A: No. Minor surgery can frequently be performed in the doctor's surgery under local anaesthetic. Operations such as the incision of an abscess, or the suturing of a wound do not require the facilities of a hospital.

Nevertheless, it is usually advisable to have even minor operations performed in an operating theatre of a hospital. The patient can then have access to professional care during the recovery phase. Operations such as removal of skin cysts, D and C (dilation and curettage), and many dental operations are performed on a day admission basis. But all hospitals require written consent before surgery is undertaken.

Q: *How is consent given for an operation?*

A: The surgeon explains what the operation entails, and asks for a Consent for Operation form to be signed. The form states that the patient agrees to the operation and that the details of the operation have been explained. The form also gives the surgeon permission to carry out any further procedure necessary if there is an unexpected complication.

Permission for an operation should be given by the patient if he or she is over the age of consent, or by a parent or guardian if the patient is under this age. But if the patient is unconscious or mentally ill, consent must be obtained from the nearest relative or legal guardian.

A surgeon may also be faced with an unconscious patient who is in need of urgent treatment and for whom permission cannot be obtained. This may be because the identity of the patient is not known or the next of kin is not available. In this situation, the surgeon has to make every effort to find someone who can give permission. If no one is

available, the surgeon is under a moral, if not legal, duty to undertake any life-saving surgery.

Q: *What treatment is given to a patient before an operation in hospital?*

A: The patient usually goes into hospital the day before an operation, so that any tests can be performed and medical and nursing staff can make sure the patient is in good health.

The patient is usually given sedation the night before an operation, and is not allowed to eat or drink for at least four hours before the operation. This ensures that the stomach is empty and that solid food will not appear if vomiting occurs.

An hour before the operation, an injection, usually of a mild sedative opiate drug combined with an atropine-like drug, is given to dry the secretions. The patient is then taken to the anaesthetic room. In this room the anaesthetist usually gives an intravenous injection of a short-acting barbiturate drug. This puts the patient to sleep before any further form of anaesthetic is given.

Q: *What can a patient expect to occur after an operation?*

A: After an operation, the patient is usually kept in a recovery room or, in the case of major surgery, taken to an intensive care unit. As soon as the patient's general condition is good enough, he or she is returned to the ward or room.

On recovering consciousness from a

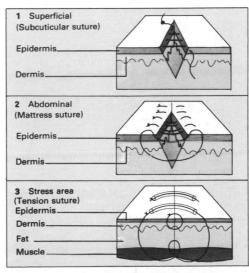

Sutures used to close incisions: (1) superficial, (2) abdominal, and (3) stress areas.

Suture

major abdominal operation, the patient is given an intravenous infusion of salts or blood into the vein of one arm. A naso-gastric tube may have been passed through one nostril and into the stomach to keep it empty of fluid. In addition to a dressing over the wound, a drain (frequently a tube) may extend from it to a suction bottle. This prevents the collection of blood or serous fluid in the operation area. In patients who have gynaecological or genitourinary operations, a catheter has usually been put in the bladder. This is connected to a bottle at the side of the bed.

During the first few hours after an operation, a nurse takes frequent recordings of blood pressure and pulse rate as well as keeping close observation of the amount of intravenous fluid and the measurement of urinary flow.

As soon as the intestine is starting to work again, the patient is allowed to have sips of liquid and the naso-gastric tube and intravenous infusion are removed.

Q: *How quickly does a patient recover after surgery?*

A: This depends on the type of operation and the patient's previous state of health. But even with major surgery, most patients are able to leave hospital within two weeks.

Q: *Are there any general precautions that a patient should take after surgery?*

A: Yes. It is important that patients who have had abdominal or thoracic surgery should not lift heavy weights for at least two months, and should not drive a car until the surgeon has given permission. It is advisable to avoid crowded situations, such as parties or theatres, where respiratory infections may be caught, because coughing can impose a strain on wounds.

A high protein diet is necessary, with additional vitamins as well as adequate rest, both at night and during the day.

Q: *Do all operations leave a scar?*

A: Any operation that involves an incision leaves a scar; there is no way of avoiding it. However, many surgeons try to position the scar to run in the natural skin folds so that it is not obvious when the scar has fully healed.

Suture is the technique of uniting parts of the body by stitching them together. The term has several other meanings, including the material with which a wound is stitched together, or the stitch that is left after the wound has been sutured. A suture is also a joint between two bones formed by fibrous tissues, as between the bones of the skull.

The materials most commonly used for surgical sutures are silk, cotton, or nylon, but steel wire may also be used for additional strength. Some sutures are made of materials such as catgut or synthetic substances that are slowly destroyed by the body. The tissues are finally held together by scar formation.

Swab is a piece of cotton that is used to collect pus or suppurating fluid for bacteriological culture and examination, or the gauze used by a surgeon to soak up blood and body secretions when cleaning a wound during an operation.

Swallowing is the movement of food from the mouth, through the pharynx, into the upper part of the oesophagus, and down to the stomach. It is a complex, co-ordinated movement of various muscles. The tongue forces the food backwards and the glottis closes, blocking the windpipe and preventing food from passing into the lungs. The food passes down the oesophagus by peristalsis, a series of waves of muscular contractions.

Q: *What disorders cause difficulty in swallowing?*

A: Difficulty in swallowing is known medically as dysphagia. It may be caused by a disorder of the throat, or it may be a symptom of a more general disease.

Q: *What disorders of the throat produce dysphagia?*

A: A common cause is a foreign body, such as a bone or fruit stone, that blocks the oesophagus and prevents

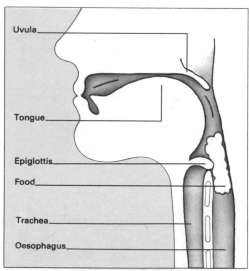

Uvula

Tongue

Epiglottis

Food

Trachea

Oesophagus

Swallowing closes the epiglottis over the trachea to prevent food entering the windpipe.

swallowing. If the pharynx becomes infected, it results in pain as well as dysphagia. TONSILLITIS and QUINSY are examples of such infection.

ACHALASIA, a lack of the normal muscle co-ordination of swallowing, can produce dysphagia.

Occasionally, cancer of the pharynx, larynx, or oesophagus is the cause of problems with swallowing.

Q: What general diseases cause dysphagia?

A: It may be caused by a muscle disorder, such as MYASTHENIA GRAVIS; a neurological disorder, such as MOTOR NEURON DISEASE or POLIOMYELITIS; or an infection, such as DIPHTHERIA, which causes both muscle weakness and nerve damage. Sometimes iron deficiency ANAEMIA can be associated with dysphagia.

Q: How is dysphagia treated?

A: The treatment depends on the cause, which must be diagnosed by a doctor.

Sweat. *See* PERSPIRATION.

Swelling is an abnormal enlargement of any part of the body. *See* OEDEMA.

Sydenham's chorea. *See* CHOREA.

Sympathectomy is an operation in which the nerves of the SYMPATHETIC NERVOUS SYSTEM are inactivated, either by surgically cutting them or by destroying them chemically.

Sympathectomy may be performed on the sympathetic nerves in the neck to relieve the symptoms of RAYNAUD'S PHENOMENON. It may also be done in the lumbar region to improve the blood circulation in the legs. This may be used to treat INTERMITTENT CLAUDICATION or GANGRENE of the feet.

Sympathetic nervous system is part of the autonomic nervous system. It operates in conjunction with the parasympathetic nervous system. The sympathetic nervous system prepares the body for action by dilating the pupils of the eyes, cooling the skin, and raising the blood pressure and pulse rate. The blood is diverted from the intestines to the skeletal muscles, and the adrenal glands are stimulated to produce the hormone adrenaline, which enhances these actions.

The smooth muscle in the bronchi relaxes, allowing more air to enter the lungs; muscular movement in the intestines slows down; and sweating occurs.

All of this activity increases the basic metabolic rate of the body, increasing the use of glucose released from the liver, and prepares the body for immediate physical and mental activity.

See also AUTONOMIC NERVOUS SYSTEM; NERVOUS SYSTEM; PARASYMPATHETIC NERVOUS SYSTEM.

Symphysis is a cartilage joint between two bones. An example is the joint between the two bones at the front of the pelvis (pubic symphysis).

Symptom is a disruption of the normal functioning of the body that a patient notices, and which may indicate an underlying disorder. A pathognomonic symptom is characteristic of one specific disorder.

See also SYNDROME.

Syncope is a sudden, temporary loss of consciousness that is caused by an inadequate flow of blood to the brain. It is the medical term for a faint. *See* FAINTING.

Syndactyly is webbing between the fingers and toes. In most cases the condition is inherited, and usually affects both hands or feet. Syndactyly of the toes does not require treatment. Syndactyly of the fingers can be corrected by surgery.

See also POLYDACTYLISM.

Syndrome is a group of signs and symptoms that collectively indicate a particular disease or disorder.

Synovitis is inflammation of the synovial membrane, the layer of smooth, slippery membrane that lines the joints, surrounds tendons, and forms protective bags over bony protuberances (bursa).

Synovitis may be caused by injury to a joint; infection; or by various joint disorders, such as arthritis. The affected joint becomes swollen and painful, especially when the joint is moved. Treatment is directed toward the underlying cause.

See also ARTHRITIS; BURSITIS; CAPSULITIS; TENOSYNOVITIS.

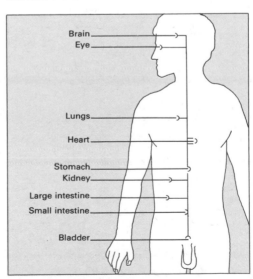

Brain
Eye
Lungs
Heart
Stomach
Kidney
Large intestine
Small intestine
Bladder

Sympathetic nervous system controls all the involuntary movements of the body.

Syphilis

A talk about Syphilis

Syphilis, also known as lues, is a contagious venereal disease that is caused by infection with spiral-shaped bacteria called *Treponema pallidum.* It can affect any tissue in the body, causing a wide variety of symptoms and complications.

The infection enters the body through the mucous membranes, such as the vagina and male urethra, or through grazes in the skin. It is usually transmitted by sexual intercourse. The infection can also pass through the placenta to a foetus, causing syphilis in the unborn child.

After infection, there is an incubation period before any symptoms appear. This may vary from a week to three months, but is usually about three or four weeks. Then the disease progresses through three stages, known as primary, secondary, and tertiary syphilis.

Q: *What are the symptoms of primary syphilis?*

A: A small red spot appears at the site of infection and ulcerates to form a CHANCRE that has a hard base. The chancre is usually painless and does not bleed but, when cut, exudes a clear fluid that contains the syphilis bacteria. The local lymph glands may become swollen. The chancre usually occurs on the penis, anus, or rectum in men, and on the vulva, cervix, or anal area in women. Occasionally, the chancre may appear on the lips, tongue, or even the tonsils.

Characteristic symptoms of syphilis	
Primary stage 2 to 4 weeks	Chancres appear on lip, tongue, nipples, or genitals. Painless swelling of lymph glands near genitals.
Secondary stage 6 weeks	Mild rash appears. Eruption of skin, reddish brown coppery spots, recurring possibly at a later stage.
Latency period	No obvious symptoms
Tertiary stage up to 20 years later	Heart, blood vessels, and central nervous system may be involved. Insanity and various types of psychoses may develop.

Syphilis is characterized by various symptoms at different stages of its development.

The chancre heals spontaneously in about one or two months, often leaving a scar. In a few cases, there is no chancre and the disease passes directly to secondary syphilis.

Q: *What are the symptoms of secondary syphilis?*

A: The symptoms of secondary syphilis usually appear about two months after infection. There is generalized illness with fever, headache, tiredness, aching of limbs, and a rash. Flat ulcers with raised edges often form in the mouth, vulva, penis, or rectum at the junction of the mucous membranes and the skin. These ulcers are known as condylomata lata and are extremely infectious.

Secondary syphilis may also cause enlargement of the liver, spleen, and lymph glands.

Secondary syphilis may persist for several months before the symptoms disappear. It is followed by a latent stage, after which tertiary syphilis may develop.

Q: *What are the symptoms of tertiary syphilis?*

A: It may take as long as twenty years before tertiary syphilis develops, or it may never occur. It may affect any part of the body, and may simulate almost any disease.

Tertiary syphilis may affect the central nervous system (neurosyphilis); the heart and blood vessels (cardiovascular syphilis); or it may produce swelling in the skin, bones, and intestinal organs (benign tertiary syphilis).

Neurosyphilis may cause general paralysis of the patient, with delusions, personality deterioration, and insanity, or it may cause TABES DORSALIS in which the normal reflexes are lost. If the spinal cord is affected, there may be sudden paralysis of the legs, and either urinary retention or incontinence.

Cardiovascular syphilis damages the aorta, causing it to become dilated (aneurysm). This swelling may compress adjacent organs, resulting in difficulty in swallowing, difficulty in talking, or collapse of part of the lungs. The aneurysm may rupture, causing sudden death. The heart valves may also be damaged, causing angina pectoris or heart failure.

Benign tertiary syphilis is characterized by the formation of gummas, which are swollen areas of firm, scar-like tissue. They may affect any part of the body, but usually produce only minor symptoms caused by localized swelling.

Q: How is syphilis treated?

A: Penicillin is effective in treating all stages of syphilis. Primary and secondary syphilis can be completely cured, but tertiary syphilis can only be arrested because the tissue damage cannot be repaired.

It is important for the patient to have regular medical checks to ensure that the treatment has been effective. The sexual contacts of the patient should be traced, and treated for syphilis if necessary.

Q: What are the symptoms of congenital syphilis?

A: Some infants with congenital syphilis never develop any symptoms throughout their lives. Others show symptoms at or shortly after birth, with blisters on the palms and soles; thickened, raised patches around the mouth and nappy area; and bloodstained nasal discharge. Within the first three months of life, the child's bones may become infected, causing weakness or apparent paralysis in one or more limbs. There may also be meningitis, epilepsy, or mental retardation.

In some children, the symptoms do not develop for several months or even years. When the symptoms do become apparent, there may be abnormalities of the incisor teeth (Hutchinson's teeth); infection of the eye (keratitis); gradual deafness; and neurosyphilis. Gummas may also develop particularly in the nose, producing a flattened nose because of the destruction of the nasal septum.

Q: How is congenital syphilis treated?

A: Congenital syphilis is usually treated with penicillin. If the mother is treated before the fourth month of pregnancy, the foetus is not affected. Treatment later in pregnancy usually cures both the mother and the foetus but, in some cases, the child may be born with some indication of infection.

If syphilis is not diagnosed until the child has been born, treatment prevents any further damage from occurring. It is important that other children in the family are examined to ensure that they do not have congenital syphilis. Both the mother and the child should be regularly examined after the infection has been treated.

Syringe is an instrument for injecting fluids into the body, or for washing out cavities or wounds. A hypodermic syringe consists of a glass or plastic tube, a fine nozzle, and a tightly fitting plunger. A needle is attached to the nozzle, and the complete assemblage is sterilized before use.

An irrigating syringe has a large rubber bulb instead of a plunger. It is used to wash out wax from the ears, and to cleanse wounds and body cavities.

See also INJECTION.

Syringomyelia is a rare congenital anomaly of the spinal cord or the lower part of the brain involving the central canal. Cavities slowly form in the substance of the cord in the region of the lower neck, but do not produce symptoms until late adolescence or early adulthood.

Q: What are the symptoms of syringomyelia?

A: The area involved is in the centre of the spinal cord, and the nerve fibres that are closest to the cord are the ones that are first affected. These fibres carry pain and temperature sensations, so that the first symptom may be a painless cut or burn on the hands or arms.

There is a gradual loss of sensation over the shoulders and arms, accompanied by weakness of the legs, as the disorder slowly progresses. If the lower part of the brain is involved, dizziness (vertigo) and problems with speech (dysarthria) and swallowing (dysphagia) may occur.

The condition slowly progresses over many years, causing increasing loss of sensation and paralysis, first of the legs and later of the rest of the body.

Q: What is the treatment for syringomyelia?

A: There is no effective form of treatment.

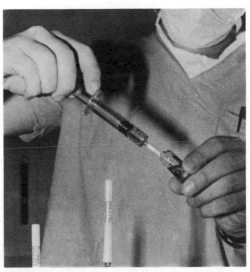

Syringe is an instrument used to draw up fluid and inject it into tissues or vessels.

Systole

Surgery has been attempted and may, in very few cases, be successful.

Systole is the contraction of the heart muscle that causes the forceful ejection of blood into the arterial system.

See also DIASTOLE.

T

Tabes dorsalis, also known as locomotor ataxia, is a syphilitic infection of the nerves in which there is progressive degeneration of the nerve fibres of the spinal cord. Tabes dorsalis may not develop until ten or twenty years after the original infection and is more common in men than in women.

The initial and the most characteristic symptom is an intense stabbing pain in the legs; this is known as a lightning pain. There may also be a loss of sensation in the limbs and a lack of awareness of their position.

As the disease progresses, the patient may walk unsteadily, with a typical high-stepping gait. There may also be a loss of sensation in the bladder, causing retention of urine and, eventually, incontinence. In the late stages of the disease, there may be lightning pains in the abdomen, and vomiting.

The treatment for tabes dorsalis is the same as that for syphilis. *See* SYPHILIS.

TAB vaccine is a combined vaccine that provides partial immunity to typhoid, paratyphoid A, and paratyphoid B fevers. *See* IMMUNIZATION.

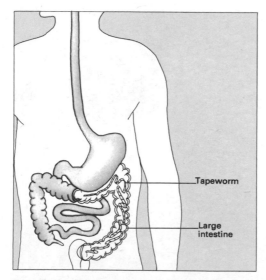

Tapeworm infests the descending section of the large intestine, where it rapidly grows.

Tachycardia is a rapid heart rate of more than one hundred beats a minute when the patient is at rest. Tachycardia may be caused by excessive exercise; an emotional response, such as fear; or an increase in the metabolic rate, which may occur with hyperthyroidism, fever, or infection. Tachycardia may also result from anaemia, haemorrhage, or the use of certain drugs.

See also ARRHYTHMIA; BRADYCARDIA.

Talipes is the medical term for clubfoot. *See* CLUBFOOT.

Talus is one of the seven tarsal bones of the foot. It articulates with the lower ends of the tibia and fibula to form part of the ankle joint. *See* FOOT.

Tampon is a plug of absorbent material, such as cotton wool or gauze, that may be inserted in the vagina to absorb menstrual bleeding. *See* MENSTRUATION.

Tapeworms (cestodes) are parasitic worms that are shaped like long, flat pieces of tape. Three main species of tapeworm infest human beings: *Taenia saginata* (beef tapeworm); *Taenia solium* (pork tapeworm); and *Diphyllobothrium latum* (fish tapeworm). Occasionally, another species, *Echinococcus granulosus*, may infest people, causing cysts to form in the liver (*see* HYDATID CYST).

The adult worms live in the human intestine. At one end of the worm is a head (scolex) with small hooks that attach it to the intestinal wall. Behind the scolex are hundreds of segments in which eggs develop. The segments break off, pass out of the body in the faeces, and are eaten by the primary host (cattle, pigs, or fish). The eggs hatch into larvae in the primary host. The larvae penetrate the intestinal wall and are carried by the blood circulation to the muscles, where they form cysts.

People become infested when they eat undercooked meat. The cysts mature into adult worms in the human intestine, thereby perpetuating the cycle.

Q: *What are the symptoms of an infestation with tapeworms?*

A: The most common symptom is the presence of tapeworm segments in the faeces. If a person is heavily infested, there may also be abdominal pain and loss of weight.

Q: *How are tapeworm infestations treated?*

A: In most cases, treatment with worm-killing drugs such as niclosamide is effective. Tapeworm infestation can be prevented by thoroughly cooking all meat and fish.

See also CYSTICERCOSIS.

Tarsus is the back of the foot between the metatarsal bones and the tibia and fibula.

The tarsus consists of seven tarsal bones. One of these, the TALUS, forms part of the ankle joint. *See* FOOT.

Tartar is a deposit on the teeth that consists of calcium salts and the remains of food. If the layer of tartar is allowed to accumulate, it may irritate the gums and cause GINGIVITIS or PERIODONTITIS.

Taste is the sensation that is obtained when specialized sensory nerve endings (the taste buds) detect soluble substances. The taste buds can register four fundamental tastes, either singly or in combination: sweet, bitter, sour, and salty. The sense of taste can be affected by a disorder of the mouth or nose.

Taste buds are sensory nerve endings on the surface of the tongue. They detect tastes and send impulses to the brain, where the perception of taste occurs. *See* TASTE.

Tay-Sachs disease is an inherited disorder in which there is a deficiency of a specific enzyme that breaks down fatty substances called lipids in the nervous system. The lipids accumulate in the brain cells, which gradually degenerate. The disease is more common in families of Jewish descent than in others.

Q: What are the symptoms of Tay-Sachs disease?

A: An affected child appears to be normal for the first few months after birth. But as the brain cells degenerate, there is a gradual onset of spasticity; convulsions; blindness; and a progressive loss of physical and mental abilities. Tay-Sachs disease is invariably fatal; the child usually dies before the age of four years.

Q: Can Tay-Sachs disease be prevented?

A: Yes. All potentially affected parents should obtain genetic counselling. Screening tests can be performed that can identify carriers of Tay-Sachs disease.

It is also possible to detect the disorder in a foetus by using AMNIOCENTESIS.

TB is an abbreviation for TUBERCULOSIS.

Tears are watery, slightly alkaline secretions that protect and lubricate the eyes. They contain salt and also an antibacterial enzyme (lysozyme) that prevents the eye from becoming infected. Tears are secreted by special glands around the eye (*see* LACRIMAL APPARATUS).

Teeth. Adult humans have thirty-two teeth, sixteen in each jaw; children have twenty milk, or deciduous, teeth. The outer layer of a tooth consists of hard, white enamel. Under the enamel is dentine, which is an ivory-like substance. Dentine forms the major part of a tooth. In the centre of a tooth is a soft pulp layer, which contains blood vessels, nerves, and odontoblasts (cells that can form more dentin if a tooth is damaged).

Q: What are the functions of the teeth?

A: There are four different types of teeth: incisors, canines, premolars, and molars. The incisors are used for cutting; the canines are used for gripping and tearing; and the back teeth, the premolars and molars, are used for grinding and chewing.

Q: How should teeth be cared for?

A: The teeth can be kept healthy by careful diet, with as little sugar as possible; regular brushing; and visits to the dentist every six months.

See also DENTAL DISORDERS; TEETHING; TOOTH DECAY.

Teething is the natural process by which a baby's teeth erupt through the gums. Teething may cause a slight increase in salivation; rubbing of the gums; and general restlessness.

In most babies, there is no need for any specific treatment for teething.

Telangiectasis is a disorder in which the small blood vessels become abnormally dilated, producing a type of angioma (*see* ANGIOMA). Telangiectases usually occur as red spots on the face and thighs. They are more common in the elderly; people exposed to the sun; people with varicose veins; and people treated with corticosteroid drugs. In most cases, the cause of the disorder is unknown.

Temperature is a measurement of the amount of heat in an object. The normal body temperature of a healthy person (taken with a thermometer placed under the tongue) is 37°C (98.4°F). *See* BODY TEMPERATURE; FEVER.

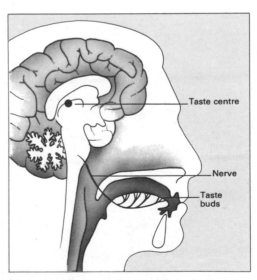

Taste stimuli are received by the taste buds on the tongue and transmitted to the brain.

Temper tantrum

Temper tantrum is a common occurrence in children between one and three years old, when the child is trying to assert his or her individuality. Temper tantrums usually last only a minute or two, but may recur if the child is unable to get what he or she wants.

Q: How should a child with temper tantrums be treated?

A: Parents should be firm and consistent in attitude toward the child, and should try to avoid any major conflict. It is advisable not to show anxiety and stress during a temper tantrum or, if possible, to ignore it.

Temporal lobe epilepsy is a form of epilepsy in which the seizures originate in the temporal lobe of the brain. *See* EPILEPSY.

Tendinitis is inflammation of a tendon. It is usually accompanied by tenosynovitis (inflammation of the membrane around a tendon). *See* TENOSYNOVITIS.

Tendon is the thick, strong, inelastic band of fibrous tissue that attaches a muscle to a bone. A tendon may be strained by excessive use, or, occasionally, ruptured. A tendon and its surrounding synovial membrane may also become inflamed (*see* TENOSYNOVITIS).

Tenesmus is painful straining to urinate or defecate. Straining to urinate may be a symptom of CYSTITIS; a bladder stone; or disorders of the prostate gland in which the flow of urine is obstructed. Straining to defecate may be a symptom of CONSTIPATION; an anal FISSURE; an anal FISTULA; an anal abscess; or, rarely, cancer of the rectum.

Tennis elbow is strain of the tendons of muscles to the forearm near the region of the outer side of the elbow. It is caused by repeated stress, particularly stress produced by sudden twisting movements.

Q: What are the symptoms of tennis elbow?

A: Pain on gripping, tenderness at the outer side of the elbow, and aching in the muscles of the outer side of the forearm, are the usual symptoms.

Q: How is tennis elbow treated?

A: Treatment may not be needed in mild cases. If the pain persists or becomes worse, injections of corticosteroid drugs and a local anaesthetic may be effective. If this fails, physiotherapy with massage and heat treatment may help.

Tenosynovitis is an inflammation of the synovial membrane that surrounds a tendon. It is often accompanied by inflammation of the underlying tendon (tendinitis). The cause of tenosynovitis is not known, but it may result from strenuous exercise; infection from an overlying wound; or from various diseases, such as rheumatoid arthritis, gout, or Reiter's disease.

Teratoma is a usually malignant tumour that consists of several different types of tissue, none of which originates in the area in which the tumour occurs. Treatment is by surgical removal, followed by radiotherapy and chemotherapy.

Termination means the end of an event. It commonly refers to the termination of a pregnancy (ABORTION).

Testicle. *See* TESTIS.

Testis is one of the two primary male reproductive organs (gonads) that lie in the scrotum. Each testis is about 4 centimetres (1.5 inches) long, and is partly surrounded by a protective bag that contains a small amount of fluid.

Q: What are the functions of the testes?

A: After puberty, the testes produce the male hormone TESTOSTERONE, and the reproductive cells (SPERM). From the testis, the sperm pass along special ducts to the EPIDIDYMIS. The epididymis leads to the VAS DEFERENS, through which the sperm are carried to the SEMINAL VESICLES where they are stored.

Q: What conditions affect the testis?

A: The testis may not reach the correct position after passing out of the abdomen and into the scrotum of a foetus; this condition is known as an UNDESCENDED TESTICLE. Excessive fluid may accumulate in the small bag next to the testis and form a HYDROCELE. The testis may become infected and inflamed (ORCHITIS) which may lead eventually to STERILITY. Occasionally, cancer of the testis (SEMINOMA teratoma) may develop.

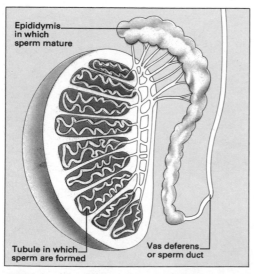

Epididymis in which sperm mature

Tubule in which sperm are formed

Vas deferens or sperm duct

Testis manufactures sperm in the tubules, and they mature in the epididymis.

Test meal is a standardized meal that is given to test the gastric secretion of the stomach. A test meal may be used in the diagnosis of various disorders. Modern methods of testing acid secretion are done without giving a test meal.

Testosterone is the male sex hormone produced principally by the TESTIS. The amount of testosterone produced is controlled by the follicle-stimulating hormone (FSH), and luteinizing hormone (LH), both of which are secreted by the front lobe of the pituitary gland. At the onset of puberty there is an increase in the production of testosterone, particularly in boys.

Q: What are the effects of testosterone?

A: Testosterone stimulates the development of male secondary sexual characteristics. These include facial and pubic hair; enlargement of the larynx, which produces deepening of the voice; enlargement of the penis and testes; alteration of body shape; and an increase in muscle strength. Testosterone is also thought to influence the development of balding.

Although women produce only a small amount of testosterone, it occasionally affects hair growth after menopause. Rarely, overproduction of testosterone by the adrenal glands may result in the development of male secondary sexual characteristics in women (*see* VIRILISM).

Tetanus, also known as lockjaw, is caused by the toxin of the bacterium *Clostridium tetani.*

The bacteria are usually found in soil, and can remain alive for many years in the form of spores. The microorganisms grow in dead or damaged tissue that does not have an adequate blood supply and therefore has a low oxygen level. Infection may result from any wound that is contaminated by infected soil.

Q: What are the symptoms of tetanus?

A: There is an incubation period that may vary between four and fourteen days, but can last as long as seven weeks. The initial symptoms include stiffness of the jaw; slight difficulty in swallowing; restlessness; and stiffness of the arms, legs, and neck.

As the disease progresses, the patient may run a fever and may have difficulty opening the mouth (trismus or lockjaw). This may be accompanied by stiffness of the face muscles, which may contract to produce a characteristic fixed grin. As the stiffness of the muscles increases, there may be painful convulsions, which may be fatal.

Q: How is tetanus treated?

A: Hospitalization in a quiet room is necessary. A tracheostomy, a temporary

opening in the windpipe, may be performed, and the patient may be given mechanical artificial respiration to aid breathing. An intravenous infusion may also be necessary to correct the patient's fluid balance.

Antitoxin in the form of gamma globulin is given to reduce the effect of the toxin. Muscle relaxant drugs will reduce the muscle spasms, and drugs that cause complete paralysis may be used when the patient is maintained on artificial respiration.

Q: Can tetanus be prevented?

A: Yes. An attack of tetanus itself does not confer immunity, but tetanus can be prevented by immunization.

See also IMMUNIZATION.

Tetany is a spasm of the muscles producing contractions in the hands, feet, and face (TRISMUS). Sometimes flexing of the arms and legs, with cramp-like pain may occur. Occasionally, seizures may occur.

Tetany may result from an abnormally low concentration of calcium in the blood (HYPOCALCAEMIA). Temporary hypocalcaemia may be caused by hyperventilation (resulting from temporary lowering of calcium when carbon dioxide is lost from the body); prolonged hypocalcaemia may be caused by a deficiency of the parathyroid hormones. Vitamin D deficiency may also cause tetany.

Q: How is tetany treated?

A: If tetany is caused by hyperventilation, the patient should breathe into a paper bag. This normalizes the carbon dioxide concentration of the blood. Tetany that is

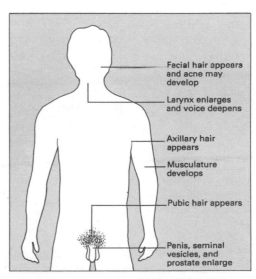

Facial hair appears and acne may develop

Larynx enlarges and voice deepens

Axillary hair appears

Musculature develops

Pubic hair appears

Penis, seminal vesicles, and prostate enlarge

Testosterone stimulates the development of male sexual characteristics during puberty.

Tetracyclines

caused by prolonged hypocalcaemia may be treated with intravenous injections of calcium salts. Tetany resulting from vitamin D deficiency disappears when the deficiency is corrected.

Tetracyclines are a group of antibiotics that are produced by certain species of the fungus *Streptomyces*. Tetracycline drugs are effective against many bacterial infections. They are commonly prescribed to treat urinary infections; streptococcal infections; pneumonia; brucellosis; and rickettsial diseases, such as typhus. Tetracyclines may also be used to treat bacterial infections in patients who are sensitive to penicillin. Bacteria may become resistant to tetracyclines, but this does not usually occur during a short course of treatment.

Q: Can tetracyclines produce adverse side effects?

A: Yes. Treatment with tetracyclines may produce nausea, vomiting, and diarrhoea. Allergic reactions are extremely rare. Prolonged treatment may lead to moniliasis and deficiency of the B vitamins. Occasionally, the skin may become abnormally sensitive to light. In children, tetracyclines may discolour the teeth, so should not be taken by children under the age of seven.

Tetraplegia, also known as quadriplegia, is paralysis of all four limbs. *See* PARALYSIS.

Thalamus is a collection of nerve cells that is situated above the hypothalamus and is part of the forebrain. There are two thalami, one on each side of the midline of the brain. The thalami act as co-ordinating centres for nerve

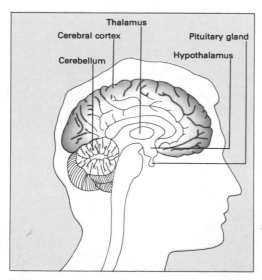

Thalamus receives all the sensory impulses except those from the nose.

impulses from all of the senses. The impulses are then relayed to other areas in the brain, such as the cerebral cortex and hypothalamus.

Thalassaemia is the name given to a group of haemolytic anaemias, which are disorders that affect the red blood cells. Cooley's anaemia and Mediterranean anemia are types of thalassaemia.

Q: What are the symptoms of thalassaemia?

A: Symptoms of thalassaemia usually occur only in those who have inherited an abnormal gene from both parents; this is called thalassaemia major. When only one gene is inherited (thalassaemia minor), there are usually no symptoms.

The symptoms of thalassaemia major vary in severity. The common symptoms include breathlessness, pallor, and fatigue. There may also be jaundice; leg ulcers; enlargement of the spleen; and the formation of gallstones. The skull bones may thicken, and other bones may fracture easily.

Iron that is released from damaged red blood cells is deposited in the tissues (haemosiderosis), which may damage the heart muscle and ultimately result in heart failure.

Q: How is thalassaemia treated?

A: There is no effective treatment other than blood transfusion.

See also ANAEMIA; HAEMOCHROMATOSIS; SIDEROSIS.

Thalidomide is a sedative drug that was prescribed extensively in Europe during the late 1950s and early 1960s.

When it was taken by pregnant women thalidomide was found to cause foetal deformities, especially of the limbs, and the drug was withdrawn. It was also discovered that thalidomide caused a permanent form of peripheral neuritis.

Thermogram is a record of the infra-red heat waves that are emitted by the body. It gives a visual display of the hot and cold areas of the whole body. The technique of obtaining a thermogram is known as thermography; it involves photographing or televising the body with a special camera that is sensitive to heat.

Thermography may be used in detecting breast cancer because the tumour is slightly hotter than the surrounding body tissues. It may also be used to study the flow of blood throughout the body.

Thermometer is an instrument for measuring temperature. A clinical thermometer is used to measure body temperature; its range of measurement is from 34.5°C (94°F) to 42°C (108°F).

See also BODY TEMPERATURE.

Thiamine is a vitamin (vitamin B_1) that occurs naturally in such foods as dried yeast; wheat germ; liver; pulses; and brown rice. Thiamine is essential for the normal metabolism of fats and carbohydrates, and also the functioning of nerves and heart muscle. Thiamine deficiency may result from an inadequate diet; impaired absorption of nutrients, as may occur with sprue or alcoholism; or from increased bodily demands, which may result from hyperthyroidism or pregnancy. Thiamine deficiency may cause BERI-BERI or, rarely, KORSAKOFF'S SYNDROME.

See also VITAMINS.

Thirst is the desire for fluid, especially water. The sensation of thirst is caused by, among many other factors, an increase in sodium concentration in the blood, and by loss of potassium from the body cells.

Thirst may be a symptom of various conditions, such as haemorrhage; profuse sweating; vomiting; diarrhoea; or excessive urination, as in diabetes mellitus or diabetes insipidus. Patients with heart failure may suffer from extreme thirst, but if they drink too much water, oedema of the legs may develop.

Thoracic duct is the largest lymphatic vessel in the body and joins the superior vena cava. It extends from the second lumbar vertebra up to the root of the neck. It receives lymph from all of the lower body, including the legs.

See also LYMPHATIC SYSTEM.

Thoracoplasty is a surgical operation in which several ribs are removed. The chest wall then collapses onto the underlying lung, causing the lung itself to collapse. This operation was frequently used in the treatment of tuberculosis.

Thoracotomy is any surgical operation that involves opening the chest wall.

Thorax (chest) is the part of the trunk between the neck and the abdomen. It is enclosed by the thoracic spine at the back; twelve pairs of ribs on either side; the breast-bone (sternum) in front; and the diaphragm muscle at the bottom.

The thorax contains the two lungs; the heart; the main blood vessels – the aorta and pulmonary artery and their branches, and the venae cavae and pulmonary veins; and the oesophagus (gullet). Other structures include the thoracic duct; the thymus; the sympathetic ganglia and nerves; and the pleura (the membrane surrounding the lungs). The central part of the thorax that contains the heart and oesophagus is the mediastinum.

The muscles of the thorax include the intercostal muscles between the ribs; and the muscles that attach the shoulder girdle, the shoulder bone (scapula), the collar-bone (clavicle), and the bone of the upper arm (humerus) to the chest wall.

Threadworm is a small, parasitic nematode worm that infests the intestine. British authorities use this term to refer to the worm *Enterobius vermicularis* (*see* OXYURIASIS); Americans use it to refer to the worm *Strongyloides stercoralis* (*see* STRONGYLOIDES).

Throat is the common name for the pharynx and the fauces, the opening that leads from the back of the mouth into the pharynx. The front part of the neck is also referred to as the throat.

Throat, lump in, is a symptom of many disorders, such as a mild throat infection, and laryngitis. It is often accompanied by inflammation of the throat and slight discomfort on swallowing. A lump in the throat may also be caused by pressure on the throat from an enlarged thyroid gland (goitre) or from swollen lymph glands. Emotional states may cause the sensation of a lump in the throat that varies in severity, and this condition is known as globus hystericus.

If the sensation of a lump in the throat persists, a doctor should be consulted.

Throat abscess is a localized accumulation of pus in the throat. Throat abscesses occur most commonly around the tonsils. This condition is known as quinsy or peritonsillar abscess. *See* QUINSY.

Thromboangiitis obliterans, also known as Buerger's disease, is a chronic disease of the blood vessels in which there is a narrowing of the arteries and veins. *See* BUERGER'S DISEASE.

Thrombocytopenia is a decrease in the normal number of platelets, which are the

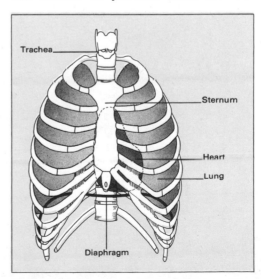

Thorax is the area of the body from the trachea to the diaphragm, including the lungs.

457

Thrombolysis

particles in the blood that are essential for clotting. The condition may result from decreased platelet production, caused by leukaemia, cancer, drugs, aplastic anaemia, or irradiation. Thrombocytopenia may also result from increased platelet destruction, which may be caused by drugs, such as sulphonamides, or poisons. Injuries and burns may cause the body to use platelets faster than they can be replaced, which may cause a temporary platelet deficiency. The commonest cause of thrombocytopenia is called idiopathic thrombocytopenic purpura (ITP). This is a type of autoimmune disease in which platelets are destroyed in the spleen.

Q: *What are the symptoms of thrombo-cytopenia?*

A: The main symptom is bleeding, which may occur in any part of the body. Usually, bleeding occurs just below the skin, producing bruises and small haemorrhages (petechiae). Anaemia may result from excessive bleeding.

Q: *How is thrombocytopenia treated?*

A: Treatment is directed toward the underlying cause. Transfusions of platelets may be given until the treatment takes effect or until the patient recovers naturally. In patients with idiopathic thrombocytopenic purpura, treatment with corticosteroid drugs may be effective. In severe cases, removal of the spleen may be necessary.

Thrombolysis is the destruction of a clot in a blood vessel (thrombus) by means of an intravenous infusion of enzymes that dissolve the thrombus. The technique involves a con-

tinuous infusion of enzymes into a vein for at least two days. This is followed by treatment with ANTICOAGULANT drugs to prevent further blood clots from forming.

Thrombophlebitis. *See* VENOUS THROMBOSIS.

Thrombosis is the formation of a blood clot (thrombus) in an artery or vein. When a thrombus becomes detached from its original site of formation, it is called an embolus.

See also ARTERIOSCLEROSIS; EMBOLISM; GANGRENE; STROKE; VENOUS THROMBOSIS.

Thrombus is a blood clot in a blood vessel. *See* BLOOD CLOT; VENOUS THROMBOSIS.

Thrush is an infection caused by the fungus *Monilia albicans*. *See* MONILIASIS.

Thumb is the first digit of the hand. It contains only two bones (phalanges), unlike the fingers, which have three. *See* HAND.

Thumb sucking is a common habit in almost all babies and children. It occurs as frequently in breast-fed babies as in bottle-fed babies. Thumb sucking becomes less frequent after the age of three years and seldom continues after the age of ten.

Excessive thumb sucking may cause blistering of the thumb, which may lead to skin infection. Continual thumb sucking may also affect the normal position of the front teeth.

Usually it is safe to let a child suck a thumb. But, if problems such as skin damage or dental deformity develop, the child should be gently persuaded to stop. The child should not be punished.

Thymus is an organ in the upper part of the chest cavity lying just behind the breastbone (sternum). It is composed largely of cells similar to lymphocytes. The thymus grows until puberty, and then gradually shrinks and is replaced by fat.

The full function of the thymus is not known. It produces lymphocytes, a type of white blood cell, and plays a part in the development of immunity.

Q: *What disorders may affect the thymus?*

A: Disorders of the thymus are uncommon. Rarely, children are born without a thymus or with a defective one. This produces a defect in immunity and the child suffers from repeated infections. Tumours of the thymus are also rare, but many patients with MYASTHENIA GRAVIS have thymic tumours and usually recover when the tumour is removed. Most thymic tumours are benign (noncancerous).

Thyroidectomy is the surgical removal of part or all of the thyroid gland. A medical thyroidectomy is the destruction of part or all of the thyroid gland by the use of drugs.

A thyroidectomy may be performed to treat overactivity of the thyroid gland (hyper-

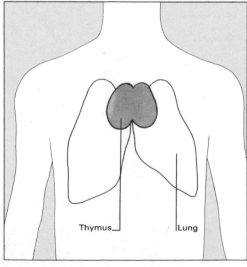

Thymus helps to combat infection during childhood by producing lymphocytes.

thyroidism), or to remove nodules that form in or on the gland. It may be necessary to remove part of the thyroid gland if it becomes greatly enlarged (goitre) and obstructs breathing.

Q: *Are there any hazards associated with a thyroidectomy?*

A: Yes, but these are rare. During surgery, great care has to be taken not to remove all four parathyroid glands, or to cut the nerves to the vocal cords. Removal of the parathyroid glands may cause HYPOCAL-CAEMIA and TETANY. If one of the nerves to the vocal cords is cut, hoarseness may result; if both nerves are cut, the patient will be unable to speak. If too much of the thyroid gland is removed, hypothyroidism eventually develops, and replacement of the deficient thyroid hormones will be necessary.

Thyroid gland is an endocrine gland in the front of the neck. It consists of two lobes, one on each side of the Adam's apple, which are joined across the front of the windpipe, just below the voice box.

The thyroid gland secretes two main hormones, thyroxine and triiodothyronine, into the bloodstream. These hormones stimulate all the cells in the body. The thyroid gland also secretes a hormone (calcitonin) that reduces the concentration of calcium in the blood.

The production of thyroid hormones is controlled by the thyroid stimulating hormone (TSH), which is secreted by the pituitary gland. This control is modified by the hypothalamus, which detects thyroid hormone levels in the blood and influences the secretion of TSH.

Q: *What disorders may affect the thyroid gland?*

A: The thyroid gland may become enlarged (goitre) because of a deficiency of iodine, overactivity (hyperthyroidism), or underactivity (hypothyroidism). Nodules may form in the thyroid gland and cause hyperthyroidism. The nodules may be either benign or malignant (cancerous).

Occasionally, the thyroid gland may become inflamed (thyroiditis). Rarely, this is caused by infection; more often, it is a form of autoimmune disease (Hashimoto's thyroiditis).

Thyroid preparations are drugs that are used to treat disorders of the thyroid gland, such as simple goitre; hypothyroidism (underproduction of thyroid hormones); hyperthyroidism (overproduction of thyroid hormones); and thyroiditis (inflammation of the thyroid gland).

Thyroid preparations are available as extracts of thyroid glands from animals, or as synthetic preparations of thyroxine or triiodothyronine.

Q: *Can thyroid preparations produce adverse side effects?*

A: Yes. Thyroid hormones may produce cramps; palpitations; and anginal pain. They may also permanently affect the heart. For this reason, thyroid hormones should be used with caution in those with heart disorders.

A talk about Thyrotoxicosis

Thyrotoxicosis, also known as Graves' disease, is a disorder caused by the overproduction of thyroid hormones by the thyroid gland (hyperthyroidism). Often the cause is not known. There seems to be a breakdown in the normal balance of the feedback mechanism between the pituitary gland and thyroid gland. This results in overstimulation of the thyroid gland by the hormone (thyroid stimulating hormone) that is produced by the pituitary gland. Rarely, the thyroid gland grows a benign tumour, and this can also cause an overproduction of thyroid hormones.

Occasionally, thyrotoxicosis starts after an emotional shock or prolonged period of anxiety.

Q: *What are the symptoms of thyrotoxicosis?*

A: The symptoms include sweating; nervousness; hunger; loss of weight; diarrhoea; trembling hands; and bulging of the eyes (exophthalmos). Often, there is a slight

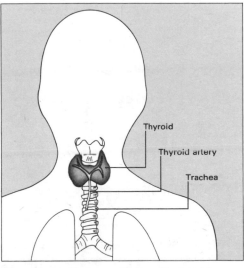

Thyroid gland is located below the Adam's apple and folds around the trachea.

Thyroxine

swelling in the neck, just below the Adam's apple, because of enlargement of the thyroid gland. In older people, there may also be depression, atrial fibrillation, and heart failure.

Q: *How is thyrotoxicosis treated?*

A: While the condition is being diagnosed, drugs (beta-blockers) may be prescribed to control the symptoms. Once the diagnosis has been confirmed, there are three possible forms of treatment. The most suitable depends on expert medical advice.

Drugs that reduce thyroid activity are usually effective. Alternatively, the patient may undergo surgery to remove part of the thyroid gland or any active nodule in the gland (thyroidectomy).

Radioactive iodine treatment is simple and effective. Both surgery and radioactive iodine treatment tend to be followed, some years later, by diminished production of the thyroid hormones (*see* HYPOTHYROIDISM).

Q: *Are there any complications of thyro-toxicosis?*

A: Yes. Occasionally, the symptoms of thyrotoxicosis suddenly become much worse in a condition called a thyroid crisis, which may be brought on by acute anxiety, childbirth, or an operation. Thyrotoxicosis can develop into a fatal condition, with fever, rapid heartbeat, and worsening of all the other symptoms. This requires urgent hospital treatment.

A more common complication is that caused by protuberance of the eyes (exophthalmos). Such eye problems sometimes become worse after treatment for thyrotoxicosis, and result in swelling of the eyelids and tissues behind the eyeball. This condition requires skilled care to prevent eye infection. Another possible complication is ophthalmoplegia (paralysis of the nerves of the eye) that results in double vision (diplopia). This condition tends to improve on its own.

Thyroxine is one of the two principal hormones that are secreted by the thyroid gland; the other main thyroid hormone is triiodo-thyronine.

The effect of both hormones is similar: they increase the metabolic rate of the body cells. Preparations of these hormones may be given to treat thyroid gland deficiency disorders, such as hypothyroidism.

See also THYROID GLAND.

Tibia, also known as the shin-bone, is the innermost and largest of the two bones of the lower leg. The fibula is the outer bone.

The upper end of the tibia forms the knee joint with the femur and is covered by two semicircular cartilages (menisci). The lower end of the tibia forms the ankle joint with the fibula and the talus bone.

See also POTT'S FRACTURE.

Tic is an habitual, involuntary spasm or twitch that usually affects the face, head, neck, or shoulder muscles.

Tics often become more frequent when a person is under emotional stress, and disappear during sleep. For this reason, they are thought to be of psychological origin.

Childhood tics usually disappear spontaneously. But tics in adults may resist treatment. Psychotherapy may help some people but it is not always successful.

See also CHOREA; TRIGEMINAL NEURALGIA.

Tic douloureux, also known as trigeminal neuralgia, is a nervous disorder that causes severe facial pain. *See* TRIGEMINAL NEURALGIA.

Ticks are small, blood-sucking parasites that are related to the mites. Soft-bodied ticks (*Argasidae*) may transmit the spiral-shaped bacteria that cause RELAPSING FEVER. Hard-bodied ticks (*Ixodidae*) may transmit the rickettsial bacteria that cause African tick typhus, Rocky Mountain spotted fever, and Q FEVER. Ticks may also play a part in the transmission of TULARAEMIA.

Some species of ticks can cause tick paralysis. This condition is characterized by lethargy; muscle weakness; loss of co-ordination; and paralysis, which may affect the respiratory muscles. Hospital treatment is necessary for tick paralysis.

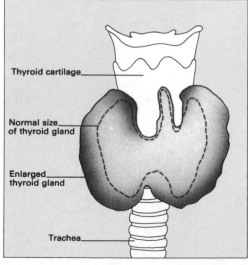

Thyroid cartilage

Normal size of thyroid gland

Enlarged thyroid gland

Trachea

Thyrotoxicosis results from overactivity of the thyroid gland, which may become enlarged.

Tietze's syndrome is a rheumatic disorder that is characterized by pain and tenderness on the front of the chest, although it is more common on the left side than on the right. The underlying cause of the condition is not known. The pain results from swelling of the rib cartilages where they join the breastbone.

Treatment for Tietze's syndrome is seldom necessary. It usually disappears spontaneously within about eight weeks. In severe cases, treatment with antirheumatic or painkilling drugs may be necessary.

Tinea is a fungal disease of the skin. The term usually refers to RINGWORM.

Tinea versicolor is a mild fungal skin infection that produces pale brown, slightly scaly areas on the chest, abdomen and neck. These affected areas may appear as pale patches on darker or sunburnt skins. Selenium shampoo usually cures the condition.

Tine test is a test for tuberculosis. It is performed using an instrument with several prongs (tines) that penetrate the skin and introduce a solution of dead tuberculosis organisms (tuberculin). This test is not as sensitive as the MANTOUX TEST.

See also HEAF TEST; TUBERCULIN TEST.

Tinnitus is the subjective sensation of noises in the ear without there being any external sound. It may be experienced as a buzzing, ringing, hissing, or roaring noise, or as a series of more complex sounds. Tinnitus may be continuous or intermittent, and is usually associated with varying degrees of deafness.

Any disorder of the ear may cause tinnitus, such as wax in the outer ear; MÉNIÈRE'S DISEASE; OSTOSCLEROSIS; and OTITIS. It may also result from a head injury; nerve disorders; arteriosclerosis; smoking; and drugs.

Tocopherol is a general term for several compounds that are chemically related to vitamin E (alpha tocopherol). Vitamin E plays a part in the metabolism of fats in the body cells and also helps to maintain the stability of the cell membranes. It occurs naturally in wheat germ and can also be artificially synthesized.

See also VITAMINS.

Toe is a digit of the foot. Each toe has a protective nail at the end. The big toe (hallux) has two phalangeal bones; the other four toes each have three phalangeal bones. Movement of the toes is controlled by muscles in the foot and leg.

The toes help to distribute the weight of the body evenly along the heads of the main bones of the foot (the metatarsal bones). The toes also help to balance the body.

Q: What disorders can affect the toes?

A: Various generalized bone and joint disorders may affect the toes, such as osteoarthritis; rheumatoid arthritis; and gout, which usually affects the first joint of the big toe. These disorders may cause deformities of the toes, such as HALLUX VALGUS, HALLUX RIGIDUS, and HAMMERTOE. Rarely, a child may be born with more than the normal number of toes (polydactylism).

See also TOE, CLAW.

Toe, claw, is a foot deformity in which one or more toes are abnormally curled. It is most commonly caused by poorly fitting shoes. In such cases treatment is seldom necessary until adulthood, when minor surgery to straighten the toes may be required.

Toilet training. Learning to control the bladder and bowels is an important stage in a child's development. Children cannot control their bladder and bowels until the nervous system has developed sufficiently. This normally occurs between the ages of eighteen months and two years. Bowel control is usually achieved first. But, by the age of about two-and-a-half years, most children have learned bladder control as well. Girls usually attain this stage before boys.

Q: How should a child be toilet trained?

A: There are no firm rules about toilet training. One method of toilet training involves gradually establishing a daily routine. The parent should sit the child on the potty immediately after breakfast. After a few minutes, the baby should be lifted from the potty. If there is anything in the potty, the parent should express obvious approval. If not, the parent should not punish the child.

See also BED-WETTING.

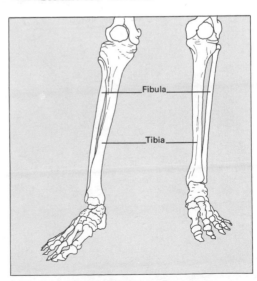

Tibia is the inner bone of the lower leg; it articulates with the ankle and the femur.

Tomogram

Tomogram is an X-ray image of one plane of the body, rather like a cross-sectional view. A tomogram is obtained by using a special technique in which the X-ray apparatus is rotated around the patient while the X-ray picture is being taken. *See* CAT SCANNER.

Tongue is the movable muscular organ that lies partly on the floor of the mouth and partly in the pharynx. It is attached to the hyoid bone above the larynx, to the base of the skull below the ears, and to the lower jaw. The tongue's surface is covered with a special mucous membrane that contains numerous TASTE BUDS which can detect salt, sour, bitter and sweet tastes. The tongue also manipulates food, and helps in the production of speech.

Q: What disorders can affect the tongue?

A: The most common disorder is inflammation of the tongue (*see* GLOSSITIS). Ulcers may form as a result of rubbing against broken teeth, or of the spread of a mouth ulcer (*see* COLD SORE).

An ulcer or a lump on the tongue may be caused by cancer; it occurs most commonly in those who smoke. Cancer of the tongue may be treated by inserting radioactive needles into the tongue, or by surgical removal of the cancer.

Q: Why may the tongue become discoloured or furred?

A: Discoloration or furring of the tongue is not always a sign of disease. It may result from smoking; a course of antibiotics; indigestion; a respiratory infection; or tonsillitis.

A bright red tongue may be a symptom of vitamin B deficiency, either PELLAGRA or PERNICIOUS ANAEMIA. A black tongue is often due to excessive smoking, but it may also appear for no apparent reason then disappear spontaneously.

Tonic is the medical term for a continuous muscle contraction, as opposed to clonic contractions in which the muscles alternately contract and relax. As a general term, tonic refers to a preparation that is supposed to restore a person to normal health.

Tonsil is an almond-shaped mass of sponge-like lymphoid tissue. The two palatine tonsils are situated at the entrance to the pharynx, one on each side, below the soft palate and above the base of the tongue. The lingual tonsil is a similar mass of lymphoid tissue that is situated on the back of the tongue and which, with the adenoids and the tonsils, forms a ring of lymphoid tissue that protects the entrance to the throat. The tonsils and adenoids become smaller as children grow older.

Q: What are the functions of the tonsils?

A: The tonsils have two functions: they trap and destroy micro-organisms that enter the throat; and they play a part in the body's immune system by producing antibodies.

Q: What disorders may affect the tonsils?

A: The most common disorders that affect the tonsils are TONSILLITIS and GLANDULAR FEVER.

Tonsillectomy is the surgical removal of the tonsils. The adenoids are often removed (adenoidectomy) at the same time. The tonsils are not usually removed unless the patient has suffered several attacks of otitis media or tonsillitis. A doctor may also recommend a tonsillectomy if complications, such as QUINSY (peritonsillar abscess), develop from tonsillitis.

Q: Can a tonsillectomy cause complications?

A: Yes, but these are rare. Middle ear infections, such as otitis media, may occur, but the most serious complication is haemorrhage. For this reason it is advisable to stay in hospital until the surgeon is certain the area is healing well.

Q: What happens at the operation, and how long is it necessary to stay in hospital?

A: For four hours before the operation the patient must not eat or drink. Two hours later a sedative is given. Generally, a parent is allowed to stay with a child until the anaesthetist is ready to inject an anaesthetic into a vein in the arm.

After the operation the patient is sleepy for several hours, but apart from some bloodstained saliva there should be no painful complications. Next day the

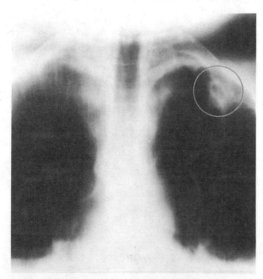

Tomogram is a type of X-ray used to study organs at certain depths within the body.

patient may complain of a sore throat. This is easily controlled with aspirin, iced drinks, ice cream, and jelly, which can be consumed without too much discomfort. In most cases the patient returns home within five days.

Tonsillitis is an inflammation of the tonsils. It is usually caused by a viral infection, but may also result from infection with streptococcal bacteria. Tonsillitis occurs most commonly during early childhood.

Q: What are the symptoms of tonsillitis?

A: Tonsillitis is characterized by a sore throat; difficulty in swallowing; head-ache; and high fever. In very young children, the main symptoms may be abdominal pain; vomiting; and diarrhoea.

Q: How is tonsillitis treated?

A: The treatment of viral tonsillitis is directed toward relieving the symptoms. It is not usually necessary to remove the tonsils surgically (tonsillectomy) unless tonsillitis recurs, or complications arise.

   Tonsillitis that is caused by streptococcus infection is treated with antibiotics, usually penicillin. Aspirin may also be prescribed to relieve the symptoms. The patient should drink plenty of fluids to prevent dehydration.

Q: What complications can result from tonsillitis caused by streptococcus?

A: A type of allergic reaction may occur, causing RHEUMATIC FEVER, acute NEPHRITIS, SCARLET FEVER, or ERYTHEMA NODOSUM. OTITIS, middle ear infection, and QUINSY may complicate any kind of tonsillitis.

Toothache (for EMERGENCY treatment, see First Aid, p.595) is pain in a tooth, or in the area around a tooth. It can be a symptom of almost any dental disorder but is most commonly caused by caries (*see* TOOTH DECAY). Other common causes of toothache include GINGIVITIS; PERIODONTITIS; and an abscess at the root of the tooth.

   A dentist should be consulted as soon as possible so that the underlying cause can be treated. Painkilling drugs, such as aspirin or paracetamol, may give temporary relief.

Tooth decay, also known as dental caries, is disintegration of a tooth because of bacterial action. Tooth decay begins with the formation of jelly-like PLAQUE on the surface enamel of the teeth. Bacteria in the plaque produce acid, which erodes the enamel and exposes the underlying dentine. The acid may also irritate the gums and cause GINGIVITIS. If the decay is not stopped by dental treatment, it spreads to the central pulp, and eventually reaches the root canals. Bacteria may penetrate the decayed teeth and produce a

a dental abscess, which may cause toothache.

Q: How is tooth decay treated?

A: Tooth decay requires expert dental treatment. If the decay is relatively minor, the damaged area of the tooth is drilled out, then filled with a special metal amalgam. Severely decayed teeth may need to be extracted.

Q: How may tooth decay be prevented?

A: Tooth decay may be prevented by a correct diet and good dental hygiene. The teeth should be cleaned thoroughly with TOOTHPASTE after every meal. Dental floss should also be used to remove plaque and food from between the teeth.

Toothpaste is a form of dentifrice that consists of a mild abrasive, a detergent, and, usually, flavouring and colouring.

   Good dental hygiene depends more upon correct brushing than the type of toothpaste or dentifrice used. But toothpastes that contain fluoride help to prevent tooth decay.

Tophus is a gritty deposit that consists of the salts of uric acid. It may be found in the ears, and joints in people with gout. *See* GOUT.

Torn cartilage. *See* CARTILAGE; MENISCUS.

Torpor is a state of drowsiness or numbness in which there is no response to any stimulation except the most insistent or painful.

Torticollis is the medical name for wryneck. *See* STIFF NECK.

Touch, sense of, is the sense by which pressure on the skin is perceived. There are many thousands of sensory nerve endings throughout the surface of the skin that detect different levels of pressure and vibration. Some of the nerve endings are concentrated

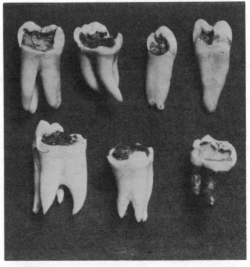

Tooth decay is a progressive breakdown of the structure of the enamel, dentine, and root.

Tourniquet

in particular parts of the body, such as the fingertips and lips. The nerve endings send impulses to the brain, where they are deciphered into various touch sensations.

Tourniquet is a constricting band that is placed around a limb to stop the blood flow.

It is extremely dangerous for an unskilled person to use a tourniquet in the treatment of severe bleeding. If a tourniquet is applied for too long, the tissues in the limb die, and the limb may need to be amputated. A tourniquet must be released at least every thirty minutes.

Toxaemia is a general illness that is caused by the absorption of poisonous bacterial toxins. Toxaemia may also refer to a complication of pregnancy that is commonly known as PRE-ECLAMPSIA.

Toxic means poisonous. The term is also used to describe an illness that is caused by poisonous substances.

Toxin is any poisonous substance of plant or animal origin. For example, venom is the toxin of a snake. The term usually refers to poisons that are produced by bacteria.

Many bacterial toxins can cause diseases, such as bacterial dysentery; diphtheria; food poisoning; gas gangrene; and tetanus. Long-term immunity against some toxins can be produced by injections of toxoid, which is a modified form of a toxin (*see* IMMUNIZATION).

Toxocariasis is a parasitic disease that is caused by infestation with the larvae of two species of roundworm, *Toxocara canis* or *Toxocara cati*. The adult worms live in the intestines of dogs and cats. The worms produce eggs, which are excreted in the faeces.

Humans become infested when they eat the eggs.

Toxocariasis occurs most commonly in children, as a result of sucking objects that are contaminated with the eggs. The eggs hatch into larvae in the intestine, penetrate the intestinal wall, and then spread throughout the body in the bloodstream. The larvae can affect most tissues in the body.

Q: What are the symptoms of toxocariasis?

A: The symptoms include fever; coughing or wheezing; and, occasionally, a skin rash. The liver and spleen may be enlarged, and there may be inflammation of the back of the eye. The larvae may affect the lungs, causing pneumonia. The disease is usually mild, and rarely causes prolonged illness.

Q: How is toxocariasis treated?

A: Toxocariasis may be treated with one of several drugs, such as thiabendazole or diethylcarbamazine.

Toxoid is a bacterial toxin that has been modified by chemical treatment so that it has lost its poisonous properties, but can still stimulate the formation of antibodies. Injections of toxoids can induce immunity against various diseases, such as diphtheria and tetanus (*see* IMMUNIZATION).

Toxoplasmosis is infection with the parasitic protozoan *Toxoplasma gondii*. This microorganism can infect any warm-blooded animal, but it requires a member of the cat family as its main host. In cats, the microorganism produces infectious cysts (oocysts), which are shed in the cat's faeces. In other animals, the microorganisms form cysts in the muscles. Humans become infected by exposure to oocysts in cat faeces, or by eating undercooked meat that contains the muscle cysts. The microorganisms then reproduce within the body cells. But, as immunity develops, reproduction stops and the parasites form cysts in the body tissues. The microorganisms can also infect an unborn child (congenital toxoplasmosis).

Q: What are the symptoms of toxoplasmosis?

A: In most cases, toxoplasmosis does not produce any symptoms. When symptoms do occur, they include slight fever; tiredness; muscle pains; and enlargement of the lymph glands.

Toxoplasmosis may cause prolonged illness in those whose resistance to infection is low. In such people, there may be weakness; headaches; diarrhoea; weight loss; and, sometimes, a severe eye infection (choroiditis). Rarely, it causes high fever and meningitis.

Congenital toxoplasmosis may cause a spontaneous abortion if the infection

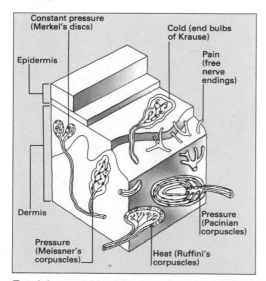

Touch is sensed by a combination of specialized nerves that relay information to the brain.

Constant pressure (Merkel's discs)

Cold (end bulbs of Krause)

Epidermis

Pain (free nerve endings)

Dermis

Pressure (Pacinian corpuscles)

Pressure (Meissner's corpuscles)

Heat (Ruffini's corpuscles)

occurs early in pregnancy. Infection later in pregnancy may cause a miscarriage or stillbirth, or the child may be born with the infection.

At birth, the symptoms may be severe and rapidly fatal. Alternatively, symptoms may be absent at birth but may develop within a few months. In such cases, there may be choroiditis, which may lead to blindness; jaundice; skin rashes; and enlargement of the spleen and liver. There may also be brain damage.

Q: *How is toxoplasmosis treated?*

A: Drug treatment with a combination of pyrimethamine (an antimalarial drug) and sulphonamides is usually effective when the toxoplasmosis organisms are reproducing. There is no effective treatment for destroying organisms in the cyst stage. However, toxoplasmosis is rarely fatal in adults.

Trachea, also known as the windpipe, is the tube that extends from the voice box (larynx) to a point above the heart, where it divides into two tubes (bronchi) that lead to the lungs. The trachea is composed of C-shaped cartilage rings, which are held together by fibrous tissue. It is lined with a layer of moist, mucous membrane.

Food and liquid are both prevented from entering the trachea by a hinged flap of tissue (epiglottis) that diverts the food from the back of the tongue toward the oesophagus.

Tracheitis is an inflammation of the trachea (windpipe). It is commonly associated with an infection of the larynx (*see* LARYNGITIS) or bronchial tubes (*see* BRONCHITIS).

Tracheostomy is the surgical operation of cutting into the front of the trachea (windpipe) to relieve an obstruction and maintain a clear airway. The trachea is opened, and a double tube is placed in the hole. The outer tube remains permanently in place, but the inner tube can be removed for cleaning.

A tracheostomy may be performed if infection or injury causes problems with breathing in the throat (larynx), or after a patient has undergone a major operation on the lungs.

Tracheotomy is a surgical incision that is made through the skin and trachea (windpipe) when performing a TRACHEOSTOMY.

Trachoma is an infection of the thin membrane that covers the front of the eye (conjunctiva). It is a common cause of blindness in tropical countries.

Trachoma is caused by infection with the microorganism *Chlamydia trachomatis*. It is highly infectious and can be transmitted either directly by close contact, or indirectly by infested clothing.

Q: *What are the symptoms of trachoma?*

A: After an incubation period of about ten days, the symptoms of severe CONJUNCTIVITIS appear, with sore, watering eyes, and abnormal sensitivity to light (photophobia).

The symptoms gradually disappear but leave the conjunctiva red, inflamed, and covered with small lumps. These lumps eventually scar, causing blurring of vision and finally blindness. The scarring may also affect the eyelids, causing the edges to turn inward.

Q: *How is trachoma treated?*

A: Treatment with antibiotics is usually effective. Early diagnosis and treatment is essential to prevent scarring and possible blindness. If these have already occurred, a CORNEAL GRAFT operation may be necessary. Surgery may also be necessary to correct ingrowing eyelids.

Traction is the act of pulling or drawing. This is the method by which a baby may be delivered with forceps; a fracture reduced; or a fracture reduction maintained. Weight traction is a system of weights and pulleys that are attached to a fractured limb so that the broken bones remain in the correct position. Traction is also used in manipulative and osteopathic treatment.

A talk about Tranquillizers

Tranquillizers are drugs that are used to reduce mental stress without disturbing normal mental activities. There are two main

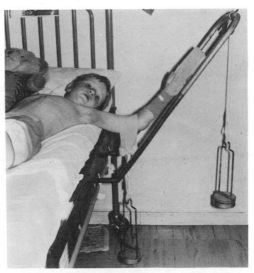

Traction is a method of treatment which holds fractured bones in position by using weights.

Transference

groups of tranquillizing drugs: minor tranquillizers and major tranquillizers. The minor tranquillizers are used to treat acute anxiety. They may also be combined with antidepressant drugs to treat patients who are both anxious and depressed. The major tranquillizers are used to treat psychotic mental illnesses, such as schizophrenia.

Q: What are the different types of minor tranquillizers?

A: The benzodiazepine group of drugs are the most commonly prescribed minor tranquillizers. They produce four main effects: sedation; alleviation of anxiety; prevention of convulsions; and muscle relaxation.

Various other drugs are also used as minor tranquillizers, such as hydroxyzine and loxapine.

Q: Can minor tranquillizers produce adverse side effects?

A: Yes. The main side effects include dizziness, drowsiness, and lack of co-ordination. Care should be taken when driving or operating machinery, and alcohol should be avoided. Minor tranquillizers may produce physical dependence during a long course of treatment, so a doctor may limit their use.

Q: What are the different types of major tranquillizers?

A: The major tranquillizers include the phenothiazines, thioxanthine derivatives, and butyrophenones. The phenothiazines are the most commonly prescribed of these drugs. All the groups of major tranquillizers produce similar effects, which include sedation; relaxation of the muscles; reduction of aggression; and prevention of nausea.

The major tranquillizers are extremely effective in controlling the symptoms of serious mental illnesses. Their use has enabled many patients to lead relatively normal lives.

Q: Can major tranquillizers produce adverse side effects?

A: Yes. Patients who are highly sensitive to these drugs may develop skin rashes and jaundice. The production of hormones may also be affected, which may cause irregular menstruation. Large doses may cause trembling and muscle rigidity.

Transference is the redirection of emotion from important figures, such as parents, to another person, usually to a psychiatrist or a doctor who is treating the person.

Transfusion is the infusion of blood or plasma into the veins of a person. *See* BLOOD TRANSFUSION.

Transfusion reaction is a dangerous reaction that occurs between the blood of a donor and the recipient. Such reactions are rare when the blood types of the donor and the recipient are properly cross-matched. The severity of transfusion reactions varies greatly. The onset of the reaction is usually rapid, with breathlessness; chest pain; vomiting; and symptoms similar to those of shock.

Q: What causes a transfusion reaction?

A: A transfusion reaction is usually caused by an incompatability between the blood of the donor and that of the recipient. The recipient has antibodies that destroy the red blood cells of the transfused blood. This reaction may cause jaundice and disorders of the kidneys, which may become blocked, resulting in haemoglobin in the urine, and kidney failure.

In most cases, such complications are temporary, and are usually followed by a complete recovery.

See also BLOOD TRANSFUSION.

A talk about Transplant surgery

Transplant surgery is the transference of a tissue or organ from one person to another, or from one site to another in the same person. The main difficulty with transplantation is to prevent the body from treating the new organ as a foreign substance and destroying it (tissue rejection).

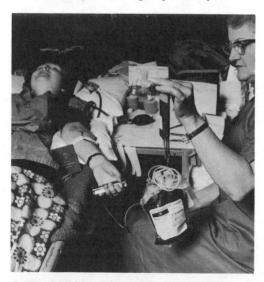

Donor gives blood that will be used in the future for a blood transfusion.

Q: When is transplant surgery performed?

A: Transplant surgery is performed when it is considered the most effective form of treatment. For example, a kidney transplant may be performed to stop the need for regular KIDNEY DIALYSIS. Corneal transplants may be performed to restore the sight of a person with severe corneal scarring. Heart valves may be transplanted to treat valvular heart disease. Diseased blood vessels may be replaced to treat arteriosclerosis. The technique has been performed successfully with tendons, nerves, bones, and skin.

Transplants between different people have been performed with the heart, liver, kidneys, and bone marrow. Other organs, such as the lungs, fallopian tubes, and pancreas have also been transplanted, but such transplants are still experimental.

Q: Are transplant operations successful?

A: There is no guarantee that a transplant operation will be successful. The success rate depends to some extent on the tissue being transplanted.

Up to seventy per cent of patients with heart and kidney transplants survive for at least two years after the operation.

Q: Why isn't transplant surgery always successful?

A: The relatively few transplantations that fail usually do so because of tissue rejection. Every person, unless an identical twin, has a characteristic set of proteins in the body (tissue type), rather like a fingerprint. The better the match between tissue types of the transplanted organ and the recipient, the lower the chances of rejection. Identical twins have the same tissue type, so rejection is extremely unlikely.

Q: Can rejection be prevented?

A: Yes, although the technique is not always successful. Several drugs reduce the ability of the transplant recipient to produce antibodies by suppressing the immune system of the recipient. These drugs are called immunosuppressive drugs.

Because these drugs suppress the immune system, they also prevent the body from reacting to infection so that even the mildest infection may be fatal. However, new immunosuppressive drugs are being developed, and rejection is becoming less of a problem.

Q: Which transplants need immuno-suppressive drug treatment?

A: Kidney, heart, and liver transplants usually require immunosuppressive

treatment for several years. The dosage is reduced slowly when a doctor is satisfied that rejection is unlikely.

Q: Which transplants do not need immunosuppressive drug treatment?

A: Corneal and tendon transplants can be performed without the problem of rejection. Transplantation of blood vessels and heart valves is usually successful without drug treatment because the transplanted tissues are replaced by the recipient's tissues.

Q: What happens if the transplanted organ is rejected?

A: The result of rejection depends, to some extent, on the organ that has been transplanted. If a vital organ, such as the heart or liver, is rejected, the patient usually dies unless another transplant can be performed. Most kidney transplant patients can be kept alive by kidney dialysis until another kidney is available for transplantation.

Transvestism is the desire to dress in the clothing of the opposite sex as a means of obtaining sexual excitement. A transvestite is not necessarily homosexual.

Trauma is the medical term for an injury. It usually refers to a physical injury but may also refer to a psychological shock.

Traveller's diarrhoea is a mild intestinal disorder that causes abdominal cramps, diarrhoea, and also vomiting. The combination of a bland diet, antispasmodic drugs, and kaolin usually controls the symptoms. *See* DIARRHOEA.

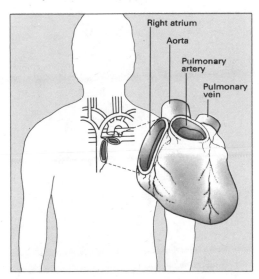

Transplant surgery involving the heart enables the surgeon to implant a healthy donor organ.

Travel sickness

Travel sickness. *See* MOTION SICKNESS.

Trematodes, also known as liver flukes, are parasitic flatworms that require a member of the snail family as an intermediate host before causing various infections in man. *See* FLUKES; SCHISTOSOMIASIS.

Trembling. *See* TREMOR.

Tremor is an involuntary quivering of the muscles. There are several different types of tremor: a coarse tremor is one in which the movements are slow; a fine tremor produces rapid movements; and an intention tremor appears only when voluntary movements are attempted. Tremors may be present all the time or they may occur irregularly.

Tremors may be associated with shivering, excitement, or fear, or they may be a symptom of a more serious underlying disorder. Tremors may be caused by acute anxiety; poisoning; overactivity of the thyroid gland; or failure of the liver or kidneys. Other underlying causes of tremors include nervous disorders, such as Parkinson's disease; multiple sclerosis; Huntington's chorea; general paralysis of the insane (caused by syphilis of the brain); and Friedrich's ataxia, which is degeneration of the spinal cord.

Trench foot is a condition resembling frostbite of the foot. *See* IMMERSION FOOT.

Trench mouth is a painful ulceration of the mucous membranes of the mouth and throat. *See* VINCENT'S ANGINA.

Trephine is a small cylindrical saw that is used to make a circular hole in the skull, thereby exposing the brain for surgery.

Treponema is a genus of spiral-shaped bacteria. Many of these bacteria are parasitic,

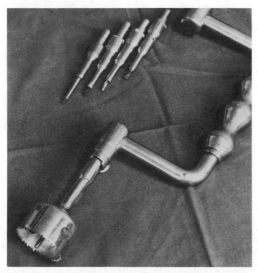

Trephine is a surgical instrument used for cutting circular pieces of bone from the skull.

and cause various diseases, such as PINTA, SYPHILIS, and YAWS.

Trichiasis is a condition in which the eyelashes grow inward and rub against the cornea of the eye. This causes irritation, watering of the eyes, and a feeling of a foreign body in the eye.

Trichiasis may result from various eye disorders, such as trachoma; inflammation of the eyelids (blepharitis); or entropion, in which the eyelids turn inward. It is treated by removing the inturned eyelash, or by surgical out-turning of the eyelids.

Trichinosis is a disorder that is caused by infestation with the parasitic roundworm *Trichinella spiralis*. People become infected by eating raw or undercooked pork that contains cysts of the parasite. The cysts break open in the stomach and they release larvae, which penetrate the wall of the small intestine, mature into adult males and females, and mate. After mating, the female worms discharge larvae which spread to the muscles and form small cysts that eventually calcify.

Q: What are the symptoms of trichinosis?

A: The symptoms vary according to the number of infecting larvae. Diarrhoea, nausea, and vomiting may occur within a few days of infection. About two weeks later there may be swelling of the eyelids; conjunctivitis; and abnormal sensitivity to light (photophobia). These symptoms may be followed by aching of the muscles, intermittent fever, and increasing weakness.

A variety of further symptoms develop, depending on the organs that are infected. Pneumonia and pleurisy, encephalitis and meningitis and sometimes heart muscle involvement (myocarditis) may all occur. If the myocarditis is severe, heart failure will develop. These severe and serious symptoms may last for between one and two months before gradually improving, leaving a vague aching of the muscles.

Q: How is trichinosis diagnosed and treated?

A: In the initial stages it is difficult to make a definite diagnosis, but the history of eating raw pork may be suggestive. The larvae may be found on muscle biopsy, and a skin test will become positive after about four weeks of the infection.

Treatment with thiabendazole is usually effective. Corticosteroid drugs may also be necessary to prevent an allergic reaction to the infection.

Trichinosis can be prevented by thoroughly cooking all pork.

Trichomonas vaginalis is a parasitic protozoan that is found in the vagina and in the male urethra. It seldom causes any symptoms in men, but the trichomonas may be transmitted to sexual partners. In women, it usually causes symptoms only after it has been disturbed by sexual intercourse, menstruation, or, rarely, vaginal surgery. The protozoan may cause VAGINITIS, with an offensive vaginal discharge and painful urination.

Treatment with drugs, such as metronidazole, is usually effective. The patient's sexual partner should also be treated.

Trichuriasis is infestation with the parasitic roundworm *Trichuris trichiura* (whipworm). It results from eating food that is contaminated with the worm's eggs. The eggs hatch into larvae in the small intestine, and migrate to the large intestine. By the time the larvae have reached the colon, they have matured into adult roundworms. The adults attach themselves to the lining of the colon and produce more eggs, which pass out of the body in the faeces.

Q: What are the symptoms of trichuriasis?

A: Symptoms usually appear only with heavy infestations. In such cases, there may be abdominal pain and diarrhoea. Extremely heavy infestations, particularly in children, may cause intestinal bleeding; anaemia; weight loss; and rectal prolapse.

Q: How is trichuriasis treated?

A: Treatment with mebendazole is usually effective. Trichuriasis may be prevented by careful personal hygiene.

See also ROUNDWORMS.

Trigeminal neuralgia, also known as tic douloureux, is a disorder of the trigeminal nerve, which supplies the face with sensory and some motor functions. The disorder occurs most commonly in the elderly. The cause is not known.

Q: What are the symptoms of trigeminal neuralgia?

A: The only common symptom is a severe, brief pain on one side of the face. This pain is often triggered by a light touch, cleaning the teeth, or by chewing.

Q: How is trigeminal neuralgia treated?

A: Treatment with some anticonvulsant drugs, such as carbamazepine and phenytoin, or with anti-migraine drugs is often effective. If such treatment is not successful, a doctor may recommend a surgical operation to cut the trigeminal nerve.

Triglyceride is a type of lipid that is formed from a combination of fatty acids and glycerol. Most animal and vegetable fats are triglycerides.

The relationship between triglycerides, cholesterol, and lipoproteins is complex, but there is evidence to associate high levels of these three substances in the blood with an increased incidence of arteriosclerosis.

Excessive saturated animal fat in the diet causes a long-term increase in the concentration of triglycerides and cholesterol in the blood. A high triglyceride blood concentration may be associated with alcoholism; diabetes mellitus; the nephrotic syndrome; hypothyroidism; pregnancy; and also use of the contraceptive pill.

A diet that is low in animal fats and regular exercise can help to reduce the level of triglycerides in the blood.

Trismus is a spasm of the jaw muscles causing difficulty in opening the jaws. It may be caused by a fracture or dislocation of the jaw; a throat infection; or irritation of the nerves that control the jaw muscles, as occurs with tetanus. *See* TETANUS.

Trocar is a surgical instrument for piercing the walls of a cavity. It consists of a tube with a sharp, pointed central part, that can be removed, leaving the outer tube in place. A form of trocar is used for intravenous transfusions and for piercing the abdominal wall to remove ASCITES. TRACHEOSTOMY tubes often contain a central trocar.

Tropical diseases are those that occur almost exclusively in tropical climates. This is mainly because (1) the organisms that cause the diseases are able to survive only in tropical conditions; (2) the diseases are transmitted by insects or animals that are found only in the tropics; and (3) poor sanitation and health care are common in many tropical countries.

Travellers can be immunized against some

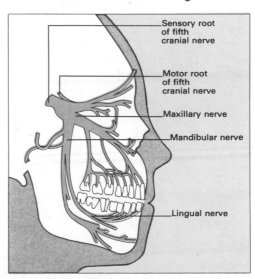

Trigeminal neuralgia can affect any part of the face supplied by the fifth cranial nerve.

Labels in figure:
Sensory root of fifth cranial nerve
Motor root of fifth cranial nerve
Maxillary nerve
Mandibular nerve
Lingual nerve

Tropical sore

tropical diseases. The use of insect-repellent creams may help to prevent insect-borne diseases. Diseases that are transmitted by body contact can usually be prevented by careful personal hygiene.

Air travel has introduced some tropical diseases to temperate climates where such diseases do not usually occur. Any fever or disorder that occurs within about two months of returning from the tropics should be reported to a doctor immediately.

Tropical sore, also known as Delhi boil and Oriental sore, is a skin ulcer that is caused by infection with parasitic microorganisms of the genus *Leishmania. See* LEISHMANIASIS.

Truss is a device that is used to hold a hernia (rupture) in place. A truss is usually used only when surgical treatment of a hernia is not possible. *See* HERNIA.

Trypanosomiasis is a general term for any of several related diseases that are caused by parasitic protozoa of the genus *Trypanosoma. See* CHAGAS' DISEASE; SLEEPING SICKNESS.

Trypsin is an enzyme produced by the pancreas that digests proteins in the small intestine.

Tsetse fly is a bloodsucking insect that transmits sleeping sickness. *See* SLEEPING SICKNESS.

TSH test is performed to assess the activity of the thyroid gland. It involves measuring the concentration of radioactive iodine in the thyroid gland both before and after the administration of thyroid-stimulating hormone (TSH).

Tubal pregnancy is a pregnancy that takes place in a fallopian tube instead of in the womb. *See* ECTOPIC PREGNANCY.

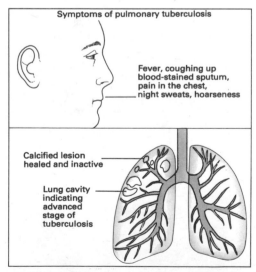

Tuberculosis can affect many parts of the body; pulmonary tuberculosis is the most common.

Tuberculin test is a skin test to determine whether a person has ever been infected with tuberculosis or related bacteria. A small amount of tuberculin, which is a preparation of dead tuberculous bacteria, is injected into the skin. A red swelling indicates previous infection with tuberculosis or immunization with BCG vaccine. A tuberculin test does not reveal whether the infection is active or inactive. *See* BCG; HEAF TEST; MANTOUX TEST; TINE TEST; TUBERCULOSIS.

A talk about Tuberculosis

Tuberculosis is an infectious disease that is usually caused by the bacteria *Mycobacterium tuberculosis.* Rarely, it may be caused by other species of *Mycobacterium,* such as *Mycobacterium bovis* which is found predominantly in cattle.

Infection may result from inhalation of minute droplets of infected sputum or, less commonly, from drinking infected milk. If the infected person is not immune, the bacteria grow freely within the body and spread from the lungs to other parts of the body.

Eventually the patient develops immunity and the bacteria stop spreading. They become surrounded by scar tissue and may not cause further tissue damage.

At a later stage, the protective layer of scar tissue may break down. This may be due to the development of another disorder; a reduction in immunity, which may occur with old age; the use of corticosteroid drugs; or malignant diseases, such as leukaemia and Hodgkin's disease.

Symptoms of tuberculosis occur when the body's immunity does not develop fast enough to prevent the infection from spreading to various parts of the body, or when immunity is interrupted by old age or certain drugs or diseases. The symptoms of tuberculosis in children usually differ from those in adults.

Q: *What are the symptoms of tuberculosis in children?*

A: The main symptoms of childhood tuberculosis include fever; weight loss; and swelling of the lymph glands. If the primary site of infection is in the lungs, the lymph glands in the chest become enlarged; if it is in the gastrointestinal tract, the lymph glands in the neck or abdomen are affected.

The enlarged lymph glands may ulcerate, causing bronchial irritation, with coughing and the collapse of parts of the lung. There may also be ulceration into the bronchial tubes, causing tuberculous pneumonia. If the lymph glands in the neck are affected, they may discharge pus through the skin. Swelling of the lymph glands in the abdomen may result in a slow form of PERITONITIS.

Q: *What are the symptoms of tuberculosis in adults?*

A: There is often a period of many months before symptoms appear. In most cases, the infection primarily involves the top of one of the lungs, although it may spread to other parts of the body. The initial symptoms include tiredness; weight loss; fever during the evening; and profuse sweating at night.

As the infection progresses, the patient begins to cough up blood-stained sputum, which may be infectious. If a large area of the lung is affected, pleurisy may develop, causing breathlessness and chest pain.

In some patients, particularly the elderly and those with silicosis, the progress of the disease is extremely slow and is accompanied by a large amount of lung scarring. In such cases, the main symptoms are usually breathlessness and coughing.

Q: *In what other ways can tuberculosis affect the body?*

A: Tuberculosis may affect any organ in the body. It may cause infection of the membranes round the brain (meningitis), which is characterized by headache, drowsiness, and intermittent vomiting. This usually affects children and is often fatal unless treated rapidly. In miliary tuberculosis, the infection spreads extremely rapidly, and small abscesses develop in most organs. Tuberculosis may also affect the bones, most commonly the spine (Pott's disease); the kidneys; or the epididymis. The infection may spread from the abdominal organs or the lungs, which may result in tuberculous peritonitis or inflammation of the fallopian tubes (salpingitis). Rarely, tuberculosis may affect the adrenal glands, causing ADDISON'S DISEASE.

More commonly, tuberculosis involves the membrane surrounding the lungs (pleura), causing an accumulation of tuberculous fluid between the layers of the pleura (pleural effusion). This may cause a serious illness, particularly if the fluid contains a large amount of pus.

Most people who become infected with tuberculosis do not develop symptoms of the disease: they become immune and the infection remains dormant in scar tissue.

Q: *How is tuberculosis diagnosed?*

A: Tuberculosis may be diagnosed with X-rays and examination of the sputum for the tuberculosis bacteria. Blood tests and a positive TUBERCULIN TEST may be used to confirm the diagnosis.

In children, X-rays are usually not helpful, and the doctor must obtain a history to determine if there has been exposure to tuberculosis.

Q: *How is tuberculosis treated?*

A: Most patients respond quickly to chemotherapy and are discharged from hospital after two or three weeks. Patients who are seriously ill may require hospitalization for two or three months.

Drugs are prescribed until the sensitivity of the bacteria to antibiotics and the response of the patient are determined. Thereafter, the drugs may be changed to suit the individual patient. They should be taken for many months. The drugs most commonly used are isoniazid (INH) in combination with rifampicin or ethambutol and, occasionally, streptomycin by injection.

Tuberculous meningitis requires specialized treatment. Early diagnosis is extremely important.

Q: *Can tuberculosis be prevented?*

A: Yes. Vaccination with BCG, which is a preparation of attenuated tuberculosis bacteria, has been shown to confer lifetime immunity in certain populations.

Q: *What are the "open" and "closed" forms of tuberculosis?*

A: "Open" tuberculosis refers to the stage in the disease when a person is producing

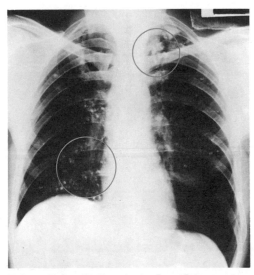

Tuberculosis affecting the lungs may be revealed by an X-ray examination.

Tularaemia

infectious sputum. "Closed" tuberculosis refers to the noninfectious stage, in which the tuberculosis bacteria are surrounded by scar tissue. Patients with "open" tuberculosis should be isolated until sputum tests for the bacteria are negative.

Q: *What precautions should be taken by people who have been in contact with tuberculosis?*

A: Those who have been in contact with an infectious case of tuberculosis should be examined for infection by a doctor. If the person has been in very close contact, or has had a tuberculin test that indicates recent infection with tuberculosis, treatment with antituberculous drugs for at least a year is needed. Other contacts should be kept under regular observation, with chest X-rays, after being vaccinated with BCG if the tuberculin test is negative. Contacts of patients with "closed" tuberculosis should also be examined.

Tularaemia, also known as rabbit fever, is a disorder that is caused by the bacterium *Francisella tularensis.* The bacteria can penetrate unbroken skin, and most cases of tularaemia result from handling infected wild animals, particularly rabbits. Occasionally, infection may result from eating undercooked meat, or from the bite of an infected tick.

Q: *What are the symptoms of tularaemia?*

A: After an incubation period of about a week, there is a sudden onset of high fever; headache; nausea; vomiting; and extreme weakness. A day or two later, an inflamed nodule appears at the site of infection. The nodule ulcerates rapidly, and further ulcers may appear near the mouth or eye. The lymph glands around the site of infection may become swollen; they may also ulcerate and discharge pus.

The patient may develop a skin rash or pneumonia at any time during the illness, which usually lasts three or four weeks.

Q: *How is tularaemia treated?*

A: Treatment with streptomycin or tetracycline is effective in most cases. The patient should undergo the full course of treatment to prevent a relapse.

Tumour is any swelling of the body tissues, such as an abscess, a cyst or a tissue growth. The term usually refers to a spontaneous new growth (neoplasm), which may be either malignant (cancerous) or benign (noncancerous). A malignant tumour is a neoplasm that grows and spreads throughout the body. A benign tumour is a neoplasm that does not spread or infiltrate other tissues of the body.

Most tumours are benign and are not life-threatening. However, malignant tumours may spread and cause extensive damage. *See* CANCER; SARCOMA.

Turner's syndrome is a CHROMOSOME anomaly of females in which one of the two X chromosomes is absent, so that there are forty-five instead of the normal forty-six chromosomes.

A person with Turner's syndrome has the physical appearance of an immature female. The characteristic features include short stature; webbing of the neck; multiple birthmarks; and underdeveloped or absent ovaries. There may be swelling of the hands and feet during infancy. Some patients have congenital heart defects, and a few are mentally retarded. At puberty, the breasts fail to develop normally, and menstruation does not occur.

There is no effective treatment for Turner's syndrome until the patient reaches puberty. After puberty, oestrogen and progesterone drugs can be given to replace the deficiency of ovarian hormones. Normal secondary sexual characteristics and menstrual periods can then occur.

Twilight sleep is a condition of impaired consciousness that is produced by a combination of painkilling drugs and inhaled anaesthetic gases. Twilight sleep is often induced in order to reduce the pain of childbirth, while keeping the mother sufficiently aware to be co-operative during labour (*see* PREGNANCY AND CHILDBIRTH).

Twins. There are two types of twins: fraternal twins (dizygotic or binovular twins), and identical twins (monozygotic or monovular

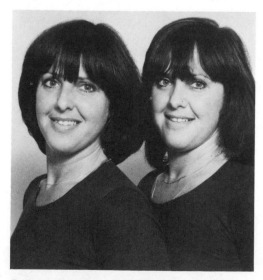

Twins formed from one fertilized ovum that splits are identical, or monozygotic.

twins).

Fraternal twins result from the fertilization of two separate eggs that are usually released simultaneously. They may be the same sex or different sexes. Each has a separate placenta within the womb, and each develops independently of the other.

Identical twins result from the fertilization of a single egg that later divides into two. They are the same sex, and share a single placenta. Rarely, the egg may not divide completely and the two foetuses remain joined (SIAMESE TWINS).

Twins occur in about one in eighty pregnancies, but the frequency varies slightly from country to country.

Fraternal twins are more common in families with a history of twins; in mothers who are older than average; and in mothers who have had more than the average number of babies.

Q: Can a twin pregnancy cause problems?
A: Yes. The initial difficulty is that of diagnosis. About one in ten twin pregnancies may go unnoticed until the onset of labour. A twin pregnancy may be confirmed by ultrasonic testing, or, if necessary, by an X-ray examination to show both foetuses.

Pre-eclampsia, anaemia, and premature labour occur more commonly with twin births. But, the main problem of a twin pregnancy is delivery. The first baby usually causes little difficulty, but the second may be in the wrong position and may require turning for a normal delivery. Another problem is survival of both twins without brain damage caused by a rapid delivery.

Due to the problems of pre-eclampsia and prematurity, there is a greater incidence of infant mortality during the latter half of pregnancy, during labour, or within a few days of birth. There is also a greater risk of haemorrhage in the mother after birth.

See also PREGNANCY AND CHILDBIRTH.

Twitching is an involuntary muscle contraction that produces a small, spasmodic jerking movement. It may occur as a TIC, as restless legs, or as a symptom of TETANY. Twitching may be a symptom of various neurological disorders, but occasional twitching in a healthy person is not serious.

Tympanum is the anatomical name for the eardrum. See EAR.

Typhoid fever, also known as enteric fever, is an intestinal disease that is caused by infection with the bacterium *Salmonella typhi*. Typhoid is the most serious of the salmonella infections. Similar, but milder infections with other salmonella bacteria cause PARATYPHOID fever.

Most cases of typhoid result from eating infected food or from drinking contaminated water. Food and water may become contaminated by direct contact with the urine or faeces of an infected person. Flies may carry the infection from faeces to food. When the bacteria have been swallowed, they penetrate the small intestine and spread throughout the body in the bloodstream.

Q: What are the symptoms of typhoid?
A: After an incubation period of about one or two weeks, there is a gradual onset of headache; loss of appetite; fatigue; and constipation.

During the following week, the patient's temperature rises gradually to about 40°C (104°F). This is accompanied by abdominal pain, nosebleeds, and slow pulse rate. Pale, rose-coloured spots may appear on the chest and abdomen; they usually last for about three or four days.

The high fever usually lasts for about a week, and the patient may become delirious. Diarrhoea may develop toward the end of the second week, by which time the fever starts to disappear. In most cases, the fever disappears completely by the end of the third week of illness.

Q: Can typhoid cause any complications?
A: Yes, pneumonia is the most common complication. More serious complications may occur in patients who develop diarrhoea. In such cases, the intestine may ulcerate and bleed. Severe bleeding from an ulcer may lead to anaemia, or may even

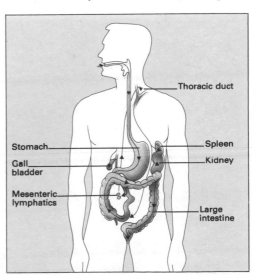

Typhoid bacteria enter the body orally then infect the bloodstream via the thoracic duct.

Typhus

be fatal. Perforation of the ulcer will cause peritonitis. Relapses occasionally occur, but they are usually minor.

Q: *How is typhoid diagnosed and treated?*

A: A positive diagnosis may require a test to culture the bacteria spreading in the blood and to detect a rise in the antibodies (Widal test). The patient's urine and faeces may be cultured for the typhoid bacteria.

Typhoid is usually treated with antibiotics. Chloramphenicol is generally the most effective antibiotic, but bacterial strains have developed that are resistant to it. In such cases, ampicillin or trimethoprim-sulphamethoxazole drugs will be prescribed.

In addition to drug therapy, the patient may require a blood transfusion and intravenous infusions of fluid to prevent dehydration. Patients with perforation or haemorrhage of the intestine usually need an emergency operation to repair the ulcerated area. If the patient suffers a relapse, a further course of antibiotics is necessary.

It is essential that all patients who have had typhoid should have at least six specimens of faeces cultured and examined to ensure that the bacteria have been killed. Until this has been done, the patient should not be allowed to handle food, and should take great care with personal hygiene.

Q: *What is a carrier of typhoid?*

A: A typhoid carrier is a person who has made a complete recovery from the

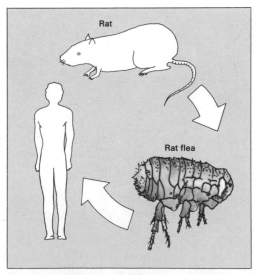

Endemic typhus is a disease transmitted by a flea that infests rats and humans.

disease, but who continues to excrete typhoid bacteria in the urine and faeces. Such people can transmit the infection to others.

Q: *Can typhoid be prevented?*

A: No, but it is possible to reduce the likelihood of infection. All drinking water should be purified, if necessary by boiling, and milk should be pasteurized. Carriers of typhoid should not be allowed to handle food. Immunization with typhoid vaccine gives partial protection against infection, and may reduce the severity of the symptoms in those who contract typhoid.

See also IMMUNIZATION; SALMONELLA.

Typhus is a general term for any of several related diseases caused by various species of *Rickettsia,* which are microorganisms that resemble both bacteria and viruses.

The typhus group is generally considered to consist of a range of similar diseases, including epidemic typhus; endemic typhus; and scrub typhus. Some authorities consider Rocky Mountain spotted fever and Q fever to be forms of typhus. Although these diseases are also caused by *Rickettsia,* they are often classified as forms of spotted fever.

Epidemic typhus is caused by *Rickettsia prowazeki.* The infection may result from contamination of a bite by the faeces of the human body louse, or from inhalation of louse faeces. Endemic typhus is caused by *Rickettsia mooseri,* which is transmitted by fleas from infected rats or mice. Scrub typhus is caused by *Rickettsia tsutsugamushi,* which is transmitted by a mite that normally lives on rodents.

Q: *What are the symptoms of epidemic typhus?*

A: After an incubation period of between ten and fourteen days, there is a sudden onset of a severe headache and fever. The fever rises to about 40°C (104°F) and usually lasts for about two weeks. Between four and six days after the onset of symptoms, pink spots appear on all parts of the body except the face, hands, and feet. The spots may darken as a result of bruising. The patient may also vomit, and be in a state of delirium or shock. Epidemic typhus has a high mortality rate, particularly among untreated patients. Rarely, the symptoms of epidemic typhus may recur without the patient being reinfected. This is called Brill-Zinsser disease.

Q: *What are the symptoms of endemic typhus?*

A: The symptoms of endemic typhus are similar to those of epidemic typhus, but are usually much milder. The mortality rate is low.

Q: *What are the symptoms of scrub typhus?*

A: The symptoms are similar to those of epidemic typhus, but scrub typhus may also cause a red nodule at the site of the mite bite. The nodule ulcerates and forms a black scab (eschar). A skin rash and cough may also develop. The rash is usually less clearly defined than the rash of epidemic typhus. Some patients may also develop complications, such as pneumonia and, rarely, inflammation of the heart muscle (myocarditis).

Q: *How is typhus treated?*

A: For all forms of typhus, treatment with antibiotics is usually effective. Patients who are seriously ill may also require hospitalization and treatment with intravenous infusions of fluid.

Q: *Can typhus be prevented?*

A: Yes. Effective vaccines are available against epidemic and endemic typhus, but not against scrub typhus.

The control of mites, lice, and rodents are also effective preventive measures. It is advisable to use insecticides and mite-repellent creams when visiting areas in which typhus is common.

See also RICKETTSIA.

U

Ulcer is an open sore that may occur on the skin or the internal mucous membranes of the body. For example, an ulcer may develop inside the mouth (aphthous ulcer); around the lips (cold sore); on the cornea; or in the stomach and duodenum (PEPTIC ULCER).

Q: *What causes ulcers?*

A: Ulcers may be caused by relatively minor disorders, such as a burn or abrasion. They also may result from more serious disorders. For example, ulcerative colitis produces ulceration of the colon; scrub typhus produces a skin ulcer called an eschar; and syphilis produces a chancre sore. Cancer may produce an ulcer in almost any part of the body.

Ulcers are particularly likely to develop in parts of the body where there is poor blood circulation, which may be caused by varicose veins. Reduced sensation in a particular part of the body may be caused by nervous disorders, and may also lead to ulceration.

See also BEDSORE; PEPTIC ULCER; RODENT ULCER; ULCERATIVE COLITIS.

Ulcerative colitis

Ulcerative colitis is a disorder of the large intestine in which the colon becomes inflamed and ulcerated. It usually occurs in people between fifteen and thirty-five years old. The underlying cause of the disorder is not known.

Q: *What are the symptoms of ulcerative colitis?*

A: The most common symptom is a series of attacks of bloody diarrhoea that vary in severity and duration from one person to another, and from one attack to another. They may start suddenly or gradually, and may occur as frequently as ten or fifteen times in twenty-four hours. The attacks are often accompanied by pain and spasms of the bowel (tenesmus). Attacks also may cause fever, loss of appetite, and weight loss.

With mild attacks, the symptoms are less alarming. The patient may feel tired but usually there are no signs of generalized illness.

The symptoms usually disappear between attacks, although some patients may suffer from mild diarrhoea.

Q: *Can ulcerative colitis cause complications?*

A: Yes. The most serious complications are associated with a sudden attack of bloody diarrhoea with perforation of the intestine, peritonitis, and intestinal bleeding.

People with ulcerative colitis also may develop anaemia; arthritis; inflammation of the eyes; or tender nodules under the skin. If ulcerative colitis persists for longer than about ten years, there is a much greater than average chance of

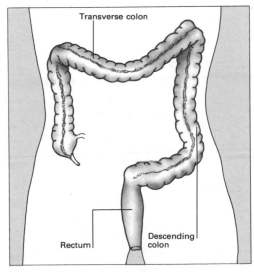

Ulcerative colitis first affects the rectum, then progresses to involve the colon.

Ulna

developing cancer of the colon.

Q: How is ulcerative colitis diagnosed and treated?

A: A positive diagnosis may require an internal examination (endoscopy) of the colon and a barium enema X-ray.

Mild attacks of ulcerative colitis are usually treated with antidiarrhoeal drugs and rest. A special sulphonamide drug may control the symptoms of a severe attack and prevent recurrences. Treatment with corticosteroids, by mouth and as enemas, may also be necessary.

Persons who suffer an extremely severe attack may require hospital treatment. If complications develop, such as peritonitis or intestinal bleeding, emergency surgery may be necessary.

The outcome of ulcerative colitis is variable. However, most patients suffer repeated attacks over many years, and about thirty per cent eventually require some form of surgery. Patients with recurrent ulcerative colitis should have regular internal examinations of the colon to check for early signs of intestinal cancer. In many such cases, it is necessary to remove the colon and make an ILEOSTOMY, an opening in the abdominal wall for the small intestine.

Ulna is the slightly smaller of the two bones of the forearm. The other bone is the radius. At its upper end, the ulna articulates with the radius and humerus to form the elbow joint. At its lower end, the ulna joins with the radius to form the inner side of the wrist joint. *See* ELBOW; WRIST.

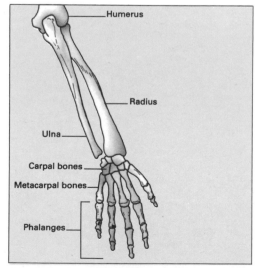

Ulna is able to twist round the radius, allowing a 180° turn of the wrist and hand.

Ultrasound techniques involve the use of high frequency sound waves (ultrasound) for diagnostic and therapeutic purposes.

Ultrasound is much too high-pitched to be audible (above about 20,000 cycles per second). It is focused into a thin beam, which is passed into the body. When ultrasound hits bone or air in the body, most of it is reflected while other tissues absorb the sound to varying degrees. When ultrasound is used for diagnosis, the echo is converted into a visual image. This image requires skilled interpretation by a specialist.

By using ultrasound techniques, it is possible to distinguish between different tissues in the body, measure the organs, and detect movement in the body.

Q: Is ultrasound dangerous?

A: No. It seems to be entirely safe. The amount of energy in ultrasound is too low to cause damage.

Q: Can ultrasound techniques be used anywhere in the body?

A: No. The skull reflects ultrasound, thereby preventing investigation of the brain. Ultrasound recordings of parts of the body that contain air, such as the lungs, are difficult to interpret.

Q: Are there any special uses of ultrasound?

A: Yes. Ultrasound is especially useful in investigating pregnancy because it does not harm the foetus or the mother. It may be used to measure the skull of a foetus, thereby giving an indication of the foetus's age; to detect foetal movements; to determine the position of the placenta; and to detect multiple pregnancies.

With ultrasound techniques, pregnancy can be detected as early as five weeks after conception. Abnormalities of the mother's womb, such as placental abnormalities or a hydatidiform mole, may be revealed. Foetal abnormalities, such as anencephalus, can also be detected early in pregnancy.

Ultrasound is particularly useful during AMNIOCENTESIS, because it can show the position of the placenta inside the mother's body.

Q: What other uses of ultrasound are there?

A: Ultrasound may be used to distinguish between a solid tumour and a cyst, to discover the cause of liver enlargement, to investigate kidney disorders, and to aid a biopsy of the liver. It may also help to diagnose thyroid, pancreatic, and gynaecological disorders, and to locate devices within the body, such as an intrauterine device.

Echocardiography is a form of ultrasound technique that may be used to diagnose heart disorders.

Ultrasound techniques may also be used to detect narrowing of the arteries and arterial thrombosis by recording alterations in the blood flow.

In the treatment of disease, a beam of ultrasound can be focused on a specific area within the body, where the energy of the beam changes into heat. This technique is used for relieving muscle and joint pains. A very powerful beam of ultrasound can be used to destroy small areas of body tissue.

Umbilical cord is the flexible, rope-like structure that connects the foetus with the PLACENTA. It is usually about eighteen inches (45cm) long. The umbilical cord consists of two umbilical arteries and one umbilical vein, which are surrounded by a thick layer of jelly (Wharton's jelly) and a thin membrane. The umbilical vein transports oxygen and nutrients to the foetus. The umbilical arteries carry waste products from the foetus.

Soon after childbirth, the umbilical cord is tied and then cut by an obstetrician. The part of the cord that is still in the womb is expelled with the afterbirth. The stump that remains attached to the baby shrivels and falls off after a few days, leaving a small scar called the umbilicus (navel).

Unconsciousness (for EMERGENCY treatment, *see* First Aid, p.573) is a state of reduced awareness. It may vary in depth from a state of stupor, in which a person responds to painful stimulation, to a state of coma, in which a person cannot be roused by any form of stimulation.

The unconscious is a psychiatric term for the part of the mind that is believed to operate without the individual's immediate awareness or control.

See also COMA; STUPOR; TORPOR.

Undescended testicle is a condition in which a testis has not moved into the scrotum. *See* CRYPTORCHIDISM.

Undulant fever is another name for brucellosis. *See* BRUCELLOSIS.

Upper respiratory tract infection (URTI or URI) is any infection of the nose (rhinitis), throat (pharyngitis), or larynx (laryngitis). The most common form of upper respiratory tract infection is the common cold.

Uraemia is a toxic condition in which waste products of protein digestion, such as urea, are retained in the blood instead of being excreted in the urine. Uraemia is associated with kidney failure.

Q: What conditions can cause uraemia?

A: Uraemia may be caused by any condition that reduces the flow of blood through the kidneys, such as haemorrhage,

vomiting, diarrhoea, or a serious illness. Kidney disease, such as nephritis, prevents the excretion of waste products which accumulate in the blood, causing uraemia. Disorders of the prostate gland or bladder stones block urine flow from the bladder and cause back pressure of urine into the kidneys, resulting in kidney failure and uraemia. Bacterial infections may also cause uraemia.

Q: What are the symptoms of uraemia?

A: The symptoms vary according to the underlying cause. Generally, the symptoms of acute uraemia include headaches, high blood pressure, confusion, dry mouth, and reduced urination.

The symptoms of chronic uraemia develop gradually. The first symptom is usually frequent urination (polyuria). Later, fatigue, loss of appetite, twitching muscles, confusion, and coma develop.

Because of the combination of illness, vomiting, and vitamin deficiency, the patient may also develop malnutrition.

Q: How is uraemia treated?

A: The treatment of uraemia is directed toward the underlying cause. A doctor may recommend a special diet that is low in protein, salts, and water to reduce the symptoms. Patients with high blood pressure may require special treatment to prevent heart failure.

If kidney failure is likely to develop, a specialist may advise kidney dialysis or, in suitable cases, a kidney transplant.

Q: Can uraemia cause complications?

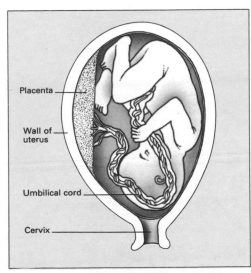

Umbilical cord carries nutrients and waste products between the mother and the foetus.

Ureter

A: Yes. Uraemia may cause heart failure, disturbance of calcium metabolism, abnormal bone formation, nerve damage, and bleeding, which may occur anywhere in the body. Uraemia may also affect the immune system, leaving the patient vulnerable to infection.

If the condition is not treated, the patient becomes comatose and may die.

Ureter is one of a pair of thin, muscular tubes that drain urine from each kidney into the bladder. The urine is passed down the ureter by alternate contraction and relaxation (peristalsis) of the muscles in the ureter.

Several disorders may affect the ureter. For example, HYDRONEPHROSIS, which is accumulation of urine in the pelvis of the kidney, may be caused by obstruction of the ureter, or by a failure of normal peristalsis. The ureter may also become blocked by a stone (NEPHROLITHIASIS) or a tumour.

Urethra is the tube through which urine is discharged from the bladder.

In women, the urethra is short; it opens between the vagina and clitoris. The urethra is longer in men and also serves as the passage for semen. It passes through the prostate gland where it is joined by the sperm ducts, and opens at the end of the penis.

Various disorders may affect the urethra. It may open on the lower surface (hypospadiasis) or on the upper surface (epispadiasis) of the penis. Both these abnormalities are relatively common birth defects in boys.

The urethra may become infected and inflamed (URETHRITIS), which may result in scarring and narrowing of the urethra in men, or CYSTITIS in women. PROSTATE PROBLEMS may also deform the urethra, which may lead to difficulty in urination.

Urethritis is inflammation of the urethra, the tube through which urine passes from the bladder and out of the body. It may be caused by venereal disease, such as GONORRHOEA or NONSPECIFIC URETHRITIS, or by the spread of infection from the local skin, as in honeymoon CYSTITIS.

The symptoms of urethritis include a painful discharge from the penis in men or from the urethra in women, and frequent urination.

Treatment depends upon the underlying cause. Usually, antibiotics are curative.

Uric acid is one of the waste products of the metabolism of certain proteins that is usually excreted in the urine. Uric acid crystallizes in the tissues when it is present in excessive amounts, resulting in GOUT.

Other conditions that increase the production of uric acid include blood disorders; psoriasis; and lymphomas (growths in the lymphatic system). Excessive uric acid in the body does not always result in gout, but the greater the excess, the greater the likelihood of developing gout.

Too much uric acid in the urine may result in the development of kidney stones.

See also URICOSURIC AGENTS.

Uricosuric agents are drugs that reduce the amount of uric acid in the body. They are used to treat GOUT.

Probenecid is a uricosuric agent that works by increasing the excretion of uric acid in the urine. It is usually necessary to continue treatment with probenecid for life. Another drug, called allopurinol, works by preventing the formation of uric acid. Allopurinol is among the safest of the urincosuric agents for the long-term treatment of gout.

Most uricosuric agents should be used with caution during an acute attack of gout. They may temporarily aggravate the condition by causing crystals of uric acid in the body tissue to dissolve in the blood.

See also URIC ACID.

Urinalysis is the detailed analysis of urine. It may be performed to detect alterations in the composition of the urine, which may help in the diagnosis of many disorders, particularly those of the kidney and urinary tract.

Q: What tests may be performed in a urinalysis?

A: Various chemical tests may be performed on the urine to detect abnormal substances. For example, the presence of glucose is a typical, but not conclusive, sign of DIABETES MELLITUS.

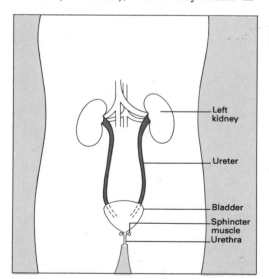

Left kidney
Ureter
Bladder
Sphincter muscle
Urethra

Ureter conveys urine to the bladder, from where it is expelled through the urethra.

The urine may also be tested for acidity and the presence of ketones to confirm a preliminary diagnosis of diabetes mellitus. Albumin in the urine (albuminuria) may indicate NEPHRITIS. Bilirubin in the urine may be a sign of JAUNDICE. The presence of blood in the urine (HAEMATURIA) may be caused by a urinary tract infection, a stone, polyp, cancer, or some other abnormality. An abnormal protein in the urine may be a feature of MYELOMA.

The specific gravity, concentration, and volume of urine produced in twenty-four hours may be measured to assess kidney function.

Most of these tests can be performed in a doctor's surgery. Special tests may require laboratory analysis of the urine, for example, to detect hormones, and the concentration of various other chemicals.

Urinary abnormalities are usually symptoms of disorders of various parts of the urinary system. The following table lists urinary abnormalities with their possible underlying disorders. Each abnormality has a separate entry in the A–Z section of this book. Any of these abnormalities should be reported to a doctor.

Disorder	Abnormality
Bladder disorder	DYSURIA (painful urination)
	INCONTINENCE
Cystitis	Nocturnal enuresis (*See* BED-WETTING)
	STRANGURY (extremely painful urination)
Kidney disease	ALBUMINURIA (albumin in the urine)
	ANURIA (lack of urine)
	GLYCOSURIA (sugar in the urine)
	HAEMATURIA (blood in the urine)
	HAEMOGLOBINURIA (haemoglobin in the urine)
	MELANURIA (dark urine)
	NOCTURIA (urination at night)
	OLIGURIA (reduced production of urine)
	POLYURIA (excessive production of urine)
	RETENTION (inability to urinate)

Urinary acidifiers are drugs or chemicals, such as ammonium chloride and ascorbic acid, that make the urine acidic. They may be used to increase the effectiveness of certain drugs, or to increase the rate at which the kidneys eliminate some drugs from the body.

Urinary tract consists of all the organs and ducts that are involved in the production and elimination of urine. It comprises the two kidneys (*see* KIDNEY) and ureters (*see* URETER), the BLADDER, and the URETHRA.

Urine is a fluid that is produced by the kidneys, carried to the bladder by the ureters, and out of the body through the urethra. Urine consists mainly of water, but it also contains waste products that are filtered from the blood by the kidneys. The elimination of waste products in the urine helps to keep the body fluids at the optimum concentration.

The principal waste products are urea, uric acid, creatine, and other nitrogen compounds that are produced by various metabolic processes, mainly by the digestion of proteins. Urine also contains sodium chloride and other salts, and a few body cells.

Normal urine is amber in colour and has a faint but distinctive odour. Occasionally, urine contains abnormal substances, such as sugar or blood. Analysis of the urine may help to diagnose a large number of disorders.

See also URINALYSIS.

Urogenital means concerning the urinary and reproductive systems.

Urology is the branch of medicine that is concerned with the male and female urinary tract, and the male genital organs.

Urticaria, also known as hives or nettle rash, is a skin condition that is characterized by the eruption of welts and itching. *See* HIVES.

Uterus is the medical name for the womb. *See* WOMB.

Uveitis is inflammation of the uveal tract,

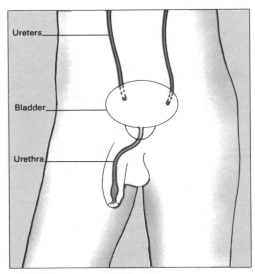

Urinary tract includes the ureters to the bladder, the bladder, and the urethra.

479

Uvula

which is the part of the eye that comprises the iris, the ciliary body, and the choroid. In most cases, uveitis occurs without apparent cause. The symptoms differ according to whether the front or the back of the eye is affected. Uveitis that affects the front of the eye causes IRITIS; uveitis that affects the back of the eye causes CHOROIDITIS.

Uvula is a small, fleshy mass of tissue. The term usually refers to the structure that hangs from the soft palate at the back of the mouth. This is called the palatine uvula.

Vaccination is inoculation with infectious microorganisms or some part of them (a vaccine) to confer immunity against a specific disease.

See also IMMUNIZATION.

Vaccine is a preparation of disease-producing (pathogenic) microorganisms, or some part of them, that is given to induce immunity. There are three main types of vaccine: those that contain specially treated living organisms, such as measles vaccine; those that contain dead organisms, such as whooping cough vaccine; and those that contain specially prepared toxins, such as diphtheria vaccine.

See also IMMUNIZATION.

Vaccinia is a contagious viral disease that primarily affects cattle, but which also may cause a mild pustular infection in humans. *See* COWPOX.

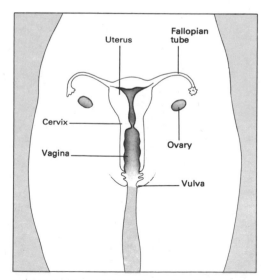

Vagina is the passage between the uterus and the external surface of the body at the vulva.

Vacuum extractor (ventouse) is an alternative to FORCEPS for use in assisting the delivery of a baby. It is a suction cap that is placed over the baby's head. The suction allows an obstetrician to gently pull the child during delivery. It is easier to attach than forceps, and pressure is applied over a larger area of the skull. There is no evidence that this reduces the chances of brain damage to the baby, but it does cause less damage to the mother than the use of forceps.

Vagina is the part of a female's genital tract that extends upward and backward from the vulva to the cervix (neck of the womb). The walls of the vagina are composed of fibrous and elastic tissue, so that it is normally a closed, flattened structure lying between the urethra in front and the rectum at the back.

An adult's vagina is about 7cm (three inches) long when relaxed, but it can stretch considerably during sexual intercourse. The size of the vagina is controlled by the surrounding muscles. During intercourse and childbirth, the muscles relax and contract. The ridged skin lining the vagina (epithelium) changes with the hormonal variations that occur during the menstrual cycle. The amount of mucous secretions also varies during the cycle.

Vaginal discharge, known medically as leucorrhea, is not necessarily abnormal; many women experience a slight discharge. However, it may be a symptom of VAGINITIS (inflammation of the vagina) or cervicitis. Other causes include a foreign body in the vagina, such as a bead in an infant girl or a forgotten tampon in a woman.

The discharge usually consists of secretions from the cervix (neck of the womb) and vagina. The amount of these varies from time to time during the menstrual cycle, because of the hormonal response of the cells that line the vagina and cervix. A day or two after menstruation has ended there is a slight increase in secretions. Another noticeable increase occurs in the middle of the cycle at about the time of OVULATION.

Sexual stimulation, physical or psychological, also causes an increase in secretions.

Newborn females usually have a swollen vulva and a slight vaginal discharge because of the presence of maternal hormones in their bloodstream. *See* LOCHIA.

Vaginismus is an extreme spasm of the muscles surrounding the lower end of the vagina, which causes pain and makes sexual intercourse extremely difficult (dyspareunia).

Q: What causes vaginismus?

A: The cause is usually of psychological origin, often fear. Other causes include inflammation of the vagina.

Q: How is vaginismus treated?

A: A doctor checks for any physical cause of pain before psychiatric treatment is recommended. Overcoming fear of intercourse may take a long time.

    See also SEXUAL PROBLEMS.

Vaginitis is inflammation of the vagina. It produces vaginal discharge.

Q: What causes vaginitis?

A: Many women, probably fifteen to twenty per cent, have infectious organisms in the vagina that can cause inflammation, but only a sudden change in environment triggers them into action. Such infection may be stimulated by such diverse factors as the use of antibiotics, the contraceptive pill, vaginal douching, or sexual intercourse. The common microorganisms that infect the vagina are MONILIASIS (thrush) and TRICHOMONAS VAGINALIS.

Q: What are the symptoms of vaginitis?

A: Vaginitis causes soreness and a discharge. Typically, moniliasis causes an intense irritation, soreness, and a thick, white discharge, whereas trichomonas produces a more offensive, greenish watery discharge with less irritation.

Q: How is vaginitis treated?

A: Moniliasis is more common in women who are pregnant or who are taking contraceptive pills (because of their hormonal effect on the vaginal cells), but it is seldom necessary to stop taking the pills. Patients who develop moniliasis following a course of antibiotics treatment for some other condition, usually improve rapidly once the appropriate treatment is given.

    Moniliasis is treated with suppositories or creams inserted into the vagina each night for at least a week. Trichomonas is treated with pills taken orally. The patient's sexual partner also should be treated. Other forms of vaginitis, such as nonspecific bacterial vaginitis, can be treated with a combination of suppositories, creams, or appropriate antibiotic drugs by mouth.

Q: Is vaginitis sexually transmitted?

A: Moniliasis may be sexually transmitted. If the woman has recurrent attacks, it is often advisable for the man to use a cream to be applied to the end of the penis at night. *See* CERVICITIS; SALPINGITIS; VAGINAL DISCHARGE; VULVITIS.

    In cases of trichomonas, the man usually has the infection without any symptoms, and he should be given treatment at the same time as the woman.

Vagotomy is an operation to cut the VAGUS NERVE. Usually both branches of the nerve are cut at a point adjacent to the oesophagus where they pass through the diaphragm muscle. This greatly reduces the secretion of hydrochloric acid by the stomach. The operation frequently is done at the same time as a partial gastrectomy in the treatment of a PEPTIC ULCER, or a pyloroplasty, used to repair the pylorus.

Vagus nerve (tenth cranial nerve) is the principal nerve of the parasympathetic nervous system. It arises from the lower part of the brain stem (the medulla oblongata), passes through the base of the skull, down the neck, and through the chest to the abdomen.

    The vagus nerve sends out branches to various parts of the body, including the outer ear, the throat, the vocal cords, the heart and lungs, and the digestive organs. The sensory fibres of the vagus nerve transmit sensations of stretch from the lungs, and of pressure from the heart. The motor fibres constrict the bronchi and stimulate the digestive organs. Both these types of fibres are part of the parasympathetic nervous system. The vagus nerve also contains fibres that are not part of this system. These ordinary fibres help to control speech and swallowing.

    See also AUTONOMIC NERVOUS SYSTEM; PARASYMPATHETIC NERVOUS SYSTEM.

Valgus is any deformity in which part of the body is bent outwards from the midline. For example, talipes valgus is a form of clubfoot in which the heel is turned outwards.

    See also VARUS.

Valley fever, also known as coccidioidomycosis, is an infectious disease that is caused by the fungus *Coccidioides immitis.*

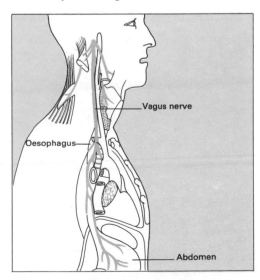

Vagus is one of the most widely distributed nerves with a motor and sensory function.

Valve

It occurs mainly in the southwest United States. Valley fever usually produces relatively mild symptoms that are similar to those of a feverish cold or acute bronchitis. Rarely, it may cause a form of pneumonia in which the brain also may be affected, producing a form of meningitis.

Treatment of the mild form of valley fever usually is not necessary because most patients recover spontaneously. The severe form of the disease is treated with the antifungal drug amphotericin, but even with treatment, the mortality rate is high in severe cases.

Valve is a fold of tissue within a tube in the body that prevents the backflow of fluid. Valves occur in the heart, veins, and lymphatic vessels. The ileocaecal valve is situated between the caecum and the small intestine. It helps to prevent digested food from moving backward in the intestine.

Valvotomy is a surgical operation in which a valve is cut. It most commonly is performed to repair a heart valve that has become deformed by scarring.

Valvular disease is a relatively common disorder of the heart in which there is deformity of the heart valves, lack of the usual number of flaps that form the valves, or constriction or dilation of the opening.

RHEUMATIC FEVER causes scarring of the valves and may lead to narrowing (stenosis) or dilation of the passages. It usually affects the mitral valve between the left atrium and left ventricle of the heart, but other valves, such as the tricuspid, aortic, and pulmonary valves, also may be damaged. Sometimes more than one valve is affected.

Valvular disease causes additional strain on the heart muscle and frequently leads to HEART FAILURE later in life. The distortion of the heart valves causes an alteration in blood flow through the heart, resulting in a HEART MURMUR. The type, timing, and position of the murmur help a doctor to determine the particular valve that is affected. Special diagnostic techniques, such as echocardiography and angiocardiography, may be necessary.

Apart from heart failure, the major complication of valvular disease is infection of the damaged valves resulting in SUBACUTE BACTERIAL ENDOCARDITIS.

In most cases, the deformed valves can be corrected surgically, either by a VALVOTOMY to remove the scarred tissue, or by replacement of the defective valve.

See also HEART DISEASE; HEART SURGERY; MITRAL VALVE DISEASE.

Vaporizer is a device that converts a fluid into a vapour spray. This is an effective method of administering medication for disorders of the lungs and bronchial tubes, such as asthma, bronchitis, and croup.

Varicella is the medical name for chickenpox. *See* CHICKENPOX.

Varicocele is varicose veins around the testes. The enlargement of the veins of the spermatic cord, which causes varicocele, is more common on the left side than the right in adolescent males. It seldom causes more than a slight ache that can be relieved, if necessary, by a scrotal support.

The increased blood flow and warmth in a varicocele occasionally may be a factor in reducing sperm production, leading to sterility in a man.

A varicocele may sometimes occur in a woman's vulva.

A talk about a Varicose vein

Varicose vein is a vein that is abnormally swollen and twisted. Varicose veins result from increased blood pressure in the veins, and damage or absence of the normal valves.

Damage to the valves may be caused by VENOUS THROMBOSIS. Absence of the normal valves may be due to a congenital defect. Increased blood pressure may result from an abdominal tumour, such as a fibroid in the womb, an ovarian cyst, pregnancy, or obesity. Varicose veins are more common in women than men. The condition also occurs in some families more than others, which suggests a hereditary factor.

Q: Where do varicose veins occur?

A: Varicose veins usually occur in the legs, but they also may occur around the anus,

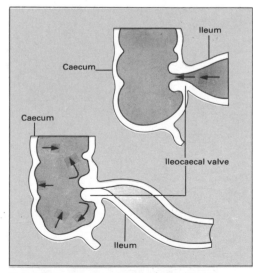

Valve between the ileum and the caecum allows food to pass in one direction only.

causing piles (haemorrhoids); around the testes (varicocele); or in the vulva of a pregnant woman.

The veins at the lower end of the oesophagus may also become enlarged as a result of CIRRHOSIS of the liver when there is an increase in venous pressure in the hepatic portal vein.

Q: What are the symptoms of varicose veins?

A: The most obvious symptom is the appearance of the affected veins. Varicose veins are blue and snake-like. They occur near the skin in the legs and may stand out from the legs. The patient also may suffer from aching of the legs and swelling of the ankles at the end of the day.

Q: How are varicose veins treated?

A: In the early stages, or for those who are elderly or unfit, an elastic stocking may relieve the aching and swelling. But it does not cure the condition.

Varicose veins also may be treated by injecting a fluid that inflames the vein wall, and then bandaging the leg tightly for about six weeks to keep the walls of the vein close together. The resultant scarring causes the walls of the vein to stick together.

Surgical treatment involves cutting and tying the varicose veins, passing a wire instrument down the length of the vein, and then removing the vein by pulling on the wire. This technique is known as stripping.

Q: What complications occur with varicose veins?

A: The most common complication is phlebitis, which has the same inflammatory effect on the vein as injection treatment. The vein becomes tender and eventually scarred, resulting in a nodule under the skin. Severe phlebitis may require antibiotics and tight bandaging. Rarely, anticoagulants may be necessary if a deep vein has also become thrombosed.

Bleeding from a varicose vein may result from injury (for EMERGENCY treatment, *see* First Aid, p.516).

Variola is the medical name for smallpox. *See* SMALLPOX.

Varus is a deformity in which a part of the body bends inwards from the midline.

Vas deferens, or sperm duct, is the tube that carries the sperm from the epididymis of the testes to the seminal vesicles (alongside the prostate gland), where sperm is stored. *See* TESTIS; VASECTOMY.

A talk about Vasectomy

Vasectomy is a form of sterilization for men in which a section of each of the two sperm ducts (vas deferens) is removed surgically. This operation prevents sperm from reaching the urethra.

Q: How is a vasectomy performed?

A: The operation can be done under a local or general anaesthetic. An incision is made at a site that overlies the point at which each sperm duct leaves the scrotum. The two sperm ducts are cut, and the ends are tied firmly with a material that does not dissolve, such as silk. The two incisions are then closed.

Q: How soon after a vasectomy does a man become sterile?

A: The man is fertile for about two or three months after the operation until sperm that were in the seminal vesicles when the operation was performed have either died or been ejaculated.

Q: Are there any immediate problems with a vasectomy?

A: There may be slight local discomfort over the groin wounds for two or three days, but this should not interfere with normal activities. Sexual intercourse may be uncomfortable, so it is advisable to abstain until the stitches are removed or are absorbed by the body, which normally takes about four or five days.

Q: Can a vasectomy cause long-term problems?

A: Long-term problems are extremely rare.

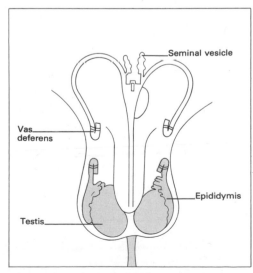

Vasectomy is a surgical operation in which parts of the two sperm ducts are removed.

Vasoconstrictor

There may be a dull ache in the testes for several weeks after the operation, but this slowly disappears.

The most common long-term problems usually are psychological in origin. The only difference a vasectomy makes is to stop the production of sperm. A man's sex drive (libido) usually is undiminished after the operation; it may even increase because the fear of an unwanted pregnancy is removed. A vasectomy does not reduce the production of sex hormones, nor should it affect a man's feelings of masculinity.

See also STERILIZATION.

Vasoconstrictor is any agent that causes constriction of the blood vessels. This effect usually is brought about by drugs, but it also may be the result of nervous stimulation.

Vasodilator is any agent that produces a dilatation of the blood vessels. It usually is a drug but also may be the result of nervous stimulation.

Vasomotor rhinitis is a condition affecting the mucous membranes that line the nose. It causes symptoms of runny nose, sneezing, postnasal drip and, occasionally, headache. The symptoms are similar to those of hay fever, but no allergic cause can be found.

Q: What causes vasomotor rhinitis?

A: In most cases, there is no obvious cause. Sometimes anxiety, changes in room temperature, or hormonal changes associated with adolescence, menstruation, or menopause may be factors.

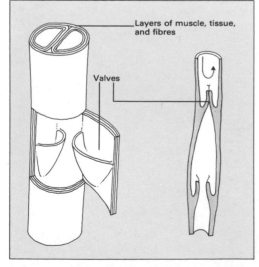

Veins frequently contain valves that prevent the backward flow of blood.

Occasionally, a similar condition occurs as a side-effect of some drugs used to treat high blood pressure, or as a result of overuse of nasal sprays or drops.

Q: How is vasomotor rhinitis treated?

A: Treatment is difficult. The symptoms are thought to be caused partly by overactivity of the parasympathetic nervous system, and so loss of weight, regular exercise, and the stopping of smoking may all help. Treatment with corticosteroid nasal sprays is effective in some cases.

Vasopressor is anything that stimulates the contraction of blood vessels, causing an increase in blood pressure. *See* VASOCONSTRICTOR.

Vasovagal syncope is the medical name for fainting induced by the sudden dilatation of the blood vessels (vasodilatation). This can happen because of either nervous stimulation, or a fall in heart rate because of vagal effects on the heart. *See* FAINTING.

VD. *See* VENEREAL DISEASES.

Vector is a person or an animal, but usually an insect, that carries an infection from one person to another, or from an infected animal to a person. For example, mosquitoes may be vectors of malaria and yellow fever. *See* FLEAS; MITES; MOSQUITO; TICKS.

Vegan is a person who does not eat meat, fish, or any type of animal or fish products. Vegans may suffer from vitamin B_{12} deficiency unless the vitamin is obtained from yeast. *See* VEGETARIAN; VITAMIN.

Vegetarian is a person who does not eat meat or fish. Most vegetarians, however, do eat some animal products, such as milk, eggs, and cheese. A carefully-planned vegetarian diet can provide all the nutrients that are essential for good health.

See also DIET; VEGAN; VITAMINS.

Vein is a thin-walled blood vessel that carries blood from the body tissues back to the heart. All veins, except the pulmonary veins and the umbilical vein, carry blood with a low concentration of oxygen and a high concentration of carbon dioxide.

Like the arteries, the walls of the veins consist of three layers, but the muscle and middle layers are thinner than in the arteries and cannot keep the vein open if the blood pressure is low.

Veins start as capillaries within the body tissues. The capillaries unite to form veins, which themselves ultimately join to form two major veins (the venae cavae) that drain into the heart. The four pulmonary veins drain directly into the left atrium of the heart.

There are two veins that begin and end in

capillaries. These are known as portal veins. The hepatic portal vein drains blood from the gastrointestinal tract to the liver. The hypophyseoportal vein connects the hypothalamus in the brain to the anterior lobe of the pituitary gland and conveys hormones that stimulate the production of pituitary hormones.

See also PORTAL VEIN; VARICOSE VEIN; VENA CAVA; VENOUS THROMBOSIS.

Vena cava is one of the two veins (superior vena cava and inferior vena cava) that drain venous blood from all parts of the body, except the heart, into the right atrium of the heart. The superior vena cava returns blood from the head, neck, and arms to the heart. The inferior vena cava returns blood from the chest, abdomen, and legs to the heart.

A talk about Venereal diseases

Venereal diseases, known as VD, are infections that are contracted through sexual intercourse or by close body contact.

Q: What symptoms are indicative of venereal disease?

A: Any discharge from the penis or vagina, painful urination, or development of an ulcer on the sexual organs following intercourse may indicate venereal disease. These symptoms usually are obvious in men, but in women they may be so mild as to be unnoticeable. People who notice these symptoms should inform their sexual partners and both should consult a doctor immediately.

Q: What are the different types of venereal disease?

A: The different venereal diseases have separate entries in the A-Z section of this book. *See* CHANCROID; GONORRHOEA; GRANULOMA INGUINALE; LYMPHOGRANULOMA VENEREUM; NONSPECIFIC URETHRITIS; SYPHILIS.

Q: Are there other diseases that may be transmitted by sexual intercourse?

A: Yes. Scabies commonly is transmitted during sexual intercourse. Trichomonas vaginalis often is transmitted to women by men, although it usually does not produce symptoms in men.

A virus infection known as herpes genitalis is probably the most common cause of painful ulceration of the genital organs. The ulcers may take a long time to heal and may reappear several times.

Genital warts are caused by a virus infection that commonly occurs in conditions of poor hygiene. The genital area becomes covered with moist, pink swellings which have a tendency to recur, despite treatment.

Moniliasis, a fungal infection, is a common problem in women. It may be stopped, only to return after intercourse with a partner who has penile moniliasis.

Q: What should a person do who may have a venereal disease?

A: It is important to consult a doctor or to attend a venereal disease clinic. A definite diagnosis of venereal disease may require a physical examination and samples of any penile or vaginal discharge. Blood tests to detect the presence of antibodies to syphilis also may be performed.

If the patient has a venereal disease, appropriate treatment is needed. The patient must regularly attend a clinic, usually every two weeks at first, then once a month for six months. This is necessary to ensure that the disease has been cured and that more than one venereal disease was not contracted at the same time.

Q: Should a patient with VD take any other precautions?

A: Yes. It is essential to abstain from sexual intercourse until it is certain that the infection has been cured. All sexual contacts of an infected person should receive medical attention.

Q: Can venereal disease be cured?

A: Yes. The common forms of venereal disease usually can be cured with antibiotics. However, people with nonspecific urethritis or herpes genitalis

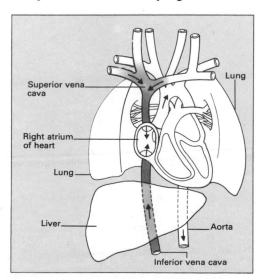

Vena cava connects the right atrium with the lungs and the body's venous system.

Venerology

may have to wait for the condition to improve naturally, which may take several months.

In order to cure venereal disease, it is essential that the patient's disease should be diagnosed early and treated correctly. People who suspect that they have the symptoms of venereal disease must consult a doctor as soon as possible.

Q: Can venereal disease be prevented?

A: Yes, but only by complete sexual abstinence. In men and women the use of a condom may help to reduce the likelihood of catching a venereal disease.

Q: Is it possible to immunize against VD?

A: No. There are no vaccines that are effective against any form of venereal disease.

Venerology is the specialty of medicine concerned with the diagnosis and treatment of venereal diseases. The doctor who practises this specialty is called a venerologist.

Venipuncture is the act of puncturing a vein with a needle. It may be done to obtain a sample of blood for testing, or during an intravenous infusion, when the needle is left in the vein.

Venogram is a procedure in which a dye is injected into a vein so that an X-ray photograph will reveal the shape, size, and extent of the vein. *See* ANGIOGRAM.

Venom is a poisonous substance from a snake, insect, or other animal that can be injected through the skin by a bite or sting. It contains a variety of poisons and toxic

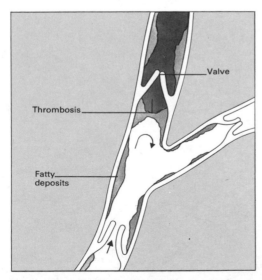

Venous thrombosis is more likely to occur near a valve where the flow of blood is sluggish.

enzymes. *See* ANTIVENIN; SNAKEBITE.

A talk about Venous thrombosis

Venous thrombosis is the formation of a blood clot (thrombus) in a vein. Clotting that is associated with inflammation of a vein (phlebitis) is known as thrombophlebitis; clotting that occurs without venous inflammation is called phlebothrombosis.

Q: What causes venous thrombosis?

A: Venous thrombosis may be caused by any of several factors. These include damage to the wall of a vein, either as a result of injury, infection, or some form of autoimmune disorder in which the body reacts against itself, causing venous inflammation. Sometimes thrombosis may develop because of the combination of an increase in the clotting factors within the blood and slowing of the normal blood circulation.

The use of hormones, particularly oestrogen, may predispose a person to blood clotting.

Q: What are the symptoms of venous thrombosis?

A: Symptoms vary according to whether a superficial or deep vein is involved. The most common type of venous thrombosis is associated with superficial veins. With varicose veins, a combination of poor blood circulation, mild skin inflammation and, sometimes, ulceration may cause thrombophlebitis of the leg. This may result in local tenderness and swelling of the vein, and redness and swelling of the nearby skin.

If a deep vein has thrombosed, the symptoms may include swelling of the ankles, slight tenderness when the calf is pressed, and discomfort when the foot is pulled upwards. Deep vein thrombosis in areas other than the leg may be impossible to detect, and the diagnosis of deep vein thrombosis may require special techniques such as X-rays of the veins (*see* VENOGRAM), ultrasound techniques, and a variety of blood tests.

Q: Can venous thrombosis cause complications?

A: Yes. The most serious complication occurs when a piece of the blood clot breaks off to form an embolus (*see* EMBOLISM). This is potentially fatal. Emboli, however, are relatively rare.

The long-term consequence of venous thrombosis is usually degeneration of the valves in the affected veins. This may result in swelling of the ankles, and skin disorders, such as dermatitis and ulcers.

Superficial venous thrombosis seldom causes serious complications.

Q: *How is venous thrombosis treated?*

A: If a deep thrombosis is diagnosed, hospital treatment with anticoagulant (blood-thinning) therapy is required. Initially, injections of heparin usually are given. Later, other anticoagulant drugs are administered orally.

Anticoagulant treatment usually is continued for about six months. If an embolus develops, surgery may be necessary to tie off the affected vein.

Superficial venous thrombosis usually is treated with painkillers and tight bandaging of the leg to maintain an adequate blood supply.

If ankle swelling or other complications develop after deep vein thrombosis, the patient should wear elastic support stockings for his or her lifetime.

Q: *Can venous thrombosis be prevented?*

A: Yes. Some persons are more likely than others to develop venous thrombosis. Those at risk include the elderly; those with diabetes; those with blood disorders, such as polycythaemia vera; women who take contraceptive pills that contain oestrogens; people with a history of thrombosis; and patients who have undergone gynaecological surgery. In such cases, anticoagulant treatment may be necessary before surgery is performed. This may prevent venous thrombosis from occurring.

Before surgery is performed, the patient should do special calf and leg exercises. After surgery, he or she should resume physical activity as soon as possible. Such measures reduce the likelihood of venous thrombosis.

See also BUDD-CHIARI SYNDROME; WHITE LEG.

Ventral is the front (abdominal) surface of the body, also called the anterior surface, as opposed to the dorsal, or posterior, surface.

Vermiform appendix is the full anatomical name for the appendix. *See* APPENDIX.

Verruca is a wart on the foot. Verrucas commonly are called plantar warts; they are caused by a virus. *See* WART.

Vertebra is any of the thirty-three bones of the spinal column. The flexible part of the spinal column consists of seven cervical vertebrae in the neck; twelve thoracic vertebrae at the back of the chest; and five lumbar vertebrae in the small of the back. The five

vertebrae below the lumbar vertebrae are fused to form the SACRUM. The lowest four vertebrae form the COCCYX.

Q: *What is the structure of a vertebra?*

A: A typical vertebra consists of two main parts: an inner, front part called the body; and an outer, back part called the vertebral arch. These two parts surround a central space through which the spinal cord passes.

The body is roughly cylindrical in shape, with flattened upper and lower surfaces. The bodies of adjacent vertebrae are separated by tough discs of fibrocartilage (intervertebral discs). The vertebral bodies increase in size down the length of the spine.

The vertebral arch consists of seven bony outgrowths. There are two pedicles that project backward from the body. The two laminae form connecting processes between the pedicles. The spinous process is a bony outgrowth that projects backward and downward. The two traverse processes project sideways and provide sites for the attachment of muscles and ligaments.

On the lower surfaces of the pedicles of each vertebra are two areas that form joints with similar surfaces on the upper parts of the pedicles of the vertebra below.

The seven cervical vertebrae differ from the others. The cervical vertebrae are smaller; the spinous process divides into two parts; and the transverse processes each contain a hole through

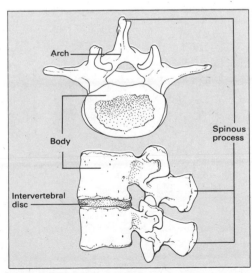

Arch

Body

Spinous process

Intervertebral disc

Vertebrae are separated by intervertebral discs, which allow the spinal cord to bend.

Vertigo

which the vertebral arteries to the brain pass. The top two bones of the cervical spine are completely different from typical vertebrae. The top bone, called the atlas, articulates with the skull. The atlas is a ring-like structure, without a vertebral body. This shape makes nodding movements of the head possible. The second cervical vertebra is called the axis. It has an upwards projection (the odontoid process) that fits into the part of the atlas where its vertebral body normally would be. The odontoid process enables the head to rotate.

The twelve thoracic vertebrae each bear a pair of ribs, which articulate with the sides of the vertebral bodies and the transverse processes.

See also SLIPPED DISC; SPINE; SPONDYLITIS; SPONDYLOSIS.

Vertigo is a disorder of balance which gives a person the sensation of spinning around in space when at rest. Alternatively, objects may appear to be spinning around the person. It is different from DIZZINESS, which is a vague sensation of unsteadiness.

Q: What causes vertigo?

A: Any disorder that affects the ear, the auditory nerve, or the centre in the brain concerned with balance may be responsible. Other causes include toxic compounds such as drugs, alcohol, or food poisoning, and also sudden disturbances of eye function.

Q: What ear disorders cause vertigo?

A: Blockage of the Eustachian tube or wax in the external ear may cause vertigo.

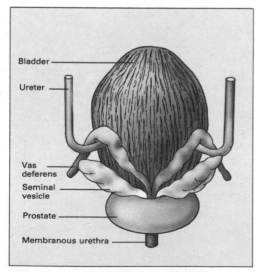

Vesicle is a pouch-like sac or bladder that contains fluid, such as the seminal vesicle.

Infections of the middle ear and inner ear, such as OTITIS media and LABYRINTHITIS or involvement by other disorders, such as OTOSCLEROSIS and MÉNIÈRE'S DISEASE, also cause vertigo.

Q: How does the auditory nerve become involved?

A: Vestibular neuronitis infections, in which the nerve cells become inflamed, are the most common cause. A tumour of the auditory nerve may produce vertigo as well as increasing deafness.

Q: What conditions affecting the brain cause vertigo?

A: The centres that co-ordinate balance are in the brain stem, and have connections with the cerebellum and temporal lobes of the cerebral hemispheres. These may be disturbed by a STROKE or ARTERIOSCLEROSIS, particularly in the elderly. Disorders such as MULTIPLE SCLEROSIS, EPILEPSY, and a brain TUMOUR may cause vertigo.

Q: What is benign paroxysmal positional vertigo?

A: Symptoms of vertigo may occur when the head is moved quickly, but they last for only a few seconds. It is thought to be a minor disturbance of the organ of balance and often spontaneously improves after several months.

Q: Are there any other symptoms that may accompany vertigo?

A: Yes. Nausea and vomiting commonly accompany vertigo, and walking may be difficult with a tendency to fall over sideways. The eyes may flicker (nystagmus), and there may be buzzing in the ears (tinnitus).

Q: How is vertigo treated?

A: The immediate treatment is to lay the person down, in a comfortable position, with the eyes closed. A doctor must be consulted, because antinauseant drugs can be prescribed to help to control the symptoms until a diagnosis is made.

Vesicle is either (1) a bladder or sac containing fluid, such as the gall bladder or urinary bladder; or (2) a blister on the skin containing serous fluid, as occurs in chickenpox and shingles.

See also BLISTER; PAPULE; RASH.

Vestibulitis. *See* LABYRINTHITIS.

Viable means capable of living. A foetus is considered to be viable when it has reached a stage at which it can be kept alive outside the womb. Usually this is when the foetus is at least twenty-eight weeks old.

Vibrio is a genus of motile, curved, rod-shaped bacteria. There are more than thirty different species of *Vibrio* of which three cause disease. *Vibrio cholerae* causes CHOLERA. There are two strains of this species – the normal strain, and a more resistant strain that is known as the El Tor strain. *Vibrio fetus* and *Vibrio parahemolyticus* rarely cause disease.

Villus is a small finger-like protrusion from the surface of a membrane in the body. The lining of the small intestine is covered with millions of villi that provide a large surface area for the secretion of intestinal enzymes and the absorption of digested food. Chorionic villi help the placenta to adhere to the lining of the womb.

Vincent's angina, also known as trench mouth, is a form of STOMATITIS (inflammation of the mouth). It is caused by bacteria which infect the gums, mucous membranes, tonsils, and pharynx. This disorder may develop when oral hygiene is neglected, if nutrition is poor, or in some serious illness such as leukaemia.

Q: What are the symptoms of Vincent's angina?

A: The chief symptom is a sudden onset of painful, bleeding gums (GINGIVITIS), with ulceration inside the cheeks and on the tongue. The patient has a foul-smelling breath and sometimes develops a fever.

Q: How is Vincent's angina treated?

A: Antiseptic oxygenating mouthwashes and dental care produce a rapid improvement. A dentist or doctor may prescribe an antibiotic drug and, if necessary, extra vitamins. Smoking should be avoided.

Virilism is the development of masculine characteristics in women or children. In boys, it is associated with the bodily changes of puberty. The early development of male secondary sex characteristics is caused by excessive secretion of the male sex hormone testosterone by the adrenal glands.

Q: What symptoms may occur in women?

A: Male-type distribution of body hair develops, with deepening voice and the onset of baldness. Acne may appear, and the woman's periods may become irregular or cease (AMENORRHOEA). There is usually an increase in sex drive (libido).

Q: How is the condition diagnosed and treated?

A: A diagnosis is made after examination of the patient's urine for breakdown products of testosterone, and X-rays to detect the presence of an adrenal gland tumour. Corticosteroid drugs will reduce the adrenal gland activity in mild cases. But an operation usually is necessary to remove a part of the adrenal glands, or a tumour if it is present.

Virulent means extremely poisonous. The term is applied to any infection that causes a rapid onset of severe symptoms because of its poisonous effects. Virulent infections are more likely to be fatal than indolent, benign infections.

Virus is one of a group of minute infectious organisms that are visible only under an electron microscope. They are much smaller than bacteria. Viruses consist only of a strand of either DNA or RNA, which are complex proteins that carry genetic information, and an outer coat of protein. Viruses cannot provide their own energy, nor can they grow outside living cells. For this reason, all viruses are parasitic. They alter the functions of the cells they infect so that these cells supply the viruses with energy and with the means of reproducing themselves.

Q: Do viruses infect all of the body tissues?

A: Yes, but individual viruses show a preference for particular tissues. For example, the poliomyelitis virus preferentially infects part of the nervous system, the rabies virus infects the brain, and the chickenpox virus infects the skin. Any viral infection may cause generalized symptoms of muscle aching and fever.

Not all viruses cause disease. Some remain within the body cells without disordering them, but can be activated by an alteration in the body.

Q: What diseases do viruses cause?

A: Many common diseases are caused by viruses; for example, chickenpox, German measles, influenza, measles, mumps, and many respiratory diseases.

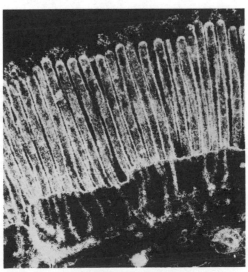

Villus, a short, finger-like projection, increases the absorbing surface of the gut.

Viscera

Other viral diseases include dengue fever, encephalitis, shingles, smallpox, and yellow fever. At least thirty different viruses can cause the symptoms of the common cold.

Some diseases are caused by slow viruses that remain in the body for several years before producing any symptoms. Multiple sclerosis may be caused by an alteration in a person's immunity to a slow virus.

Q: How does the body react to viral infections?

A: At the onset of a virus infection, the body has little resistance to the virus, apart from the presence of lymphocytes, which are a type of white blood cell, and a small amount of INTERFERON, which is a substance that helps to destroy viruses. Within a few days of infection, the body's immune system is stimulated by the viruses to produce antibodies and larger amounts of interferon.

Q: Is it possible to prevent virus infections?

A: Yes. Vaccines have been produced against some of the common virus infections. Vaccines to combat German measles, measles, and poliomyelitis usually are given routinely in early childhood. It also is possible to vaccinate against influenza, rabies, smallpox, typhus, yellow fever, and mumps.

Antibiotics are ineffective against most virus infections, but new drugs are available to help to combat smallpox and shingles.

Q: Can viruses cause tumours?

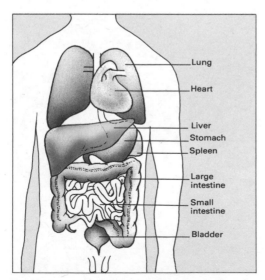

Viscera is a collective term for the internal organs of the chest and abdomen.

A: Yes. Viruses may cause benign (non-cancerous) growths, such as warts and the skin tumours that occur with molluscum contagiosum.

See also IMMUNITY; IMMUNIZATION.

Viscera is a general term for the internal organs in the abdominal and chest cavities. The viscera includes the heart, lungs, liver, spleen, gastrointestinal tract, womb, and bladder.

Visceroptosis is a downward displacement of the visceral organs. In most cases, no cause for the condition can be found. Visceroptosis may affect any of the internal organs, but it most commonly occurs in the abdomen.

Vision. *See* EYE.

Vitamins are chemical substances that are essential for the normal working of the human body. They are effective in extremely small amounts and act mainly as regulators of the body's metabolic processes. Most vitamins must be obtained from food but some, such as biotin and vitamin K, can be synthesized in the body by intestinal bacteria. Vitamin D can be synthesized directly by the body from the action of sunlight on the skin.

Vitamins are classified as either water-soluble or fat-soluble. Fat-soluble vitamins are vitamin A (retinol), vitamin D (calciferol), vitamin E (tocopherol), and vitamin K (phytomenadione). Water-soluble vitamins are vitamin C (ascorbic acid) and the vitamin B group: vitamin B_1 (thiamine), vitamin B_2 (riboflavine), vitamin B_6 (pyridoxine), vitamin B_{12} (cyanocobalamin), biotin, folic acid, and pantothenic acid.

Q: Is a daily intake of vitamins essential?

A: No. The body can store fat-soluble vitamins for many months and water-soluble vitamins for several weeks. A balanced diet should contain sufficient vitamins to maintain these stores. Growing children need proportionately more vitamins than adults. The body's vitamin requirements are also increased during illness, pregnancy, and breast-feeding.

Q: What are the effects of excessive vitamins in the diet?

A: Most vitamins do not produce any effects when taken in large amounts. But, vitamins A, D, and K may produce adverse effects if excessive amounts are taken continually for a long period. An overdose of vitamin A may cause hair loss, peeling of the skin, joint pains, and liver damage. Excessive vitamin D may cause kidney damage and the formation of calcium deposits in the body tissues. Excessive vitamin K in the newborn may cause kernicterus, which is a form of

Name	Source	Functions	Effects on deficiency	Additional information
Vitamin A (retinol)	Fish liver oils, eggs, butter, milk, cheese, liver, apricots, broccoli, cabbage, carrots.	Essential for night vision, healthy skin, and mucous membranes.	Night blindness, dry eyes (xerophthalmia), dry skin.	Excessive intake may cause hair loss, peeling of the skin, joint pains, and liver damage.
Vitamin B₁ (thiamine)	Yeast, whole grains, pork, liver, nuts, peas and beans, potatoes.	Essential for normal functioning of nerve cells, heart muscle, and carbohydrate metabolism.	Beriberi.	Increased amount needed during growth, pregnancy, and breast feeding.
Vitamin B₂ (riboflavine)	Yeast, eggs, milk, cheese, liver, kidney, green vegetables.	Essential for normal protein and carbohydrate metabolism, and for maintaining mucous membranes.	Cracked lips (cheilosis), skin rashes, dim vision.	Increased amount needed during growth, pregnancy, and breast feeding.
Vitamin B₆ (pyridoxine)	Yeast, whole grains, fish, liver, peas and beans.	Essential for general functioning of body cells and amino acid metabolism.	Convulsions in infants, anaemia, nerve disorders.	Increased amount needed during growth, pregnancy, breast-feeding.
Vitamin B₁₂ (cyanocobalamin)	Eggs, milk, cheese, butter, liver, beef, pork.	Essential for growth of red blood cells and normal functioning of nerve cells.	Pernicious anaemia, dim vision, peripheral neuritis.	Deficiency is especially likely in total vegetarians (vegans), and persons with sprue, or following a total gastrectomy.
Niacin (nicotinic acid)	Yeast, meat, fish, whole grains, peas and beans.	Essential for cell metabolism, absorption and carbohydrates, and healthy skin.	Pellagra.	Resists most cooking and preserving processes.
Biotin	Present in all common foods.	Essential for energy production from fats and carbohydrate, and for formation of hormones.	Deficiency does not occur naturally.	Biotin can be produced by bacteria in the intestine.
Folic acid	Yeast, liver, kidney, green, leafy vegetables; fruit.	Essential for growth of red blood cells.	Anaemia and peripheral neuritis.	Increased amount needed during growth, pregnancy, and breast-feeding. Deficiency is particularly likely in people with sprue.
Pantothenic acid	Whole grains, eggs, liver, kidney, peanuts, cabbage.	Essential for normal functioning of enzymes inside the body cells.	Deficiency does not occur naturally.	Pantothenic acid can be produced by bacteria in the intestine.
Vitamin C (ascorbic acid)	Citrus fruits, tomatoes, potatoes, green vegetables.	Essential for normal tissue growth and repair, and normal functioning of blood vessels.	Scurvy.	Vitamin C is easily destroyed by cooking and ultraviolet light.
Vitamin D (calciferol)	Fish liver oils, eggs, butter, liver, yeast.	Essential for normal absorption of calcium and phosphorus, and for normal bone formation.	Rickets in children, osteomalacia in adults.	Increased amount needed during growth, pregnancy, and breast-feeding. Excessive intake may cause kidney damage and calcium deposits in the body tissues.
Vitamin E (tocopherol)	Eggs, vegetable oils, wheat germ, green vegetables.	Essential for stability of cell membranes.	Decreased resistance to rupture of red blood cells.	May also play a part in fertility. Produced by intestinal bacteria.
Vitamin K (phytomenadione)	Vegetable oils, pork, liver, leafy vegetables.	Essential for normal blood clotting.	Bleeding, particularly in premature babies.	Vitamin K can be produced by intestinal bacteria. Deficiency is rare in adults.

Vitiligo

jaundice that occurs in children and which damages the brain.

Q: *What are the effects of insufficient vitamins in the diet?*

A: Prolonged vitamin deficiency leads to depletion of the vitamin stores in the body. This, in turn, results in various deficiency diseases (*see* DEFICIENCY DISEASES).

Q: *Are vitamin supplements necessary?*

A: Additional vitamins are unnecessary if a person is healthy and is eating a balanced diet. Certain vitamins, particularly the fat-soluble vitamins, may be harmful if taken in excessive amounts.

Additional vitamins may be needed during an illness or following a surgical operation. Those with disorders in which there is insufficient absorption of vitamins in the intestine may require vitamin supplements until the underlying disorder has been cured. Other disorders that increase the metabolic activity of the body's cells, such as an overactive thyroid gland, may increase the body's vitamin needs. A doctor will recommend vitamin supplements if they are necessary.

Q: *Are vitamins affected by cooking and storing?*

A: Yes. Some vitamins are unstable substances and can easily be destroyed by incorrect storing and cooking of food.

The fat-soluble vitamins can withstand normal cooking, but vitamins A and E are gradually destroyed by exposure to the air.

The amount of water-soluble vitamins is greatly reduced by boiling food because the vitamins dissolve in the water. Vitamin B_1, vitamin B_6, folic acid, and pantothenic acid are destroyed by heat; vitamin B_2 is destroyed by light; and vitamin C is destroyed by heat, light, and air. For these reasons, food should be used when fresh and should not be overcooked.

Certain food preservatives also destroy the vitamins in food. This may affect the vitamin content of canned foods.

Vitiligo is a relatively common skin disorder that affects about one per cent of the population. It involves the loss of normal skin pigment in irregular patches because melanin (the chemical that produces pigment) fails to be produced. About ten per cent of those affected recover spontaneously.

The condition may start at any age, but it commonly appears before the age of twenty. It generally is thought to be an auto-immune disease with an inherited component.

Vitiligo is more common in patients with some form of auto-immune disorder, such as pernicious anaemia, diabetes mellitus, and alopecia areata.

Q: *How is vitiligo treated?*

A: There are few drugs available to aid patients with vitiligo. Methyoxy psoralen has been found to help recolouring of the skin if it is exposed to sunlight. People with small patches of vitiligo can use special make-up to camouflage the area.

Vitreous humour is the jelly-like substance that fills the part of the eye behind the lens. See HUMOUR.

Voice box is a common name for LARYNX.

Volvulus is a twisting of the intestine around itself. This not only creates an intestinal obstruction, but also blocks the blood vessels that serve it. A volvulus most commonly occurs in the small intestine, caecum, and the sigmoid colon.

Q: *Why does a volvulus occur?*

A: A volvulus may be the result of an anomaly present at birth. One loop of bowel is larger than usual, and there is a longer membranous fold (mesentery). Another cause may be the looping of part of the intestine around an adhesion, a scar left by inflammation or surgery.

Q: *What are the symptoms of a volvulus?*

A: The symptoms of a volvulus are similar to the symptoms of intestinal obstruction: abdominal pain, and vomiting. A volvulus of the large intestine causes vomiting, and invariably involves complete constipation and abdominal pain, with swelling of the abdomen.

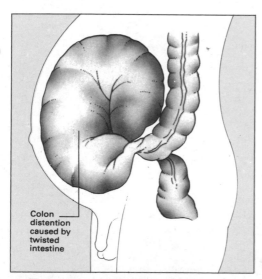

Colon distention caused by twisted intestine

Volvulus occurs when the intestine twists over itself, causing abdominal distention.

Q: How is a volvulus treated?

A: In most cases, an abdominal operation is needed to untwist the volvulus and, if the intestine has become gangrenous, to remove the damaged part of the intestine. It often is necessary to have a temporary colostomy while the intestine returns to normal.

See also INTESTINAL OBSTRUCTION.

A talk about Vomiting

Vomiting, known medically as emesis, is the forceful throwing up of some or all of the stomach contents by reversal of peristalsis, the normal muscular contractions of the stomach. For EMERGENCY treatment, *see* First Aid, p.597.

Vomiting may be a symptom of various disorders, some local to the stomach and some more generalized disorders. It usually is preceded by a loss of appetite and nausea.

Q: What are the local causes of vomiting?

A: The most common cause of vomiting is acute or chronic GASTRITIS (inflammation of the stomach). Vomiting sometimes occurs with a PEPTIC ULCER, particularly if there is PYLORIC STENOSIS (narrowing of the stomach exit). Vomiting also is a symptom of any form of INTESTINAL OBSTRUCTION.

Babies may vomit for a great variety of reasons. Some babies vomit more easily than others but, provided there is a general weight gain and the baby is obviously well, it is not a serious symptom.

Q: What generalized disorders may cause vomiting?

A: The onset of high fever and any condition that affects the sense of balance, such as a virus infection of the inner ear (labyrinthitis) result in vomiting.

Vomiting is a common symptom if the vomiting centre in the thalamus of the brain is disturbed by a MIGRAINE or by increased brain pressure associated with a brain TUMOUR. This takes place also in MENINGITIS and ENCEPHALITIS. Hormone changes in pregnancy alter the sensitivity of the vomiting centre, and this accounts for MORNING SICKNESS and also the excessive vomiting that may occur with HYPEREMESIS gravidarum.

Vomiting can occur for psychological reasons, such as an emotional shock or a nauseous sight or smell.

Vomiting also occurs in serious metabolic disorders; for example kidney failure and the onset of diabetic coma.

Q: Is vomiting always a serious symptom?

Von Recklinghausen's disease

A: No. Occasional vomiting at the start of a generalized illness is part of that disorder. But prolonged and continued vomiting is a serious symptom because it leads to dehydration, which is usually an indication of a severe underlying disorder.

Q: How should vomiting be treated?

A: Until medical help is available, lay the patient down, supported by one or two pillows. Do not allow the patient to drink anything. Bathing the patient's face with a cool, damp flannel is often soothing.

Vomit should be collected in a bowl or other receptacle, in case the doctor wishes to examine it.

If vomiting ceases with these simple measures, and if there are no other symptoms, it may not be necessary to call a doctor. Keep the patient lying still for at least an hour, and do not allow any fluid to be drunk for two hours. Begin drinking by taking small sips of liquid to avoid starting another attack of vomiting.

Continued vomiting always is a more serious problem in small babies than in adults, because dehydration occurs more quickly. This is particularly the case if there also is diarrhoea.

Von Recklinghausen's disease, also known as neurofibromatosis and molluscum fibrosum, named after the German pathologist, is an inherited condition in which multiple freckle-

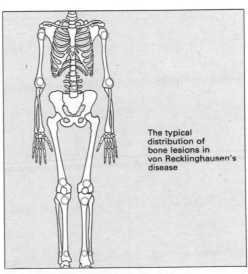

The typical distribution of bone lesions in von Recklinghausen's disease

Von Recklinghausen's disease is associated with destructive lesions of the bones.

493

Vulva

like spots appear on the skin. Nodules (fibromas) also occur and can be felt through the skin. The nodules also occur on nerves (neurofibroma).

Von Recklinghausen's bone disease is also an alternative name for hyperparathyroidism (*see* PARATHYROID GLANDS.)

Q: What are the symptoms of von Recklinghausen's disease?

A: The nodules may be noticeable at birth or may gradually develop later. Often, the skin spots are present at birth. As the child grows, curvature of the spine (scoliosis) may develop and, occasionally, become severe.

The nodules may occur anywhere in the body and cause pressure on adjacent tissues. The neurofibroma cause neurological symptoms, such as neuralgia and paralysis. Therefore, a variety of symptoms may occur. Any symptoms that do develop need careful assessment by a specialist familiar with this disease.

Q: How is von Recklinghausen's disease treated?

A: Treatment is necessary only if the symptoms are severe. Scoliosis may need orthopaedic treatment, and nodules may require surgical removal.

Vulva is the female external genital organ that surrounds the outside opening of the vagina and clitoris. In front, there is a soft padded area covered with hair (mons pubis), and sweeping back from this are the two large folds of the labia majora enclosing two smaller folds, the labia minora. These folds contain lubricating glands, the largest of which (Bartholin's glands) lie at the back.

The vulva extends into the firm, fibrous tissue of the perineum, which is in front of the anus. Between the labia minora lies the fold of skin called the hymen, which partly closes the entrance to the vagina until it is broken by sexual intercourse or by the use of internal tampons.

Inflammation of the vulva is common (*see* VULVITIS). Other disorders are rare.

Vulvitis is inflammation of the VULVA. Its symptoms are soreness and itching.

Q: What causes vulvitis?

A: Any of the causes of inflammation of the vagina (vaginitis) may produce vulval itching. These commonly result from moniliasis (thrush) or trichomonas vaginalis infections, but vulvitis also may occur in diabetes mellitus or general skin diseases such as psoriasis and scabies.

In about one third of cases with vulval irritation, the cause is psychological. But continued scratching produces inflammation that may become infected and cause vulvitis.

Q: What other vulval infections may occur?

A: Other vulval infections include venereal diseases such as syphilis, granuloma inguinale, chancroid, lymphogranuloma venereum, and a viral infection producing warts that may develop on any part of the vulva. Infection with a herpes virus may develop into painful, shallow ulcers.

Q: How is vulvitis treated?

A: The patient must be examined to discover the cause of the irritation. Swabs may be taken for culture to identify an infection; the appropriate treatment can then be given.

Corticosteroid creams usually are soothing and often are prescribed until a firm diagnosis has been made.

See also BARTHOLIN'S CYST; LEUKO-PLAKIA; MONILIASIS; TRICHOMONAS VAGINALIS; VAGINITIS; VENEREAL DISEASES; WARTS.

Vulvovaginitis is inflammation of both the vulva (vulvitis) and the vagina (vaginitis). It commonly is caused by moniliasis (thrush) and trichomonas vaginalis infections. *See* VAGINITIS; VULVITIS.

W

Warts are skin growths caused by virus infection. They are most common in children between seven and twelve years of age.

Q: Are there different kinds of warts?

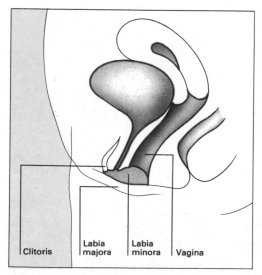

| Clitoris | Labia majora | Labia minora | Vagina |

Vulva, the female external genital organ, includes the clitoris and the labia.

A: Yes. The common wart is a small, raised rough lump on the skin made up of small columns of tissue arising from the base. They vary in colour from normal flesh tint to dark brown-black. Common warts usually occur on the hands, knees, and less frequently on the face or eyelids. They may also appear around the edges of the nails.

Plantar warts (verruca) are the same as the common wart, but are flat because of the different texture of the skin of the sole of the foot. They may be painful because the nodule presses into the flesh.

Venereal or genital warts (condylomata acuminata) are a typical wart infection, sometimes transmitted by sexual intercourse (*see* VENEREAL DISEASES).

Q: How are warts treated?

A: Warts usually disappear spontaneously. Treatment with solid carbon dioxide (dry ice) or liquid nitrogen destroys the wart and the surrounding tissue, leaving a small blister. There are various chemical solutions that can destroy warts, but these have to be used with care. It is advisable to remove any skin application after one or two days and then to rub away the dead tissue before reapplying the medication.

More radical methods of removing warts, such as by cautery, surgery, or X-rays, frequently leave a small scar which may itself produce a small, tender nodule.

Genital warts require special treatment due to their position and possible association with other venereal diseases

Q: Are there any other kinds of warts?

A: Yes. Many people describe any small lump or nodule on the skin as a wart. Although these are not necessarily true warts, the appearance may be similar.

Changes in the skin, occurring with age, may produce slightly raised pigmented areas (senile keratosis), frequently in people who have spent years in the sun.

Seborrhoeic keratosis causes slightly raised darkened areas in the skin that appear as though stuck on the skin surface. These occur most commonly on the trunk but do not need treatment unless they are disfiguring.

See also CYST; RODENT ULCER; MOLLUSCUM CONTAGIOSUM.

Wasp sting venom is composed of various proteins and enzymes (for EMERGENCY treatment, *see* First Aid, p.515). The venom is rarely fatal unless the victim is allergic to it. In this case, ANAPHYLAXIS closely followed by death may occur.

Wasserman Reaction (W.R.) is a blood test that is used in the diagnosis of SYPHILIS.

Wasting, known medically as phthisis, is a gradual loss of body tissue and bulk. *See* STARVATION.

Watering eyes usually are caused by an emotional state, although blockage of the LACRIMAL APPARATUS or inflammation of the eyes also cause excessive production of tears.

See also EYE DISORDERS.

Water on the knee is a form of bursitis. *See* BURSITIS.

Wax, known medically as cerumen, is a soft substance produced by special glands in the ear canal. There is a large variation in the amount of wax produced by different people. Wax usually drains out by itself.

This production and discharge of wax is responsible for the continual cleansing of the ear canal of potentially harmful organisms and debris.

Q: What conditions cause increased wax production?

A: Two conditions that may cause increased production are chronic otitis externa and Parkinson's disease.

Q: How is hardened wax removed?

A: It should first be softened with warm olive oil or bicarbonate of soda solution for a few days before visiting a doctor. It may then be syringed out with warm water. Do not use any object to scrape out the wax, because of the danger of damaging the eardrum.

Q: Can wax formation be prevented?

A: No. It is a perfectly normal secretion.

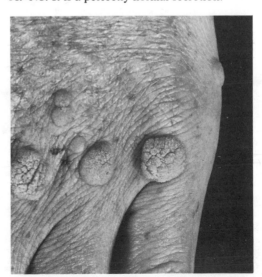

Warts on the hands usually form as many small growths.

Weakness

Hard wax can be prevented by using warm olive oil once every two to three weeks to keep the wax soft.

Q: Are commercial wax softening mixtures safe to use?

A: Yes, provided they are used with care, especially by people who have had OTITIS externa. Some mixtures may soften the skin and allow infection to occur.

Weakness, or debility, is the sensation of loss or partial loss of strength and vigour. It is a symptom of a number of conditions and disorders, and a person who continues to feel weak should consult a doctor.

Weal is a red, swollen area of skin.

Weaning is the period in infancy when feeding gradually is changed from being entirely milk-based to include other foods, such as cereal, fruit, and vegetables. It also is used as an expression to describe the time at which a baby is taken off the breast and given milk feeding by bottle.

The age at which the weaning takes place varies widely from mother to mother, and is a matter for discussion between the mother and the doctor. New foods usually are introduced for the first time between the ages of two to three months, but this is often delayed until later. Breast-feeding may continue for many months, even when other foods are being given.

Weight problems. Many people may think that they are overweight when, in fact, their weight may be normal for their height, age, and sex. They are worried because their own shape or figure does not conform to the currently fashionable ideal. But very few people are able to achieve this shape, and it may even be abnormal in a biological and anatomical sense for some individuals.

Apart from such shape problems, there are genuine weight problems. A person may be overweight or underweight compared to the average or desirable weight. This can cause a physical disorder or anxiety.

Q: How is average weight calculated?

A: Weight tables are compiled by taking the weights of a large number of people and working out an average. The average weight varies because of many factors. For example, races vary in physical proportions; and some families are heavier than others, and their children inherit this characteristic. Weight also varies with occupation. Manual workers, athletes, and military personnel, for example, tend to be better developed and heavier than those who do light work.

Q: How does the body normally regulate weight?

A: Most people stay about the same weight throughout adult life, or gain weight only slowly. The appetite centre, in the hypothalamus of the brain, regulates the amount that is eaten. A slight imbalance results in a gradual weight gain. Even an extra slice of bread a day may cause a gain of 0.25kg (half-a-pound) a month, and about 3kg (seven pounds) in a year.

Q: When should a person consider there is a weight problem?

A: Average expected weights should not be considered ideal weights. The correct weight varies from ten per cent below to ten per cent above the average weight, and is still normal. Weight well above or below this is probably abnormal.

Q: What should be done if a person is below the normal weight?

A: A person may decide that he or she is underweight, but this may be because of racial or inherited characteristics. If, however, there has definitely been a weight loss, a doctor should be consulted and the cause found.

Q: How do underweight people gain weight?

A: This is a matter for a doctor, who first makes sure that there is no disorder that needs treatment. Some people become dangerously underweight by starving themselves. ANOREXIA NERVOSA is an extreme form of self-starvation common in adolescent girls and needs specialized drug and psychiatric treatment. Depression, anxiety, and general fatigue are other factors in weight loss.

Q: Why do people become overweight?

A: Nearly always because they eat too much.

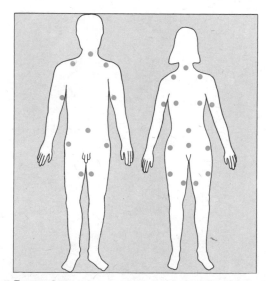

Excess fat tends to accumulate in certain areas, which differ between men and women.

When people eat more than they need for the amount of energy they expend, they tend to get fat.

But some people may be overweight because of a physical disorder, and some gain weight because of compulsive eating, often a sign of underlying anxiety or depression. Weight gain also may follow a long illness.

Q: *Why do some people gain weight much more easily than others?*

A: The reasons for weight gain are not fully understood, but the answer may lie in an individual's metabolism. Babies who are fed excessive amounts of food become fat babies and often grow into fat adults.

Q: *Are some foods more likely to produce obesity than others?*

A: Yes. Foods rich in carbohydrates, particularly those containing sugar, that exceed the body's carbohydrate requirement, get converted into fat. Proteins, such as meat and fish, fruit, and vegetables, are less likely to cause obesity. Alcohol has a high calorie content and, apart from other damage it may cause, is a factor in obesity.

Q: *Are there any hazards in being overweight?*

A: Yes. Overweight people have a greater chance of getting coronary thrombosis and strokes because of arteriosclerosis. Such people are more likely to develop diabetes mellitus; are more likely to hurt themselves seriously in accidents; develop osteoarthritis, particularly of the knees, hips, and ankles; and have more complications following surgery, such as venous thrombosis and chest infections.

Q: *How should an obese person lose weight?*

A: Anyone who is more than twenty per cent over the expected average weight for his or her age, sex, and height should discuss weight loss and dieting with a doctor. Sudden weight changes may cause extreme fatigue and exhaustion. Crash diets can be dangerous and may lead to vitamin deficiency diseases.

A gradual reduction in the amount of food eaten can result in a weight loss of 1 to 1.5kg (two to three pounds) a week, an overall loss of 5kg (ten pounds) a month. The doctor will probably recommend fewer carbohydrate foods, alcohol, and wheat products, and more protein foods and fresh salads.

Regular exercise is of value because it increases the body's metabolic rate and gives the person a sense of well-being and relative freedom from fatigue.

Once the ideal weight has been achieved, there can be a slight relaxation in the detail of the diet so that the ideal weight is maintained. It is, however, essential to keep to the same basic diet for life, to avoid a return to the original eating habits that caused obesity.

Q: *Can drugs help in the treatment of obesity?*

A: Yes. If obesity is caused by anxiety or depression, treatment with tranquillizers and antidepressant drugs can be a great help in reducing compulsive eating. Diuretic drugs, however, help to lose only 1 to 1.5kg (two to three pounds) of water from the body. Appetite suppressant drugs are only moderately effective, and do not help the obese person to learn new ways of eating. When such drugs are stopped, the weight usually increases again. Hormones, such as thyroid pills, have little effect unless taken in excessive amounts. Pep pills, such as amphetamines, reduce the appetite but are dangerous, not only because of the hazard of addiction, but also because of the effect on blood pressure and increased mental activity.

Q: *Should vitamins be taken while dieting?*

A: No. There should be no need for additional vitamins if the person is in good health and keeps to a sensible, balanced new diet.

Q: *How can people help themselves if their weight is normal and they are dissatisfied with their shape?*

A: Regular exercise helps to increase muscle tone and decrease waist measurements, as well as producing a slight slimming of

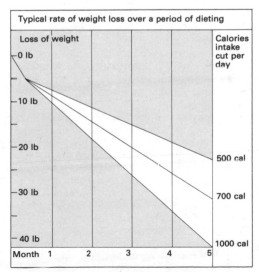

Dieting often causes weight to decrease dramatically at first, then more gradually.

the thighs. Weight may increase slightly due to extra muscle, but the figure will improve.

Q: Can disorders reduce body weight?

A: Yes. Any long-term illness, such as tuberculosis, sprue, untreated diabetes, or cancer, is accompanied by loss of weight. Fevers, operations, or accidents cause an increase in metabolic rate. Thus the body tissues are used faster than they can be replaced, and there is a loss of weight. Another cause of increased metabolic rate is hyperthyroidism.

Q: Can any disorders produce an increase in weight?

A: Yes. Heart, kidney, and liver failure are accompanied by retention of fluid in the body (oedema), and this results in a weight gain. An underactive thyroid gland (hypothyroidism) is often accompanied by an increase in weight.

Drug treatment of some mental disorders may be associated with a weight gain because of an effect on the hypothalamus.

Weil's disease. *See* LEPTOSPIROSIS.

Wen. *See* CYST.

Wharton's jelly is a layer of jelly-like substance that surrounds the umbilical arteries and veins in the UMBILICAL CORD.

Wheezing is a rasping or whistling sound heard with some breathing disorders.

See also STRIDOR.

Whiplash injury occurs when a sudden jerking forward of the body throws the head backward, resulting in injury to the neck. A whiplash injury commonly occurs in a car accident or as a sports injury. All such injuries must be treated by a doctor.

Q: What are the symptoms of a whiplash injury?

A: Momentary loss of consciousness may occur, usually followed by acute spasm and pain in the long muscles in the back of the neck. Almost always the victim has a STIFF NECK.

Sometimes there may be a partial dislocation of one of the cervical vertebrae, or an acute prolapsed intervertebral disc (*see* SLIPPED DISC).

In rare cases, a fracture occurs, or a disc may press on the spinal cord and cause weakness and loss of sensation in the areas of the body below this level in the neck. Paralysis may follow.

Whipworm. *See* WORMS.

White blood cells, also known as leucocytes, are relatively large, colourless cells in the blood that play a major part in combating infection. Unlike RED BLOOD CELLS, white blood cells contain a nucleus. There are three

main categories of white blood cells: polymorphonuclear leucocytes, which have granules in the cell fluid; monocytes; and lymphocytes. Polymorphonucleocytes (polymorphs) are also known as granulocytes.

Polymorphs are subdivided into neutrophils, eosinophils, and basophils according to their reaction to a special dye. They are produced in the bone marrow.

The other leucocytes are subdivided into monocytes and lymphocytes. They are produced in the bone marrow, lymph nodes, spleen, and thymus gland.

There are between 4,000 and 10,000 white blood cells per cubic millimetre of blood in a healthy person. Bacterial infections usually result in an increase in the number of white blood cells; viral infections may result in a decrease in the number of white blood cells.

Q: How do white blood cells combat infection?

A: When the body is injured or infected, white blood cells pass through the walls of the capillary blood vessels and congregate at the site of injury or infection. Then they engulf and destroy invading bacteria and other foreign bodies. In doing so, the white blood cells themselves are destroyed, and form pus.

The lymphocytes also produce antibodies (*see* IMMUNITY). Lymphocytes are found in most body tissues and play a major part in the body's reaction to prolonged infections, such as tuberculosis. *See* AGRANULOCYTOSIS; LEUKAEMIA; PLATELET; RED BLOOD CELL.

Whiteleg is a condition that occurs after deep vein thrombosis in a leg. *See* THROMBOSIS.

Whitlow. *See* PARONYCHIA.

Whooping cough, or pertussis, is a disease of the respiratory tract. Infection is by the microorganism called *Bordetella pertussis*; the microorganism is transported by droplets. The disease is commonest in infancy. Incubation period is ten to twenty-one days, and the infectious period from the onset of symptoms until three weeks after the beginning of the paroxysmal stage.

Q: What are the symptoms of whooping cough?

A: The three stages of the disease begin with (1) the catarrhal. The patient develops common cold symptoms, slight fever, sneezing, rhinitis, irritability with loss of appetite, and a dry cough which increases in violence after two weeks, becoming a series of short coughs followed by a long dragging in of breath, during which the "whoop" is heard.

Vomiting is common in (2) the paroxysmal stage. As this is the most serious stage, a watch must be kept for complications such as pneumonia, possibly leading to bronchiectasis and emphysema in later life. Severe coughing can cause haemorrhage of membranes in the nose and eyes. Mental retardation can result from cerebral haemorrhage, as can spastic paralysis.

The third stage (3), the decline, begins after about four weeks. The coughing bouts subside and food intake improves. Recovery may take several months.

Q: *How is whooping cough treated?*

A: The antibiotic erythromycin may prevent the onset of paroxysmal coughing if given early in the catarrhal stage. If not arrested at this stage, isolation and normal cough treatment combined with sedatives for sleep are recommended.

Q: *Can whooping cough be prevented?*

A: Yes. A vaccine of killed *Bordetella pertussis* organisms must be given to an infant in three doses, usually at the age of 5, 6, and 12 months, and combined with diphtheria and tetanus vaccine.

Whooping cough is uncommon and a milder disease in later life.

Widal test is a blood test performed in the investigation of TYPHOID FEVER.

Wilson's disease is a rare, hereditary disorder in which there is an abnormal accumulation of copper in the body, particularly in the liver and brain. This causes cirrhosis, anaemia, and a form of chorea. Wilson's disease is caused by an abnormal recessive gene that controls copper metabolism in the body. Death usually occurs unless treatment with penicillamine, a drug which increases the excretion of copper, is successful.

Wind. *See* FLATULENCE.

Windpipe. *See* TRACHEA.

Wisdom teeth are the third and last molar teeth on each side of the upper and lower jaw. They may not come through until after the age of twenty-five. *See* TEETH.

If the jaw is not large enough to accommodate them, the wisdom teeth may become impacted. When this happens, they are extracted by a dentist under a general or a local anaesthetic.

Witches' milk is a common name for the small amount of rather watery milk produced for a few days after birth by the breasts of a newborn baby of either sex. This action is stimulated by maternal hormones in the baby's bloodstream.

Womb, or uterus, is a thick muscular organ about the size of a clenched fist located in the abdomen of females. It is lined with a layer of cells (the endometrium) that respond to the varying hormonal stimulus of the menstrual cycle (*see* MENSTRUATION). During pregnancy the womb is the organ that surrounds the developing foetus.

The womb is a pear-shaped organ with two fallopian tubes (oviducts) that extend from each side of the upper end to the ovaries. At the lower end, the cervix (neck of the womb) leads into the vagina. The womb is supported below by a combination of ligaments that stretch from the side of the cervix to the pelvic bones.

See also CERVICITIS; ENDOMETRITIS; FIBROID; GYNAECOLOGICAL DISORDERS; HYSTERECTOMY; MENSTRUAL PROBLEMS; POLYP; PROLAPSE.

Woolsorter's disease is a fatal lung disorder caused by ANTHRAX.

Worms are primitive animals, many species of which cause parasitic infections. Worms are classified into three main groups: tapeworms (Cestoda); roundworms (Nematoda); and flukes (Trematoda).

Tapeworms that infest the intestine include the beef tapeworm (*Taenia saginata*) and the fish tapeworm (*see* DIPHYLLOBOTHRIUM LATUM). The most common tapeworm that infests human beings is the sheep tapeworm (*Echinococcus granulosus*), causing hydatid disease (*see* HYDATID CYST). The pork tapeworm (*Taenia solium*) can cause CYSTICERCOSIS.

Roundworms that infest the intestine include *Ascaris lumbricoides* (*see* ROUNDWORMS); threadworms, such as *Enterobius vermicularis* (*see* OXYURIASIS); hookworms, such as *Ancylostoma duodenale* (*see* ANKYLOSTOMIASIS); other worms, such as *Strongyloides stercoralis* (*see* STRONGYLOIDES); and whipworms, such as *Trichuris trichuria* (*see* TRICHURIASIS). Roundworms that infest the body tissues include *Wuchereria bancrofti*, which causes Bancroftian filariasis (*see* ELEPHANTIASIS); *Brugia malayi*, which causes Malayan filariasis (*see* ELEPHANTIASIS); *Dracunculus medinensis*, which causes dracontiasis (*see* GUINEA WORM); *Loa loa*, which causes loiasis (*see* LOA LOA); *Onchocerca volvulus*, which causes river blindness (*see* ONCHOCERCIASIS); *Toxocara canis* and *Toxocara cati*, which cause TOXOCARIASIS; and *Trichinella spiralis*, which causes TRICHINOSIS.

Flukes that infest the body tissues include various species of *Schistosoma* (*see* SCHISTOSOMIASIS); *Clonorchis sinensis*; *Fasciola hepatica*, also known as the liver fluke; and the lung fluke, *Paragonimus westermani* (*see* PARAGONIMIASIS).

See also FLUKES; ROUNDWORMS; TAPEWORMS.

Wound is any injury that causes damage by cutting or tearing tissues. A surgeon's incision is an aseptic (without infection) wound.

Wrist

A contusion (bruise) is a wound in which the skin is not broken. A penetrating wound is small, but the underlying structures are damaged far more than the punctured layer.

See also BLEEDING.

Wrist, known medically as the carpus, is the joint between the arm and the hand. There are eight bones in the wrist, located in two rows. The SCAPHOID, lunate, triquetral, and pisiform bones form a joint with the radius and ulna bones of the forearm. The trapezium, trapezoid, capitate, and hamate bones form joints with the five metacarpal bones of the hand. Each of the wrist bones forms a joint with each of the others. All of the bones are surrounded by synovial membranes and ligaments.

See also CARPAL TUNNEL SYNDROME.

Wrist drop is caused by paralysis of the muscles of the forearm, so that the wrist remains flexed ("dropped") and is unable to extend backward. Wrist drop usually follows injury to the radial nerve in the upper arm, or paralysis of muscles in the forearm.

Writer's cramp is stiffness of the thumb, first two fingers, and forearm muscles.

Wryneck. *See* STIFF NECK.

Xanthelasma is a condition in which small, yellow flat spots form in the inner corners of the upper and lower eyelids. It is most commonly seen in the elderly.

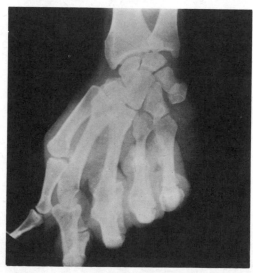

Wrist, the area between the forearm and the hand, contains eight carpal bones.

Q: What causes xanthelasma?

A: It may occur spontaneously for no obvious reason. But the condition often is associated with increased amounts of CHOLESTEROL in the blood, with LIPAEMIA, and with the appearance of a XANTHOMA elsewhere in the body.

Q: What is the treatment of xanthelasma?

A: Xanthelasma does not cause discomfort or disease, and so does not require treatment other than any that may be prescribed for lipaemia.

Xanthoma is a deposit or lump of yellow fatty substance (lipids) in the skin and tendons. The condition is most common in the ACHILLES TENDON, in the tendons of the hand and foot, and it occurs with LIPAEMIA, an inherited disorder in which there are excessive amounts of lipids in the blood. XANTHELASMA, a yellowish tumour on the upper and lower eyelids found in elderly people, also may occur. Individuals with xanthoma have an increased chance of developing coronary heart disease.

Q: How is xanthoma treated?

A: Treatment includes a low cholesterol diet (without saturated fats) and drugs that further decrease the lipids in the blood. The nodules of fatty substances sometimes ulcerate through the skin and have to be removed surgically.

X chromosome is one of the two types of human sex chromosomes. The other is called the Y chromosome. If two X chromosomes are present, the person is a female. If an X and a Y chromosome are present, the person is a male. The X chromosome usually is of a shape and size similar to the other twenty-two pairs of chromosomes present in the nucleus of every cell in the human body. *See* CHROMOSOME; GENE; Y CHROMOSOME.

Xenophobia is a psychiatric term for an abnormal dread or hatred of strangers or foreigners.

See also PHOBIA.

Xenopus test is a PREGNANCY TEST in which a female African toad (*Xenopus laevis*) is injected with urine from a woman who suspects that she is pregnant. If the woman is pregnant, the toad produces eggs within twelve hours of the injection. The xenopus test may give false results in some cases, and has been replaced by more reliable tests.

Xeroderma is a condition in which the skin is abnormally dry and rough.

Q: Why does the skin become abnormally dry?

A: The skin may become abnormally dry because of sunburn; the gradual dryness that occurs with increasing age; vitamin A deficiency; or ichthyosis, a mild type of dry skin disorder present at birth.

Q: How is xeroderma treated?

A: Often the problem is a minor one and it is only the mild irritation that makes the patient visit a doctor. The doctor usually prescribes a cream to keep moisture and fat in the skin, and advises against using soap. Vitamin A is prescribed only if there is evidence of deficiency.

    See also ICHTHYOSIS.

Xerophthalmia is a disorder that results in dry eyes and reduced tear production, or a roughness of the conjunctiva often associated with night blindness.

Q: What causes xerophthalmia?

A: Vitamin A deficiency may be one cause; HYPOTHYROIDISM or a form of SARCOID also may be responsible for the condition.

Q: How is xerophthalmia treated?

A: Vitamin A produces an immediate improvement, and hypothyroidism can be treated with THYROXINE. If dryness continues, special eye solutions containing cellulose preparations can be used as artificial tears.

X-rays are a form of electromagnetic radiation that can penetrate body tissues to varying degrees. This variation in the amount of X-rays absorbed by different tissues can be recorded on film to produce an X-ray photograph.

    See also RADIATION; RADIOGRAPHY; RADIOLOGY; RADIOTHERAPY.

Yaws is an infectious tropical disease caused by the spiral-shaped bacterium *Treponema pertenue*. This bacterium is indistinguishable from that which causes syphilis (*Treponema pallidum*) and pinta. Yaws is spread by direct contact between the infectious swellings of a diseased person and a break in the skin of another person. The bacterium that causes yaws cannot penetrate unbroken skin, nor can it pass through the placenta.

Q: What are the symptoms of yaws?

A: After an incubation period of about a month, a swelling appears at the site of infection; this may ulcerate and then heal. While it is healing, further soft swellings appear on the lips, elbows, buttocks, and knees. They are highly infectious, but rarely produce any irritation. Occasionally, the soft swellings may affect the underlying bones, particularly in the hands and feet. This may cause a limp in children.

When the soft swellings have healed, there often is an interval of several years before any further symptoms occur. After this interval, nodules appear on the skin. They may ulcerate and often affect underlying tissues. The ulcers heal slowly, forming scars that may be greatly disfiguring. The bones also may become distorted, and there may be shortening of the ligaments in the joints.

Q: How is yaws treated?

A: Yaws can be cured by treatment with penicillin. Surgery also may be necessary to correct any disfigurement or bone deformity.

    See also PINTA; SYPHILIS; TREPONEMA.

Y chromosome is one of the two types of human sex chromosomes; the other is called the X chromosome. If a Y chromosome is paired with an X chromosome, the person is a male. If two X chromosomes are paired, the person is a female. The Y chromosome is so called because its shape is markedly different from the other forty-five chromosomes, which all resemble the X chromosome. *See* CHROMOSOME; GENE; X CHROMOSOME.

Yeast is a general term for any of the single-celled fungi of the genus *Saccharomyces*. Yeast is used for leavening bread and for brewing (brewer's yeast). Brewer's yeast is a rich source of vitamin B. Some species of yeast may cause disorders (such as MONILIASIS) or may be poisonous.

Yellow fever is a virus infection transmitted to humans by the bite of the mosquito *Aedes aegypti*. The disorder is common in tropical climates, particularly in Africa and South

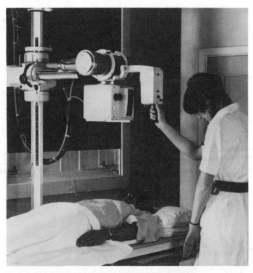

The patient lies over a photographic plate as the radiographer adjusts the X-ray equipment.

Yellow jaundice

America. There is an incubation period of three to six days after infection and then symptoms appear.

Q: *What are the symptoms of yellow fever?*

A: Symptoms appear suddenly and include a shivering attack (rigor), high fever, severe headache and bone pains, vomiting, mild confusion, signs of meningitis, and photophobia (sensitivity to bright light).

The patient's temperature returns to normal in about four days and he or she appears to be recovering. But after a few hours, jaundice begins to appear, the fever returns, and there is bleeding into the urine, from the mouth, and into the skin.

The organs that are particularly involved are the liver (causing hepatitis), kidneys (kidney failure) and, to a lesser extent, the heart (heart failure), as well as the brain (encephalitis). The symptoms become increasingly severe, and death may occur within a week after a few hours in coma.

In people who live in the endemic areas and who have some immunity, the illness is much less severe and of shorter duration. In such people, yellow fever does not cause any permanent damage to the body, but full recovery may be attained only after several weeks or even months.

Q: *What is the treatment for yellow fever?*

A: There is no cure for yellow fever. The only treatment available is the administration of intravenous fluids, antinauseant drugs and, if necessary,

kidney dialysis, as well as skilled medical and nursing care in hospital.

Q: *Is there any protection against yellow fever?*

A: Yes. Immunization with an extremely mild yellow fever virus gives protection for ten years. It should not be done within three weeks of a smallpox vaccination, and not given to children under the age of one year because there is a slight risk of causing encephalitis. It also is advisable not to immunize during pregnancy, even though foetal damage has not been detected.

An international certificate stating that a person has received immunization against yellow fever is valid from ten days after the injection for ten years. Such a certificate is legally required of travellers to countries where the disease is prevalent.

Preventive measures include mosquito control by screening, spraying, and destruction of breeding areas. Mass immunization also helps to decrease the incidence of the disease.

Yellow jaundice. *See* JAUNDICE.

Z

Zinc oxide is a white odourless powder that may be prepared in paste, lotion, cream, or powder form. It is used alone or combined with other substances as a soothing preparation in the treatment of eczema, varicose veins, and haemorrhoids, and around colostomies and ileostomies. It also is used as dusting powder for prickly heat and, combined with mild antiseptics, as a cement used as a temporary packing for holes in the teeth (caries).

Zinc oxide often is used in preparations on special bandages that are applied to ulcerated or eczematous areas of the skin. The bandages are left in place for some days, or even weeks, for as long as it takes for the underlying condition to heal.

Zoonosis is any disease of animals that can be transmitted to humans under natural conditions.

See also ANTHRAX; BRUCELLOSIS; CAT-SCRATCH FEVER; DENGUE; ENCEPHALITIS; GLANDERS; LASSA FEVER; MALARIA; PLAGUE; PSITTACOSIS; RABIES; ROCKY MOUNTAIN SPOTTED FEVER; SLEEPING SICKNESS; TYPHUS.

Zygote is the cell that is formed when a sperm fertilizes an egg (ovum). *See* FERTILIZATION.

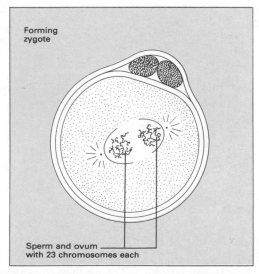

Forming zygote

Sperm and ovum with 23 chromosomes each

Zygote is formed when a sperm passes into an ovum and a new cell nucleus is formed.